Register Now for Online Access to Your Book!

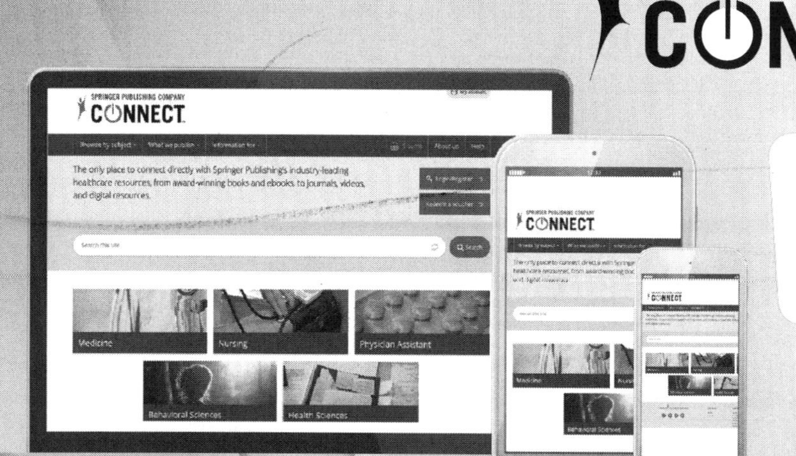

Your print purchase of *Translation of Evidence Into Nursing and Healthcare, Third Edition,* **includes online access to the contents of your book**—increasing accessibility, portability, and searchability!

Access today at:

http://connect.springerpub.com/content/book/978-0-8261-4737-0
or scan the QR code at the right with your smartphone and enter the access code below.

0JXGB945

Scan here for quick access.

If you are experiencing problems accessing the digital component of this product, please contact our customer service department at cs@springerpub.com

SPRINGER PUBLISHING COMPANY

View all our products at springerpub.com

Kathleen M. White, PhD, RN, NEA-BC, FAAN, is a professor at the Johns Hopkins University School of Nursing. She holds a joint faculty appointment in the Hopkins Carey School of Business and the Hopkins School of Education. Dr. White also holds a joint appointment as a clinical nurse specialist (CSN) at Johns Hopkins Hospital, where she was a member of a collaborative team that developed the widely published, award-winning Johns Hopkins Nursing Evidence-Based Practice Model and guidelines. Dr. White was a senior advisor at the Health Resources and Services Administration from 2010 to 2013, where she worked in the National Center for Health Workforce Analysis and the Office of Performance Management. Her numerous practice policy and leadership roles have included serving as the chairperson of the American Nursing Association Congress on Nursing Practice and Economics from 2006 to 2010, as a member of the Maryland Governor's Health Quality and Cost Council from 2009 to 2015, and the Maryland Patient Safety Center's board of directors, where she served as their inaugural chairperson until 2011. She currently serves on the Maryland Health Care Commission's Hospital Performance Evaluation Guide Advisory Committee and is the vice-chairperson of the Johns Hopkins Howard County General Hospital Board of Trustees.

Sharon Dudley-Brown, PhD, RN, FNP-BC, FAAN, is an associate professor and Director, Doctor of Nursing Practice Program at the University of Delaware. She also holds an appointment at the Johns Hopkins University School of Medicine, where she sees patients as well as conducts research on patients with inflammatory bowel disease. Dr. Dudley-Brown has held several academic appointments, both nationally and internationally, and has worked as a nurse practitioner at several institutions over the past 25+ years. She has published numerous peer-reviewed papers and abstracts in the fields of nursing, inflammatory bowel disease, Crohn's disease, and ulcerative colitis, and is currently a member of several editorial boards, including that of *Gastroenterology Nursing*, where she is the online editor. She is an active member of the Crohn's and Colitis Foundation (CCF) and serves on the National Nurse and Advanced Practice Provider Committee as well as on her local medical advisory committee.

Mary F. Terhaar, PhD, RN, ANEF, FAAN, is the Arline H. and Curtis F. Garvin Professor and Associate Dean for Academic Affairs at the Frances Payne Bolton School of Nursing at Case Western Reserve University. She is responsible for the quality and integrity of academic programing, global nursing, recruitment, student services, and accreditation. Formerly, Dr. Terhaar served as director of the DNP program and was an associate professor at Johns Hopkins University School of Nursing. Based on over 35 years' experience in perinatal, neonatal, pediatric and administrative nursing, she has led performance improvement and translation efforts in large academic healthcare institutions, community hospitals, and educational programs. Dr. Terhaar leads faculty preparing clinical scholars who will transform practice and care through the meticulous translation of evidence toward the solution of significant practice challenges. She teaches across the baccalaureate, graduate, and doctoral programs. Dr. Terhaar designed the Scholarly Project sequence, as well as the Foundations for Scholarship course, which prepares students for the return to academics, for the rigor of scholarly writing, and for impactful dissemination. She has published and presented the curriculum, the multimodal approach to evaluation, which involves performance-improvement activities designed to increase the rigor of the education provided to the DNP, and the outcomes that have resulted from the work of both the faculty and students.

Translation of Evidence Into Nursing and Healthcare

THIRD EDITION

Kathleen M. White, PhD, RN, NEA-BC, FAAN

Sharon Dudley-Brown, PhD, RN, FNP-BC, FAAN

Mary F. Terhaar, PhD, RN, ANEF, FAAN

Editors

SPRINGER PUBLISHING COMPANY

Springer Publishing Company, LLC
11 West 42nd Street
New York, NY 10036
www.springerpub.com
http://connect.springerpub.com/home

Acquisitions Editor: Adrianne Brigido
Compositor: Exeter Premedia Services Private Ltd.

ISBN: 978-0-8261-4736-3
ebook ISBN: 978-0-8261-4737-0
PowerPoints ISBN: 978-0-8261-4738-7
DOI: 10.1891/9780826147370

Qualified instructors may request supplements by emailing textbook@springerpub.com

20 21 22 23 / 5 4 3 2

Library of Congress Cataloging-in-Publication Data

Names: White, Kathleen M. (Kathleen Murphy), 1953- editor. | Dudley-Brown, Sharon, editor. | Terhaar, Mary F., editor.
Title: Translation of evidence into nursing and healthcare / Kathleen M. White, Sharon Dudley-Brown, Mary F. Terhaar, editors.
Other titles: Translation of evidence into nursing and health care
Description: Third edition. | New York, NY : Springer Publishing Company, LLC, [2020] | Preceded by Translation of evidence into nursing and health care / [edited by] Kathleen M. White, Sharon Dudley-Brown, Mary Terhaar. Second edition. 2016. | Includes bibliographical references and index.
Identifiers: LCCN 2019043554 (print) | LCCN 2019043555 (ebook) | ISBN 9780826147363 (paperback) | ISBN 9780826147370 (ebook) | ISBN 9780826147387 (PowerPoints)
Subjects: MESH: Evidence-Based Nursing—organization & administration | Diffusion of Innovation | Translational Medical Research—methods
Classification: LCC RT51 (print) | LCC RT51 (ebook) | NLM WY 100.7 | DDC 610.73—dc23
LC record available at https://lccn.loc.gov/2019043554
LC ebook record available at https://lccn.loc.gov/2019043555

Publisher's Note: **New and used products purchased from third-party sellers are not guaranteed for quality, authenticity, or access to any included digital components.**

Printed in the United States of America.

This book is dedicated to our students,
who embrace the tremendous challenge of exploring the issues,
weighing the evidence, and transforming practice.

It is essential that each and every one of us
question the status quo, expect better ways to care, and collaborate always.
Society demands better outcomes:
Together, we have the ability and the responsibility to deliver.

Contents

Contributors

Carla Aquino, DNP, RN, Nursing Program Director, Clinical Quality and Magnet Office of the Nursing Professional Practice, The Johns Hopkins Hospital, Baltimore, Maryland

Judith A. Ascenzi, DNP, RN, APRN-CNS, CCRN, Pediatric Intensive Care Unit, The Johns Hopkins Hospital, Baltimore, Maryland

Jemma Ayvazian, DNP, ANP-BC, AOCNP, Director, Nursing Education, Office of Academic Affiliations, Department of Veterans Affairs, Washington, DC

Suzanne M. Cowperthwaite, DNP, RN, NEA-BC, Director of Nursing, University of Maryland Medical Center, Greenebaum Comprehensive Cancer Center, Baltimore, Maryland

Rachael Crickman, DNP, ARNP-CNS, AOCNS, OCN, Oncology Clinical Nurse Specialist, Swedish Medical Center, Seattle, Washington

Deborah S. Croy, DNP, RN, ANP-BC, AGPCNP-BC, CLS, AACC, Nurse Practitioner, Bland County Medical Clinic, Bastian, Virginia

Maria M. Cvach, DNP, RN, FAAN, Director of Policy Management and Integration, Johns Hopkins Health System, and Clinical Safety Specialist, Armstrong Institute for Patient Safety and Quality, Johns Hopkins Medicine, Baltimore, Maryland

Charlene M. Deuber, DNP, NNP-BC, CPNP, Neonatal Nurse Practitioner, Children's Hospital of Philadelphia Neonatal Network, Einstein Medical Center Montgomery, East Norriton, Pennsylvania

Christina DiNapoli, DNP, FNP, Nurse Practitioner, Weill Cornell Medical College, New York, New York

Sharon Dudley-Brown, PhD, RN, FNP-BC, FAAN, Associate Professor and Director, Doctor of Nursing Practice Program, University of Delaware, School of Nursing, Newark, Delaware

Deborah S. Finnell, DNS, CARN-AP, FAAN, Professor Emerita, Johns Hopkins School of Nursing, Baltimore, Maryland

Juliane Jablonski, DNP, RN, CCRN, CCNS, Hospital of the University of Pennsylvania, Philadelphia, Pennsylvania

Mariam Kashani, DNP, CRNP, Director, Clinical Programs at Integrative Cardiac Health Project, Walter Reed National Military Medical Center, Bethesda, Maryland

Mary Marshman, DNP, RN, Assistant Vice President of Nursing Services, WellStar Kennestone Regional Medical Center, Marietta, Georgia

Lorenzo T. Nava, DNP, CNP, FNP-C, Nurse Practitioner Residency Program Director, Medical Staff, Crownpoint Healthcare Facility, Crownpoint, New Mexico

Scott M. Newton, DNP, MBA, RN, Vice President, Care Model Solutions, TeleTracking Technologies, Inc., Pittsburgh, Pennsylvania

Judy Phillips, DNP, FNP-BC, AOCN, CCRN, Assistant Professor of Nursing, Lenoir-Rhyne University, Hickory, North Carolina, and Nurse Practitioner, Cancer Care of Western North Carolina, Asheville, North Carolina

Lisa Groff Reuschling, DNP, RN, Director, Women and Children's Services, Greater Baltimore Medical Center, Towson, Maryland

Suzanne Rubin, DNP, MPH, CRNP-P, Nurse Practitioner, Full Term Nursery, Johns Hopkins Hospital, Baltimore, Maryland

Lisa M. Sgarlata, DNP, MSN, RN, FACHE, Chief Patient Care Officer/Chief Nurse Executive, Lee Health System, Fort Myers, Florida, and RWJF Executive Nurse Fellow

Julie Stanik-Hutt, PhD, ACNPC, GNP-BC, CCNS, FAANP, FAAN, Professor (Clinical) and Director, AG-ACNP Program, University of Iowa College of Nursing, Iowa City, Iowa

Nancy Sullivan, DNP, RN, Assistant Professor/Simulation Director, Johns Hopkins School of Nursing, Baltimore, Maryland

Martha Sylvia, PhD, MBA, RN, Associate Professor, Medical University of South Carolina, Charleston, South Carolina

Mary F. Terhaar, PhD, RN, ANEF, FAAN, Professor and Associate Dean for Academic Affairs, Frances Payne Bolton School of Nursing, Case Western Reserve University, Cleveland, Ohio

Kathleen M. White, PhD, RN, NEA-BC, FAAN, Professor, Johns Hopkins University School of Nursing, Johns Hopkins University, Baltimore, Maryland

Joyce P. Williams, DNP, AFN, FAAN, Professor, Adjunct Faculty, Stevenson University, Pikesville, Maryland

Marisa L. Wilson, DNSc, MHSc, RN-BC, CPHIMS, FAMIA, FAAN, Associate Professor, Director of Nursing Health Services Leadership Pathway, Coordinator, University of Alabama at Birmingham School of Nursing, Birmingham, Alabama

Laura J. Wood, DNP, MS, RN, NEA-BC, Senior Vice President, Patient Care Operations and Chief Nursing Officer, Sporing Carpenter Chair for Nursing, Boston Children's Hospital, Boston, Massachusetts

Rhonda Wyskiel, MSN, RNc, Director of Performance Improvement and Innovation at Greater Baltimore Medical Center, Armstrong Institute for Patient Safety and Quality, Johns Hopkins Medicine, Baltimore, Maryland

Lina A. Younan, DNP, MSN, RN, Clinical Associate Professor, Hariri School of Nursing, American University of Beirut, Lebanon

Jenelle M. Zambrano, DNP, CNS, RN Clinical Nurse Specialist, Los Angeles County Harbor–UCLA Medical Center, Los Angeles, California

■ CONTRIBUTORS TO THE PREVIOUS EDITION

Judith A. Ascenzi, DNP, RN, CCRN

Jemma Ayvazian, DNP, ANP-BC, AOCNP Nursing Education Program Evaluation Manager, Office of Academic Affiliations, Department of Veterans Affairs, Washington, DC

Rachael Crickman, DNP, RN, AOCNS Oncology Clinical Nurse Specialist, Virginia Mason Medical Center, Seattle, Washington

Deborah S. Croy, DNP, RN, ANP-BC, AGPCNP-BC, CLS, AACC Adult Cardiovascular Nurse Practitioner, Bland County Medical Clinic, Bastian, Virginia

Maria M. Cvach, DNP, RN, FAAN

Charlene Deuber, DNP, CPNP, NNP-BC Neonatal Nurse Practitioner, Division of Neonatology, Children's Regional Health Center, Cooper Health, Camden, New Jersey

Christina DiNapoli, DNP, FNP-BC

Sharon Dudley-Brown, PhD, RN, FNP-BC, FAAN Assistant Professor, Johns Hopkins University Schools of Medicine and Nursing, Baltimore, Maryland

Deborah S. Finnell, DNS, PHMHP-BC, CARN-AP, FAAN Associate Professor, Director of the Master's and Doctor of Nursing Practice Programs, Johns Hopkins School of Nursing, Acute and Chronic Care Department, Baltimore, Maryland

Barbara B. Frink, PhD, RN, FAAN

Juliane Jablonski, DNP, RN, CCRN, CCNS

Mariam Kashani, DNP, CRNP

Mary Marshman, DNP, RN, CNRN Director of Nursing & Critical Care Services, Disease Specific Certification Coordinator, Centra Health, Lynchburg, Virginia

Lorenzo T. Nava, DNP, FNP Medical Staff, Crownpoint Healthcare Facility, Crownpoint, New Mexico

Scott M. Newton, DNP, RN, MHA, EMT-P Director of Nursing, Johns Hopkins Hospital, Department of Emergency Medicine & Lifeline Critical Care Transport Team, Johns Hopkins University School of Nursing; Lecturer, Baltimore, Maryland

Lisa Groff Paris, DNP, RNC-OB, C-EFM

Judy Phillips, DNP, FNP-BC, AOCN, CCRN Nurse Practitioner, Cancer Care of Western North Carolina; Assistant Professor of Nursing, Lenoir-Rhyne University, Hickory, North Carolina

Suzanne Rubin, DNP, MPH, CRNP-P Pediatric Nurse Practitioner, Newborn Nursery, Johns Hopkins Hospital, Baltimore, Maryland

Cynda Hylton Rushton, PhD, RN, FAAN

Lisa M. Sgarlata, DNP, MSN, MS, RN, FACHE Robert Wood Johnson Foundation Executive Nurse Fellow, Chief Administrative Officer, Lee Memorial Hospital; Robert Wood Johnson Foundation Executive Nurse Fellow, Fort Meyers, Florida

Julie Stanik-Hutt, PhD, CRNP, CCNS, FAANP, FAAN Professor and Director, Adult/Geriatric Acute Care Nurse Practitioner Track, Doctor of Nursing Practice Program, University of Iowa College of Nursing, Iowa City, Iowa

Nancy Sullivan, DNP, ARNP Instructor, Director of Clinical Simulation, Department of Acute and Chronic Care, Johns Hopkins University School of Nursing, Baltimore, Maryland

Martha Sylvia, PhD, MBA, RN

Mary F. Terhaar, DNSc, RN, FAAN Professor and Associate Dean for Academic Affairs, Frances Payne Bolton School of Nursing, Case Western Reserve University, Cleveland, Ohio

Kathleen M. White, PhD, RN, NEA-BC, FAAN Associate Professor, Clinical Nurse Specialist, Johns Hopkins University School of Nursing; Hopkins Carey School of Business, Director of Entry Into Practice Program, Track Coordinator of the MSN Health Systems Management/MSN-MBA Tracks, Johns Hopkins University, Baltimore, Maryland

Joyce Williams, DNP, AFN-BC, FAAFS, FAAN Assistant Professor, Graduate and Professional Studies–Nursing, Stevenson University, Owings Mills, Maryland

Marisa L. Wilson, DNSc, MHSc, RN-BC, CPHIMS Associate Professor, Specialty Track Coordinator, Nursing Informatics, School of Nursing/Family, Community, and Health Systems, University of Alabama School of Nursing, The University of Alabama at Birmingham, Birmingham, Alabama

Laura J. Wood, DNP, MS, RN Senior Vice President, Patient Care Services and Chief Nursing Officer, Spring Carpenter Chair for Nursing, Boston Children's Hospital, Boston, Massachusetts

Rhonda Wyskiel, MSN, RNc

Lina A. Younan, DNP Clinical Assistant Professor, Hariri School of Nursing, American University of Beirut, Beirut, Lebanon

Jenelle M. Zambrano, DNP, CNS, RN, CCRN, CCNS Clinical Nurse Specialist, Los Angeles County Harbor–UCLA Medical Center, Los Angeles, California

Preface

We are excited to share with you the third edition of this text, which is intended to serve as an introduction to and a comprehensive resource for the work of translation. Consistent with the first edition, we use the language of translation because our focus is more precisely on the planning, execution, and achievement of important outcomes rather than the development of the science of implementation. We intend to encourage and facilitate broad adoption of translation as a means to achieve the Quadruple Aim and to ground the work solidly in theory and evidence. Ultimately, this approach contributes to the scholarship and rigor of the DNP as well as the advancement of implementation science.

In recent years, the frameworks, approaches, and analytics that are useful for translation have become more plentiful and more diverse. Familiar structures, processes, and approaches to collaboration have been refined and new ones have been developed to promote success. More important, many innovative and effective translation projects have been reported in the literature. All are useful as a means to guide the novice as well as inspire and challenge the practiced translator to achieve greater impact.

Since the first text was published, so much has changed in the area of translation and the body of related work has both expanded and matured. Many resources are now available. This text can form the scaffold for DNP education and the scholarly project. It can also serve as a playbook for DNPs as they begin to practice nursing at the highest level and transform healthcare and the health of society.

This third edition presents refreshed and expanded content to describe the work of translation. Examples of successful translation projects are presented to demonstrate the process of working from a problem; through meticulous prosecution of the evidence; to careful planning, execution, evaluation, and finally, broad dissemination. The exemplars presented here demonstrate high-impact, sustainable change that transforms culture and practice. This content is provided in six discrete but compatible sections introduced here.

■ PART I: TRANSLATION OF EVIDENCE

Part I contains three chapters that describe the process of translation from a theoretical perspective. Part I will be familiar to those who used earlier editions, but the content represents recent developments in practice and the literature. **Chapter 1**, Evidence-Based Practice, serves as a primer on the topic. This chapter reviews the key tenets of evidence-based practice, presents a historical view of the work, and introduces a select few frameworks that have demonstrated impact over time. **Chapter 2**, The Science of Translation and Major Frameworks, provides a detailed overview of many frameworks that help to organize and facilitate the process of translating science into practice. In this edition, you will find new frameworks and an emphasis on improvements and revisions to the originals. **Chapter 3**, Change Theory and Models: Framework for Translation, describes the major theories and models as they relate to the process of translation. After all, translation is a powerful approach to accomplishing change, therefore, understanding the change process is essential.

■ PART II: USE OF TRANSLATION

Part II contains four chapters that describe the application of translation to select practice foci, including outcomes management, safety and quality, leadership, and health policy. Each chapter presents refreshed content related to the important topics covered in the first edition. **Chapter 4**, Translation of Evidence to Improve Clinical Outcomes, focuses on the use of evidence to support practice guidelines across the discipline in support of improving outcomes that matter. **Chapter 5**, Translation of Evidence for Improving Safety and Quality, describes the fast growing evidence base for safety and quality work. **Chapter 6**, Translation of Evidence for Leadership, describes the body of knowledge about leadership that applies to the work of translation to achieve the Quadruple Aim, attain professional success, and ensure practice excellence. **Chapter 7**, Translation of Evidence for Health Policy, provides a guide to help the DNP influence health policy through the application and dissemination of evidence.

■ PART III: METHODS AND PROCESS FOR TRANSLATION

Part III contains five chapters that describe a reliable and rigorous approach to the process of translation. The focus here is practical, and much is new in this edition. **Chapter 8**, Methods for Translation, describes 15 commonly applied methods used to translate evidence into practice and explores the best fit and utility of each. This chapter is intended to help those engaged in the work to consider the many approaches to translation and to select the approach that is best suited to the practice environment and clinical challenge at hand. **Chapter 9**, Project Management for Translation, provides a tactical and pragmatic approach that can be used to ensure that the work achieves faithful translation of evidence as well as appropriate adaptation to the individual practice setting. The unfolding case describes application of project management tools to plan for and manage the execution of a single, high-impact translation project. **Chapter 10**, Ethical Responsibilities of Translation of Evidence and Evaluation of Outcomes, describes the responsibilities of the DNP engaged in translation and explains the processes to follow when preparing for institutional review board review. **Chapter 11,** Data Management and Evaluation of Translation, serves two purposes: It promotes reliable and rigorous evaluation of translation efforts and, in so doing, increases the successful dissemination of improvement work. In **Chapter 12,** Dissemination of Evidence, the authors strongly encourage high-quality dissemination of the work of translation, and this chapter is a guide to help the reader accomplish that goal.

■ PART IV: ENABLERS OF TRANSLATION

Part IV is new to this edition. In it you will find content to support effective translation. The processes described here are necessary but not sufficient for successful translation. **Chapter 13,** Education: An Enabler of Translation, describes approaches that support adoption of evidence in teaching in order to change the knowledge, skills, attitudes, and behaviors of caregivers and patients. **Chapter 14,** Information Technology: A Foundation for Translation, serves as a guide to help the reader understand how information technology and informatics techniques both support the translation process and serve as a medium for a translation itself. **Chapter 15,** Interprofessional Collaboration and Teamwork for Translation, provides an overview of the body of evidence to guide effective interprofessional collaboration in support of high-impact translation. The final chapter in this section, **Chapter 16,** Creating a Culture That Promotes Translation, describes best practices for building strong culture that has a significant impact.

■ PART V: ISSUES IN TRANSLATION

Part V contains two chapters to promote successful translation. **Chapter 17,** Best Practices in Translation: Challenges and Barriers in Translation, provides an experience-based guide to the potential impediments to successful translation in order to support effective planning, surveillance for early warning signs, and proactive problem-solving, and describes best practices in translation. **Chapter 18,** Legal Issues in Translation, provides an environmental scan of the potential risks and threats to success when teams undertake a program of improvement.

■ PART VI: TRANSLATION EXEMPLARS

This section was added in the second edition. It contains three chapters in which examples of successful translation projects are presented. **Chapter 19** presents five population health exemplars, **Chapter 20** presents eight specialty practice exemplars, and **Chapter 21** presents eight healthcare system exemplars. Fifteen exemplars relate to a method presented in Chapter 8. The remaining six relate to the education strategies presented as enablers to translation in Chapter 10. All projects presented

TABLE P.1 Practice Innovation Spectrum

	Research	Evidence-Based Practice	Quality Improvement
Nature of knowledge	Discovery	Application	Problem-solving
Nature of the result	New knowledge	Fidelity and fit	Fast fix
Level of control	High	Moderate	Low
Context	Precise	Expanded	Untidy
Scope	Variable	Local	Local
Adaptation	Rigorous control	Adaptability	Practicality
Applicability	Generalizable findings	Population specific and site specific	Problem focused
Analytics	Qualitative and quantitative	Qualitative and quantitative *or* Statistical process control	Statistical process control
Statistical power	Essential	Optional	Optional
Goal	Precision	Replication applicability impact	Impact
Leadership	PhD and IP team	DNP and IP team	DNP and IP team

IP, interprofessional.

in Part VI were conducted by DNP students in collaboration with interdisciplinary teams and all have been formally disseminated. All exemplars come from a broad range of practice areas, and all accomplished clinically relevant, measurable, sustainable improvement. Reference to the primary source is contained within each. *Qualified instructors may obtain access to supplementary material (PowerPoints) by emailing textbook@springerpub.com.*

■ CONCLUSIONS

The conversation in nursing and the health professions has historically emphasized the distinctions between the scholarship of the PhD and that of the DNP. It has become generally accepted recently that discovery is the domain of the former and translation the work of the latter. At the time of publication of this third edition, it remains useful to frame these efforts on a continuum of innovation (Table P.1). On the one hand, research seeks to discover new knowledge—where none is available—to support effective practice and care. On the other hand, quality improvement seeks to address problems encountered in the provision of that care. In between these two poles, translation seeks to bring evidence to bear on challenges in the real world of practice using reliable and valid evidence to improve care and robust analytics to evaluate the impact. All the work represented on this continuum is essential to improving outcomes and attaining the Quadruple Aim.

Whereas different curricula develop in students and graduates the competencies required to lead efforts at different points along that continuum, in fact, it will be diverse teams that accomplish innovation. Both sets of competencies will be essential. But it will be diverse interprofessional teams, whose members possess these skill sets and this knowledge, that will achieve the greatest success and highest impact. So this book provides a description of the resources and processes that DNPs will rely on to drive translation, which are the same ones that teams can rely on and practice to guide and support that work.

The editors and contributors hope you find this to be a useful and practical, yet scholarly guide and resource. We encourage you to visit the primary sources to deepen your understanding of projects that interest you. As the body of evidence to support and direct translation grows, your contribution is much needed and encouraged.

Mary F. Terhaar

Acknowledgments

Dr. White would like to thank her family for their continuing support and encouragement for her work over the years.

Dr. Dudley-Brown would like to acknowledge her husband and friends, who provided unwavering support and encouragement during this journey.

Dr. Terhaar would like to thank Dennis, Colin, Hannah, and Aidan for their patience, good humor, and unfailing support.

Together, we recognize the contributions of the team members who contributed to the first and second editions. We thank the faculty of the Johns Hopkins University School of Nursing, who grow nurse scholars, scientists, and clinicians for the world; we recognize our colleagues at Johns Hopkins Hospital, who help to keep the patients at the center of all we do; and Denise Rucker, who always keeps the students in focus.

Introduction

■ TRANSLATION OF EVIDENCE INTO PRACTICE AND IMPLEMENTATION SCIENCE

In today's healthcare, there is a widely accepted emphasis on evidence-based practice (EBP) that focuses on growing an environment where evidence supports clinical and administrative decision-making to ensure the highest quality of care, promotes optimal outcomes, and creates a culture of critical thinking and accountability. Since the development of the EBP movement, much attention has centered on how to successfully implement evidence into practice and facilitate the spread of those EBPs. The translation of evidence into practice requires strategy. Many and varied translation frameworks and models have emerged to guide implementation efforts and ensure the adoption of evidence into routine practice. These models include key elements for consideration in the evidence translation process, such as the type of evidence, the practitioners and stakeholders involved in the translation, organizational behaviors and their internal and external environments, the type of intervention to be used, and the process design for the translation. The process usually involves introducing the new evidence and strategies to change behavior and performance. These strategies are based on different assumptions using theories of change, organizational design, leadership, decision-making, and social ecology. Practice professionals play a major role in the translation of new evidence into practice efforts in order to improve the effectiveness and efficiency of the delivery of healthcare.

Implementation science, a field concerned with how to successfully implement new evidence, has rapidly developed out of a need to understand the successes and failures of evidence adoption because of the emphasis on EBP in our healthcare settings. The most commonly used definition of implementation science is "the scientific study of methods to promote the systematic uptake of research findings and other evidence-based practices into routine practice, and, hence, to improve the quality and effectiveness of health services and care" (Eccles & Mittman, 2006). Implementation research focuses on testing how interventions work in real settings, the role of organizational culture, and other aspects of the implementation process such as how to improve the uptake of evidence and promote sustainability. Implementation research study designs include evaluation of and testing of implementation strategies in relationship to the type of evidence, the practitioners involved, and organizational characteristics such as culture, learning, leadership, communication patterns, centralized versus decentralized processes, and availability of resources. The research often uses mixed methods, combining qualitative and quantitative techniques. Implementation science seeks to understand how and why change processes work, and by rigorously studying methods of systems improvements it attempts to answer the question: What are the best methods to facilitate the uptake of evidence into practice?

Over the last 20 years, there is concern that local success in translating evidence into practice is often challenging to replicate, spread, and/or sustain over time. Factors that facilitate the change in practice may work in one setting, but not in another. These local successes are not generalizable because the translation is performed in a single setting of convenience without considering other critical organizational contributing or confounding factors. In addition, simplistic impact measures are often used, and spread and sustainability are rarely part of the translation strategy.

Finally, you may be wondering why I have written this introduction for a book on translation of evidence into practice. There is ongoing concern about the use of appropriate terminology by healthcare professionals to describe our improvement work. The translation of evidence into practice involves processes of evidence appraisal, synthesis, and dissemination by practitioners. These processes take place within complex organizations, the focus of both the translation teams and implementation science. Implementation science focuses on the research that is necessary to generate evidence about how to facilitate translation of EBPs and the rigorous testing of improvement strategies essential to the understanding of when, where, why, and how an intervention for translation of evidence is effective. Well-designed and effective implementation strategies affect the sustainability of those efforts. Critical to this discussion is the role for researchers, practitioners, and administrators who collaborate to understand how successful implementation occurs. The business case for both EBP and implementation science is clear: safe, timely, effective, efficient, and equitable evidence-based healthcare practices that maximize value for the patient.

Kathleen M. White
Professor, Johns Hopkins School of Nursing
Co-editor, *Translation of Evidence Into Nursing and Healthcare*, Third Edition

■ REFERENCE

Eccles, M. P., & Mittman, B. S. (2006). Welcome to implementation science. *Implementation Science, 1*(1). doi:10.1186/1748-5908-1-1

Translation of Evidence Into Nursing and Healthcare

PART ONE

Translation of Evidence

CHAPTER ONE

Evidence-Based Practice

Kathleen M. White

Let whoever is in charge keep this simple question in her head (not, how can I always do this right thing myself, but), how can I provide for this right thing to be always done?
—Florence Nightingale (1860)

Evidence-Based Practice (EBP) Is Not New. In fact, most contemporary literature credits Dr. Archie Cochrane, a British epidemiologist, who in the 1970s was the impetus for moving medicine toward EBP. Cochrane criticized the medical profession and its use of findings from medical research: "It is surely a great criticism of our profession that we have not organized a critical summary, by specialty or subspecialty, updated periodically, of all randomized controlled trials" (Cochrane, 1972).

The implementation of EBP in healthcare has moved us from a "do something . . . anything" framework of patient care to "Why do we do these things when we don't really know what works?" The Evidence-Based Medicine Working Group (1992), in promoting a new paradigm for medical practice, is often quoted as saying:

> Evidence-based medicine de-emphasizes intuition, unsystematic clinical experience, and pathophysiologic rationale as sufficient grounds for clinical decision making and stresses the examination of evidence from clinical research. Evidence-based medicine requires new skills of the physician, including efficient literature searching and the application of formal rules of evidence [in] evaluating the clinical literature. (p. 2420)

However, the nursing profession also lays claim to the origins of EBP based on Florence Nightingale's collection of epidemiological data that were used to change practice (Titler et al., 2001). Nightingale emphatically taught her nurses that the foundation of clinical practice was to use evidence to guide clinical decision-making. Stetler and Marram (1976), in their earliest work on research utilization for nursing, noted that even though tools are available to critique research design, there are no criteria to help the nurse—from critique to application—to decide whether and how to use the findings in the nurse's specific work environment. For nursing, the framework for decision-making has long been the nursing process: a systematic problem-solving methodology that has served us well. However, this process does not include the step of questioning one's own practice and being able to say "I don't know if what I am doing is really improving the patient's outcome." The evaluation step of the nursing process takes the nurse only halfway to maximizing quality and effectiveness of care. This chapter discusses the importance of EBP for nursing and presents a summary of key EBP nursing models in use today.

■ WHY EBP AND WHY NOW?

Nurses can no longer rely solely on their clinical experience to provide quality care. Nurses routinely need to question their practice and look for alternative methods to improve the processes of care. As the nurse evaluates patient care processes and their outcomes as part of everyday care, he or she must ask whether the best and the most current practices are being used and whether those interventions are producing the best outcomes for the patient. This critical thinking is the foundation for EBP and should be guided by a systematic approach to the evaluation of current practice. EBP in healthcare today uses a formal process with specific criteria to appraise emerging evidence and methods for incorporating that evidence to inform and change practice.

Why has the emphasis for the use of evidence in practice gained so much momentum? The Institute of Medicine's report, *Health Professions Education* (2003), called for all health professional educational programs to include competency in five areas: patient-centered care, quality improvement, interprofessional collaborative practice, health information technology, and emphasizing EBP. In addition, a U.S. Department of Health and Human Services report (2012) defined a national quality strategy, an important element of the Affordable Care Act, to improve the quality and delivery of healthcare services, patient health outcomes, and population health. This quality strategy began with three aims—better care, healthy people/healthy communities, and affordable care—for quality improvement. It has developed into a road map for quality with a consensus-based set of core principles to guide the quality strategy and all efforts to improve health and healthcare delivery. These 10 principles are based on the implementation of evidence-based interventions that have been shown to have positive benefit and impact the health and health outcomes of individuals and populations (Agency for Healthcare Research and Quality [AHRQ], 2010).

The increasing complexity of the healthcare delivery systems has seen five important factors that challenge clinicians to seek and use evidence to guide their practice. The first factor is the high visibility of the *quality and safety movement* in healthcare. In the midst of ever-increasing healthcare choices, clinicians want to know what works to increase the quality of care delivered, including the best practices to improve and optimize patient outcomes, the satisfaction with care to optimize the patient experience throughout the continuum of care, and implementation of safer systems of care to protect patients from medical error. It has been recommended recently that consumers should be included in discussions and implementation of safety and quality initiatives at local levels, and this challenges clinicians to consider the role of patients in these initiatives. For example, proper hand-washing before and after patient contact has been consistently shown to decrease the spread of infections. Empowering patients to ask their physician or nurse when they enter their hospital room or clinic suite, "Have you washed your hands?" directly involves the patient in implementing evidence at the point of care.

The second factor is the *tremendous growth of new knowledge* available to today's healthcare clinician. As of April 5, 2018, 5,235 journals are currently indexed for MEDLINE. MEDLINE includes journals that are cited as *Index Medicus* as well as other non-*Index Medicus* journals. There are 4,946 journals indexed as *Index Medicus* and 289 additional non-*Index Medicus* journals, on topics such as dentistry, nursing, healthcare administration and delivery, healthcare technology, history of medicine, consumer health, and HIV/AIDS (National Library of Medicine, 2018). The Cumulative Index to Nursing and Allied Health Literature (CINAHL; EBSCO *host*, n.d.) now includes more than 4,000 journals in its index for nursing and allied health professionals. In 1995, when there were fewer journals than are available to clinicians today, it was estimated that clinicians would need to read 19 articles a day, 365 days a year to stay abreast of the explosion of new information (Davidoff, Haynes, Sackett, & Smith, 1995). The challenge to be updated with new knowledge in healthcare is even greater today. Evidence-based practice is a way for nurses to bridge the research–practice gap (International Council of Nurses, 2012).

The third factor is the research in healthcare that has shown that there is a *considerable delay in incorporating new evidence into clinical practice* (Balas & Boren, 2000). There are many examples of these delays in implementing knowledge into practice, too numerous to cite here; however, the most famous is that in 1973, there was good evidence for the effectiveness of thrombolytic therapy in reducing mortality in acute myocardial infarction (MI), which is still not uniformly given in a timely fashion to patients who would benefit.

The fourth factor is a result of the growth of new knowledge and the delays in implementing that new knowledge, a resultant *decline in best care knowledge for patient care*. There is so much information available to the clinician and limited time to read and evaluate it for use in practice. It is widely recognized that the knowledge of best care has a negative correlation with the year of graduation (i.e., the longer the time since graduation, the poorer a person's knowledge of best care practices). EBP techniques, such as systematic reviews of evidence, available to the clinician at websites—such as the Cochrane Collaboration, the AHRQ, National Guidelines Clearinghouse, and the Joanna Briggs Institute—synthesize new knowledge and make it available to clinicians to improve best care knowledge.

Finally, the *tremendous consumer pressure* created by an increasingly savvy consumer who has online healthcare information at her or his fingertips has increased consumer expectations to take part in treatment decisions. Patients with chronic health problems who often access the Internet have considerable expertise in the self-management of their healthcare. Nurses at the point of care are in important positions to provide up-to-date information to patients, incorporating the best available evidence when patients question the type and quality of care being provided.

The factors mentioned previously demand that nurses in today's healthcare system be knowledgeable about their practice and use explicit criteria and methods to evaluate their practice to incorporate appropriate new evidence. However, the research over the past 15 years has been inconsistent on nurses' use of evidence to inform and improve practice.

In one of the earliest EBP studies, Mitchell, Janzen, Pask, and Southwell (1995) investigated the use of research in practice in Canadian hospitals and found that only 15% had a research utilization/EBP program for their nurses and only 38% based changes in practice on research, but that 97% wanted assistance in teaching their nurses about the research process. They also found that only 35% of small hospitals of less than 250 beds had nursing research journals in their libraries.

In 2000, Parahoo studied nurses' perceptions of research and found that many reported a lack of skill in evaluating research and felt isolated from colleagues who might be available to discuss research findings. The study found that nurses lacked the confidence to implement change and felt that they did not have the autonomy to implement changes. Parahoo also found that organizational characteristics are the most significant barriers to research use among nurses, including lack of organizational support for EBP, noting a lack of interest; a lack of motivation; a lack of leadership; and a lack of vision, strategy, and direction among managers.

In a Cochrane review, Foxcroft and Cole (2006) examined studies that had identified organizational infrastructures that promote EBP to determine the extent of effectiveness of the organizational infrastructure in promoting the implementation of research evidence to improve the effectiveness of nursing interventions. They found only seven case study designs to review. They concluded that there were no studies rigorous enough to be included in the review and recommended that conceptual models on organizational processes to promote EBP need to be researched and evaluated properly.

Pravikoff, Tanner, and Pierce (2005) studied the EBP readiness of RNs in a geographically stratified random sample of 3,000 RNs (n = 1,097) obtained from a nationwide publishing company. The purpose of the study was to examine the nurses' perceptions of their skills in obtaining evidence and their access to tools to obtain that evidence. Of the RNs, 760 were currently in clinical practice. Among that group, the study team found that 61% of the respondents said they needed to seek information at least once per week; however, 67% of those nurses always or frequently sought information from a colleague instead of a reference text, and only 46% were familiar with the term *EBP*. In addition, 58% reported not using research reports at all to support their practice, 82% reported never using a hospital library, and 83% reported rarely or never seeking a librarian's assistance. These are large gaps in nurses' skills and knowledge that need to be closed to enable EBP.

In a study to identify the presence or absence of provider and organizational variables associated with the use of EBP among nurses, Leasure, Stirlen, and Thompson (2008) surveyed nurse executives to identify barriers and facilitators to the use of EBP. They found that facilitators to EBP are reading journals that publish original research; joining journal clubs, nursing research committees, and facility research committees; and having facility access to the Internet. However, the barriers included lack of staff involvement in projects, no communication of projects that were completed, and no knowledge on outcomes of projects.

More recent studies by Melnyk and colleagues have assessed beliefs about and the state of EBP among U.S. nurses. They found that having an organizational culture and work environment that supports EBP is positively associated with nurse satisfaction, belief in EBP, and implementation of EBP by nurses and other healthcare providers (Melnyk, Fineout-Overholt, Gallagher-Ford, & Kaplan, 2012; Melnyk, Fineout-Overholt, Giggleman, & Cruz, 2010). They also found that even though EBP is generally accepted by nurses despite differences in this acceptance by Magnet® and non-Magnet institutions, the nurses still identify barriers to positive implementation of EBP in their practices (Melnyk et al., 2012).

Importance of Using Best Available Evidence to Guide Nursing Practice

It is clear from this sampling of studies that EBP is continuing to evolve, but not to the extent that is necessary. Nurses must understand the importance of EBP, and healthcare organizations must invest in resources necessary for nurses to have access to evidence at the point of care. However, a systematic approach to using that evidence is necessary: A formal process is needed that uses specific criteria to appraise evidence to enhance efficiency and effectiveness of practice and uses methods for incorporating that evidence into practice. There are many good EBP models that have been developed to organize and assist nurses to ask clinical questions, evaluate new evidence, and to make changes in the clinical setting. Each of these models has advantages and disadvantages, and they vary in usefulness by setting and context. Gawlinski and Rutledge (2008) suggested that a deliberate process should be followed by an organization to select a model for EBP. They suggested that first a group should be developed to champion the EBP process and that this group should review models by using specific criteria and then summarize the strengths and weaknesses of the models by asking specific questions such as:

- What elements of EBP models are important to your organization?
- Is the model useful for all clinical situations and populations?
- Has the model been tested and disseminated?
- Is the model easy to use, and who will use the model?

They also suggested that once a model is chosen, the EBP champion group should educate the staff. Dearholt, White, Newhouse, Pugh, and Poe (2008) have gone further, suggesting that once the organization decides that an evidence-based foundation for nursing is needed, a model should be chosen that is easy for the staff nurse to use; the administration should also create a strategic initiative around the implementation of EBP for the nursing department, supporting the initiative with resources in terms of time, money, and people.

■ EBP CONCEPTUAL FRAMEWORKS AND MODELS

A conceptual framework or model is a guide to an empirical inquiry that is built from a set of concepts, deemed critical to the inquiry, which are related and function to outline the inquiry or set of actions. Frameworks have been used in nursing to guide research and to define the foundation for nursing practice and educational programs. Likewise, models for implementing EBP have been developed to guide the process. These models vary in detail and in explicit criteria and methods for carrying out an EBP inquiry. However, the following steps or phases are common to most models:

1. Identification of a clinical problem or question of practice
2. Search for best evidence
3. Critical appraisal of strength, quality, quantity, and consistency of evidence
4. Recommendation for action (no change, change, further study) based on the appraisal of evidence
5. Implementation of recommendation
6. Evaluation of that recommendation in relationship to desired outcomes

The chapter continues with a presentation of the key nursing EBP models in use today.

Stetler's Model of Research Utilization

Cheryl Stetler's Model of Research Utilization (Figure 1.1) was one of the original models developed as an EBP for nursing that began to receive attention. She originally developed the model in 1994 and revised it in 2001. The purpose of the model is to formulate a series of critical-thinking and decision-making steps that are designed to facilitate the effective use of research findings (Stetler, 2001; Stetler & Marram, 1976). The model is an individual practitioner-oriented model rather than an organizational-focused model. The revised model promotes the use of both internal data (such as quality improvement, operational, evaluation, and practitioner experience data) and external evidence (such as primary research and consensus of national experts). The model describes five phases of research utilization. In phase I, *preparation*, the nurse searches for and selects research to be evaluated for practice implementation. This step is driven by critical thinking about potential internal and external influencing factors. During phase II, *validation*, the nurse appraises the findings of the study using specific methodology and utilization considerations. In phase III, the *comparative evaluation* or *decision-making* phase, a decision about whether a practice change can be made is determined using four applicability criteria: (a) the substantiating evidence, (b) the fit for implementing the research findings in the setting, (c) the feasibility of implementation, and (d) the evaluation of current practice. Phase IV is when the *translation* or *application* of the research findings is implemented and the "how tos" of implementation are considered. Phase V, *evaluation*, requires that processes include different types and levels of evaluation.

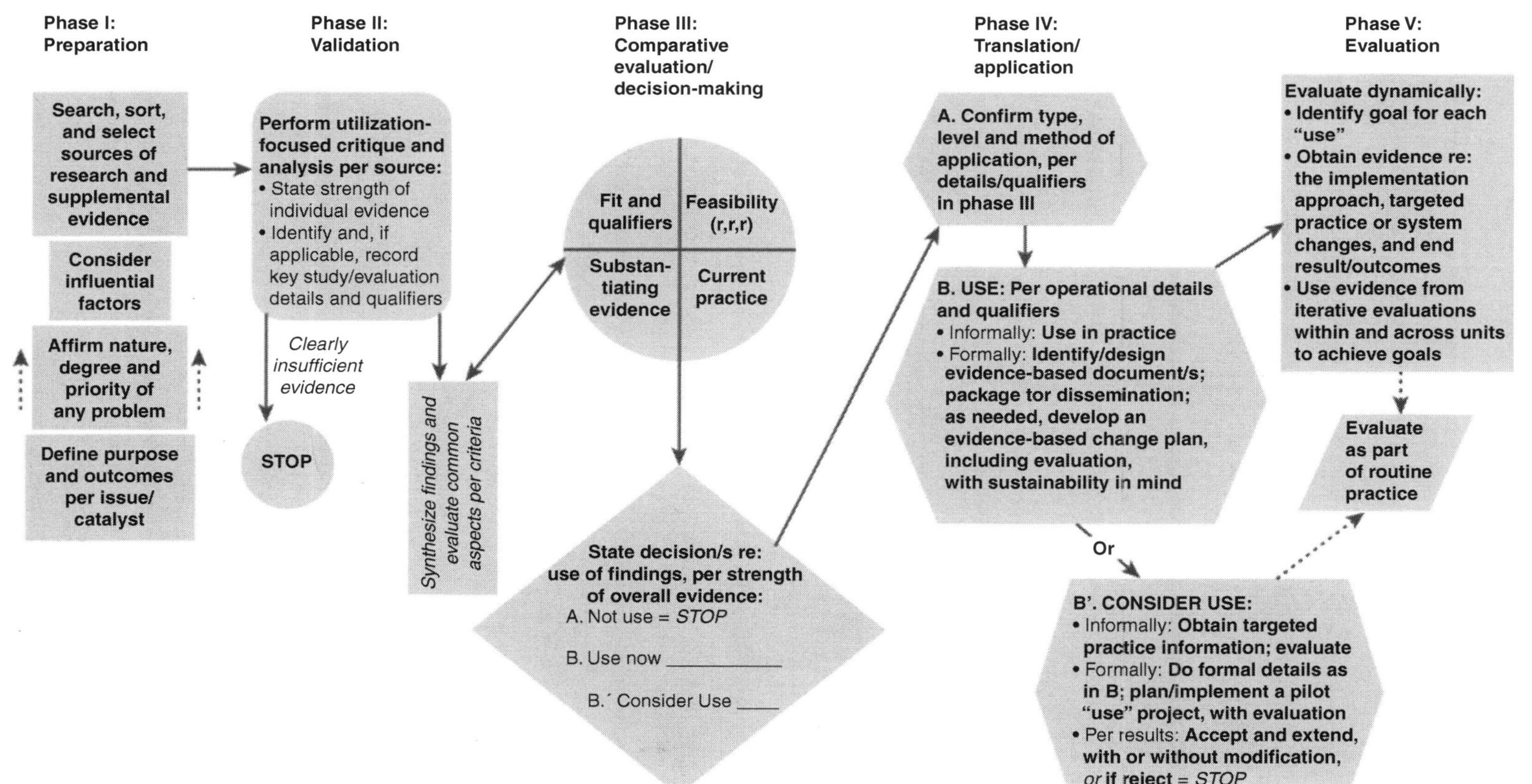

FIGURE 1.1 The Stetler model.

r, r, r, risk factors, resources, and readiness of others to be involved.

Source: From Stetler, C. (2010). Stetler model. In J. Rycroft-Malone & T. Bucknall (Eds.), *Evidence-based practice series*. Oxford, UK: Wiley-Blackwell.

Dobbins's Framework for Dissemination and Utilization of Research

In 2001, Dobbins, Cockerill, and Barnsley studied the factors affecting the utilization of systematic reviews. The purpose of their study was to determine the extent to which public health decision makers in Ontario used five systematic reviews to make policy decisions and to determine the characteristics that predict their use. The findings of the study were used to assist health services researchers in disseminating research. Informed by their own research and using Everett Rogers's Diffusion of Innovations theory, the Dobbins's framework for dissemination and utilization of research (Figure 1.2) was developed to inform policy and practice. The model illustrates that the process of adoption of research evidence is influenced by characteristics related to the individual, organization, environment, and innovation. The model includes five stages of innovation: knowledge, persuasion, decision, implementation, and confirmation. Identified

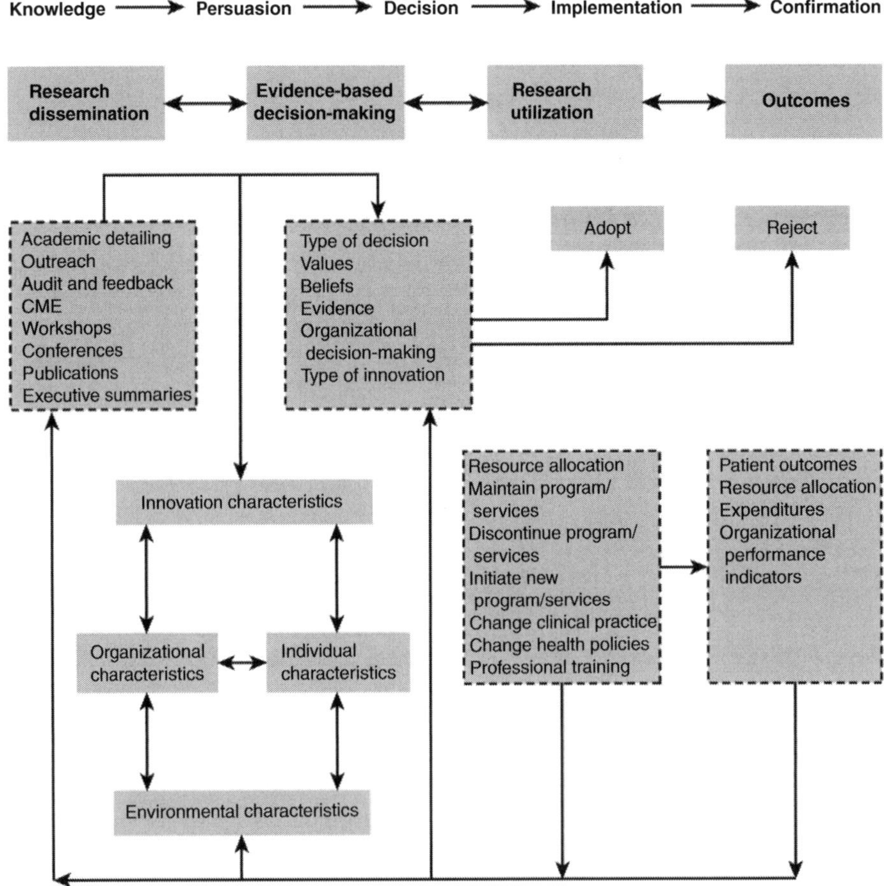

FIGURE 1.2 Framework for research dissemination and utilization.

CME, continuing medical education.

Source: Adapted with permission from Dobbins, M., Ciliska, D., Cockerill, R., & Barnsley, J. (2001). Factors affecting the utilization of systematic reviews: A study of public health decision makers. *International Journal of Technology Assessment in Health Care, 17*(2), 203–214. doi:10.1017/S0266462300105069

under each of the five stages are the considerations for transferring research to practice in healthcare (Dobbins, Ciliska, Cockerill, Barnsley, & DiCenso, 2002).

Funk's Model for Improving the Dissemination of Nursing Research

In 1987, the research team of Funk, Champagne, Tornquist, and Wiese, after concluding that there was a huge gap between the conduct of nursing research and the use of research findings to improve practice, developed the BARRIERS scale to assess the perceptions of barriers of clinicians, administrators, and academicians to the utilization of research findings in practice. Items were derived from the literature, from research data, and from the Conduct and Utilization of Research in Nursing (CURN) project's research utilization questionnaire (Crane, Pelz, & Horsley, 1977). The BARRIERS scale consisted of 28 items in four categories: characteristics of the adopter, the organization, the innovation, and the communication. The tool was tested with a sample of 1,948 RNs in clinical practice (n = 924). Standard psychometric analyses of the tool were performed and replicated. Using the results of this analysis, the team developed a model for improving research utilization. The Funk model for improving dissemination of nursing research (Figure 1.3) includes three components: the qualities of the research, characteristics of communication, and facilitation of utilization (Funk, Tornquist, & Champagne, 1989). The model delineates three mechanisms to achieve the dissemination of research: (a) hold topic-focused, practice-oriented research conferences; (b) write monographs that are based on the research conference presentations; and (c) develop an information center that provides ongoing dialogue, support, and consultation for the dissemination (Funk et al., 1989). The goal of the approach is to reach the practicing nurse with research results and to provide support and consultation to those doing the research.

Clinical Practice Guideline Implementation Model

The Registered Nurses Association of Ontario (RNAO; 2002) took the lead in Canada in developing best practice guidelines for nurses. The Nursing Best Practice Guidelines (NBPG) project was funded by the Ontario Ministry of Health and Long-Term Care and involved the development, implementation, evaluation, and dissemination of a series of clinical practice guidelines (CPGs). Early on in the project it became evident that healthcare organizations were struggling to identify ways to implement the guidelines, and little attention was being paid to implementation strategies. The RNAO established a panel of nurses and researchers, chaired by Alba DiCenso, to develop a planned, systematic approach to the implementation of the CPGs (DiCenso et al., 2002). The likelihood of success in implementing CPGs increases when:

- A systematic process is used to identify a well-developed, evidence-based CPG.
- Appropriate stakeholders are identified and engaged.
- An assessment of environmental readiness for CPG implementation is conducted.

- Evidence-based implementation strategies that address the issues raised through the environmental readiness assessment are used.
- An evaluation of the implementation is planned and conducted.
- Consideration of resource implications to carry out these activities is adequately addressed (DiCenso et al., 2002).

The panel developed an implementation model (Figure 1.4) with an accompanying tool kit for implementing CPGs (rnao.ca/bpg/resources/toolkit-implementation-best-practice-guidelines-second-edition).

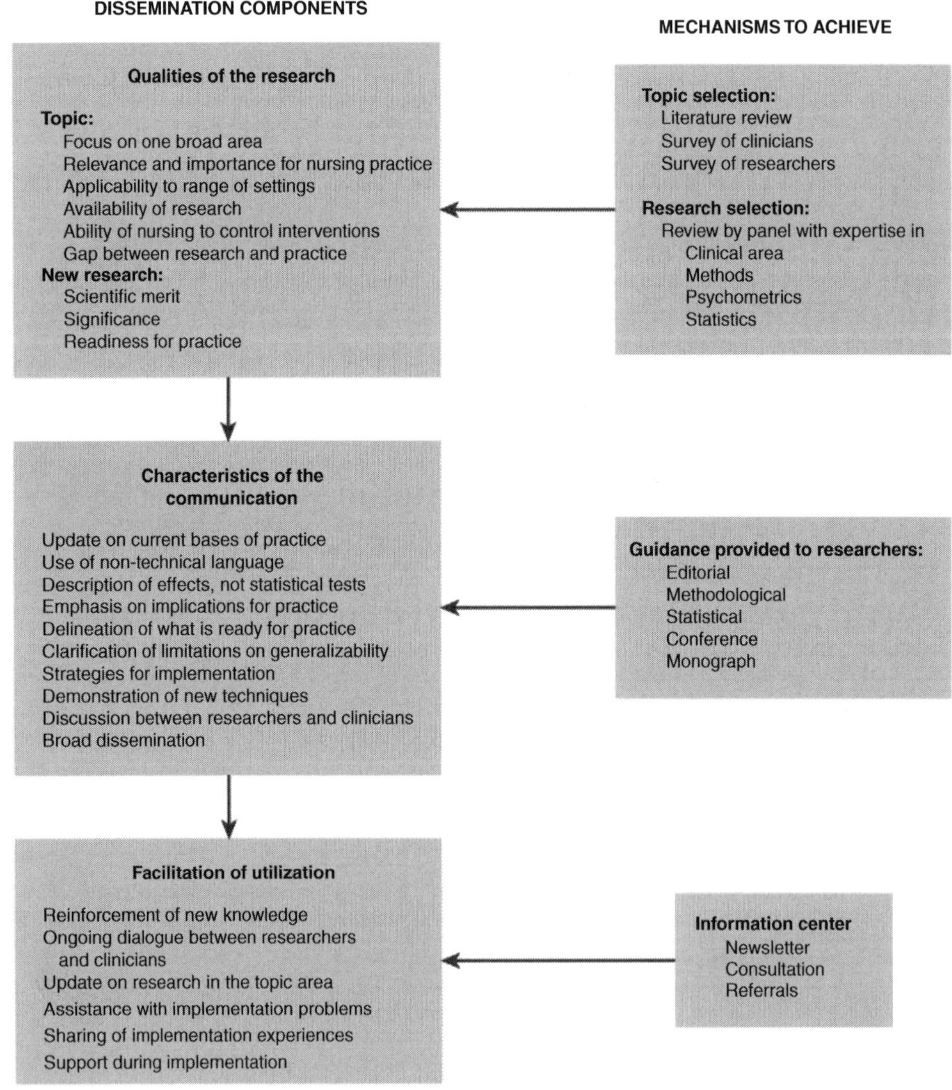

FIGURE 1.3 The Funk research dissemination model.

Source: Reprinted with permission from Funk, S. G., Tornquist, E. M., & Champagne, M. T. (1989). A model for the dissemination of nursing research. *Western Journal of Nursing Research, 11*(3), 361–372. doi:10.1177/019394598901100311. Copyright by Sage Publications, Inc.

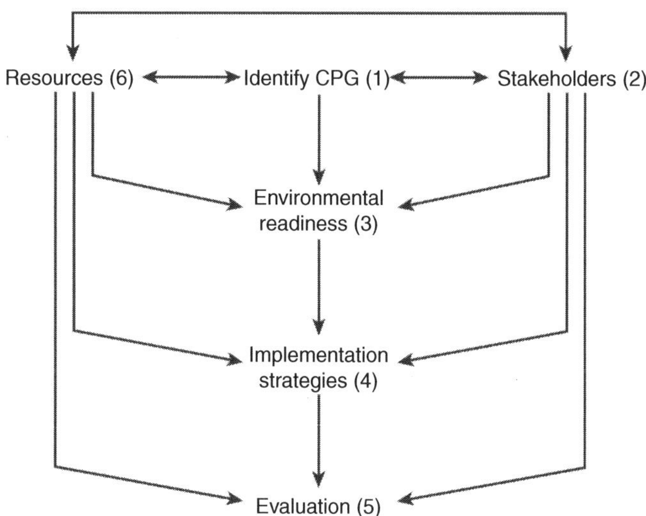

FIGURE 1.4 CPG implementation model.

CPG, clinical practice guideline.

Source: From Registered Nurses Association of Ontario. (2002). *Toolkit: Implementation of clinical practice guidelines*. Retrieved from http://rnao.ca/bpg/resources/toolkit-implementation-best-practice-guidelines-second-edition.

The Johns Hopkins Nursing EBP Model and Guidelines

The Johns Hopkins Nursing EBP (JHNEBP) Model (Figure 1.5) was developed by a collaborative team of nurse leaders from the Johns Hopkins Hospital (JHH) and

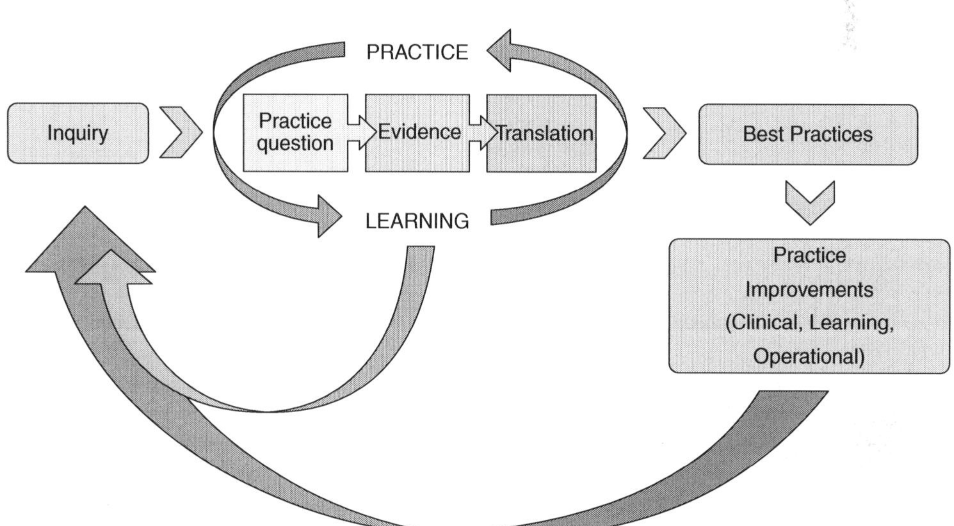

FIGURE 1.5 Johns Hopkins Nursing evidence-based practice conceptual model.

Source: From Dang, D., & Dearholt, S. (2017). *The Johns Hopkins nursing evidence-based practice model and guidelines*. Indianapolis, IN: Sigma Theta Tau International.

the Johns Hopkins University School of Nursing (JHUSON) asked to evaluate current practice, policies and procedures to ensure they were evidence-based. The team developed this practical model with accompanying guidelines and tools so that staff nurses would be able to evaluate current evidence and translate research findings into patient care. The goals of EBP at both the JHH and JHUSON are to:

- Ensure the highest quality of care.
- Use evidence to promote optimal outcomes or provide equivalent care at lower cost/time.
- Support rational decisions (including structural changes) that reduce inappropriate variation.
- Make it easier to do our job (optimal processes).
- Promote patient satisfaction and health-related quality of life (HRQOL).
- Create a culture of critical thinking and ongoing learning.
- Grow an environment where evidence supports clinical and administrative decisions.

The JHNEBP conceptual model was updated in 2017 to reflect more contemporary practice and terminology.

The JHNEBP model is defined as a problem-solving approach to clinical decision-making within a healthcare organization, which integrates the best available scientific evidence with the best available experiential (patient and practitioner) evidence, considers internal and external influences on practice, and encourages critical thinking in the judicious application of such evidence to the care of the individual patient, patient population, or system (Newhouse, Dearholt, Poe, Pugh, & White, 2005). The model also includes the three domains of professional nursing: nursing practice, education, and research.

The guidelines that accompany the model describe the three phases in getting to an EBP (Figure 1.6). These three phases are described as the "PET" process, an acronym that stands for the *practice question*, *evidence*, and *translation*.

The first phase, or "P" in PET, is the *practice* question and involves six steps:

1. Recruit an interprofessional team.
2. Define the problem.

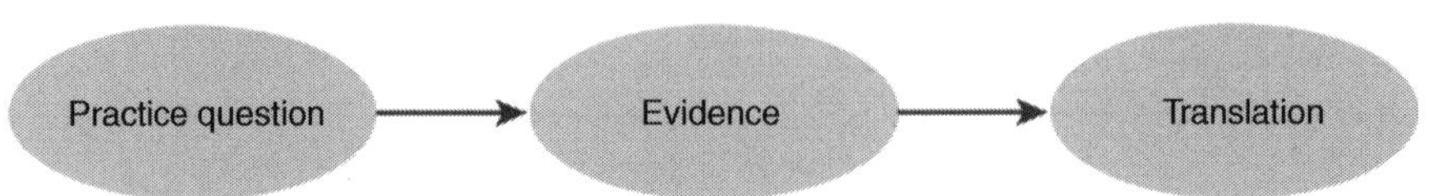

FIGURE 1.6 Evidence-based practice process.

Source: Reprinted with permission from Newhouse, R. P., Dearholt, S. L., Poe, S. S., Pugh, L. C., & White, K. M. (2005). Evidence-based practice: A practical approach to implementation. *Journal of Nursing Administration, 35*(1), 35–40. doi:10.1097/00005110-200501000-00013. Copyright by the Johns Hopkins Hospital/Johns Hopkins University.

3. Develop and refine the EBP question using the PICO format, which will help to identify key search terms for the evidence search (Richardson, Wilson, Nishikawa, & Hayward, 1995):
   P → Patient, population, or problem (age, gender, patient setting, or symptoms)
   I → Intervention (treatment, medications, education, and diagnostic tests)
   C → Comparison with other treatments (may not be applicable or may not be apparent until additional reading is done)
   O → Outcome (anticipated outcome).
4. Identify stakeholders.
5. Determine responsibility for project leadership.
6. Schedule team meetings

The second phase, or "E" in PET, is *evidence* and involves another five steps:

1. Conduct an internal and external search for evidence: Think about key search terms for the evidence search and brainstorm about what databases and other places there are to search for the evidence.
2. Appraise the level and quality of each piece of evidence.
3. Summarize the individual evidence.
4. Synthesize the overall strength and quality of the evidence.
5. Develop recommendations for change based on evidence synthesis:
   - Strong, compelling evidence, consistent results
   - Good evidence, consistent results
   - Good evidence, conflicting results
   - Insufficient or absent evidence

The third phase, or "T" in PET, is *translation*, which includes the following nine steps:

1. Determine the fit, feasibility, and appropriateness of recommendations for translation path.
2. Create an action plan.
3. Secure support and resources to implement the action plan.
4. Implement the action plan.
5. Evaluate the outcomes.
6. Report the outcomes to the stakeholders.
7. Identify the next steps.
8. Disseminate the findings.

This model includes a set of tools for use during each of the phases discussed previously and a very important project management tool that delineates the 19 steps in the PET process for the user. These tools are a critical added dimension to the model and make its use very practical for the staff nurse. The eight tools are:

1. Development of a practice question
2. Stakeholder analysis tool
3. Evidence appraisal guideline—levels of evidence and quality-rating tool

4. Review tool for scientific evidence
5. Review tool for nonscientific evidence
6. Individual evidence summary table
7. Synthesis of evidence and recommendation tool
8. Project management tool (action-planning tool)

The Iowa Model of Research-Based Practice to Promote Quality Care

The Iowa Model of Research-Based Practice was developed as a decision-making algorithm to guide nurses in using research findings to improve the quality of care (Figure 1.7). It was originally published in 1994, revised in 2001, and revised again in 2015 by the Iowa Model Collaborative. The revision was based on changes in the healthcare system, emerging evidence in implementation science, and questions from users (Cullen, Hanrahan and Kleiber, 2018). The Iowa model uses the concept of "triggers" for EBP, either clinical problem-focused or new knowledge-focused triggers often coming from outside the organization. These triggers set an EBP inquiry into motion and at each point in the algorithm, the nurse must consider the organizational context and the strength and quantity of evidence, while answering several questions:

- Is the evidence to change practice sufficient?
- Are findings across studies consistent?
- Are the type and quality of the findings sufficient?
- Do the studies have clinical (not just statistical) relevance?
- Can the studies reviewed be generalized to your population?
- Are the findings of the study feasible?
- How appropriate is the risk–benefit ratio?

This model emphasizes the use of pilot testing versus the implementation of a practice change.

Rosswurm and Larrabee's Model for EBP Change

Rosswurm and Larrabee (1999), at the University of West Virginia, developed a six-step model to facilitate a shift from traditional and intuition-driven practice to implement evidence-based changes into practice (Figure 1.8). The model has been tested in the acute care clinical setting, but the authors think it is adaptable to primary care settings. The following are the six steps in the model (Larrabee, 2009):

1. Assess the need for change in practice by comparing internal data with external data.
2. Link the problem with interventions and outcomes (standard interventions, if possible).
3. Synthesize the best evidence (research and contextual evidence).
4. Design a change in practice.
5. Implement and evaluate the change in practice, including processes and outcomes.
6. Integrate and maintain the change in practice using diffusion strategies.

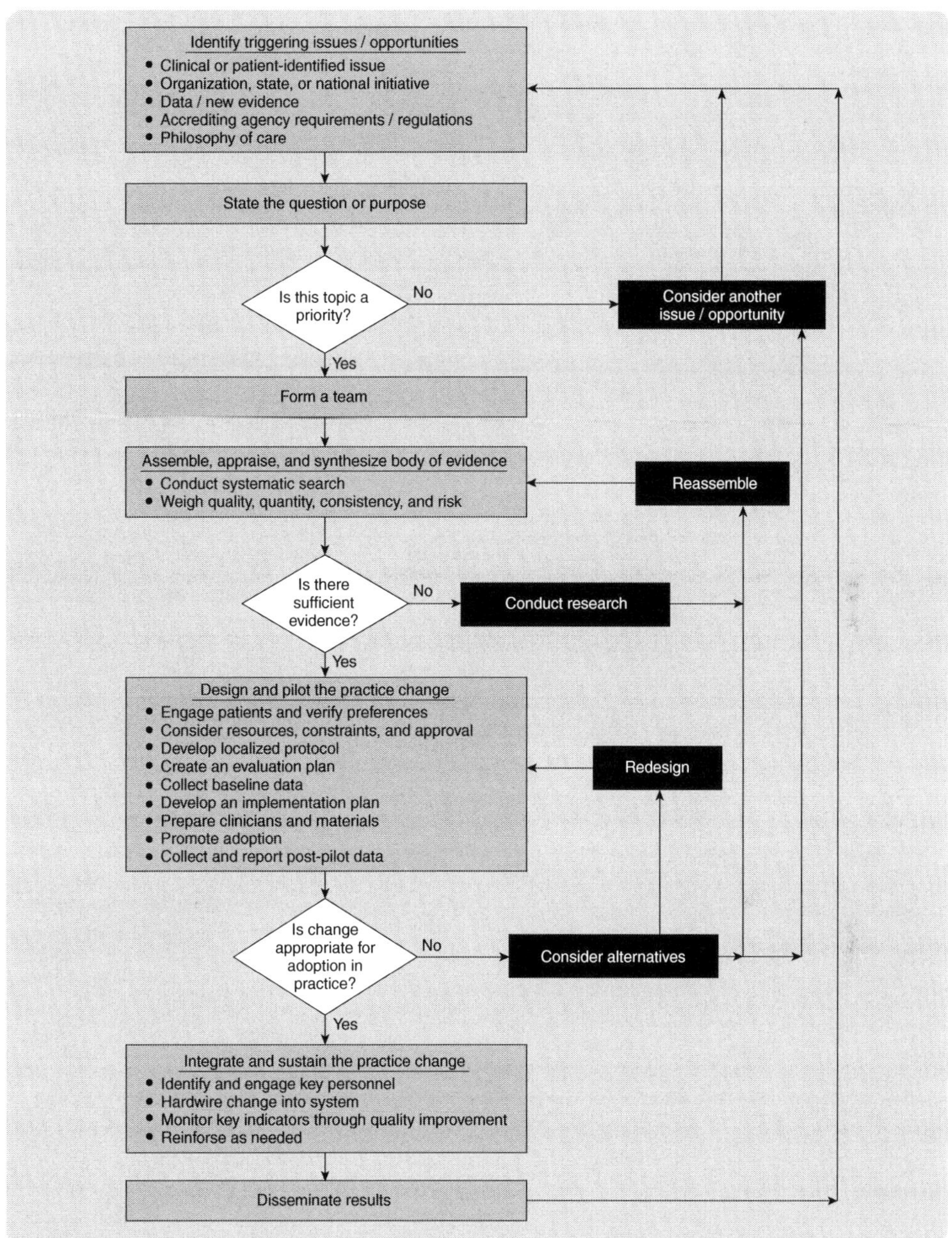

FIGURE 1.7 The 2017 Iowa Model—Revised: Evidence-based practice to promote excellence in healthcare.

Note: Used/reprinted with permission from the University of Iowa Hospitals and Clinics, Copyright 2015. For permission to use or reproduce the model, please contact the University of Iowa Hospitals and Clinics at 319-384-9098 or uihcnursingresearchandebp@uiowa.edu.

Source: From Iowa Model Collaborative. (2017). Iowa Model of evidence-based practice: Revisions and validation. *Worldviews on Evidence-Based Nursing, 14*(3), 175–182. doi:10.1111/wvn.12223

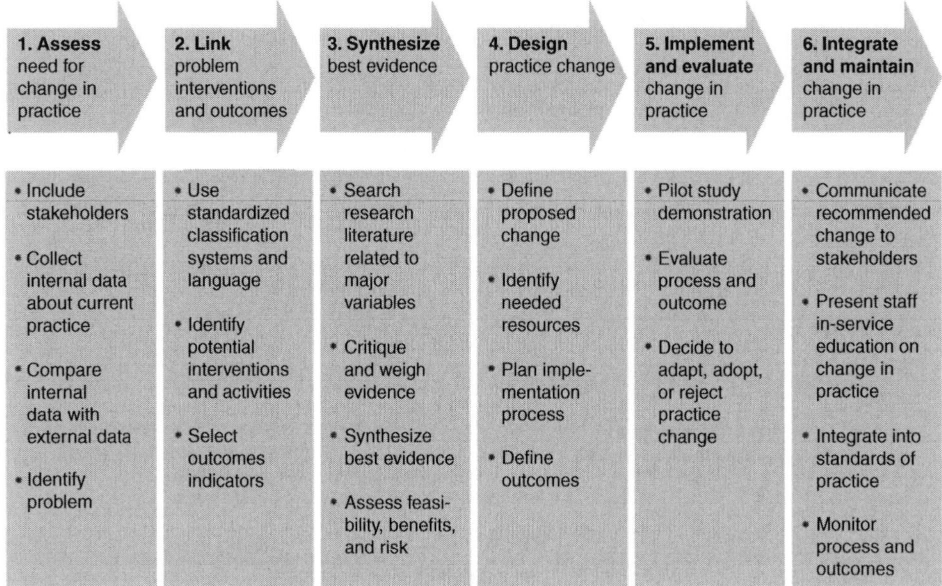

FIGURE 1.8 A model for change to evidence-based practice.

Source: Reprinted with permission from Rosswurm, M. A., & Larrabee, J. H. (1999). A model for change to evidence-based practice. *Journal of Nursing Scholarship, 31*(4), 317–322. doi:10.1111/j.1547-5069.1999.tb00510.x. Copyright by Blackwell Publishing.

The ACE Star Model of Knowledge Transformation

The Academic Center for Evidence-Based Practice (ACE; n.d.) Star Model of Knowledge Transformation (Figure 1.9) was developed by Kathleen Stevens and staff at the University of Texas Health Science Center in San Antonio to provide a framework for understanding the cycles, nature, and characteristics of knowledge that are used in EBP processes (http://nursing.uthscsa.edu/onrs/starmodel/institute/su08/starmodel.html; Stevens, 2013). The goal of the process is knowledge transformation that is defined as "the conversion of research findings from primary research results, through a series of stages and forms, to impact on health outcomes by way of [evidence-based] care" (Stevens, 2004). The model promotes EBP by stressing the identification of knowledge types (from research to integrative reviews to translation). This model does not discuss the use of nonresearch evidence. The ACE Star Model is depicted using a five-pointed star for the five stages of knowledge transformation:

Point 1: Knowledge discovery (knowledge generation)
Point 2: Evidence summary (single statement from systematic review)
Point 3: Translation into practice (repackaging summarized research—clinical recommendations)
Point 4: Integration into practice (individual and organizational actions)
Point 5: Evaluation (effect on targeted outcomes)

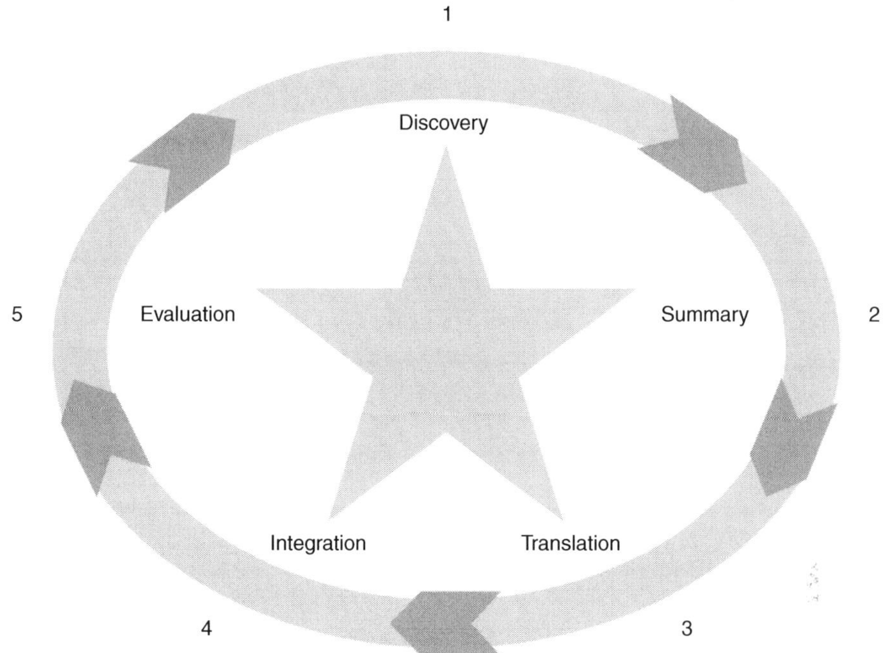

FIGURE 1.9 The ACE Star Model of Knowledge Transformation.

Source: Adapted from Stevens, K. R. (2004). *ACE Star model of EBP: Knowledge transformation*. San Antonio, TX: Academic Center for Evidence-Based Practice, The University of Texas Health Science Center at San Antonio. Retrieved from http://nursing.uthscsa.edu/onrs/starmodel/institute/su08/starmodel.html. © Stevens, 2015. Used with expressed permission.

Advancing Research Through Close Clinical Collaboration

The Advancing Research and Clinical Practice Through Close Collaboration (ARCC) Model (Figure 1.10) was originally developed by Fineout-Overholt, Melnyk, and Schultz (2005) at the University of Rochester Medical Center.

The goals of the ARCC Model are as follows:

- Promote the use of EBP among advanced practice nurses (APNs) and nurses.
- Establish the network of clinicians who are supporting EBP.
- Obtain funding for ARCC.
- Disseminate the best evidence.
- Conduct an annual conference on EBP.
- Conduct studies to evaluate effectiveness of the ARCC Model on process and outcomes of clinical care (Melnyk & Fineout-Overholt, 2005).

This model was originally developed to create a link between a college of nursing and a medical center. It is referred to as a *clinical scholar model* and relies on mentors with in-depth knowledge of EBP and expert clinical and group facilitation skills. The following are the five steps in the model:

Step 1: Ask the clinical question.
Step 2: Search for the best evidence

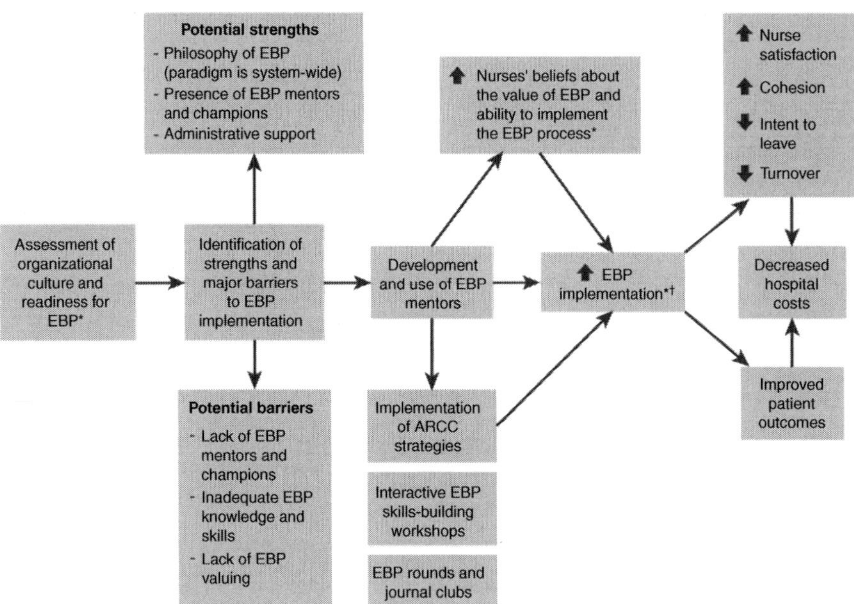

FIGURE 1.10 The Advancing Research and Clinical Practice Through Close Collaboration Model.

*Scale developed.

†Based on the EBP paradigm and using the EBP process.

ARCC, Advancing Research and Clinical Practice Through Close Collaboration; EPB, evidence-based practice.

Source: Adapted from Melnyk, B. M., Fineout-Overholt, E., Giggleman, M., & Cruz, R. (2010). Correlates among cognitive beliefs, EBP implementation, organizational culture, cohesion and job satisfaction in evidence-based practice mentors from a community hospital system. *Nursing Outlook, 58*(6), 301–308. doi:10.1016/j.outlook.2010.06.002

Step 3: Critically appraise the evidence.
Step 4: Address the sufficiency of the evidence: to implement or not to implement?
Step 5: Evaluate the outcome of evidence implementation.

Melnyk and Fineout-Overholt (2005) conducted a pilot study to test the ARCC Model at two acute care sites. The pilot study examined what must be present for a successful implementation of EBP in the acute care setting. These essentials include identifying EBP champions, redefining nurses' roles to include EBP activities, allocating time and money to the EBP process, and creating an organizational culture that fosters EBP. In addition, practical strategies for implementing EBP are presented to encourage implementation of EBP (Melnyk & Fineout-Overholt, 2005).

The Clinical Scholar Model

The Clinical Scholar Model is attributed to work facilitated by Alyce Schultz and a team of nurses at the Maine Medical Center in Portland, Maine (see Figure 1.11). The model is based on the assumption that "knowledge users produce better patient outcomes," and is a grassroots approach to developing a core group of point-of-care

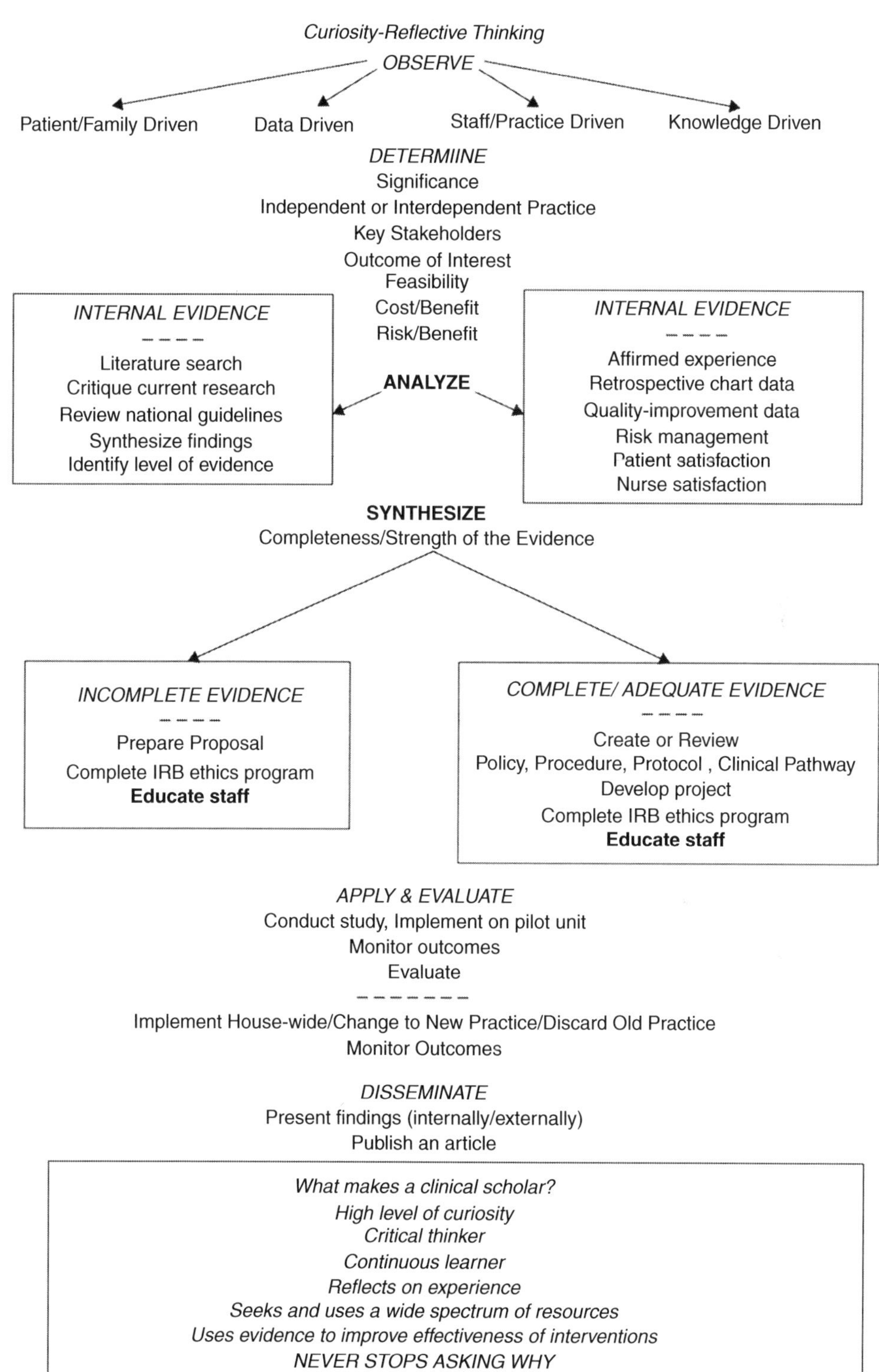

FIGURE 1.11 The Clinical Scholar Model.

IRB, institutional review board.

Source: Courtesy of Alyce A. Schultz RN, PhD, FAAN, Chandler, Arizona.

nurses who become clinical scholars and are committed to improving patient care through research, evidence-based practice, and quality improvement (Strout, Lancaster, & Schultz, 2009). The model uses an inductive approach to promote interdisciplinary EBP teamwork at the point of care by developing bedside nurses who mentor their colleagues to critique, integrate, implement, and evaluate evidence and build a cadre of innovators necessary to develop and sustain an EBP culture. The model proposes five major steps to the use of evidence in practice: observation, analysis, synthesis, application/evaluation, and dissemination.

Honess, Gallant, and Keane (2009) reported on three EBP projects that started at the point of care by staff nurses who questioned traditional practices; used the model to guide the identification, implementation, and evaluation of their current clinical practice; and used internal and external evidence to develop sound EBP changes.

Veterans Administration's Quality Enhancement Research Initiative Model

The Quality Enhancement Research Initiative (QUERI) Model (Figure 1.12) was developed by the Department of Veterans Affairs in 1998 to improve the quality of healthcare throughout the veterans system through the use of research-based best practices (Stetler, Mittman, & Francis, 2008). The program had a quality-improvement focus and included a redesign of organizational structures and policies and implementation of new information technology and a performance accountability system (Perrin & Stevens, 2004). The QUERI process model includes six steps (Stetler et al., 2008):

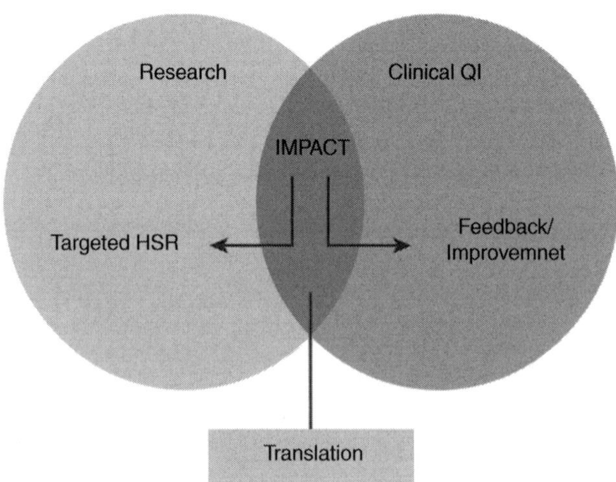

FIGURE 1.12 Quality Enhancement Research Initiative Model.

HSR, health services research; QI, quality improvement.

Source: From Feussner, J. R., Kizer, K. W., & Demakis, J. G. (2000). The Quality Enhancement Research Initiative (QUERI): From evidence to action. *Medical Care, 38*(6, Suppl. 1), I1–I6. doi:10.1097/00005650-200006001-00001

1. Select conditions per patient population that are associated with a high risk of disease and/or disability and/or burden of illness for veterans.
2. Identify evidence-based guidelines, recommendations, and best practices.
3. Measure and diagnose the quality and performance gaps.
4. Implement improvement programs.
5. Assess improvement program feasibility, implementation, and effects on patient, family, and healthcare system processes and outcomes.
6. Assess improvement program effects on HRQOL.

The program has been implemented in a four-phase pipeline framework that begins with pilot projects for improvement and feasibility, then advances to small clinical trials, and moves to regional rollouts, and, finally, the improvement based on research becomes a national effort (Department of Veterans Affairs, 2011a, 2011b). The QUERI Model is highlighted graphically showing an intersection between research and practice, and showing that the translation of research is accomplished through clinical and quality-improvement (QI) activities and enhanced by feedback in the system.

■ CONCLUSIONS

The EBP movement has made a tremendous impact on nursing clinical, administrative, and educational practices. As full partners in designing and transforming our healthcare system, nurses are critical to providing evidence-based, safe, effective, and efficient healthcare. The key to making these important contributions in today's complex healthcare environment is to understand the challenges and opportunities involved in developing, implementing, and sustaining EBP at every level of practice and setting. However, there is a lot to be learned about how those interventions are implemented and how evidence is translated into practice. The next two chapters in this book present translation frameworks that can be used to guide the implementation of evidence into practice and explore the key interrelationships within organizations that drive or restrain the translation.

■ REFERENCES

Academic Center for Evidence-Based Practice, University of Texas Health Science Center at San Antonio. (n.d.). *ACE Star model*. Retrieved from http://nursing.uthscsa.edu/onrs/starmodel/institute/su08/starmodel.html

Agency for Healthcare Research and Quality. (2010). *Principle for the National Quality Strategy (NQS)*. Retrieved from http://www.ahrq.gov/workingforquality

Balas, E. A., & Boren, S. A. (2000). Managing clinical knowledge for health care improvement. In J. van Bemmel & A. T. McCray (Eds.), *Yearbook of medical informatics 2000: Patient-centered systems* (pp. 65–70). Stuttgart, Germany: Schattauer Verlagsgesellschaft.

Cochrane, A. L. (1972). *Effectiveness and efficiency: Random reflections on health services*. London, UK: Nuffield Provincial Hospitals Trust.

Crane, J., Pelz, D. C., & Horsley, J. A. (1977). *CURN. Project research utilization questionnaire*. Michigan, MI: School of Nursing, University of Michigan.

Cullen, L., Hanrahan, K., & Kleiber, C. (2018). Nursing and EBP: From asking questions to evaluating results. Reflections on Nursing Leadership. Retrieved from https://www.reflectionsonnursingleadership.org/features/more-features/nursing-and-ebp-from-asking-questions-to-evaluating-results

Dang, D., & Dearholt, S. (2017). *The Johns Hopkins nursing evidence-based practice model and guidelines*. Indianapolis, IN: Sigma Theta Tau, International.

Davidoff, F., Haynes, B., Sackett, D., & Smith, R. (1995). Evidence-based medicine. *British Medical Journal, 310*(6987), 1085–1086. doi:10.1136/bmj.310.6987.1085

Dearholt, S. L., White, K. M., Newhouse, R. P., Pugh, L. C., & Poe, S. (2008). Educational strategies to develop evidence-based practice mentors. *Journal for Nurses in Staff Development, 24*(2), 53–59. doi:10.1097/01.NND.0000300873.20986.97

Department of Veterans Affairs. (2011a). *QUERI implementation guide*. Retrieved from http://www.queri.research.va.gov/implementation

Department of Veterans Affairs. (2011b). *Quality Enhancement Research Initiative* [Brochure]. Retrieved from http://www.queri.research.va.gov

DiCenso, A., Virani, T., Bajnok, I., Borycki, E., Davies, B., Graham, I., . . . Scott, J. (2002). A toolkit to facilitate the implementation of clinical practice guidelines in healthcare settings. *Hospital Quarterly, 5*(3), 55–60. doi:10.12927/hcq..16515

Dobbins, M., Ciliska, D., Cockerill, R., & Barnsley, J. (2001). Factors affecting the utilization of systematic reviews: A study of public health decision makers. *International Journal of Technology Assessment in Health Care, 17*(2), 203–214. doi:10.1017/S0266462300105069

Dobbins, M., Ciliska, D., Cockerill, R., Barnsley, J., & DiCenso, A. (2002). A framework for the dissemination and utilization of research for health-care policy and practice. *Worldviews on Evidence-Based Nursing, 9(7)*, 149–160. doi:10.1111/j.1524-475X.2002.00149.x

Dobbins, M., Cockerill, R., & Barnsley, J. (2001). Factors affecting the utilization of systematic reviews: A study of public health decision makers. *International Journal of Technology Assessment in Health Care, 17*(2), 203–214. doi:10.1017/S0266462300105069

EBSCO *host*. (n.d.). *Cumulative Index to Nursing and Allied Health Literature*. Retrieved from https://health.ebsco.com/products/the-cinahl-database

Evidence-Based Medicine Working Group. (1992). Evidence-based medicine: A new approach to teaching the practice of medicine. *Journal of the American Medical Association, 268*(17), 2420–2425. doi:10.1001/jama.268.17.2420

Feussner, J. R., Kizer, K. W., & Demakis, J. G. (2000). The Quality Enhancement Research Initiative (QUERI): From evidence to action. *Medical Care, 38*(6, Suppl. 1), I1–I6. doi:10.1097/00005650-200006001-00001

Fineout-Overholt, E., Melnyk, B. M., & Schultz, A. (2005). Transforming health care from the inside out: Advancing evidence-based practice in the 21st century. *Journal of Professional Nursing, 21*(6), 335–344. doi:10.1016/j.profnurs.2005.10.005

Foxcroft, D. R., & Cole, N. (2006). Organisational infrastructures to promote evidence-based nursing practice. *Cochrane Database of Systematic Reviews, 2006*(3), CD002212. doi:10.1002/14651858.CD002212

Funk, S. G., Tornquist, E. M., & Champagne, M. T. (1989). A model for the dissemination of nursing research. *Western Journal of Nursing Research, 11*(3), 361–372. doi:10.1177/019394598901100311

Gawlinski, A., & Rutledge, D. (2008). Selecting a model for evidence-based practice changes: A practical approach. *AACN Advanced Critical Care, 19*(3), 291–300. doi:10.1097/01.AACN.0000330380.41766.63

Honess, C., Gallant, P., & Keane, K. (2009). The clinical scholar model: Evidence-based practice at the bedside. *Nursing Clinics of North America, 44*(1), 117–130. doi:10.1016/j.cnur.2008.10.004

Institute of Medicine. (2003). *Health professions education: A bridge to quality*. Washington, DC: National Academies Press.

International Council of Nurses. (2012). Closing the gap: From evidence to action. Retrieved from www.old.icn.ch/publications/2012-closing-the-gap-from-evidence-to-action

Iowa Model Collaborative. (2017). Iowa model of evidence-based practice: Revisions and validation. *Worldviews on Evidence-Based Nursing, 14*(3), 175–182. doi:10.1111/wvn.12223

Larrabee, J. H. (2009). *Nurse to nurse: Evidence-based practice* (p. 22). New York, NY: McGraw-Hill.

Leasure, A. R., Stirlen, J., & Thompson, C. (2008). Barriers and facilitators to the use of evidence-based best practices. *Dimensions of Critical Care Nursing, 27*(2), 74–82. doi:10.1097/01.DCC.0000311600.25216.c5

Melnyk, B. M., & Fineout-Overholt, E. (Eds.). (2005). *Evidence-based practice in nursing and healthcare: A guide to best practice*. Philadelphia, PA: Lippincott Williams & Wilkins.

Melnyk, B. M., Fineout-Overholt, E., Gallagher-Ford, L., & Kaplan, L. (2012). The state of evidence-based practice in US nurses: Critical implications for nurse leaders and educators. *Journal of Nursing Administration, 42*(9), 410–417. doi:10.1097/NNA.0b013e3182664e0a

Melnyk, B. M., Fineout-Overholt, E., Giggleman, M., & Cruz, R. (2010). Correlates among cognitive beliefs, EBP implementation, organizational culture, cohesion and job satisfaction in evidence-based practice mentors from a community hospital system. *Nursing Outlook*, *58*(6), 301–308. doi:10.1016/j.outlook.2010.06.002

Mitchell, A., Janzen, K., Pask, E., & Southwell, D. (1995). Assessment of nursing research utilization needs in Ontario health agencies. *Canadian Journal of Nursing Administration*, *8*(1), 77–91.

National Library of Medicine. (2018, April 5). *Number of titles currently indexed for Index Medicus and MEDLINE on PubMed*. Retrieved from https://wayback.archive-it.org/org-350/20180406174949/https://www.nlm.nih.gov/bsd/num_titles.html

Newhouse, R. P., Dearholt, S. L., Poe, S. S., Pugh, L. C., & White, K. M. (2005). Evidence-based practice: A practical approach to implementation. *Journal of Nursing Administration*, *35*(1), 35–40. doi:10.1097/00005110-200501000-00013

Parahoo, K. (2000). Barriers to, and facilitators of, research utilization among nurses in Northern Ireland. *Journal of Advanced Nursing*, *31*(1), 89–98. doi:10.1046/j.1365-2648.2000.01256.x

Perrin, R., & Stevens, J. (2004). Information technology: Facilitating the translation of research into practice. *QUERI Quarterly*, *6*(1), 1–4.

Pravikoff, D. S., Tanner, A. B., & Pierce, S. T. (2005). Readiness of U.S. nurses for evidence-based practice. *American Journal of Nursing*, *105*(9), 40–51. doi:10.1097/00000446-200509000-00025

Registered Nurses Association of Ontario. (2002). *Toolkit: Implementation of clinical practice guidelines*. Retrieved from http://rnao.ca/bpg/resources/toolkit-implementation-best-practice-guidelines-second-edition

Richardson, W. S., Wilson, M. C., Nishikawa, J., & Hayward, R. S. (1995). The well-built clinical question: A key to evidence-based decision. *ACP Journal Club*, *123*(3), A12–A13.

Rosswurm, M. A., & Larrabee, J. H. (1999). A model for change to evidence-based practice. *Journal of Nursing Scholarship*, *31*(4), 317–322. doi:10.1111/j.1547-5069.1999.tb00510.x

Stetler, C. B. (2001). Updating the Stetler model of research utilization to facilitate evidence-based practice. *Nursing Outlook*, *49*(6), 272–279. doi:10.1067/mno.2001.120517

Stetler, C. B., & Marram, G. (1976). Evaluating research findings for applicability in practice. *Nursing Outlook*, *24*(9), 559–563.

Stetler, C. B., Mittman, B. S., & Francis, J. (2008). Overview of the VA quality enhancement research initiative (QUERI) and QUERI theme articles: QUERI series. *Implementation Science*, *3(1)*, 8. doi:10.1186/1748-5908-3-8

Stevens, K. R. (2004). *ACE Star model of EBP: Knowledge transformation*. San Antonio, TX: Academic Center for Evidence-Based Practice, The University of Texas Health Science Center at San Antonio. Retrieved from http://nursing.uthscsa.edu/onrs/starmodel/institute/su08/starmodel.html

Stevens, K. R. (2013). The impact of evidence-based practice in nursing and the next big ideas. *Online Journal of Issues in Nursing, 18*(2), 1.

Strout, T., Lancaster, K., & Schultz, A. (2009). Development and implementation of an inductive model for evidence-based practice: A grassroots approach for building evidence-based practice capacity in staff nurses. *Nursing Clinics of North America*, *44*(1), 93–102. doi:10.1016/j.cnur.2008.10.007

Titler, M. G., Kleiber, C., Steelman, V. J., Rakel, B. A., Budreau, G., Everett, L. Q., . . . Goode, C. J. (2001). The Iowa model of evidence-based practice to promote quality care. *Critical Care Nursing Clinics of North America*, *13*(4), 497–509. doi:10.1016/S0899-5885(18)30017-0

U.S. Department of Health and Human Services. (2012). *National strategy for quality improvement in health care*. Retrieved from http://www.ahrq.gov/workingforquality/nqs/nqs2012annlrpt.pdf

CHAPTER TWO

The Science of Translation and Major Frameworks

Kathleen M. White

Research is only a beginning, and not an end in itself.
—Carolyn Clancy, Director, Agency for Healthcare Research and Quality

Transferring Research Knowledge Into Action Is an extremely important task and it is widely accepted that successfully doing so can contribute to the delivery of better health services. However, there is still wide variation in the rate at which research and other evidence is used in practice. The gap between what is known and what is done contributes to poor health outcomes and ultimately results in inefficient use of resources.

THE DEVELOPMENT OF THE KNOWLEDGE TRANSLATION MOVEMENT

The ability to translate research evidence into routine clinical practice is fundamental to ensuring quality healthcare. However, despite the large number of well-designed clinical intervention studies in healthcare today, it is well documented that it often takes 17 or more years for research findings to be implemented by clinicians and healthcare organizations into their clinical settings (Balas & Boren, 2000). For example, a 1998 review of published studies on the quality of care received by Americans found that some people are receiving more care than they actually need, whereas some are receiving less. According to the findings, taking simple averages from many studies indicated that 70% of people received recommended acute care, 60% received recommended chronic care, 50% received recommended preventive care, 30% received contraindicated acute care, and 20% received contraindicated chronic care (Schuster, McGlynn, & Brook, 1998). Similar findings have been reported globally in both developed and developing healthcare systems.

The Agency for Healthcare Research and Quality (AHRQ) identified that this translational hurdle exists despite a wide range of strategies for implementing research into practice, which includes provider reminder systems, use of local opinion leaders, new computer decision-support systems, and even financial incentives (AHRQ, 2001).

To decrease the time from discovery to translation of evidence at the bedside, the AHRQ began a program in 1999 called *Translating Research Into Practice (TRIP)* to evaluate different strategies for translating research findings into clinical practice, primarily using randomized controlled trials. Fourteen projects were funded in the TRIP-I program. The purpose was to generate new knowledge about approaches that promoted the utilization of rigorously derived evidence to improve patient care and to enhance the use of research findings, tools, and scientific information that would work in diverse practice settings, among diverse populations, and under diverse payment systems (AHRQ, 2001).

The following year, the AHRQ funded 13 more projects as part of TRIP-II, which continued building on the first program and then focused on implementation techniques and factors, such as organizational and clinical characteristics that were associated with successfully translating research findings into diverse applied settings. The TRIP-II program was aimed at applying and assessing strategies and methods that were developed in idealized practice settings or that were in current use but had not been previously or rigorously evaluated. The aim of these 3-year cooperative agreements was to identify sustainable and reproducible strategies to accelerate the impact of health services research on direct patient care and improve the outcomes, quality, effectiveness, efficiency, and/or cost-effectiveness of care through partnerships between healthcare organizations and researchers (AHRQ, 2001). Special areas of interest included reducing disparities that disproportionately affect minority and vulnerable populations, such as diabetes and cardiovascular disease, and using information technology to accelerate more rapidly the implementation of research throughout organizations and to evaluate how computer-based interventions contribute to translating research findings into healthcare improvements and health policy.

Farquhar, Stryer, and Slutsky (2002) studied the 27 TRIP projects funded by the AHRQ and looked at several dimensions of successful programs, including provider focus, patient population, vulnerable populations, methodologies, interventions for change, outcomes measured, and conceptual frameworks used. They found that the most common TRIP intervention that was used for translation was educational, and that the most common framework that was used to organize for the translation was either adult learning theory or organizational theory. Other implementation strategies that were used in the projects were continuing education, self-instructed learning, academic detailing, audit and feedback, provider reminder systems, incentives, local opinion leaders, outreach visits, continuous quality improvement, clinical information systems, and computer decision support systems. Farquhar et al. (2002) concluded that the challenge for the TRIP projects was to find a balance between rigor and generalizability, because it was often necessary to make trade-offs between optimal study design to maintain internal validity and the need for relevance. However, even noting this challenge, most TRIP projects used randomized controlled designs. Kirchhoff (2004) reported that nursing investigators responded to this review of the TRIP projects, but noted that questions remain about the reproducibility of the intervention, the dependent-variable selection and measurement, and the manner in which the intervention interacts with the environment.

In 2005, as part of the National Institutes of Health (NIH) Road Map for Medical Research, three themes emerged (Westfall, Mold, & Fagnan, 2007). The third theme resulted in the development of a program of translational research that created the Institutional Clinical and Translational Science Awards (CTSA) program, designed to support the clinical and translational science at academic health centers (Zerhouni, 2005). The NIH defined *translational research* in two ways along the research continuum. The first, or type I translational research, is the process of applying discoveries made in the laboratory, testing them in animals, and then developing trials and studies for humans for treatment and prevention approaches. The second, or type II translational research, is research aimed at enhancing the adoption of best treatment practices by the medical community with a goal of institutionalizing effective programs, products, and services. The goals of these NIH TRIP-II translational research studies are to (a) identify community, patient, physician, and organizational factors that serve as barriers and facilitators to translation; (b) develop novel intervention and implementation strategies to increase translation, such as quality-improvement programs or policies; and (c) evaluate the impact of strategies to increase translation of relevant healthy behaviors and processes of care (NIH, 2005).

There remain major challenges to adopting and integrating new evidence into practice with little understanding of how this adoption takes place (Green & Seifert, 2005). How do healthcare practitioners translate new knowledge into the specific actions that they put into practice? Why do healthcare practitioners and organizations not incorporate new evidence or best practices quickly and reliably into their work (Berwick, 2003)? As a report of the Health and Medicine Division (of the National Academies of Sciences, Engineering, and Medicine) *Crossing the Quality Chasm: A New Health System for the 21st Century* stated, "Between the healthcare we have and the care we could have lies not just a gap, but a chasm" (Institute of Medicine [IOM], 2001, p. 1). This failure to use new knowledge and evidence is costly, harmful, inefficient, and results in ineffective care being delivered to the American public. There is a critical need to understand the process of translating or integrating the new evidence into the existing organization or practice delivery.

Green and Seifert (2005), in an article with a very apropos title, "Translation of Research: Why We Can't 'Just Do It,'" suggested that translation of research to practice happens in three stages: (a) awareness, (b) acceptance, and (c) adoption. However, they further describe that most efforts have focused on awareness and acceptance by the clinicians and organizations, and that very little attention is paid to the adoption stage. There has been research in identifying the factors in the first two stages that affect adoption, specifically how to increase and foster awareness and acceptance, but not much on understanding how the adoption takes place and how to make it more effective. Their work embraces cognitive skill–learning research that suggests that the clinician must move from awareness and acceptance, where the new knowledge is acquired, to the adoption stage—where the knowledge becomes a part of the clinician's routine procedures in practice. Critical to this change is the implementation of strategies that support clinician learning and disrupt well-practiced procedures and rules in order to incorporate the new knowledge (Green & Seifert, 2005).

Key to this learning and adoption of new knowledge is the use of appropriate implementation strategies. Glasgow and Emmons (2007) conducted a systematic review of the literature on interventions that promote the translation of research findings into practice and found four factors that serve as barriers to the translation of new knowledge: the characteristics of the intervention, the current target setting or environment, the research or evaluation design, and the interaction among the first three factors. This attention to the connectedness of the factors is particularly important for complex interventions and multifaceted programs. They posit that the implementation will be more successful when integrated and delivered in a coordinated way that reinforces all the factors, as opposed to strategies happening in separate "silos" of unrelated activities (Figure 2.1).

In a recent integrative review of the literature, Li, Jeffs, Barwick, and Stevens (2018) identified six organizational contextual features that synergistically influence

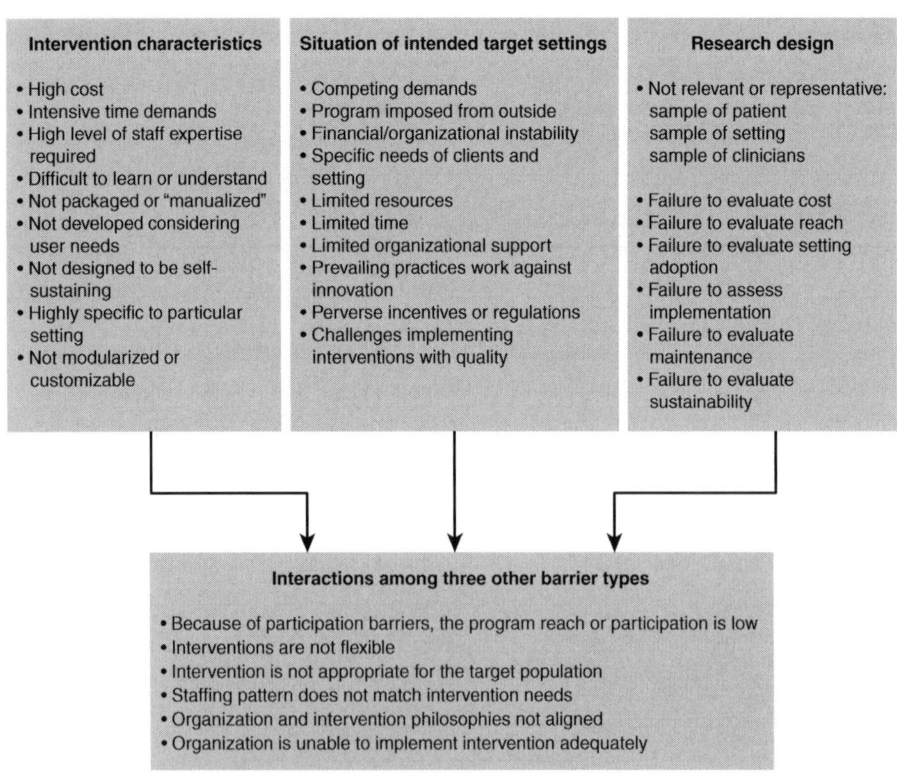

FIGURE 2.1 Glasgow and Emmons's Implementation Model.

Source: Reprinted with permission from Glasgow, R. E., & Emmons, K. M. (2007). How can we increase translation of research into practice? Types of evidence needed. *Annual Review of Public Health, 28,* 413–433. Copyright by Annual Reviews.

the implementation of evidence-based practices within an organization. These six features are the constructs in the Consolidated Framework for Implementation Research (CFIR), discussed later in this chapter. The authors concluded that the six features were interrelated and that they influenced each other in complex and dynamic ways in order to effect the implementation, thereby resulting in a change in practice. Of the six features, organizational culture was the feature most commonly reported as affecting the implementation of evidence into practice.

Newhouse and White (2011) suggest that an important strategy to enhance the uptake of research into practice is to use a systematic approach to guide the translation of the new knowledge. A conceptual model or framework will serve as a map to guide the assessment, planning, and implementation of the evidence translation and increase the chances of a successful implementation. This chapter presents a variety of translation models and frameworks from the current literature that target different innovations and contexts (Milat & Li, 2017).

Definitions of Key Knowledge Translation Words

Knowledge transfer (KT): KT is the exchange, synthesis, and ethically sound application of knowledge—within a complex system of interactions among researchers and users—to accelerate the capture of the benefits of research . . . through improved health, more effective services and products, and a strengthened healthcare system. The collaborative and systematic review, assessment, identification, aggregation, and practical application of high-quality research by key stakeholders (e.g., consumers, researchers, practitioners, policy makers) improve the lives and health of individuals (Canadian Institutes of Health Research, 2010).

Knowledge transfer: Knowledge transfer is a systematic approach to capture, collect, and share tacit knowledge in order for it to become explicit knowledge. By so doing, this process allows individuals and/or organizations to access and use essential information, which previously was known intrinsically to only one person or a small group of people (I. D. Graham et al., 2006).

Knowledge exchange: Knowledge exchange is a collaborative approach to problem-solving between researchers and decision makers that happens through linkage and exchange. Effective knowledge exchange involves interaction between decision makers and researchers that results in mutual learning through the process of planning, producing, disseminating, and applying existing or new research in decision-making (Canadian Health Services Research Foundation, 2011).

Synthesis: *Synthesis*, in this context, refers to the contextualization and integration of research findings of individual research studies within the larger body of knowledge on the topic. A synthesis must be reproducible and trans-

(*continued*)

(continued)

parent in its methods, using quantitative and/or qualitative methods. It could take the form of a systematic review (following the methods developed by the Cochrane Collaboration), result from a consensus conference or expert panel, or synthesize qualitative or quantitative results. Realist syntheses, narrative syntheses, meta-analyses, meta-syntheses, and practice guidelines are all forms of synthesis (Canadian Institutes of Health Research, 2010).

Research utilization: Research utilization is the process by which specific research-based knowledge (science) is implemented in practice (Stetler, Corrigan, Sander-Buscemi, & Burns, 1999).

Implementation: Implementation is the execution of the adoption decision, that is, the innovation or the research is put into practice (Titler, 2008).

Dissemination: Dissemination is the spreading of knowledge or research, such as is done in scientific journals and at scientific conferences. Dissemination involves identifying the appropriate audience and tailoring the message and medium to the audience. Dissemination activities can include summaries for/briefings to stakeholders; educational sessions with patients, practitioners, and/or policy makers; engaging knowledge users in developing and executing a dissemination/implementation plan; tools creation; and media engagement (Canadian Institutes of Health Research, 2010).

Diffusion: Diffusion is the process by which an innovation is communicated through certain channels, over time, among members of a social system (Rogers, 2003).

Websites for KT

www.ktclearinghouse.ca/knowledgebase/modelsandtheories

The AHRQ's TRIP program: An initiative focusing on the implementation techniques and factors associated with successfully translating research findings into diverse applied settings (www.ahrq.gov/research/trip2fac.htm)

Campbell Collaboration (C2): An international organization that conducts systematic reviews of education, social welfare, and social science research (www.campbellcollaboration.org)

Canadian Institutes for Health Research (CIHR): The major federal agency that is responsible for funding health research in Canada that has established charges for KT research, development, and dissemination (www.cihr-irsc.gc.ca/e/29529.html)

(continued)

(*continued*)

Cochrane Collaboration: An international organization that conducts systematic reviews of health and medical research (www.cochrane.org)

International Development Research Center (IDRC): The IDRC acts to initiate, encourage, support, and conduct research into the problems of the developing regions of the world and into the means for applying and adapting scientific, technical, and other knowledge to the economic and social advancement of those regions (www.idrc.ca/EN/Pages/default.aspx)

Joanna Briggs Institute (JBI): JBI is an international not-for-profit research and development center within the Faculty of Health Sciences at the University of Adelaide, South Australia, that attempts to provide the best available evidence to inform clinical decision-making at the point of care; the Institute collaborates internationally with over 70 entities across the world; the Institute and its collaborating entities promote and support the synthesis, transfer, and utilization of evidence through identifying feasible, appropriate, meaningful, and effective healthcare practices to assist in the improvement of healthcare outcomes globally (joannabriggs.org):

- Translational science
- Synthesis science
- Implementation science
- Software for health professionals
- Promoting evidence-based practice

Knowledge Network: A website that brings together information about various websites, articles, and books about KT (www.knowledge.scot.nhs.uk/home.aspx)

Knowledge Translation Program (KTP) at the University of Toronto, Canada: A multidisciplinary academic program that is developed to address the gap between research evidence and clinical practice and the need to focus on the processes through which knowledge is effectively translated into changed practices (www.stmichaelshospital.com/research/kt.php)

Knowledge Utilization Studies Program at the University of Alberta, Canada: A health research program focusing on nursing, social sciences, and research utilization in the nursing profession (www.nursing.ualberta.ca/kusp)

KT Clearinghouse, Knowledge Translation Canada: A network of Canadian experts in KT joining forces to tackle the greatest challenge in healthcare today: The fact that although there is a great deal of health research being conducted, there is a gap in applying the results at the patient's bedside and in everyday health decisions (ktclearinghouse.ca/ktcanada)

(*continued*)

(continued)

National Health Service (NHS) Centre for Reviews and Dissemination at the University of York: An organization that conducts systematic reviews of research and disseminates research-based information about the effects of interventions used in health and social care in the United Kingdom (www.york.ac.uk/inst/crd/welcome.htm)

What Works Clearinghouse (WWC): A clearinghouse established by the U.S. Department of Education's Institute of Education Sciences to provide educators, policy makers, and the public with a central, independent, and trusted source of scientific evidence of what works in education (ies.ed.gov/ncee/wwc)

World Health Organization (WHO): Produced a publication titled *Knowledge Translation Framework for Ageing and Health*; the objective of the document is to assist policy makers and decision-makers in integrating evidence-based approaches to aging in national health policy development processes, specific policies, or programs addressing older population needs and other health programs concerned with issues such as HIV, reproductive health, and chronic diseases (www.who.int/ageing/publications/knowledge_translation/en)

■ TRANSLATION THEORY AND FRAMEWORKS

Translation theory and frameworks focus on the interrelationships and complex organizational dimensions that are relevant to the translation of research or new knowledge into practice. Common among the theories are discussions of the ongoing and iterative nature of the processes; the need to determine the strength and quality of the new knowledge; the inclusion of many stakeholders; the importance of context, including culture, leadership styles, and decision-making; as well as organizational structures.

KT theories are needed to guide implementation of research-based interventions into practice. To this end, Estabrooks, Thompson, Lovely, and Hofmeyer (2006) provided an overview of perspectives that come from different disciplines and that are useful for understanding the basis of KT. As described in this book in Chapter 1, Evidence-Based Practice, these authors begin by looking at the models of research utilization and evidence-based practice from the nursing literature. In addition, they describe adjuvant theories considered to be complements, such as the theory on organizations, including the change process and decision-making; social science theory on problem-solving; political and tactical theory; and, finally, behavioral and health promotion theory from the health sciences.

The development of translation models or frameworks has been slow, but it includes many and varied approaches for introducing evidence and changing behavior and performance, which are all based on different assumptions about change. The discussion begins in the early 1990s and proceeds through the development of today's latest models.

Coordinated Implementation Model

Lomas, Sisk, and Stocking (1993), in an overview of a journal issue on translation of knowledge into practice, questioned putting effort into translation of knowledge before targeting efforts to implement science and "validated truths" (p. 405) in medicine. They argued that there is too much use of untruths and invalid facts in medicine, and that the profession has an ethical obligation to move toward appraising and using valid research in practice.

Lomas (1993) proposed an active model of dissemination, replacing the previously used diffusion models that were passive, which explores "sufficient conditions" for research translation into the practice environment. His coordinated implementation model involves the careful evaluation of (a) the research information, including synthesis, distillation, and appraisal of that research evidence for use; (b) adoption by a credible body using active dissemination strategies; (c) consideration of the competing factors in the overall practice environment; and (d) the need for coordination among external audiences, including patients, clinical policy makers, community groups, administrators, and public policy makers (Lomas, 1993). Lomas uses the Effective Care in Pregnancy and Childbirth program as a case study in which to present the model (Figure 2.2).

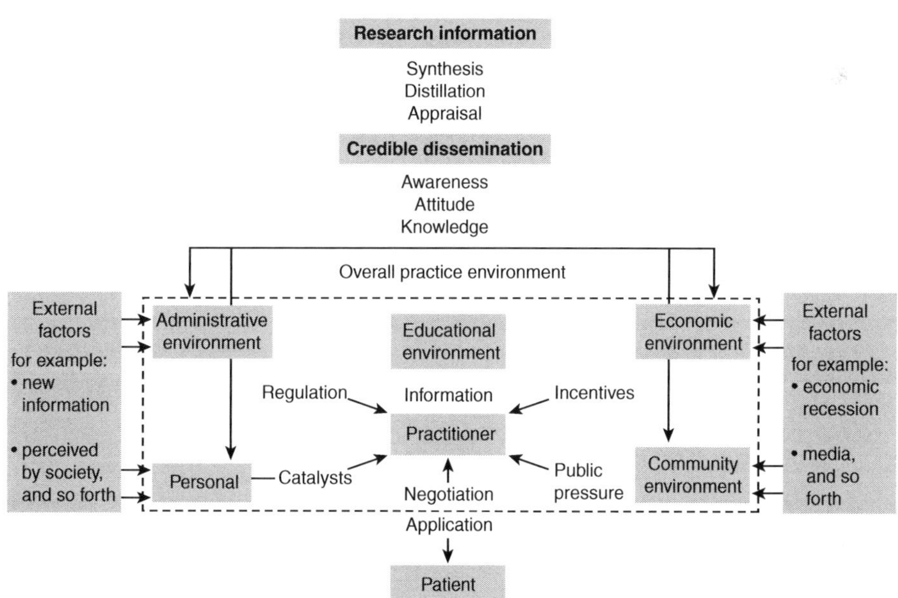

FIGURE 2.2 Lomas's Coordinated Implementation Model.

Source: Adapted from Lomas, J., Sisk, J. E., & Stocking, B. (1993). From evidence to practice in the United States, the United Kingdom, and Canada. *Milbank Quarterly, 71*(3), 405–410. doi:10.2307/3350408

Haines and Jones's Translation Model

One of the earliest translation models was described by Haines and Jones (1994), who cited unacceptable delays in implementing the findings of research into practice, which resulted in suboptimal patient care. They acknowledged that the top-down administrative, traditional education, and economic strategies used to contain cost have not been sufficient to promote change, and that the strategies for implementation must be sustainable and dynamic, taking into account the changing evidence about effectiveness. They proposed that an integrated approach using several types of dissemination strategies, the critical appraisal and use of systematic reviews and clinical practice guidelines, and adequate resources and culture change, when taken together, can speed up and increase the successful implementation of research in practice (Figure 2.3).

Rogers's Diffusion of Innovations Theory

Although not developed specifically for healthcare, the foundation for many translation models is Everett Rogers's Diffusion of Innovations theory (Rogers, 2003). Rogers discusses that change is caused by an introduction of innovation and, for translation science, this is the new knowledge or evidence. He defines "innovation" as an idea, practice, or object that is perceived as new by an individual or other unit of adoption. Time is not important to the *newness*; it is not whether the innovation is objectively newly measured by the lapse of time since its first use or discovery that is significant,

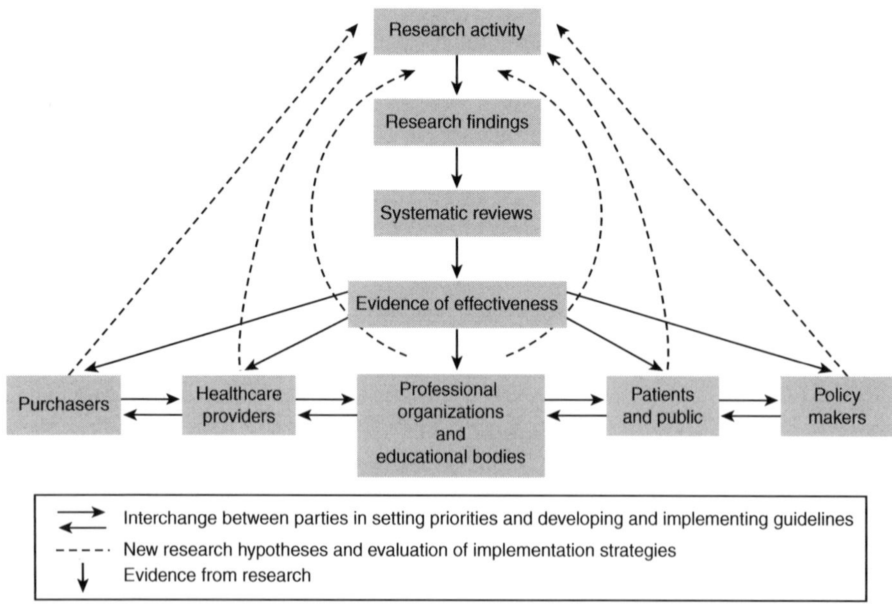

FIGURE 2.3 Haines and Jones's Translation Model.

Source: Reprinted with permission from Haines, A., & Jones, R. (1994). Implementing findings of research. *British Medical Journal, 308*(6942), 1488–1492. Copyright by BMJ Publishing Group.

but the perceived newness of the idea for the individual. This perceived newness is what determines a person's reaction to the innovation. If the idea seems new to the individual, it is considered as an innovation by the individual.

Rogers described five groups of individuals based on the characteristics of how they adopt an innovation. First are the *innovators*, who are venturesome, tolerant of risks, and like new ideas. These are estimated to comprise only about 2.5% of those involved with a change. The second group is the *early adopters*. The early adopters are usually the opinion leaders in an organization and are locally well connected; they focus on and select ideas that they like, and they like to associate with the innovators to learn, maintain, and connect to the outside. Rogers estimates that 13.5% of those involved with change are early adopters. The third group is the *early majority* of people, who are local in their perspective, learn from people they know, rely on familiarity rather than science, and are risk averse. They represent 34% or one third of the group that is involved with change. Another one third or 34% is called the *late majority*. The late majority will adopt an innovation when it finally appears to be status quo in an organization. They require and watch for local proof that the change is really going to work and stick around. The last group that Rogers identifies is the *laggards*. For this group, the point of reference is the past. They are the traditionalists in an organization and like the tried and true, not something that involves change. Unfortunately, Rogers's work shows that these individuals account for 16% of a workgroup. Each of these groups of people must be planned for and included in the change process.

The second concept that is important to Rogers's theory is *diffusion*, defined as the process by which an innovation is communicated through certain channels over time among the members of an organization. Rogers calls his model an innovation–decision process that includes information and uncertainty, views change as dynamic, and stresses the importance of commitment to and maintenance of any change.

Rogers's theory describes a five-step innovation–decision process:

1. *Knowledge:* The person becomes aware of an innovation and has some idea of how it functions.
2. *Persuasion:* The person actively seeks information about the innovation and forms a favorable or unfavorable attitude toward the innovation.
3. *Decision:* The person engages in activities that lead to a choice, benefit, or risk of adopting the innovation and makes a choice whether to accept or reject the innovation.
4. *Implementation:* The person considers the uses of the innovation and puts the innovation into practice.
5. *Confirmation:* The person evaluates the results of an innovation–decision process that was already made and makes a decision whether to continue to use the innovation or not.

The personal characteristics of those individuals involved with the innovation, as described previously, affect how early in the innovation–decision process each individual engages and begins to adopt the new idea.

Oxman, Thomson, Davis, and Haynes (1995) conducted a systematic review of methods to determine the effectiveness of different types of interventions in improving health professional performance and health outcomes. They found that dissemination-only strategies, such as conferences or the mailing of unsolicited materials, demonstrated little or no change in the behavior of health professionals when used alone, and that more complex interventions, such as the use of outreach visits or local opinion leaders, were only moderately effective, but ranged from 20% to 50% in reducing the incidence of inappropriate performance. They concluded that there were no "magic bullets" to improve a professional's practice and resulting patient outcomes.

Following up on this study, Bero et al. (1998) found that providing systematic reviews of rigorous research was helpful, but the passive dissemination of information was generally ineffective. They categorized interventions that promote behavioral changes among health professionals:

- Consistently effective interventions were reminders (manual or computerized), multifaceted interventions (a combination that includes two or more of the following: audit and feedback, reminders, local consensus processes, or marketing), and interactive educational meetings (participation of healthcare providers in workshops that include discussion or practice).
- Interventions of variable effectiveness were audit and feedback (or any summary of clinical performance), use of local opinion leaders (practitioners identified by their colleagues as influential), local consensus processes (inclusion of participating practitioners in discussions to ensure that they agree that the chosen clinical problem is important and that the approach to managing the problem is appropriate), and patient-mediated interventions (any intervention aimed at changing the performance of healthcare providers, for which specific information was sought from or given to patients).
- Interventions that have little or no effect included distributing educational materials (distribution of recommendations for clinical care, including clinical practice guidelines, audiovisual materials, and electronic publications) and didactic educational meetings (such as lectures).

This early research laid the foundation for subsequent translation discussions and modeling to emphasize the active participation and involvement of those needing to translate new knowledge into practice.

Framework for Changing Behavior

Grol and Grimshaw (1999) described lessons used for the implementation of evidence into practice by reviewing strategies to implement change. They reviewed change approaches from seven theoretical perspectives and concluded that the change approach determines the implementation plan. The seven approaches (Grol & Grimshaw, 1999) are as follows with considerations for each:

1. *Education:* Assumes that an internal motivation to improve exists, so the strategy must convey ownership of the change process

2. *Epidemiology:* Assumes the presence of sound and convincing evidence and rigorous procedures, so the strategy must include strength and quality of the evidence
3. *Marketing:* Assumes an attractive message is provided, so the strategy must adapt the message to the needs of the target group
4. *Behavior:* Assumes that human behavior can be influenced, so the strategy would include providing feedback and incentives or sanctions
5. *Social influence:* Assumes that learning and change are part of a social network, so the strategy would be to include opinion leaders and champions
6. *Organization:* Assumes there is a focus on creating conditions for change, so the strategy would be to identify areas of failure that need improvement
7. *Coercion:* Assumes that controls are needed, so the strategy would be to develop laws, regulations, policies, and procedures

They expanded their work and emphasized the importance of clinicians' decision-making using knowledge of the medical evidence, the patient-specific or social context of care, and the organizational and policy evidence, including efficiency, equity, and rationing (Grol & Grimshaw, 2003). They suggest analyzing the target setting and the target group and identifying obstacles to change; linking the interventions to the needs, facilitators, and obstacles to change; knowing the critical importance of developing a plan for change in clinical practice; implementing; and, finally, evaluating the progress toward change.

Greenhalgh's Diffusion of Innovations in Service Organizations

Following on Rogers's work, Greenhalgh, Robert, McFarlane, Bate, and Kyriakidou (2004) conducted a modified systematic review of the healthcare research literature to answer the question, "How can health service organizations spread and sustain innovations?" The review considered both the process and how to measure the diffusion of innovations in service organizations. Innovation in service delivery and organization was defined as "a novel set of behaviors, routines, and ways of working that are directed at improving health outcomes, administrative efficiency, cost effectiveness, or users' experience and that are implemented by planned and coordinated actions" (Greenhalgh et al., 2004, p. 582). They tried to distinguish among diffusion, dissemination, implementation, and sustainability.

The final review had 495 sources, including 213 empirical studies and 282 nonempirical references. Thirteen research areas relevant to the diffusion of innovations in healthcare organizations were identified. The first four areas were considered early diffusion research and included (a) rural sociology, from which Rogers first developed the concept of diffusion of innovations and the research that dealt with social networks and adoption decisions; (b) medical sociology, which studied physician clinical behavior and set a foundation for network analysis; (c) communication studies with research, which measured the speed and direction of the spread of new information; and (d) marketing research, which studied the rational analysis of costs and benefits

(Greenhalgh et al., 2004). Next, the review identified the research areas that emerged as developments from this early research and included the following:

- *Development studies:* Expanded the spread of innovations to include political, technological, and ideological contexts of innovation
- *Health promotion research:* Traditionally used as a social marketing of good ideas, but expanded to models of partnership and community development
- *Evidence-based medicine:* Research described a linear process until recently, when new developments suggested that planning had to include local context and priorities (Greenhalgh et al., 2004)

Finally, the review found relevant research in the organization and management literature, including studies that focused on the structural determinants of organizational innovation; organizational process, context, and culture; interorganizational studies; knowledge-based approaches to innovation in organizations; narrative organizational studies; and complexity studies focusing on adaptation (Greenhalgh et al., 2004).

Greenhalgh et al. (2004) developed a unifying conceptual model from the synthesis of their work to serve as a "memory aid for considering the different aspects of a complex situation and their many interactions" (p. 594). This quote sums up the main purpose for writing this book and proposing that a systematic approach, using a model or framework to translate research into practice, is the basis for the science of translation. The model of diffusion in service organizations includes nine components, but because it was synthesized from the literature, it does not necessarily include all the components that must be considered in a diffusion of innovation: (a) innovation characteristics; (b) adoption by individuals; (c) assimilation by the system (system planning and decision-making); (d) diffusion and dissemination (use of opinion leaders, champions, and type of program); (e) system antecedents for innovation (structure and culture); (f) system readiness for innovation, including tension, fit, support and advocacy, and time resources; (g) the outer context: interorganizational networks and collaborations; (h) implementation and routinization (leadership and management); and (i) the linkages among components of the model (Figure 2.4).

AHRQ: Knowledge Transfer

The AHRQ continued its work to improve the translation of research into practice as it focused its efforts on the Agency's patient safety initiative. The AHRQ Patient Safety Research Coordinating Center (PSRCC) and its steering committee developed a conceptual model to accelerate the transfer of research results from its portfolio to organizations that could benefit from the findings (Nieva et al., 2005). The AHRQ model includes three phases for knowledge transfer into practice. The first phase of the model is *knowledge creation and distillation* and includes conducting the research, followed by a process of sifting through the research results to package them in ways that will be meaningful to potential users so as to increase the likelihood that the research evidence will find its way into practice. This sifting process has been labeled *knowledge distillation* (Nieva et al., 2005). The knowledge distillation process must

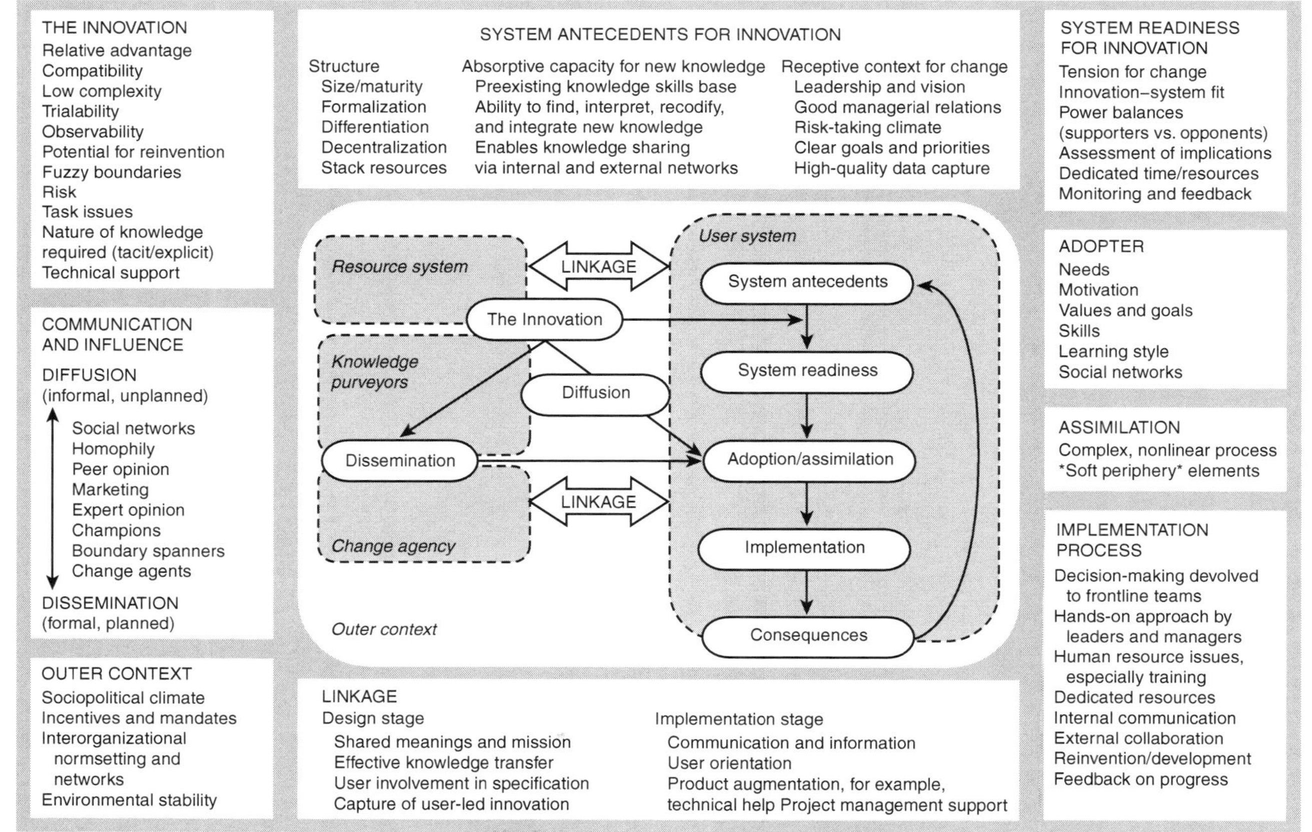

FIGURE 2.4 Conceptual model for considering the determinants of diffusion, dissemination, and innovation of implementations in health services delivery and organization, based on a systematic review of empirical research studies.

Source: From Greenhalgh, T., Robert, G., Macfarlane, F., Bate, P., & Kyriakidou, O. (2004), Diffusion of innovations in service organizations: Systematic review and recommendations. *Milbank Quarterly, 82*: 581–629. doi:10.1111/j.0887-378X.2004.00325.x

identify a broad range of users and be informed and guided by these end users of the research findings in order for the results to be implemented in care delivery. In addition to the perspectives of the end users, the criteria used in knowledge distillation should include consideration of the transportability to the real-world healthcare setting, the feasibility of translation, the volume of evidence needed by healthcare organizations and clinicians, and strength and generalizability of the evidence (Nieva et al., 2005).

The second phase is *diffusion and dissemination*, whereby efforts aimed at marketing, selecting media, and appropriate messaging are used to "get the word out" about the new knowledge in an effort to raise awareness and to garner interest in translation and replication. This phase stresses the creation of interprofessional dissemination partnerships and knowledge transfer teams in healthcare organizations to disseminate knowledge that can form the basis of action, linking researchers with intermediaries that can connect to the practitioners, healthcare delivery organizations, and professional organizations. In addition, mass diffusion efforts and targeted dissemination efforts to reach end users using specific messages to particular audiences are used (Nieva et al., 2005). This push–pull of information for diffusion and dissemination should increase the effectiveness of the efforts.

The final phase is the *end user adoption, implementation, and institutionalization*. To facilitate implementation, careful assessment of and attention to the complex interrelationships among the innovation itself, organizational structures and values, the external environment, and the individual clinicians are necessary (Nieva et al., 2005). The model focuses on the importance of the development of the intervention and recognition that changing practice takes time and considerable effort to sustain the change. Activities to increase adoption, successful implementation, and communication of the results of the implementation are identified to improve the likelihood that the innovation becomes a standard of care or "institutionalized" (Nieva et al., 2005; see Figure 2.5).

Knowledge-to-Action Model

The Canadian Institutes of Health Research (CIHR) has been at the forefront of evidence-based practice and KT efforts and is often cited as the best source of definitions to clarify confusion about the concepts of KT, knowledge exchange, research implementation, diffusion, and dissemination. I. D. Graham et al. at the University of Ottawa developed the Knowledge-to-Action (KTA) Model as an integration of knowledge creation and knowledge application (I. D. Graham, Tetroe, & KT Theories and Research Group, 2007). The KTA process uses the word *action* rather than *practice* because it is intended to be used by a wider range of users of knowledge, not just clinicians. The model visually conceptualizes the translation process or KTA as being similar to a *funnel*, in which new knowledge moves through the stages until it is adopted and used. Knowledge, at the wide mouth of the funnel, includes the broad stage of inquiry and primary research. As knowledge proceeds through the funnel, it is synthesized and, finally, tools or products that are needed to present the new knowledge are developed, so that those most likely to benefit can easily apply

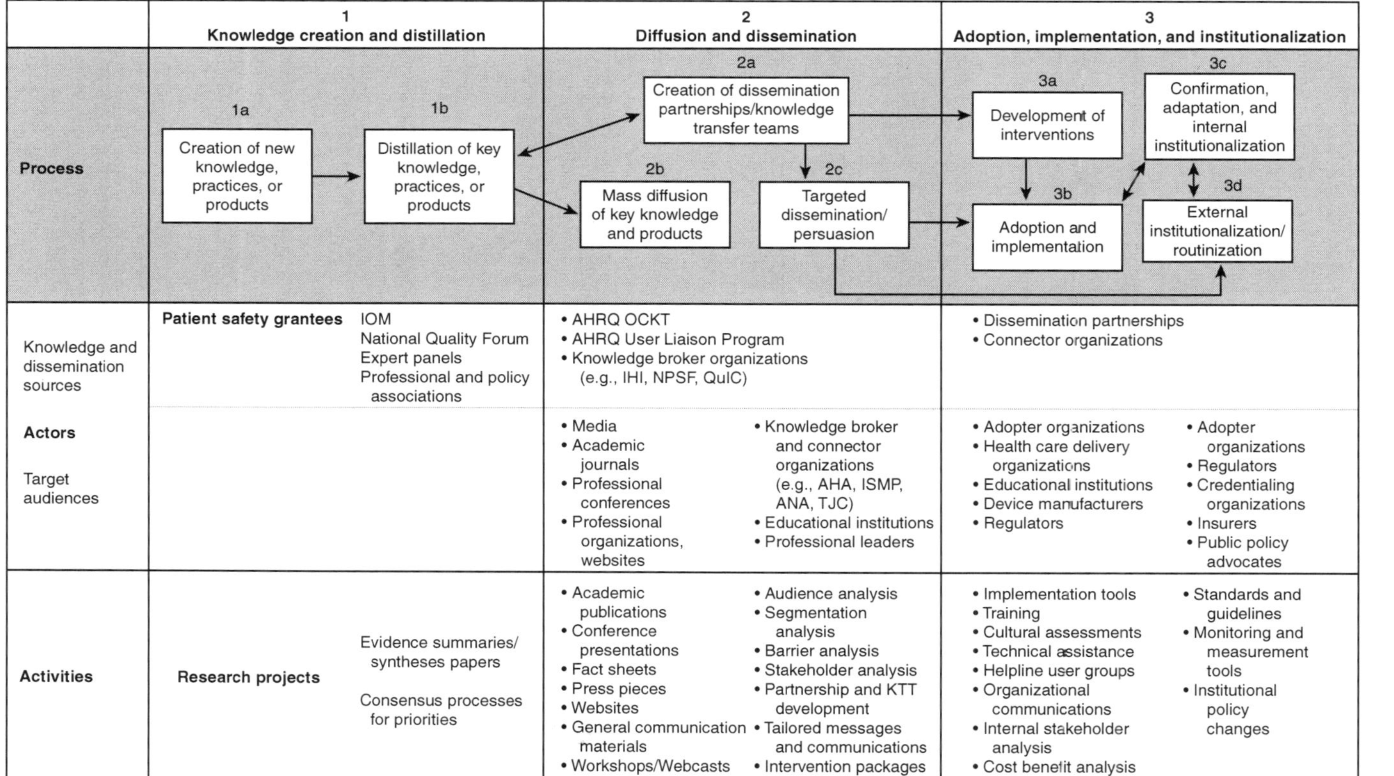

FIGURE 2.5 Knowledge transfer framework for the AHRQ patient safety portfolio and patient safety grantees.

AHA, American Heart Association; AHRQ, Agency for Healthcare Research and Quality; ANA, American Nurses Association; IHI, Institute for Healthcare Improvement; IOM, Institute of Medicine; ISMP, Institute for Safe Medication Practices; KTT, knowledge translation and transfer; NPSF, National Patient Safety Foundation; OCKT, Office of Communications and Knowledge Transfer; TJC, The Joint Commission.

Source: Adapted from Nieva, V., Murphy, R., Ridley, N., Donaldson, N., Combes, J., Mitchell, P., . . . Carpenter, D. (2005). From science to service: A framework for the transfer of patient safety research into practice. In K. Henriksen, J. B. Battles, & E. S. Marks (Eds.), *Advances in patient safety: From research to implementation* (Vol. 2, pp. 441–453). Rockville, MD: Agency for Healthcare Research and Quality. Retrieved from http://www.ncbi.nlm.nih.gov/books/NBK20521/pdf/Bookshelf_NBK20521.pdf

the knowledge. At each step in the knowledge creation process, the producer of the knowledge has the ability to tailor activities to meet specific research questions or end user needs. The action cycle of the KTA process represents the activities that implement or apply the knowledge. Planned action theories are used to develop deliberate activities that facilitate change. Feedback exists among all phases and between both the knowledge creation and the action cycles. The KTA cycle is a synthesis of work that maps commonalities in the translation process and has seven phases (Figure 2.6):

1. Identify a problem that needs to be addressed and/or reviewed, and select the knowledge or research relevant to the problem.
2. Adapt the knowledge use to the local context.
3. Assess barriers to knowledge use.
4. Select, tailor, and implement interventions to promote use of the knowledge.

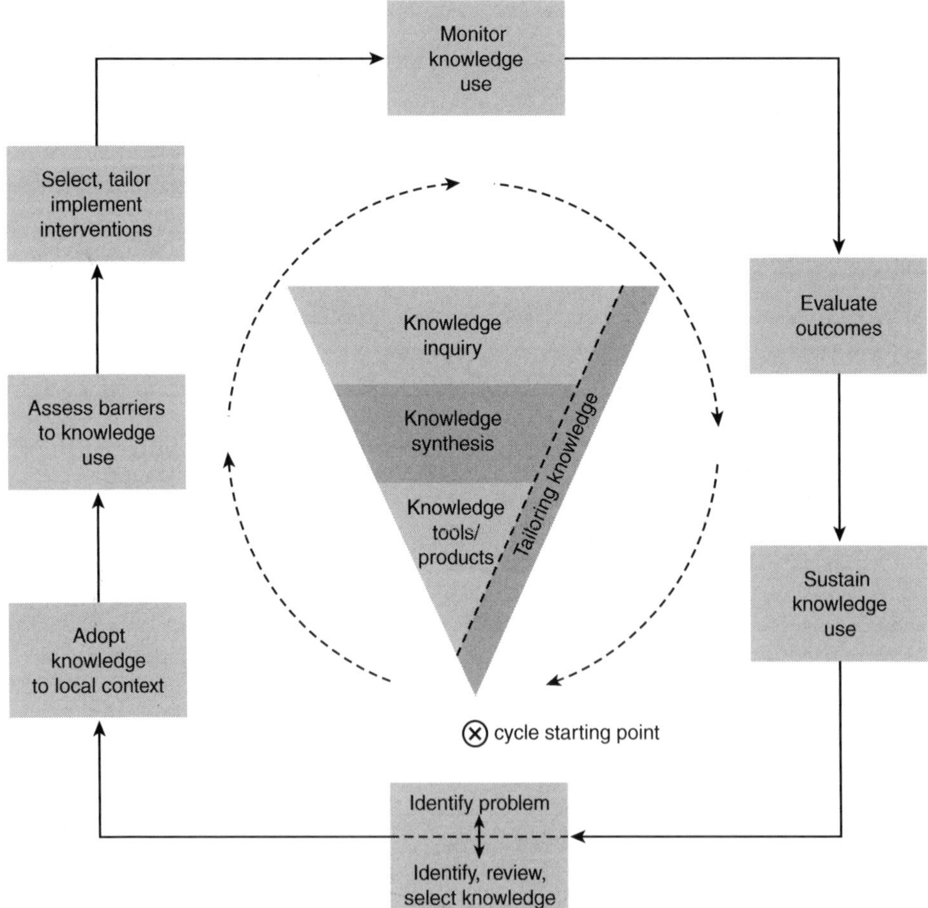

FIGURE 2.6 The knowledge-to-action cycle.

Source: Reprinted with permission from Graham, I. D., Logan, J., Harrison, M. B., Straus, S. E., Tetroe, J., Caswell, W., & Robinson, N. (2006). Lost in knowledge translation: Time for a map? *Journal of Continuing Education in the Health Professions, 26*(1), 13–24.

5. Monitor knowledge use.
6. Evaluate the outcomes of knowledge use.
7. Sustain knowledge use.

Ottawa Model of Research Use

The Ottawa Model of Research Use, developed by Logan and K. Graham (1998), views research as a dynamic process of decisions and actions that are interrelated and focuses implementation efforts on existing knowledge that is ready to be shared. The latest revision of the model (K. Graham & Logan, 2004) describes three phases and six primary elements necessary to consider when implementing research into practice. The first phase of the model is to assess the barriers and supports to the translation of the research into practice and must consider the first three elements: (a) the evidence-based innovation, (b) characteristics of potential adopters (from Everett Rogers's work), and (c) the structure and social context of the practice environment. The second phase of the model is to monitor the intervention and the degree of use, considering two more elements: implementation of interventions (considering diffusion, dissemination, and transfer strategies) and adoption of the innovation. The final phase is the evaluation and monitoring of outcomes of the translation, including patient, practitioner, and system outcomes (Figure 2.7).

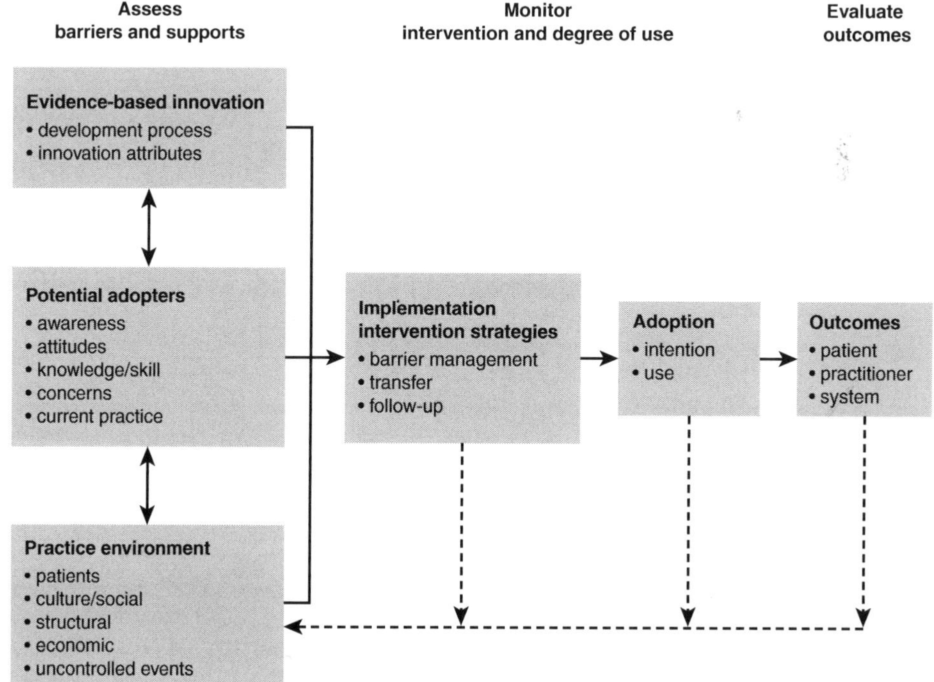

FIGURE 2.7 Ottawa Model of Research Use.

Source: Reprinted with permission from Graham, K., & Logan, J. (2004). Using the Ottawa Model of Research Use to implement a skin care program. *Journal of Nursing Care Quality, 19*(1), 18–24. doi:10.1097/00001786-200401000-00006

Promoting Action on Research Implementation in Health Services Model

The Promoting Action on Research Implementation in Health Services (PARiHS) model was developed to represent essential determinants of successful implementation of research into clinical practice, a framework to enable implementation of evidence-based practice (Kitson, Harvey, & McCormack, 1998). Kitson and colleagues were dissatisfied with the lack of attention to rational decision-making and linear processes, and failure to include the influence of context in research translation into practice (McCormack et al., 2002). The PARiHS framework posits that successful implementation is a function of three core elements: (a) the importance of clarity about the nature of the evidence being used, (b) the quality of the context, and (c) the type of facilitation needed to ensure a successful change process. Each of the three core elements has many components to consider.

Evidence is the knowledge that is derived from various sources and includes the strength and nature of the information as perceived by multiple stakeholders. It is the information that needs to be combined to be used in clinical decision-making and includes four components, corresponding to different sources of evidence: (a) research evidence from published sources or participation in formal experiments; (b) evidence from clinical experience or professional knowledge; (c) evidence from patient preferences or based on patient experiences, including those of caregivers and family; and (d) routine information derived from local practice context, which differs from professional experience, in that it is the domain of the collective environment and not the individual (Kitson et al., 2008; Rycroft-Malone, Harvey et al., 2004, Rycroft-Malone, Seers et al., 2004). Although research evidence is often treated as the most heavily weighted form, the PARiHS framers emphasize that all four forms have meaning and constitute evidence from the perspective of users.

The concept of *context* is defined as the environment or setting in which the proposed change or translation of research is to be implemented. This concept comes from the literature on learning organizations and comprises three components: (a) organizational culture, (b) leadership, and (c) evaluation (Kitson et al., 2008; McCormack et al., 2002). *Culture* refers to the values, beliefs, and attitudes shared by members of the organization and may vary at different levels of the organization. Leadership includes the elements of teamwork, control, decision-making, effectiveness of organizational structures, and issues related to empowerment. Evaluation relates to how the organization measures its performance and how (or whether) feedback is provided to people within the organization, as well as the quality of measurement and feedback.

Facilitation is defined as the "technique by which one person makes things easier for others, help others towards achieving particular goals, encourage others and promote action [distinguish from opinion leader]" and is achieved through "support to help people change their attitudes, habits, skills, ways of thinking, and working" (Kitson et al., 1998, p. 152). Facilitation is necessary to help those individuals and teams that are involved in the translation to understand what they have to change and how they are going to change it to achieve desired outcomes. Facilitation can be both internal and external. Although most prior work on the PARiHS framework focused on external facilitation, internal facilitation is important because it is a function of the organization and is therefore a constant, whereas external facilitation can be designed or developed according to the needs of the organization (Harvey et al., 2002; Kitson et al., 2008). Internal facilitators are local to the implementation team or organization and are directly involved in the implementation, usually in an assigned role. They can serve as a major point of interface with external facilitators (Stetler, Ritchie, Rycroft-Malone, Schultz, & Charns, 2007). Facilitation involves personal characteristics of those involved and styles of leadership, including openness, supportiveness, approachability, reliability, self-confidence, and the ability to think laterally and without judgment.

The PARiHS model visually depicts the relationship among evidence, context, and facilitation in four positions called the *PARiHS diagnostic and evaluative grid* (Figure 2.8).

The team has continued to define and clarify the model, performing concept analysis of each of the dimensions and studying content validity. It has hypothesized that the PARiHS framework could not only be applied by practitioners as a diagnostic and evaluative tool to successfully implement evidence into practice, but also by practitioners and researchers to evaluate such activity (Kitson et al., 2008). There are measurement challenges to this effort; however, the work continues.

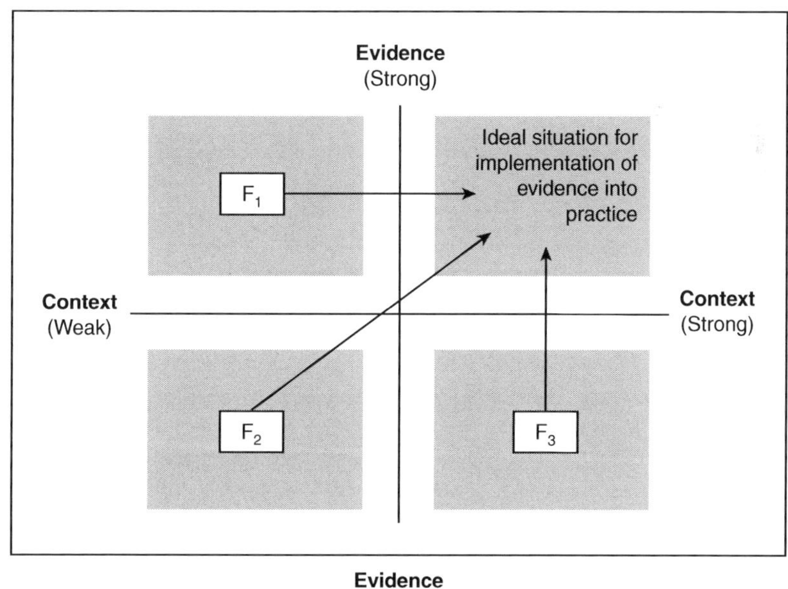

FIGURE 2.8 PARiHS diagnostic and evaluative grid.

PARiHS, Promoting Action on Research Implementation in Health Services.

Source: Adapted from Kitson, A. L., Rycroft-Malone, J., Harvey, G., McCormack, B., Seers, K., & Titchen, A. (2008). Evaluating the successful implementation of evidence into practice using the PARiHS framework: Theoretical and practical challenges. *Implementation Science, 3*, 1. Retrieved from http://www.implementationscience.com/content/pdf/1748-5908-3-1.pdf

Pathman's Pipeline

Donald Pathman, a pediatrician, and his colleagues Konrad, Freed, Freeman, and Koch (1996) studied vaccine compliance among physicians and designed a multistage model for moving from evidence to practice involving clinician uptake of the evidence, incorporation into routine practice, and patient compliance with the clinician's recommendation for the vaccine (Figure 2.9). The study concluded that the model was useful in identifying factors underlying adherence; however, they postulated that each situation in which the model is applied would have its own complexities and need for individualization. Pathman's model proposed five cognitive steps that physicians make in adhering to clinical guidelines. It also identified contextual factors that facilitate or hinder movement along these steps.

Pathman's work was tested and expanded upon, and a visual depiction was created, showing a water pipeline with faucets and leaks that represent the process of moving evidence to bedside practice. There are seven faucets or stages from evidence to action: awareness, acceptance, applicable, able, act on/adopt, agree, and adhere (Diner et al., 2007; Glasziou & Haynes, 2005). The "leaks" or barriers to implementation of new knowledge can occur at any one of the seven steps in the process (Glasziou & Haynes, 2005). Diner et al. (2007) used the Pathman Pipeline Model at a graduate medical education consensus conference to discuss the resident's uptake of research into practice. They focused on only four of the seven A's (faucets): acceptance, application, ability, and remembering to act on the existing evidence. However, the discussion quickly went to recommendations for identifying barriers for the uptake of the evidence, how to break down the barriers, how can this be incorporated into medical education, and the strategies to monitor the sustainability of implementation efforts (Figure 2.10).

Framework for Knowledge Transfer

Lavis, Robertson, Woodside, McLeod, and Abelson (2003) provide an organizing framework for knowledge transfer in the form of five questions with four specific

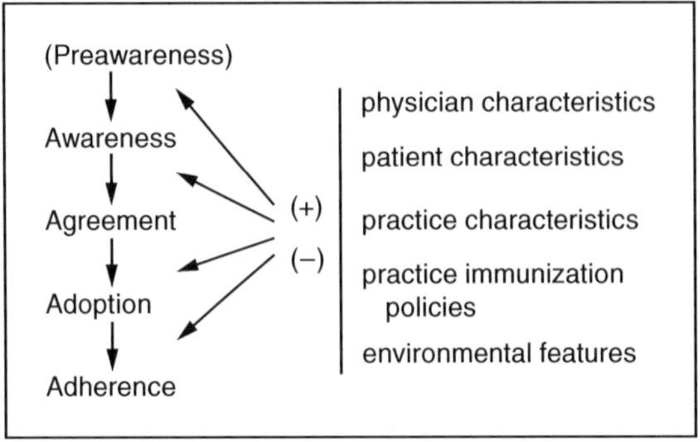

FIGURE 2.9 Multistage model for moving from evidence to practice.

Source: From Pathman, D. E., Konrad, T. R., Freed, G. L., Freeman, V. A., & Koch, G. G. (1996). The awareness-to-adherence model of the steps to clinical guideline compliance: The case of pediatric vaccine recommendations. *Medical Care*, 34(9), 873–889. doi:10.1097/00005650-199609000-00002

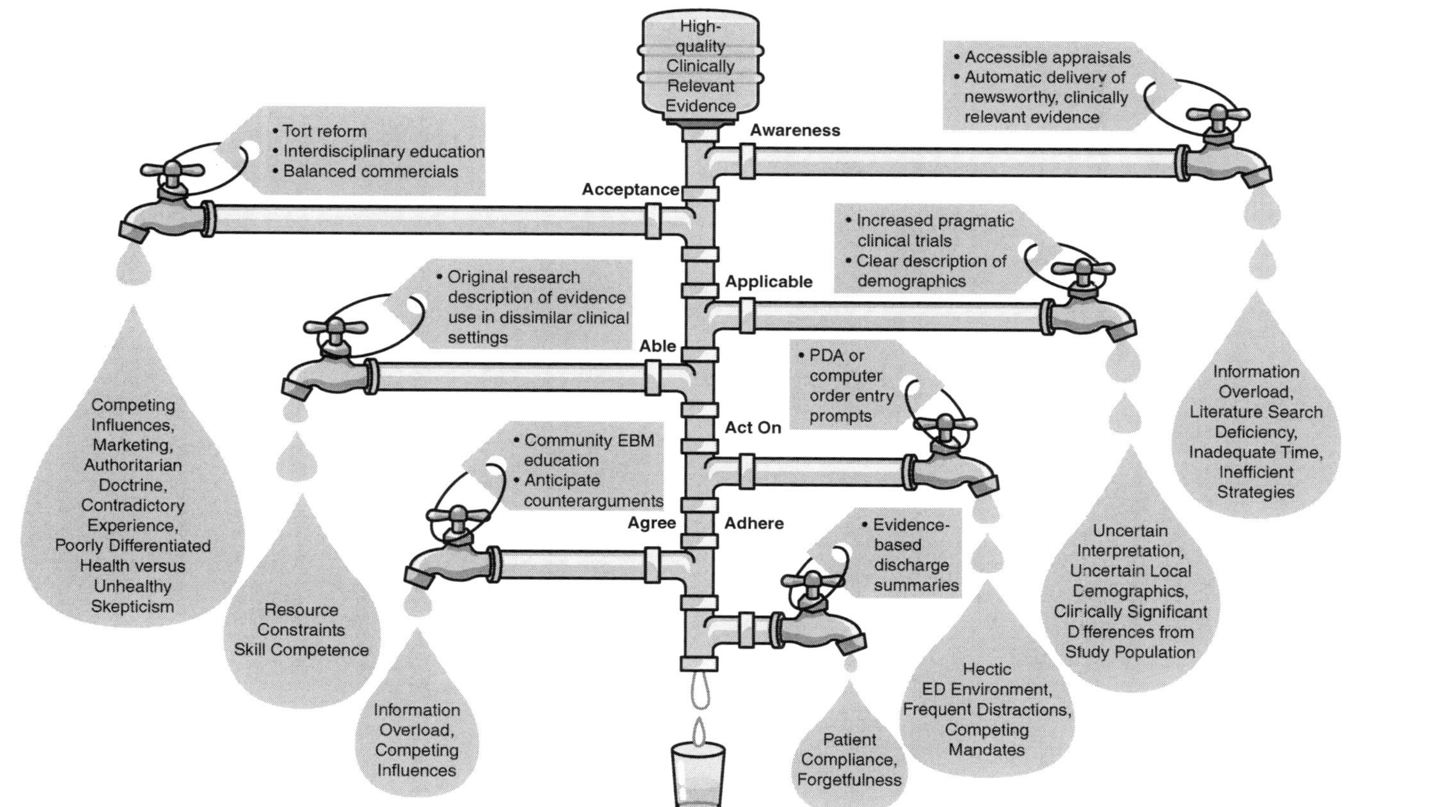

FIGURE 2.10 Pathman's Pipeline Model.

EBM, evidence-based medicine; PDA, personal digital assistant.

Source: Reprinted with permission from Diner, B. M., Carpenter, C. R., O'Connell, T., Pang, P., Brown, M. D., Seupaul, R., . . . KT-CC Theme IIa Members. (2007). Graduate medical education and knowledge translation: Role models, information pipelines, and practice change thresholds. *Academic Emergency Medicine, 14*(11), 1008–1014. doi:10.1197/j.aem.2007.07.003. Copyright by Hanley & Belfus, Inc.

audiences to consider. The four audiences are the general public, such as patients, families, citizens, and clients; service providers or the clinicians; managerial decision-makers, such as managers in hospitals, community settings, and businesses; and policy makers at federal, state, and local levels. The five questions that are the basis for the framework should be considered for each unique situation:

1. What should be transferred to the decision makers (the message)?
2. To whom should research knowledge be transferred (the target audience)?
3. By whom should research knowledge be transferred (the messenger)?
4. How should research knowledge be transferred (the KT process and support system)?
5. With what effect should research knowledge be transferred (evaluation)?

The research on this framework is discussed in Chapter 7, Translation of Evidence for Health Policy.

RE-AIM Model

The RE-AIM model was originally developed (Glasgow, Vogt, & Boles, 1999) as a framework to report research results and later to organize reviews of the health-promotion and disease-management literature. The acronym stands for reach, effectiveness, adoption, implementation, and maintenance. The goal of the RE-AIM model is to encourage planners, evaluators, funders, and policy makers to pay close attention to essential program elements, including external validity, to improve the implementation and sustainable adoption of generalizable evidence-based interventions (RE-AIM, n.d.). Since the development of the model, there have been more than 100 publications that use the model as a guide to implement new knowledge into practice in many different healthcare conditions: aging, cancer, dietary and weight loss, medication adherence, environmental change, chronic illness self-management, well-child care, eHealth, women's health, smoking cessation, and diabetes prevention. The five steps in the RE-AIM translation model are as follows:

- **Reach** the target population (How do I reach the target population?)
- **Effectiveness** of efficacy (How do I know if my intervention is effective?)
- **Adoption** by target settings or institutions (How do I develop organizational support to deliver my intervention?)
- **Implementation** consistency of the delivery of intervention (How do I ensure that the intervention is delivered properly?)
- **Maintenance** of intervention effects in individuals and setting over time (How do I incorporate the intervention so that it is delivered over the long term?)

The model stresses the importance of both the impact of and attention to the individual and institutional levels. Reach and efficacy are the first steps in the model and are more individual in impact; however, adoption and implementation occur at institutional levels of impact. Maintenance is seen as important for both levels (RE-AIM, n.d.).

TRANSLATING EVIDENCE INTO PRACTICE: A MODEL FOR LARGE-SCALE KT

Pronovost, Berenholtz, and Needham (2008) proposed a collaborative model for large-scale KT that has been shown to improve the reliability of care associated with substantial and sustained reductions in bloodstream infections associated with central lines (Pronovost et al., 2006). The integrated approach has five key components: (a) a focus on systems rather than the care of individual patients, (b) engagement of local interdisciplinary teams to assume ownership of the improvement project, (c) creation of centralized support for the technical work, (d) encouraging local adaptation of the intervention, and (e) creating a collaborative culture within the local unit of implementation and the larger system. This approach has matured into the translating evidence into practice model of the Johns Hopkins Quality and Safety Research Group; it has four phases and is intended for large-scale collaborative projects aimed at organizational change. The first phase is to summarize the evidence for improving a specific outcome. An assembled interdisciplinary team, specific to the problem, should review the evidence using standard criteria for evidence review and identify the interventions with the greatest benefit. The second phase of the model is to identify local barriers to implementation and assess the current processes and context of work, paying close attention to culture, teamwork, and communication. The third phase is to identify rigorous outcomes of the implementation and measure performance and engage in an iterative process of evaluation. The final phase is to ensure that all patients reliably receive the intervention. This is the most complex phase and must fit the organization. The model includes a "four E's" approach to improve this reliability of intervention that recognizes the importance of culture change, contextual factors, and engaging staff (Pronovost et al., 2008). The four E's are as follows (Figure 2.11):

1. *Engage* by sharing patient stories and providing an estimate of the harm that could result if the intervention is not implemented.
2. *Educate* by summarizing the scientific evidence supporting the intervention and providing the education to the staff.
3. *Execute* the intervention by standardizing care processes, creating independent checks (or checklists), and learning from the mistakes.
4. *Evaluate* the intervention by comparing baseline data against the outcomes identified to measure successful implementation.

The final translation model that is presented in this chapter is the Consolidated Framework for Implementation Research (CFIR), another model for large-scale KT (cfirguide.org/index.html). It was developed by implementation researchers affiliated with Veterans Affairs (VA) Diabetes Quality Enhancement Research Initiative (QUERI). The VA QUERI, described in Chapter 1, Evidence-Based Practice, was part of a system-wide evidence-based practice transformation aimed at improving the quality of healthcare for veterans. The CFIR provides a menu of constructs that have been associated with effective implementation and can be used in a range of applications, depending on the innovation and the context. The constructs provide a guide to systematically assess potential barriers and facilitators when planning the

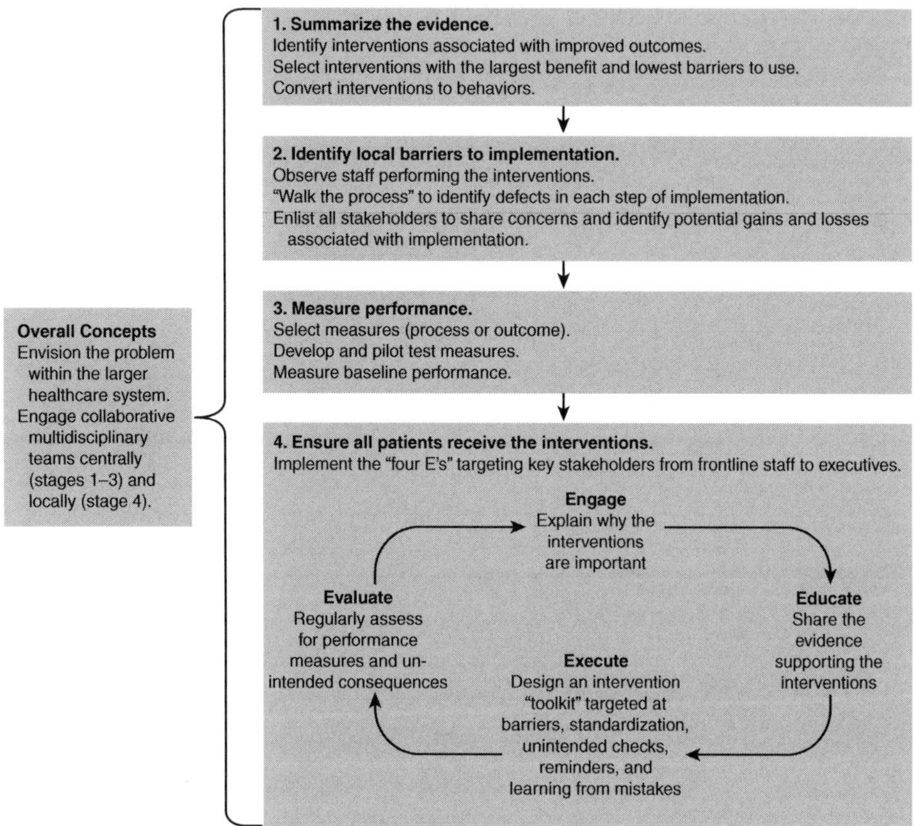

FIGURE 2.11 Strategy for translating evidence into practice.

Source: Reprinted with permission from Pronovost, P. J., Berenholtz, S. M., & Needham, D. M. (2008). Translating evidence into practice: A model for large scale knowledge translation. *British Medical Journal, 337*, a1714. doi:10.1136/bmj.a1714. Copyright by BMJ Publishing Group Ltd.

translation of an innovation (cfirguide.org). The CFIR has been found to be a practical model and has been used for both implementation and evaluation of translation of evidence to practice (Damschroder et al., 2009; Damschroder & Lowery, 2013; Powell et al., 2013). The model continues to be evaluated and recommendations continue to improve or extend its use. Table 2.1 lists the four constructs—intervention characteristics, inner setting, outer setting, and characteristics of the individuals—each of which needs to be considered when translating evidence into practice. Table 2.1 also describes the CFIR's identified steps in the translation process: planning, engaging, executing, and reflecting and evaluation.

■ CONCLUSIONS

This chapter has presented the key developments in translation theory and models over the past 15 years. With the subsequent development of each model, additional concepts were posited for consideration in the translation process. Agreed-upon

TABLE 2.1 Consolidated Framework for Implementation Research Constructs

Construct	Short Description
I. Intervention characteristics	
A. Intervention source	Perception of key stakeholders about whether the intervention is externally or internally developed
B. Evidence strength and quality	Stakeholders' perceptions of the quality and validity of evidence supporting the belief that the intervention will have desired outcomes
C. Relative advantage	Stakeholders' perception of the advantage of implementing the intervention versus an alternative solution
D. Adaptability	The degree to which an intervention can be adapted, tailored, refined, or reinvented to meet local needs
E. Trialability	The ability to test the intervention on a small scale in the organization and to be able to reverse course (undo implementation) if warranted
F. Complexity	Perceived difficulty of implementation, reflected by duration, scope, radicalness, disruptiveness, centrality, and intricacy and number of steps required for implementation
G. Design quality and packaging	Perceived excellence in how the intervention is bundled, presented, and assembled
H. Cost	Costs of the intervention and costs associated with implementing the intervention, including investment, supply, and opportunity costs
II. Outer setting	
A. Patient needs and resources	The extent to which patient needs, as well as barriers and facilitators to meet those needs, are accurately known and prioritized by the organization
B. Cosmopolitanism	The degree to which an organization is networked with other external organizations
C. Peer pressure	Mimetic or competitive pressure to implement an intervention; typically occur because most or other key peer or competing organizations have already implemented or are in a bid for a competitive edge
D. External policy and incentives	A broad construct that includes external strategies to spread interventions, including policy and regulations (governmental or other central entity), external mandates, recommendations and guidelines, pay-for-performance, collaboratives, and public or benchmark reporting
III. Inner setting	
A. Structural characteristics	The social architecture, age, maturity, and size of an organization

(continued)

TABLE 2.1 Consolidated Framework for Implementation Research Constructs (*continued*)

Construct	Short Description
B. Networks and communications	The nature and quality of webs of social networks and the nature and quality of formal and informal communications within an organization
C. Culture	Norms, values, and basic assumptions of a given organization
D. Implementation climate	The absorptive capacity for change, shared receptivity of involved individuals to an intervention, and the extent to which use of that intervention will be rewarded, supported, and expected within their organization
1. Tension for change	The degree to which stakeholders perceive the current situation as intolerable or needing change
2. Compatibility	The degree of tangible fit between meaning and values attached to the intervention by involved individuals; how those align with individuals' own norms, values, and perceived risks and needs; and how the intervention fits with existing workflows and systems
3. Relative priority	Individuals' shared perception of the importance of the implementation within the organization
4. Organizational incentives and rewards	Extrinsic incentives, such as goal-sharing awards, performance reviews, promotions, and raises in salary, and less-tangible incentives such as increased stature or respect
5. Goals and feedback	The degree to which goals are clearly communicated, acted upon, and fed back to staff, and alignment of that feedback with goals
6. Learning climate	A climate in which (a) leaders express their own fallibility and need for team members' assistance and input; (b) team members feel that they are essential, valued, and knowledgeable partners in the change process; (c) individuals feel psychologically safe to try new methods; and (d) there is sufficient time and space for reflective thinking and evaluation
E. Readiness for implementation	Tangible and immediate indicators of organizational commitment to its decision to implement an intervention
1. Leadership engagement	Leaders and managers are committed, involved, and accountable for the implementation
2. Available resources	The level of resources dedicated for implementation and ongoing operations, including money, training, education, physical space, and time
3. Access to knowledge and information	Ease of access to digestible information and knowledge about the intervention and how to incorporate it into work tasks

(*continued*)

TABLE 2.1 Consolidated Framework for Implementation Research Constructs (*continued*)

Construct	Short Description
IV. Characteristics of individuals	
A. Knowledge and beliefs about the intervention	Individuals' attitudes toward and value placed on the intervention, as well as familiarity with facts, truths, and principles related to the intervention
B. Self-efficacy	Individuals' beliefs in their own capabilities to execute courses of action to achieve implementation goals
C. Individual stage of change	Characterization of the phase an individual is in as he or she progresses toward skilled, enthusiastic, and sustained use of the intervention
D. Individual identification with organization	A broad construct related to how individuals perceive the organization and their relationship and degree of commitment with that organization
E. Other personal attributes	A broad construct to include other personal traits such as tolerance of ambiguity, intellectual ability, motivation, values, competence, capacity, and learning style
V. Process	
A. Planning	The degree to which a scheme or method of behavior and tasks for implementing an intervention are developed in advance, and the quality of those schemes or methods
B. Engaging	Attracting and involving appropriate individuals in the implementation and use of the intervention through a combined strategy of social marketing, education, role modeling, training, and other similar activities
1. Opinion leaders	Individuals in an organization who have formal or informal influence on the attitudes and beliefs of their colleagues with respect to implementing the intervention
2. Formally appointed internal implementation leaders	Individuals from within the organization who have been formally appointed with the responsibility to implement an intervention as a coordinator, project manager, team leader, or other similar role
3. Champions	Individuals who support and facilitate an implementation by overcoming indifference or resistance that the intervention may provoke in an organization
4. External change agents	Individuals who are affiliated with an outside entity and who formally influence or facilitate intervention decisions in a desirable direction
C. Executing	Carrying out or accomplishing the implementation according to plan
D. Reflecting and evaluating	Quantitative and qualitative feedback about the progress and quality of implementation accompanied with regular personal and team debriefing about progress and experience

themes are the criticality that active coordination, implementation, and dissemination of new knowledge must be guided by the evidence; the clinicians involved; the characteristics of the organization; consideration of facilitators and barriers; and the need for evaluation, monitoring, and sustainability of the implementation. The importance of planning and attention to principles of the change process for translation of research into practice have been highlighted.

■ REFERENCES

Agency for Healthcare Research and Quality. (2001). *Translating research into practice (TRIP)-II fact sheet.* Retrieved from http://www.ahrq.gov/research/trip2fac.htm

Balas, E. A., & Boren, S. A. (2000). Managing clinical knowledge for health care improvement. In J. van Bemmel & A. T. McCray (Eds.), *Yearbook of medical informatics* (pp. 65–70). Stuttgart, Germany: Schattauer Publishing.

Bero, L. A., Grilli, R., Grimshaw, J. M., Harvey, E., Oxman, A. D., & Thomson, M. A. (1998). Closing the gap between research and practice: An overview of systematic reviews of interventions to promote the implementation of research findings. The Cochrane Effective Practice and Organization of Care Review Group. *British Medical Journal, 317*(7156), 465–468. doi:10.1136/bmj.317.7156.465

Berwick, D. M. (2003). Disseminating innovations in health care. *Journal of the American Medical Association, 289*(15), 1969–1975. doi:10.1001/jama.289.15.1969

Canadian Health Services Research Foundation. (2011). *Glossary of knowledge exchange terms.* Retrieved from http://www.cfhi-fcass.ca/PublicationsAndResources/ResourcesAndTools/GlossaryKnowledgeExchange.aspx

Canadian Institutes of Health Research. (2010). *About knowledge translation.* Retrieved from http://www.cihr-irsc.gc.ca/e/29418.html

Damschroder, L., Aron, D., Keith, R., Kirsh, S., Alexander, J., & Lowery, J. (2009). Fostering implementation of health services research findings into practice: A consolidated framework for advancing implementation science. *Implementation Science, 4*(1), 50. doi:10.1186/1748-5908-4-50

Damschroder, L. J., & Lowery, J. C. (2013). Evaluation of a large-scale weight management program using the Consolidated Framework for Implementation Research (CFIR). *Implementation Science, 8(1)*, 51. doi:10.1186/1748-5908-8-51

Diner, B. M., Carpenter, C. R., O'Connell, T., Pang, P., Brown, M. D., Seupaul, R., . . . KT-CC Theme IIIa Members. (2007). Graduate medical education and knowledge translation: Role models, information pipelines, and practice change thresholds. *Academic Emergency Medicine, 14*(11), 1008–1014. doi:10.1197/j.aem.2007.07.003

Estabrooks, C. A., Thompson, D. S., Lovely, J. J., & Hofmeyer, A. (2006). A guide to knowledge translation theory. *Journal of Continuing Education in the Health Professions, 26*(1), 25–36. doi:10.1002/chp.48

Farquhar, C. M., Stryer, D., & Slutsky, J. (2002). Translating research into practice: The future ahead. *International Journal for Quality in Health Care, 14*(3), 233–249. doi:10.1093/oxfordjournals.intqhc.a002615

Glasgow, R. E., & Emmons, K. M. (2007). How can we increase translation of research into practice? Types of evidence needed. *Annual Review of Public Health, 28*, 413–433. doi:10.1146/annurev.publhealth.28.021406.144145

Glasgow, R. E., Vogt, T. M., & Boles, S. M. (1999). Evaluating the public health impact of health promotion interventions: The RE-AIM framework. *American Journal of Public Health, 89*(9), 1322–1327. doi:10.2105/AJPH.89.9.1322

Glasziou, P., & Haynes, B. (2005). The paths from research to improved health outcomes. *ACP Journal Club, 142*(2), A8–A10. doi:10.1136/ebn.8.2.36

Graham, I. D., Logan, J., Harrison, M. B., Straus, S. E., Tetroe, J., Caswell, W., & Robinson, N. (2006). Lost in knowledge translation: Time for a map? *Journal of Continuing Education in the Health Professions, 26*(1), 13–24. doi:10.1002/chp.47

Graham, I. D., Tetroe, J., & KT Theories Research Group. (2007). Some theoretical underpinnings of knowledge translation. *Academic Emergency Medicine, 14*(11), 936–941. doi:10.1197/j.aem.2007.07.004

Graham, K., & Logan, J. (2004). Using the Ottawa model of research use to implement a skin care program. *Journal of Nursing Care Quality, 19*(1), 18–24. doi:10.1097/00001786-200401000-00006

Green, L. A., & Seifert, C. M. (2005). Translation of research into practice: Why we can't "just do it". *Journal of the American Board of Family Practice, 18*(6), 541–545. doi:10.3122/jabfm.18.6.541

Greenhalgh, T., Robert, G., MacFarlane, F., Bate, P., & Kyriakidou, O. (2004). Diffusion of innovations in service organizations: Systematic review and recommendations. *The Milbank Quarterly, 82*(4), 581–629. Retrieved from http://www3.interscience.wiley.com/cgi-bin/fulltext/118784115/PDFSTART

Grol, R., & Grimshaw, J. (1999). Evidence-based implementation of evidence-based medicine. *Joint Commission Journal on Quality Improvement, 25*(10), 503–513. doi:10.1016/S1070-3241(16)30464-3

Grol, R., & Grimshaw, J. (2003). From best evidence to best practice: Effective implementation of change in patients' care. *Lancet, 362*(9391), 1225–1230. doi:10.1016/S0140-6736(03)14546-1

Haines, A., & Jones, R. (1994). Implementing findings of research. *British Medical Journal, 308*(6942), 1488–1492. doi:10.1136/bmj.308.6942.1488

Harvey, G., Loftus-Hills, A., Rycroft-Malone, J., Titchen, A., Kitson, A., McCormack, B., & Seers, K. (2002). Getting evidence into practice: The role and function of facilitation. *Journal of Advanced Nursing, 37*(6), 577–588. doi:10.1046/j.1365-2648.2002.02126.x

Institute of Medicine. (2001). *Crossing the quality chasm: A new health system for the 21st century*. Washington, DC: National Academies Press.

Kirchhoff, K. T. (2004). State of the science of translational research: From demonstration projects to intervention testing. *Worldviews on Evidence-Based Nursing, 1*(Suppl. 1), S6–S12. doi:10.1111/j.1524-475X.2004.04039.x

Kitson, A., Harvey, G., & McCormack, B. (1998). Enabling the implementation of evidence-based practice: A conceptual framework. *Quality in Health Care, 7*(3), 149–158. doi:10.1136/qshc.7.3.149

Kitson, A. L., Rycroft-Malone, J., Harvey, G., McCormack, B., Seers, K., & Titchen, A. (2008). Evaluating the successful implementation of evidence into practice using the PARiHS framework: Theoretical and practical challenges. *Implementation Science, 3*, 1. Retrieved from http://www.implementationscience.com/content/pdf/1748-5908-3-1.pdf

Lavis, J. N., Robertson, D., Woodside, J. M., McLeod, C. B., & Abelson, J. (2003). How can research organization more effectively transfer research knowledge to decision makers? *Milbank Quarterly, 81*(2), 221–248. doi:10.1111/1468-0009.t01-1-00052

Li, A., Jeffs, L., Barwick, M., & Stevens, B. (2018). Organizational contextual features that influence the implementation of evidence-based practices across healthcare settings: A systematic integrative review. *Systematic Reviews, 7*(1), 72. doi:10.1186/s13643-018-0734-5

Logan, J., & Graham, I. D. (1998). Toward a comprehensive interdisciplinary model of health care research use. *Science Communication, 20*(2), 227–246. doi:10.1177/1075547098020002004

Lomas, J. (1993). Retailing research: Increasing the role of evidence in clinical services for childbirth. *Milbank Quarterly, 71*(3), 439–475. doi:10.2307/3350410

Lomas, J., Sisk, J. E., & Stocking, B. (1993). From evidence to practice in the United States, the United Kingdom, and Canada. *Milbank Quarterly, 71*(3), 405–410. doi:10.2307/3350408

McCormack, B., Kitson, A., Harvey, G., Rycroft-Malone, J., Titchen, A., & Seers, K. (2002). Getting evidence into practice: The meaning of "context."*Journal of Advanced Nursing, 38*(1), 94–104. doi:10.1046/j.1365-2648.2002.02150.x

Milat, A., & Li, B. (2017). Narrative review of frameworks for translating research evidence into policy and practice. *Public Health Research and Practice, 27*(1), e2711704. doi:10.17061/phrp2711704

National Institutes of Health. (2005). *Fact sheet: NIH Clinical and Translational Science Awards (CTSA)*. Retrieved from https://ncats.nih.gov/files/ctsa_program_factsheet.pdf

Newhouse, R., & White, K. (2011). Guiding implementation. Frameworks and resources for evidence. *Journal of Nursing Administration, 41*(12), 513–516. doi:10.1097/NNA.0b013e3182378bb0

Nieva, V., Murphy, R., Ridley, N., Donaldson, N., Combes, J., Mitchell, P., . . . Carpenter, D. (2005). From science to service: A framework for the transfer of patient safety research into practice. In K. Henriksen, J. B. Battles, & E. S. Marks (Eds.), *Advanced in patient safety: From research to implementation* (Vol. 2, pp. 441–453). Rockville, MD: Agency for Healthcare Research and Quality.

Oxman, A. D., Thomson, M. A., Davis, D. A., & Haynes, R. B. (1995). No magic bullets: A systematic review of 102 trials of interventions to improve professional practice. *Canadian Medical Association Journal, 153*(10), 1423–1431.

Pathman, D. E., Konrad, T. R., Freed, G. L., Freeman, V. A., & Koch, G. G. (1996). The awareness-to-adherence model of the steps to clinical guideline compliance: The case of pediatric vaccine recommendations. *Medical Care, 34*(9), 873–889. doi:10.1097/00005650-199609000-00002

Powell, B., Proctor, E., Glisson, C., Kohl, P., Raghavan, R., Brouwnson, R., . . . Palinkas, L. (2013). A mixed methods multiple case study of implementation as usual in children's social service organizations: Study protocol. *Implmentation Science, 8*, 92. Retrieved from https://implementationscience.biomedcentral.com/articles/10.1186/1748-5908-8-92

Pronovost, P., Needham, D., Berenholtz, S., Sinopoli, D., Chu, H., Cosgrove, S., . . . Goeschel, C. (2006). An intervention to decrease catheter-related bloodstream infections in the ICU. *New England Journal of Medicine, 355*(26), 2725–2732. doi:10.1056/NEJMoa061115

Pronovost, P. J., Berenholtz, S. M., & Needham, D. M. (2008). Translating evidence into practice: A model for large scale knowledge translation. *British Medical Journal, 337*, a1714. doi:10.1136/bmj.a1714

RE-AIM. (n.d.). *What is RE-AIM?* Retrieved from https://www.bmj.com/content/337/bmj.a1714

Rogers, E. M. (2003). *Diffusion of innovations* (5th ed.). New York, NY: Free Press.

Rycroft-Malone, J., Harvey, G., Seers, K., Kitson, A., McCormack, B., & Titchen, A. (2004). An exploration of the factors that influence the implementation of evidence into practice. *Journal of Clinical Nursing, 13*(8), 913–924. doi:10.1111/j.1365-2702.2004.01007.x

Rycroft-Malone, J., Seers, K., Titchen, A., Harvey, G., Kitson, A., & McCormack, B. (2004). What counts as evidence in evidence-based practice. *Journal of Advanced Nursing, 47*(1), 81–90. doi:10.1111/j.1365-2648.2004.03068.x

Schuster, M. A., McGlynn, E. A., & Brook, R. H. (1998). How good is the quality of health care in the United States? *Milbank Quarterly, 76*(4), 517–563. doi:10.1111/1468-0009.00105

Stetler, C. B., Corrigan, B., Sander-Buscemi, K., & Burns, M. (1999). Integration of evidence into practice and the change process: Fall prevention program as a model. *Outcomes Management for Nursing Practice, 3*(3), 102–111.

Stetler, C. B., Ritchie, J., Rycroft-Malone, J., Schultz, A., & Charns, M. (2007). Improving quality of care through routine, successful implementation of evidence-based practice at the bedside: An organizational case study protocol using the Pettigrew and Whipp model of strategic change. *Implementation Science, 2*, 3. Retrieved from http://www.implementationscience.com/content/pdf/1748-5908-2-3.pdf

Titler, M. G. (2008). The evidence for evidence-based practice implementation. In R. G. Hughes (Ed.), *Patient safety and quality: An evidence-based handbook for nursing* (pp. i113–i161). Rockville, MD: Agency for Healthcare Research and Quality.

Westfall, J. M., Mold, J., & Fagnan, L. (2007). Practice-based research—"Blue highways" on the NIH Roadmap. *Journal of the American Medical Association, 297*(4), 403–406. doi:10.1001/jama.297.4.403

Zerhouni, E. A. (2005). Translational and clinical science—Time for a new vision. *New England Journal of Medicine, 353*(15), 1621–1623. doi:10.1056/NEJMsb053723

CHAPTER THREE

Change Theory and Models: Framework for Translation

Kathleen M. White

A butterfly is a transformation, not a better caterpillar.
—CHRIS MCGOFF

TRANSLATION MODELS, DISCUSSED IN CHAPTER 2, THE SCIENCE OF TRANSLATION AND MAJOR FRAMEWORKS, are models of change, but have been designed to guide thinking and planning specific to the translation of new knowledge into practice. In discussing the translation of research into practice it is always useful to consider change theory and models. The challenges to translating research into practice are similar to the commonly described challenges involved in any change implementation, such as gaining internal support for the change, ensuring effective leadership, integrating with existing programs, developing a supportive organizational culture, maintaining momentum while changing, and documenting and positively publicizing the outcomes of the change (Bradley, Schlesinger, Webster, Baker, & Inouye, 2004).

Change—the transformation of tasks, processes, methods, structures, and/or relationships—is necessary for organizational survival. Changes, such as the diffusion of evidence-based practice (EBP) into an organization or, more specifically, the translation of new knowledge into practice, must be planned for and managed based on how the change affects the people of the organization. When planning for change, the situation will vary widely according to the impetus for the change, the type of change needed, the personnel and clients involved, and many characteristics of the organization, agency, or practice where the change is necessary. The planning and management of change determines whether the change will be a success or a failure. Despite this well-known need for systematic planning and management of change, often guided by a model or theory, Davies, Walker, and Grimshaw (2010) found that only 6% of knowledge translation studies in their systematic review used a theory/model to guide the design or implementation of interventions to facilitate the knowledge translation.

Change has traditionally been viewed as a continual and sequential process affected by a complex set of interacting factors. The rational change approach, with its origins in economic theory, assumes that those involved in the change will have full information, act reasonably and sensibly, use sound judgment and good sense, and that the change process is predictable, linear, and static. This classical view of change does not account for today's complex and chaotic change environment (Reineck, 2007). The behavioral change approach considers that organizations and their people are goal oriented, focused on purpose, and problem driven, and that they have activities, patterns, and routines that they follow as long as they work. When those patterns and activities prove insufficient, they seek to change them. Theories of behavior change plan for and manage attitudes, norms, intentions, self-efficacy, benefits, fears, resistance, and perceived barriers to change, all concepts of human behavior (World Bank, 2010).

McConnell (2010) identified two major categories of resistance to change that must be planned for and managed as the change process is implemented. The principal cause of most resistances to change is the disturbance to the status quo or, as he describes it, a disturbance to "equilibrium," especially if the disturbance or direction for change leads into unfamiliar territory. Secondary causes of resistance are intellectual shortcomings, or the inability to conceive of certain possibilities or to think beyond the boundaries of what is presently known or believed. Both these causes of resistance to change are rooted in the EBP movement. Assessment of these causes of resistance and the development of strategies that anticipate and manage the resistance will enhance the adoption of or translation of new knowledge into practice.

This chapter discusses change theories and how they can be used to translate new knowledge into practice.

■ ORGANIZATIONAL THEORIES OF CHANGE

Lewin's Force Field Analysis

Kurt Lewin's (1951) classic theory of change is a three-phase change model that views change as a dynamic balance of forces (driving and restraining) working in opposite directions within an organization or *field* (Figure 3.1). The driving forces promote or move individuals toward the change direction, and the restraining forces inhibit or move individuals away from the change. Lewin's theory of change was developed after World War II, when he carried out research exploring how individuals change their dietary habits. He discovered that if individuals are involved in the discussion about the change and issues surrounding the change, they are able to make their own decisions to change their behavior (Lewin, 1947). The first phase of the change process is to *unfreeze* the current situation by increasing the driving forces or decreasing the restraining forces toward change. *Moving* or *changing* is the second phase during which the organization is moved toward a new equilibrium of driving and restraining forces. The final phase is *refreezing*, which must occur after the change is implemented to sustain the change within the organization. Assessment of the forces, both driving and restraining, throughout the

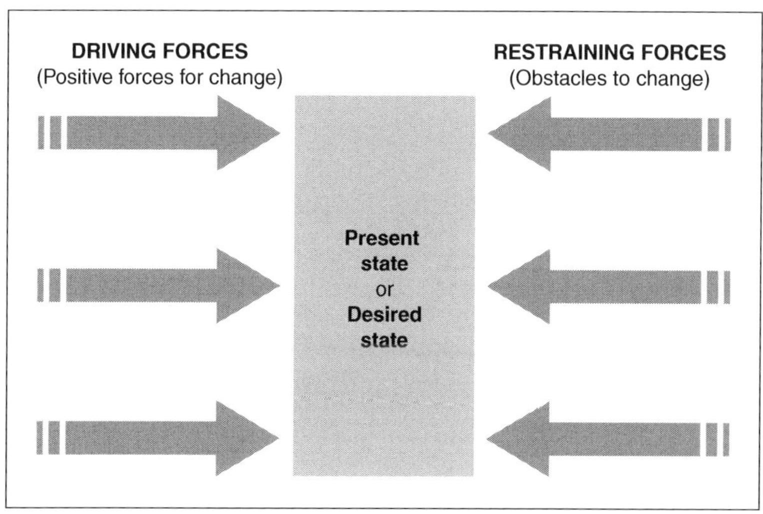

FIGURE 3.1 Lewin's force field analysis.

Source: Reprinted with permission from Lewin, K. (1947). Frontiers in group dynamics. *Human Relations, 1*(1), 5–41. doi:10.1177/001872674700100103. Copyright by Sage Publications Ltd.

change process is necessary to recognize the power of the forces and to involve the individuals in the organization, build trust, encourage a new view, and to integrate new ideas into the organization.

Lewin's theory, although often criticized as viewing change as linear and predictable, is still used to plan change in organizations, including EBP translations (Manchester et al., 2014; Shirey, 2013). Manchester et al. (2014) cite several studies and report their own application of the theory to two case studies from the Health Resources and Services Administration's Geriatric Education Center network to assert the need for planning change when dealing with contextual factors at play in the organization when implementing new evidence into practice. Instead of criticizing the linear nature of Lewin's three-step change model, they describe the "sequential anchors" of unfreezing, movement, and refreezing in the model as a way of understanding how the behaviors of health professionals become accepted and sustained in the clinical setting (Manchester et al., 2014).

Lippitt's Model of Change

Lippitt, Watson, and Westley (1958) built on the work of Lewin and developed a seven-step model of change that concentrated on the role of the leader in the change process and added the change-agent role. The seven steps are:

1. Develop need for change by diagnosing the change.
2. Establish change relationship and assess the motivation and capacity to change.
3. Clarify assessment for change and determine resources.
4. Establish goals and intentions for an action plan.

5. Examine alternatives.
6. Transform intentions into actual change and maintain the change.
7. Generalize and stabilize change and end the helping relationship of the change agent.

Havelock's Theory of Planned Change

Havelock (1976) further modified Lewin's theory of change and created a process for change agents to organize their work and implement innovation in the work environment. Havelock postulated that change is made up of cycles of action that are repeated as change advances, and that the change agent must pay attention to the steps. Havelock described six steps, but the visual of the model includes a stage 0, called *Care*, where a concern for needed change first occurs.

Care—Attention to the need for change
Relate—Build a relationship
Examine—Diagnose the problem
Acquire—Acquire the relevant sources
Try—Choose the solution
Extend—Disseminate, diffuse, and gain acceptance
Renew—Stabilize and sustain capacity

Havelock and Zlotolow (1995) created a visual of the model for change agents to use and to guide the change process. For a visual depiction of Havelock's Change Model, please go to the original source: Havelock and Zlotolow (1995).

Framework for Guiding the Process of Implementation

Howes and Quinn (1978) summarized the organizational change literature on factors related to the successful implementation of change with a "how to" list for managers to use to implement change. They described two phases and 12 levers or guidelines for change, six levers in each phase.

The first phase is to *set up an adequate orientation environment* to prepare and positively influence the change by doing the following:

- Set aside enough time for adequate introduction to the change.
- Make the relative advantage of the change easily visible.
- Show organization members (users) that their efforts will be supported.
- Show users that it will be easy to institutionalize the change and that it will be relatively nonthreatening afterward.
- Show that immediate superiors accept and support the change.
- Clearly identify the roles and responsibilities of all who will be involved in the change process.

The perceived characteristics of the change, such as the relative advantage and compatibility of the change with the present way of doing things, its simplicity, ease of understanding, and trial ability, are critically important to the user in this first phase of a change.

The second phase, to *set up adequate support networks for the implementation effort*, includes the six levers that assist the change to happen and focuses on the climate within the organization to facilitate the change:

- Produce and make supportive services available.
- Set up formal training programs to develop members' roles.
- Encourage and reward the use of horizontal and vertical communication channels.
- Relax standard operating procedures in affected (changing) units.
- Integrate change agents, managers, and users.
- Make sure users feel adequately involved.

Pettigrew and Whipp's Model of Strategic Management of Change

Pettigrew and Whipp (1991) developed a strategic model of change that involves the interaction of three essential dimensions of strategic change: context, content, and process. They also described the importance of historical, cultural, and political factors in the interaction of the essential elements. The *context* includes both external and internal factors and events that are driving the change, the *why* of change, including the organization's culture, leadership, type of clinical setting, and the characteristics of the organization. The *content* dimension describes the activities to be transformed or the *what* of change. In translation of research into practice efforts, these are the key organizational elements in the system focused on enhancing or supporting the use of evidence. The third dimension, the *process* or the *how* of change, includes the methods, strategies, and actions and interactions that will be used to make the change happen and enable the use of the new evidence (Stetler, Ritchie, Rycroft-Malone, Schultz, & Charns, 2007). The model stresses the continuous, iterative, dynamic, and uncertain nature of the change-management process.

Ferlie and Shortell: Framework for Change

Ferlie and Shortell's (1996) work is similar and proposes a model for implementing change for quality improvement in healthcare. The model focuses on the importance of context in change and describes four levels of change: (a) the individual healthcare practitioner, (b) the healthcare team, (c) the overall organization, and (d) the cultural environment of the organization.

Contemporary Change Theory

John Kotter's Eight-Step Process for Leading Change (1996) provides a contemporary view of leading change in organizations: (a) establish a sense of urgency, (b) create the guiding coalition, (c) develop a vision and strategy, (d) communicate the change vision, (e) introduce the change and empower a broad base of people to take action, (f) generate short-term wins, (g) consolidate gains and the production of even more change, and (h) institutionalize new approaches in the corporate culture to ground the changes in the culture and make them stick. Use of this model has been successful in effecting knowledge translation and large-scale transformational change in organizations, such as implementation of the electronic health record.

Kotter (1995) also describes why change efforts fail:

- Allowing too much complacency
- Failing to create a sufficiently powerful guiding coalition
- Underestimating the power of vision
- Under-communicating the vision
- Permitting obstacles to block the vision
- Failing to create short-term wins
- Declaring victory too soon
- Neglecting to anchor changes firmly in the corporate culture

Kotter (1995) acknowledges that these eight errors might be too simplistic, but that in reality, most change efforts are messy and full of surprises and need a guiding vision to reduce the failures.

This contemporary view on leading change for translation of new knowledge to practice efforts stresses the importance of the people involved in the change; their reactions to all aspects of the change, linking to context, content, and processes/facilitation; and the bigger picture or fit of the change for the organization (Kotter, 1999). Kotter's latest work (Kotter & Cohen, 2012), *The Heart of Change: Real-Life Stories of How People Change Their Organizations*, proposes that to be successful in change efforts, organizations must positively change the thinking of those involved in or affected by the change.

■ BEHAVIORAL THEORIES OF CHANGE

Social Cognitive Theory

Social cognitive theory posits that individuals learn by direct experiences, human dialog and interaction, and observation. Developed by Albert Bandura, it began as *social learning theory* and was later renamed *social cognitive theory*. Bandura (1986) indicated that the purpose of the theory is to understand and predict individual and group behavior, identify methods by which behavior can be modified or changed, and test interventions aimed at personality development, behavior pathology, and health promotion. This theory of change proposes that behavioral change is affected by personal factors, attributes of the behavior itself, and environmental influences (Robbins, 2003). Individuals must believe in their capability to change and possess the self-efficacy to change. In addition, they must perceive that there is an incentive to change, which in social learning theory is referred to as *operant conditioning*, with the positive expectations outweighing the negative consequences. Social cognitive theory is particularly useful when dealing with educational programs aimed at changing behavior, such as implementing new knowledge into practice.

Stages of Change Theory

Prochaska and DiClementi's Model of Behavior Change was originally developed for use with individual patients to change health behaviors, specifically to study smokers in therapy (DiClemente & Prochaska, 1998). The model originally had four stages and was considered linear in its original development. However, the model now has five stages (Figure 3.2) with an added stage, preparation for action, and is now viewed as a cyclical process. The model's use has also extended beyond the individual patient to include other audiences over time. The model describes five stages that people pass through when change occurs:

1. *Precontemplation* is when an individual is unaware of or does not acknowledge that a problem exists and that there is a need for change.
2. *Contemplation* is the stage when the individual becomes aware of the issue/problem and begins to think about changing his or her behavior.
3. *Preparation* for action is when the individual is ready to change and prepares to make a change. This preparation for action is defined within a 2-week period of a decision to change.
4. *Action* is when the individual engages in change activities and increases coping behaviors to deal with the change.
5. *Maintenance* is the final stage, which may take up to 6 months. The change behaviors must be reinforced to sustain the change.

Prochaska, DiClemente, and Norcross (1992) described 10 processes that predict and motivate movement through the stages: (a) consciousness raising, (b) dramatic relief, (c) environmental reevaluation, (d) self-reevaluation, (e) self-liberation, (f) social liberation, (g) reinforcement management, (h) helping relationships, (i) counterconditioning, and (j) stimulus control. This model has been used successfully in counseling patients with HIV/AIDS and sexually transmitted diseases (STDs; Centers for Disease Control and Prevention, 1993) and as a means of improving

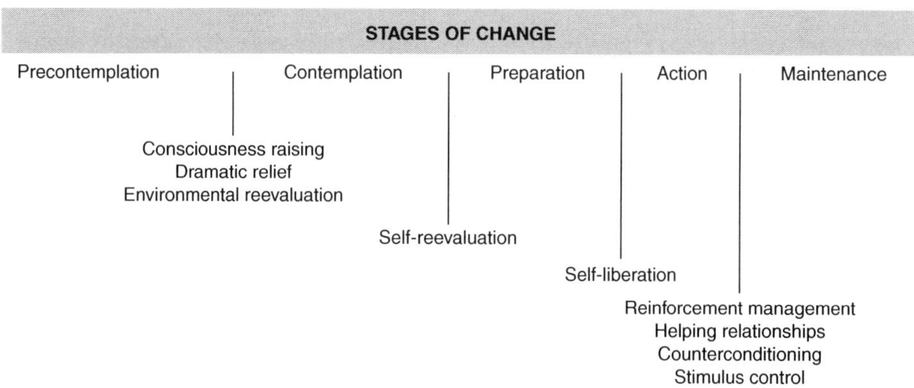

FIGURE 3.2 Stages of change theory.

Source: From Prochaska, J. O., DiClemente, C. C., & Norcross, J. C. (1992). In search of how people change—Applications to addictive behaviors. *American Psychologist, 47*(9), 1102–1114. doi:10.3109/10884609309149692

the implementation and effectiveness of interventions designed to reduce the burden of musculoskeletal injuries (Rothmore, Aylward, & Karnon, 2015; Rothmore et al., 2016). However, the influence of structure and environment are two key elements that are not specifically addressed in the model and are necessary components of planning for change or translation of new knowledge into a practice setting. In the workplace setting, individual readiness is assessed, but the intervention is aimed at the workgroup (Oakman, Rothmore, & Tappin, 2016).

Theory of Reasoned Action

This theory was developed in the late 1960s and has been used to describe an individual's intention to perform certain behaviors (Figure 3.3). The theory assumes that individuals are rational and links the individual's behavior to beliefs, attitudes, and intentions (Ajzen & Fishbein, 1980). Fishbein, Middlestadt, and Hitchcock (1994) further defined the variables:

- *Behavior*—A specific behavior that should occur so that the individual understands the needed action, for whom, when, and where
- *Intention*—The best predictor that a behavior will occur, is influenced by attitude and norms (Family Health International, 1996)
- *Attitude*—The individual's positive or negative feelings toward performing the behavior
- *Norms*—The individual's perception of others' opinions of the behavior

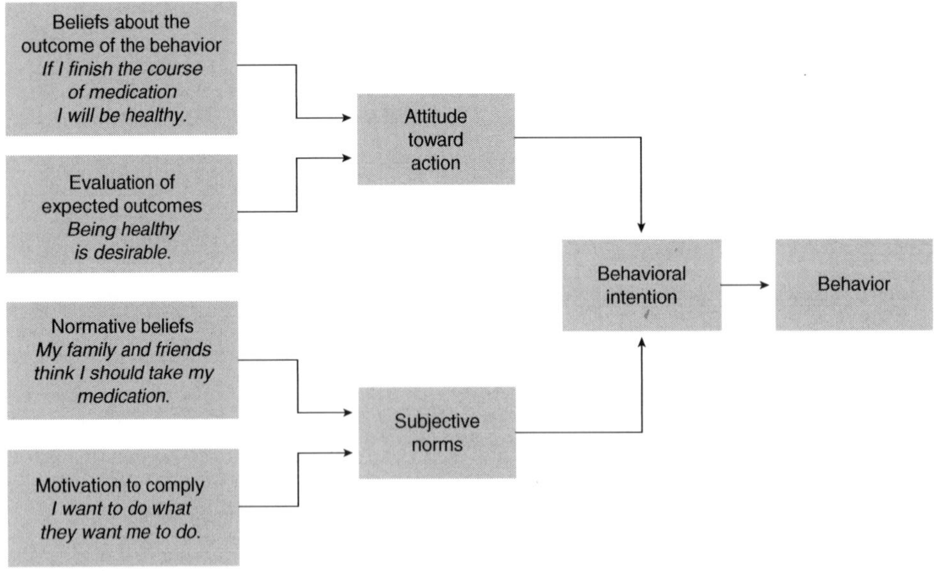

FIGURE 3.3 Theory of reasoned action.

Source: Reprinted with permission from Munro, S., Lewin, S., Swart, T., & Volmink, J. (2007). A review of health behaviour theories: How useful are these for developing interventions to promote long-term medication adherence for TB and HIV/AIDS? *BMC Public Health, 7,* 104. doi:10.1186/1471-2458-7-104. Copyright by Biomed Central, Ltd.

These variables are interrelated and describe the individual's reasoned action or intention to change. The individual must have a positive attitude toward change, and must feel that he or she has control over the change and that changing is perceived as positive by the social group. The model describes a linear change process that posits that a change in behavior is dependent on behavioral and normative beliefs. This change model has been used successfully in behavior change for individuals and groups related to smoking cessation, condom use for the prevention of STDs and HIV/AIDS nationally and internationally, dieting, exercise, seat-belt and safety-helmet use, and breastfeeding (Fishbein et al., 1994)

Social Ecological Theory

The social ecological theory offers a model to guide translation efforts that integrates multiple perspectives into the planning of interventions for behavior change, addressing the interdependencies among socioeconomic, cultural, political, environmental, organizational, psychological, and biological determinants of health (Whittemore, Melkus, & Grey, 2004). The model proposes that any individual behavior is supported and influenced by numerous systems and groups, and that any lasting behavior change requires implementation of strategies at multiple levels of influence (Emmons, 2000). Whittemore et al. (2004) described five levels of influence and the implementation strategies at each to expand diabetes prevention-and-management evidence:

- *Intrapersonal level*—Individual beliefs, values, education level, skills, and other individual factors that affect an individual's ability to change
- *Interpersonal level*—The relationships among individuals, families, groups, and communities that are part of social support to promote behavioral change
- *Institutional level*—The influence that relevant institutions have on change activities
- *Community level*—The influence that communities have on the individual, the community attitudes, and the relationship among different institutions within communities
- Public policy level and the influence of policies and regulations that affect the change intervention, the participants, and the institutions in which they function

■ THE LEARNING ORGANIZATION

Peter Senge (2006), the leading expert on learning organizations, explained that the fundamental learning units of an organization are working teams or people, who need one another to produce an outcome. He described five disciplines to becoming a learning organization. The first is to develop *systems thinking* or the ability to see the big picture, to distinguish patterns instead of conceptualizing change as isolated events, and to feel interconnected to the whole (Senge, 2006). *Personal mastery* is to focus on becoming the best person possible, to embrace lifelong learning, and to strive for a sense of commitment in one's career (Senge, 2006). The third discipline is to use *mental models*. Senge suggests that the process of using mental models begins with self-reflection, unearthing deeply held beliefs to understand how they influence the way we operate. He also believes that until there is a focus on openness, real change can never be implemented (Senge, 2006). Fourth, *building shared visions* is needed to bind an organization together and foster long-term commitment (Senge, 2006). Finally, *team learning*, critically important to today's organization, is the process of bringing team members together to develop a desire to create results in the team, to have a goal in mind, and to work together to attain it (Senge, 2006). The interaction of these five disciplines is to challenge the organization to look into its own resources and potentials, to build a collective will to learn, and to embrace change. The principles of a learning organization have great applicability to dissemination and translation of new knowledge into practice, with a focus on the team, what is necessary to implement a change, and the team's involvement in moving toward a desired new state.

Research on Change Interventions

Pascale, Millemann, and Gioja (1997) identified three concrete interventions that will change the way people change: (a) incorporating employees into the process of dealing with work challenges, (b) leading from a different place to sharpen and maintain employee involvement, and (c) instilling mental discipline to make people behave differently and then to sustain that behavior. If done properly, the proposal will create an agile organization and will shift the organization's operations or culture by altering the way people experience their own power and identity and the way they deal with conflict and learning.

Thomas et al. (1999) performed a systematic review of the evidence to evaluate strategies for successful change, specifically, the introduction of guidelines into practice. Although the evidence was insufficient, the literature suggested that essential strategies for successful change in healthcare practices included organizational commitment, active support from key stakeholders, recognition of the importance of change, a credible change agent, face-to-face contact with practitioners to promote enthusiasm, and ensuring targeted staff have ownership of the innovation and are empowered to change.

Gustafson et al. (2003) developed and tested a Bayesian model that used subjective probability estimates to predict outcomes of organizational changes, specifically, healthcare improvement projects. The model was developed with 18 factors that were identified by an expert panel and that predict implementation success. The 18 factors included (a) exploration of problem and customer needs; (b) change agent prestige, commitment, and customer focus; (c) source of ideas; (d) funding; (e) advantages to staff and customers; (f) radicalness of design; (g) flexibility of design; (h) mandate; (i) leader goals, involvement, and support; (j) supporters and opponents; (k) middle managers' goals, involvement, and support; (l) tension for change; (m) staff needs assessment, involvement, and support; (n) evidence of effectiveness; (o) complexity of implementation plan; (p) work environment; (q) monitoring and feedback; and (r) staff changes required. The model performed well on three definitions of success; however, there was no objective measure of success; only the opinions of people were involved. Identifying factors that predict success can lead to planning that increases attention to facilitators and removes barriers to the implementation of the desired change, which is similar to Lewin's classic description of the equilibrium of the force field in an organization.

Finally, Berwick (2003) studied innovations in healthcare specifically and summarized the literature, which he found to be mostly descriptive, in two ways. The first was a focus on three areas of influence that correlate with the rate of spread of change: (a) perception of the innovation (i.e., the benefit of the change, which is compatible with values, beliefs, past history, and current needs) and complexity of the innovation; (b) characteristics of the people who adopt the innovation or fail to do so; and (c) contextual factors, especially communication, incentives, leadership, and management. Second, he added that the research, although descriptive, offers seven guesses about what might help leaders to nurture good changes:

1. Find sound innovations.
2. Find and support innovators.
3. Invest in early adopters.
4. Make early adopter activity observable.
5. Trust and enable reinvention.
6. Create slack for change.
7. Lead by example.

Most recently, the debate about change management has evolved into a discussion surrounding change versus transformation. The differences are subtle, but worth discussing in a book covering change models useful for translation. William Bridges (2009) in his acclaimed work, *Managing Transitions: Making the Most of Change*, suggests that change is something that happens to people, whereas transitions or transformations are internal processes that happen within people. These transitions or transformations are about changing people's perceptions and thinking about the issue, problem, or innovation as something that needs to be "changed." The transformation involves viewing the innovation as an opportunity to let go of the status quo or traditional approach in favor of developing a new approach (Bridges, 2009; Kotter & Cohen, 2012).

As carefully described in this chapter, change management requires careful planning and implementation of change strategies and use of effective tools. Throughout the literature, there is agreement that the key elements of a carefully planned and managed change involve the following:

1. Strategic thinking and planning processes should develop the vision and strategy for the change, including mission and goals. This approach engages those affected by or involved in the change to buy-in and requires

communicating and championing the vision and mission of the change and leading the execution of the change strategy.

2. Stakeholder analysis should identify those who will be involved in, affected by, or influential in the change process. Stakeholder analysis includes understanding the role of each of those stakeholders, the level of commitment, and influence for or against the change. Understanding the stakeholders up-front when planning a change is an essential action.
3. Teamwork is critical to the success of any change. Careful assessment of the team's ability to plan, implement, and sustain the change is another essential action when planning change.
4. Development of an action plan, in the form of a project management plan, will provide the detail of goals, objectives, activities, responsibilities, time frame, and measure of success throughout the change project. The use of strategic tools for project management is detailed in Chapter 9, Project Management for Translation.
5. It is critical to deal with resistance at every stage of the change process. Barriers to the implementation of EBP are discussed in Chapter 14, Information Technology: A Foundation for Translation, and Chapter 15, Interprofessional Collaboration and Teamwork for Translation.
6. A leader who is a role model and who exemplifies the vision and mission of the change is necessary. The leadership characteristics that engender trust from those involved in the change include vision, knowledge, good listening and communication skills, being action oriented, leading by example, asking tough questions, openness, and flexibility.
7. Communication that answers the questions about which those involved or affected by the change are concerned is necessary throughout the change process: Why are we making this change? What do we have to do? When and for how long? How will it affect me? What is in it for me? How will I know it is working? Communication plans should include the use of different forms of communication and should consistently address the issues of concern for those involved or affected.

■ A FINAL ISSUE TO CONSIDER IN THE TRANSLATION OF NEW KNOWLEDGE

A final issue that needs to be considered when designing the change to translate new knowledge into practice is fidelity of implementation. *Fidelity* refers to the degree to which program providers implement programs as intended by developers/researchers (Rohrbach, Dent, Skara, Sun, & Sussman, 2007). To make programs more acceptable for translation or for the change to be accepted, the implementers/change agents may try to adapt the new knowledge/research to achieve local buy-in. The users can also choose to modify the implementation to fit the needs or improve the fit of an intervention with local conditions. However, this makes fidelity difficult to achieve, and the research has shown that the fidelity with which an intervention is implemented affects how well it succeeds (Dusenbury, Brannigan, Falco, & Hansen, 2003; Elliott & Mihalic, 2004; Rohrbach et al., 2007).

■ CONCLUSIONS

Translation of research into practice must be guided by the models and frameworks that include the process of change and the identification of critical elements or variables in the organization that affect and determine whether the new knowledge fits the organization and will be feasible to implement. In addition to fit and feasibility, consideration must be given to the varied personnel, structures, environments, leadership styles, and cultures of organizations as well as their economic, ethical, and legal environments. Graham and Tetroe (2007) cautioned against the knowledge translation imperative, translating all new knowledge into practice at any cost, but suggested that each opportunity for knowledge transfer should be judiciously evaluated for translation, with careful attention to customized planning and evaluation for the specific translation of evidence.

■ REFERENCES

Ajzen, I., & Fishbein, M. (1980). *Understanding attitudes and predicting social behavior*. Upper Saddle River, NJ: Prentice Hall.

Bandura, A. (1986). *Social foundations of thought and action: A social cognitive theory*. Upper Saddle River, NJ: Prentice Hall.

Berwick, D. M. (2003). Disseminating innovations in health care. *Journal of the American Medical Association, 289*(15), 1969–1975. doi:10.1001/jama.289.15.1969

Bradley, E. H., Schlesinger, M., Webster, T. R., Baker, D., & Inouye, S. K. (2004). Translating research into clinical practice: Making change happen. *Journal of the American Geriatrics Society, 52*(11), 1875–1882. doi:10.1111/j.1532-5415.2004.52510.x

Bridges, W. (2009). *Managing transitions: Making the most of change* (3rd ed.). Philadelphia, PA: Da Capo Press.

Centers for Disease Control and Prevention. (1993). Distribution of STD clinic patients along a stages-of-behavioral-change continuum—Selected sites, 1993. *Morbidity and Mortality Weekly Report, 42*(45), 880–883.

Davies, P., Walker, A., & Grimshaw, J. (2010). A systematic review of the use of theory in the design of guideline dissemination and implementation strategies and interpretation of the results of rigorous evaluations. *Implementtion Science, 5*(14), 1–6. doi:10.1186/1748-5908-5-14

DiClemente, C. C., & Prochaska, J. O. (1998). Towards a comprehensive transtheoretical model of change: Stage of change and addictive behaviors. In W. R. Miller & N. Heather (Eds.), *Treating addictive behaviors* (2nd ed., pp. 3–24). New York, NY: Plenum.

Dusenbury, L., Brannigan, R., Falco, M., & Hansen, W. B. (2003). A review of research on fidelity of implementation: Implications for drug abuse prevention in school settings. *Health Education Research, 18*(2), 237–256. doi:10.1093/her/18.2.237

Elliott, D. S., & Mihalic, S. (2004). Issues in disseminating and replicating effective prevention programs. *Prevention Science, 5*(1), 47–53.

Emmons, K. (2000). Health behaviors in a social context. In L. F. Berkman & I. Kawachi (Eds.), *Social epidemiology* (pp. 244–266). Oxford, UK: Oxford University Press.

Family Health International. (1996). Behavior change: A summary of four major theories. Retrieved from http://www.fhi360.org/resource/behavior-change-summary-four-major-theories

Ferlie, E. B., & Shortell, S. M. (1996). Improving the quality of health care in the United Kingdom and the United States: A framework for change. *Milbank Quarterly, 79*(2), 281–315.

Fishbein, M., Middlestadt, S., & Hitchcock, P. (1994). Using information to change sexually transmitted disease-related behaviors. In R. DiClementi & J. Peterson (Eds.), *Preventing AIDS: Theories and methods of behavioral interventions*. New York, NY: Plenum Press.

Graham, I. D., & Tetroe, J. (2007). Some theoretical underpinnings of knowledge translation. *Academic Emergency Medicine, 14*(11), 936–941.

Gustafson, D. H., Sainfort, F., Eichler, M., Adams, L., Bisognano, M., & Steudel, H. (2003). Developing and testing a model to predict outcomes of organizational change. *Health Services Research*, 38(2), 751–776. doi:10.1111/1475-6773.00143

Havelock, R. G. (1976). *Planning for innovation through dissemination and utilization of knowledge*. Ann Arbor, MI: University of Michigan, Center for Research on Utilization of Scientific Knowledge, Institute for Social Research.

Havelock, R. G., & Zlotolow, S. (1995). *The change agent's guide* (2nd ed.). Englewood Cliffs, NJ: Education Technology.

Howes, N. J., & Quinn, R. E. (1978). Implementing change: From research to a prescriptive framework. *Group & Organization Studies*, 3(1), 71–84. doi:10.1177/105960117800300107

Kotter, J. (1995). Leading change: Why transformation efforts fail. *Harvard Business Review*, 73(2), 59–67.

Kotter, J. (1996). *Leading change*. Boston, MA: Harvard Business School Press.

Kotter, J. (1999). *What leaders really do*. Boston, MA: Harvard Business School Press.

Kotter, J., & Cohen, D. (2012). *The heart of change: Real-life stories of how people change their organizations*. Boston, MA: Harvard Business School Press.

Lewin, K. (1947). Frontiers in group dynamics. *Human Relations, 1*(1), 5–41. doi:10.1177/001872674700100103

Lewin, K. (1951). Field theory in social science. In D. Cartwright (Ed.), *Selected theoretical papers*. New York, NY: Harper & Row.

Lippitt, R., Watson, J., & Westley, B. (1958). *The dynamics of planned change*. New York, NY: Harcourt, Brace, and World.

Manchester, J., Gray-Miceli, D., Metcalf, J., Paolini, D., Napier, A., Coogle, D., & Owens, M. (2014). Facilitating Lewin's change model with collaborative evaluation in promoting evidence-based practices of health professionals. *Evaluation and Program Planning*, 47(12), 82–90. doi:10.1016/j.evalprogplan.2014.08.007

McConnell, C. R. (2010). Change can work for you or against you: It's your choice. *Health Care Manager*, 29(4), 365–374. doi:10.1097/HCM.0b013e3181fa076b

Munro, S., Lewin, S., Swart, T., & Volmink, J. (2007). A review of health behaviour theories: How useful are these for developing interventions to promote long-term medication adherence for TB and HIV/AIDS? *BMC Public Health*, 7, 104. doi:10.1186/1471-2458-7-104

Oakman, J., Rothmore, P. & Tappin, D. (2016). Intervention development to reduce musculoskeletal disorders: Is the processs on target? Applied Ergonomics 56, 179–185. doi:10.1016/j.apergo.2016.03.019

Pascale, R., Millemann, M., & Gioja, L. (1997). Changing the way we change. *Harvard Business Review*, 75(6), 127–139.

Pettigrew, A., & Whipp, R. (1991). *Managing change for competitive success*. Oxford, UK: Blackwell.

Prochaska, J. O., DiClemente, C. C., & Norcross, J. C. (1992). In search of how people change—Applications to addictive behaviors. *American Psychologist*, 47(9), 1102–1114. doi:10.3109/10884609309149692

Reineck, C. (2007). Models of change. *Journal of Nursing Administration*, 37(9), 388–391. doi:10.1097/01.NNA.0000285137.26624.f9

Robbins, S. (2003). *Organizational behavior* (10th ed.). Upper Saddle River, NJ: Prentice Hall.

Rohrbach, L. A., Dent, C. W., Skara, S., Sun, P., & Sussman, S. (2007). Fidelity of implementation in project Towards No Drug abuse (TND): A comparison of classroom teachers and program specialists. *Prevention Science*, 8(2), 125–132. doi:10.1007/s11121-006-0056-z

Rothmore, P., Aylward, P., & Karnon, J. (2015). The implementation of ergonomics advice and the stage of change approach. *Applied Ergonomics, 51*, 370–76. doi:10.1016/j.apergo.2015.06.013

Rothmore, P., Aylward, P., Oakman, J., Tappin, D., Gray, J., & Karnon, J. (2016). The stage of change approach for implementing ergonomics advice—Translating research into practice. *Applied Ergonomics, 59*, 225–233. doi:10.1016/j.apergo.2016.08.033

Senge, P. M. (2006). *The fifth discipline: The art and practice of the learning organization*. New York, NY: Doubleday.

Shirey, M. (2013). Lewin's theory of planned change as a strategic resource. *Journal of Nursing Administration*, 43(2), 69–72. doi:10.1097/NNA.0b013e31827f20a9

Stetler, C. B., Ritchie, J., Rycroft-Malone, J., Schultz, A., & Charns, M. (2007). Improving quality of care through routine, successful implementation of evidence-based practice at the bedside: An organizational case study protocol using the Pettigrew and Whipp model of strategic change. *Implementation Science*, *2*, 3. doi:10.1186/1748-5908-2-3

Thomas, L. H., Cullum, N. A., McColl, E., Rousseau, N., Soutter, J., & Steen, N. (1999). Guidelines in professions allied to medicine. *Cochrane Database of Systematic Reviews*, *1991*(1). doi:10.1002/14651858.CD000349

Whittemore, R., Melkus, G. D., & Grey, M. (2004). Applying the social ecological theory to type 2 diabetes prevention and management. *Journal of Community Health Nursing*, *21*(2), 87–99. doi:10.1207/s15327655jchn2102_03

World Bank. (2010). *Theories of behavior change. Communication for Governance and Accountability Program* (CommGAP). Washington, DC: Author. Retrieved from http://siteresources.worldbank.org/EXTGOVACC/Resources/BehaviorChangeweb.pdf

PART TWO

Use of Translation

CHAPTER FOUR

Translation of Evidence to Improve Clinical Outcomes

Julie Stanik-Hutt

You ask me why I do not write something. . . . I think one's feelings waste themselves in words, they ought all to be distilled into actions and into actions which bring results.
Florence Nightingale, Notes on Nursing: What It Is, and What It Is Not

We don't see quality as just a clinical goal. It's an enterprise wide priority that encompasses customer service, compliance and wellness.
—Joseph Swedish, Past CEO, Anthem Health

Patient Outcomes Management and the Application of evidence to practice are powerful tools that can improve quality of care (The Joint Commission, 2008). The application of these symbiotic processes is the responsibility of all nurses (Foster, 2001). Since Florence Nightingale, the assessment of patient outcomes has been inextricably intertwined with nursing care. In fact, Nightingale's collection and analysis of data regarding the morbidity and mortality rates of soldiers under her care in the Crimea contributed to changes in care and, ultimately, to improved patient outcomes. Its later publication led to public and political support for the profession of nursing.

The application of the nursing process involves the identification of desired patient outcomes. Desired patient outcomes are established to direct the application of selected care interventions. Nursing interventions, based on the biopsychosocial sciences, are developed and implemented with the intention of attaining the established desired outcome. Finally, results of nursing interventions are assessed and evaluated by comparing the patient's actual outcomes to the desired outcomes. By doing so, quality and effectiveness of the delivered care are assessed, and the need for continued or altered care is determined. The application of evidence-based care is one tool nurses use to improve patient outcomes. Evidence-based practice (EBP) processes can be used to improve the care outcomes of one patient at a time or to create clinical practice guidelines (CPGs), which, when applied in practice, can improve the outcomes for groups or populations of patients. Common barriers to EBP and creation of CPG include lack of resources (number 1 barrier), time, access to evidence (research), evidence evaluation skills, and inadequate financial support (Sadeghi-Bazargani, Tabrizi, & Azami-Aghdash, 2014).

■ CLINICAL OUTCOMES

In healthcare, *quality* is defined as the "degree to which health services for individuals and populations increase the likelihood of attaining desired health outcomes and are consistent with current professional knowledge" (Institute of Medicine [IOM], 1990, p. 21). Safety is also a component of quality. Safe care is unlikely to injure or harm the patient (IOM, 2001; Newhouse & Poe, 2005). In addition, the IOM asserts that in order for care to be considered of high quality, it should also be patient centered, timely, efficient, and equitable (IOM, 2001). These characteristics clearly link patient preferences and care processes with quality (IOM, 1990). Donabedian, the "father" of healthcare quality, suggested that the quality of care could be improved by establishing standards for care structures and processes. Patient outcomes are the ultimate measures of quality as they incorporate the influence of both structures and processes of care (Donabedian, 2005; Van Driel, De Sutter, Christiaens, & De Maeseneer, 2005).

Clinical outcomes or patient outcomes are defined as the end results of care that can be attributed to services provided (treatments, interventions, and care). Donabedian (1985) referred to outcomes as "changes in the actual or potential health status of individual patients, groups, or communities" (p. 256). Clinical outcomes demonstrate the value and effectiveness of care and can be assessed for individuals, populations, and organizations (Hughes, 2008). Outcomes can be either desirable or undesirable (adverse). Outcomes are quantified or measured through the use of indicators, sometimes also called *metrics*. Outcome indicators, or metrics, gauge how patients are affected by their care. Indicators must be valid and reliable measures that are related to the outcome.

For example, to measure the adequacy of blood glucose control in a patient with diabetes, you might measure the patient's finger-stick blood glucose or glycosylated hemoglobin levels. In this case, the finger-stick blood glucose or glycosylated hemoglobin is the indicator or metric used to measure the outcome of blood glucose control. Indicators or metrics that are reported are referred to as *performance measures* (Dennison & Hughes, 2009).

Structures that support care and processes that are used to provide care are also important to care quality and can be evaluated to assess care quality (Donabedian, 1985, 2005; Hammermeister, Shroyer, Sethi, & Grover, 1995). Structure indicators assess the organization and delivery of nursing care. For example, the nurse-to-patient ratio and the skill mix of staff providing care are structure indicators. Process indicators evaluate the nature and amount of care that nurses provide. For example, documentation of patient teaching or timely reassessment of a patient's pain after the administration of an analgesic is an indicator of care processes.

Some ask, "What is the difference among goals, objectives, indicators, and outcomes?" Should they all be called *outcomes*? Outcomes are used to characterize the result (effect) of an intervention, treatment, or practitioner/provider (cause). This is essentially a cause-and-effect relationship (Parse, 2006). "Goals and objectives are something to strive for; indicators are signs of progress toward achievement of something, whereas outcomes are predictors of end-performance" (Parse, 2006, p. 189).

■ LINKING OUTCOMES TO CARE

Assessing care outcomes is not the goal in and of itself. Instead, it is important to assess outcomes in relation to the care provided (Donabedian, 1985; Heslop & Lu, 2014; Minnick, 2009). When outcome data are linked to the care environment and interventions, they provide patients, payers, and practitioners (individuals, e.g., nurses, nurse practitioners [NPs], physicians, physical therapists)/providers (organizations or agencies, e.g., hospitals, home care agencies) with information regarding the potential effect that a healthcare intervention or practitioner/provider can have on their lives. It can help patients to make decisions regarding their healthcare (Brooks & Barrett, 1998). The data can also influence a payer's decision-making regarding which services to cover or which practitioners and providers to include in the network. For example, outcome data can be used to compare one treatment for a condition with an alternative treatment or to compare care provided by different healthcare practitioners and agencies (Dennison & Hughes, 2009). The Physician Quality Reporting Initiative (PQRI), Inpatient Prospective Payment System, and Value Based Purchasing Programs at the Centers for Medicare & Medicaid Services (CMS) use outcome data to reimburse for services (CMS, 2011). Outcome data are useful to practitioners and providers because they help them to better understand the effects of the services they provide to their patients. Outcomes can also be compared with the standard levels of performance, the so-called "benchmarks" or "norms," to determine whether a service, practitioner, or provider is performing at a level that meets the established norms.

Outcomes can be used by healthcare practitioners, providers, organizations, and payers to evaluate and improve the care they provide. The best care comes from practitioners who routinely evaluate care outcomes and use that data to make adjustments to the care they provide as part of a continuous quality-improvement cycle (Mullins, Baldwin, & Perfetto, 1996). This is often called *outcomes management*. *Outcomes management* refers to the collection and analysis, in relation to the processes of care, of information that indicates the effectiveness of care. It provides a "checks and balances" process in the provision of healthcare. The use of electronic health records and "big data" allows aggregated patient care process and outcome data to be retrieved and analyzed in order to assess the quality of care. Outcome managers focus on aggregated outcome data on groups of patients with common characteristics, for example, patients with diabetes or asthma or some other health problem. By measuring and evaluating the care outcomes of groups of patients, care practices that fail to achieve desired benchmarks can be identified for improvement. Once the problems are identified, practitioners can seek out evidence-based solutions to implement and evaluate. The effectiveness of the solution is judged by the new outcomes attained. In this way, outcome measurement can be linked to EBP, and both can become "complementary, iterative processes which contribute to quality improvement" (Deaton, 2001, p. 83).

Minnick (2009) discusses the challenges encountered in the design and implementation of evidence-based outcome improvement projects. She emphasizes that the first step is the identification of the overall outcome that a project is intended to address. A population, intervention, comparison, outcome (PICO) question or other formal purpose statement can be used to start the search for evidence, benchmarks, and other data related to the desired outcome. A PICO question allows one to explore and link knowledge related to the topic with the patient population and the setting involved and the outcome of interest. This information, as well as the necessary and available resources to carry out the outcome improvement project, should be verified and reviewed with project stakeholders. Subsequently, a design for implementing and assessing the effects of the project, specifically the outcomes to be measured, should be identified.

■ NURSING OUTCOMES

In the past, the "5 Ds"—death, disease, disability, discomfort, and dissatisfaction—were the most commonly monitored outcomes of healthcare quality (Lohr, 1988). They are the outcomes that are easily measured and understood by the public and policy makers. Donabedian (2005) described the use of patient outcomes of "recovery, restoration of function and of survival" (p. 692) as indicators of care quality. However, these outcomes do not adequately represent quality and are not specific to nursing. The first challenge is to "describe what nurses do (nursing interventions) in response to what sort of patient conditions (nursing diagnoses) with what effect (nursing outcomes)" (Marek, 1997, p. 8). Researchers at the University of Iowa have provided leadership in this area by creating the Nursing Interventions Classification (NIC) and the Nursing Outcomes Classification (NOC), which link nursing interventions to diagnoses and outcomes. These systems allow the evaluation of care provided by nurses and facilitate communication regarding the same.

In 2003, 15 nursing care outcomes were selected for national reporting on nursing care performance. They included measures of patient-centered outcomes (death among surgical inpatients with treatable serious complications, pressure ulcer prevalence, falls prevalence, falls with injury, restraint prevalence, catheter-related urinary tract infections, central line-associated bloodstream infection [CLABSI], and ventilator-associated pneumonia), nursing-centered intervention processes (smoking-cessation counseling for acute myocardial infarction [AMI], heart failure [HF], and pneumonia), and system-centered structures and processes (skill mix, nursing care hours per patient day, Practice Environment Scale–Nursing Work Index, and voluntary turnover; Kurtzman & Corrigan, 2007). Later, several other patient-centered outcomes (patient satisfaction with pain management, patient education, overall care and nursing care, pediatric peripheral intravenous infiltrations, and psychiatric/physical/sexual assault) and system-centered structures and processes (nursing education and certification, nurse job satisfaction) were added to the list (Heslop & Lu, 2014). The list currently includes nursing hours per patient day, nurse turnover rate, nosocomial infections, patient falls with injury, pressure ulcer rate, pediatric pain, pediatric peripheral intravenous infiltration, nurse education and certification, restraint use, and staff mix (National Database of Nursing Quality Indicators [NDNQI], 2010). In addition to their use in performance reporting, these measures can be used in research, quality improvement, and healthcare policy activities. For example, several of the measures are included in the Robert Wood Johnson Foundation's Transforming Care at the Bedside initiative.

There are various other outcomes that are of interest to and demonstrate the broader effects of nursing care (Mitchell, 2008). These broader categories of outcomes relevant to nursing would include physiologic, psychosocial, functional, and behavioral outcomes; symptoms; quality of life; knowledge; and satisfaction. Physiologic outcomes would include pulse, blood pressure (BP), blood sugar and lipid levels, peak expiratory flow rates, weight, skin condition, and many other parameters. Psychosocial outcomes could include the individual's mood, attitudes, and abilities to interact with others. An individual's mobility, physical independence, and ability to participate in desired activities of daily living are the functional outcomes. For example, the ability of a patient with asthma to engage in physical activities, such as walking, exercising, or doing housework, is a functional outcome. Behavioral outcomes could include adequacy of coping with healthcare needs or a patient's ability to follow (adhere to) recommended care. Symptoms, such as pain, dyspnea, fatigue, and others, command attention independent of the diseases that cause them. Because symptoms interfere with a patient's physiologic, psychosocial, and functional status and quality of life, nurses are especially interested in their control. Quality of life, another natural outcome of interest for nurses, is a patient's general perception of the physical and mental well-being that can be affected by many factors, including disease and injury, stress and emotions, symptom control and functional status, as well as others. Knowledge level, an individual's understanding of health-related information, is another outcome of interest. For example, a patient's understanding of the causes of asthma and factors that can trigger and prevent exacerbations would be important to nurses because teaching patients and supporting their self-care management is a role of nursing. Although patient satisfaction is a quality indicator for all healthcare and healthcare providers, patients' satisfaction with their nursing care would be relevant to nurses.

Outcomes of interest to nurses in advanced practice roles include these broad areas as well and would also include outcomes specific to their advanced practice roles. Oermann and Floyd (2002) categorize the outcomes of APRNs into clinical, functional, cost, and satisfaction outcomes. For example, certified registered nurse anesthetists (CRNAs) might be interested in the complications of oral intubation or extubation failures, epidural catheter insertion site infections, or patient satisfaction with postoperative pain relief. Certified nurse-midwives (CNMs) might monitor perineal laceration rates or newborn Apgar scores, and certified nurse practitioners

(CNPs) would be interested in missed diagnoses or prescribing patterns. Data regarding the outcomes and impact derived from APRNs' practice support policy initiatives related to APRN education, workforce planning, recognition, regulation, and reimbursement.

Identifying the outcomes that can be clearly attributed only to nursing is a challenge. Attribution requires a high level of confidence that the outcome is a direct result of the care provided (Dennison & Hughes, 2009). When many care practitioners interact with patients and contribute to the care, it is sometimes difficult to attribute the outcome in the patient to only one practitioner or treatment. For example, a diabetic patient is consistently having high fasting blood glucose levels. The NP discusses the problem and alternative medication adjustments with the patient and then orders a new daily and sliding scale insulin dose. The RN teaches the patient the correct technique for finger-stick glucose monitoring. The registered dietitian (RD) reviews the recommended diet and helps the patient practice making better food selections. When the patient's mean fasting blood glucose levels fall to within the desired parameters, who will get the credit? To whom are these results attributed? Is it the NP, the RN, the RD, or the team?

Nurses affect patient safety outcomes by identifying and mitigating risks, monitoring patient status and communicating with others regarding changes in the patient's condition, and the surveillance activities that lead to system improvement to enhance safety. On the micro level, nurses' effect on safety variables, such as medication errors or patient falls, might be possible. However, it is again difficult to quantify nursing's effect on safety outcomes because of the multidisciplinary nature and complexity of our current healthcare systems.

Finally, patients' utilization of healthcare services, both increased and decreased, can reflect the influence of nursing care. An increased utilization might derive from nurses teaching and coaching patients regarding when, where, and how to seek care. Conversely, if nursing care increases an individual's ability for self-care management, the need for unintended office and emergency department visits—decreased utilization—could be the outcome. Examples of utilization of service outcomes are intended and unintended office visits, use of the emergency room, hospital admissions, and length of stay.

Theoretical frameworks can be used to identify and explore the factors that influence nursing's effect on patient outcomes. Joseph (2007) proposed a theoretical approach to the examination of the effect of nursing on patient and organizational outcomes. She proposed that five constructs influence outcomes, including the environment of the health facility, qualities of the nursing unit, the individual nurse, and the patient, as well as nursing care. She suggested that nursing care is affected by the qualities of the nursing unit where care is given, by the nurse providing the care, and by patient qualities associated with their needs. Joseph also proposed that the larger environment of the health facility also affects care by providing the context of care through its mission, organizational structure, and characteristics, as well as its leadership milieu. This framework is useful in identifying the variables that may influence patient as well as organizational outcomes.

TRANSLATION OF EVIDENCE TO IMPROVE OUTCOMES

Research findings support the effect of research-based nursing on patient outcomes (Heater, Becker, & Olson, 1988). A meta-analysis was used to determine the contribution that research-based nursing practice makes to patient outcomes compared with routine, procedural nursing care. Eighty-four studies (63 published, 21 unpublished) of independent nursing interventions from 1977 to 1984 were evaluated and the effect sizes were calculated. Outcomes were grouped into four content areas: behavioral, knowledge, physiological, and psychosocial. Results indicated that individuals who received research-based nursing care had better outcomes than 72% of subjects who received routine, procedural nursing care.

Unfortunately, healthcare practitioners frequently fail to integrate available evidence into day-to-day patient care (McGlynn et al., 2003). It is reported that the average time lag from discovery of knowledge to its application in practice is 17 years (IOM, 2001). Historically, care processes have been based on ritual, personal, and local institutional preferences (Ackerman, 1999; Kingston, Krumberger, & Peruzzi, 2000). For more than 25 years, attempts have been made to increase the linkage of empiric research results to practice and to narrow the "bench-to-bedside" gap to improve patient care. But very little progress has been made in synthesizing and applying the results of research to improve patient care. To bridge the bench-to-bedside gap, evidence needs to be incorporated into care protocols that are easily implemented in practice.

Probably one of the earliest examples of the creation of an evidence-based approach to care was the development in the 1970s of consistent expectations for the performance of CPR. These standards were used to train and test the competency of healthcare providers to perform external cardiac massage and rescue breathing for patients suffering from cardiopulmonary arrest. These standards were based on limited research data regarding CPR as well as expert opinion, but it standardized the process of CPR across the country and across disciplines.

Soon thereafter, many institutions developed standing orders (or order sets) to provide consistent care to specific patient populations. These documents were developed for use in one or perhaps two nursing units within an individual hospital. They simplified care by establishing one set of orders for the care of a highly selected group of patients—for example, only those admitted with specific diagnoses, usually surgical procedures. They were based on preferences and personal expertise of a single physician or a small group of physicians. They sometimes underwent institutional vetting processes.

Critical pathways began to emerge in the 1980s and 1990s as payers and institutions responded to the demands for managed care. Managed care initiatives set expectations for the provision of timely, streamlined, evidence-based care to optimize patient outcomes (Rotter et al., 2009). Care pathways were usually created by a multidisciplinary team to establish a unified but detailed care plan for a set of specific patients, with clearly described patient outcomes and timelines that could be used to implement patient care and monitor progress. Variance from the path triggered analysis and intervention. Over time, these care pathways were more likely to reflect input from all care practitioners involved with the patient population and were approved through consensus processes. These multidisciplinary teams included physicians in private practice. The pathways were used locally for all or most of the patients fitting the population and described the care they would receive and when they would receive care. They were also used in contracting with payers to provide specific services for their insured.

■ CLINICAL PRACTICE GUIDELINES

CPGs are official recommendations made by recognized authorities regarding the screening, diagnosis, treatment, and management of specific conditions. They are "systematically developed statements to assist practitioner and patient decisions about appropriate healthcare for specific clinical circumstances" (Lohr & Field, 1992, p. 27). Evidence-based CPGs may help bridge the gap between research and practice. In these CPGs, research provides the evidence that an intervention is efficacious (produces better outcomes). The CPG facilitates transfer of this intervention to everyday practice and subsequently allows evaluation of its effect on outcomes in broader patient populations (effectiveness). In this way, EBP leads to the development of practice-based evidence (Green, 2006). It allows the accumulation of evaluation data on both efficacy and effectiveness of the intervention.

In 1994, the federal government became involved in the movement to translate research to practice. At that time, the Agency for Health Care Policy and Research (AHCPR), now the Agency for Healthcare Research and Quality (AHRQ), began to develop care recommendations for common problems (acute pain, cancer pain, pressure ulcers, etc.) and published them as CPGs. These documents were developed by teams comprising experts from multiple healthcare professions, who completed exhaustive searches of the research literature related to the identified problem. The resulting body of research literature was subsequently reviewed, rated for quality, and synthesized into recommendations related to risk identification, problem assessment, prevention, and treatment. Larger groups of experts were asked to review and provide comments on the CPGs before revision and dissemination of the final versions. The Centers for Disease Control and Prevention (CDC) also got involved in establishing CPGs. For example, in 2003, they established guidelines for the prevention of healthcare-associated pneumonia (Tablan et al., 2004).

In order to close the gap between knowledge discovery and application, and thereby improve healthcare, the U.S. Department of Health and Human Services hosted the website for the National Guideline Clearinghouse from 1999 to 2018. This Clearinghouse supported the dissemination and use of CPGs by making guidelines that met stringent inclusion criteria available to healthcare professionals and organizations, payers, and patients. In 2018, the Trump administration eliminated funding to maintain this website. The impact of the loss of that valuable resource is likely to be significant, but is as yet unknown.

In 2005, the Institute for Healthcare Improvement suggested that care processes could be "bundled" together to improve patient outcomes (Resar et al., 2005). A care bundle comprises a set of three to five evidence-based care activities that are performed together in a consistent manner (Resar, Griffin, Haraden, & Nolan, 2012). In contrast to most CPGs, bundle components are limited in number and may be based on only a few research studies; inclusion of bundle components is based not only on research, but also on feasibility of use in clinical practice; and components are selected by a small group of clinical experts. At least 11 systematic reviews have examined the impact of care process bundles on care outcomes, including those related to chronic obstructive pulmonary disease (COPD), CLABSI, surgical site infections, hospital-acquired infections, sepsis, and drug errors in children. Three of these systematic reviews found that bundled care significantly reduced patients' risks associated with COPD, sepsis, and CLABSI (Damiani et al., 2015; Ista et al., 2016; Ospina et al., 2017). Another systematic review included 33 reports of the use of bundles for a variety of conditions and settings, and concluded that the largest risk reduction was produced with implementation of pressure ulcer, CLABSI, and ventilator-associated pneumonia care bundles (Lavallée, Gray, Dumville, Russell, & Cullum, 2017). It also suggested that high compliance (at least 95%) with bundles reduced infections, surgical site infections, and mortality. Care bundles seem to have found a place in clinical practice. It remains to be seen how they impact the implementation of CPG and patient outcomes.

Today, demands from patients and families, insurers, business leaders, consumer groups (the AARP, American Lung Association, American Cancer Society, etc.), and professional organizations (American Association of Critical-Care Nurses, American College of Chest Physicians, etc.) continue to promote the increased integration of available research knowledge, practitioner expertise, and patient preferences to improve patient healthcare through EBP. CPGs translate the best available research evidence into a clinically useful form that can be employed by practitioners in day-to-day practice. EBP occurs when expert healthcare providers synthesize CPG knowledge with patient needs and preferences to improve patient outcomes.

■ FACTORS THAT AFFECT ADOPTION OF CPGs

Various factors affect the adoption of CPGs. Qualities of CPGs, including ease of use, complexity, clear scientific basis, strong link between evidence and recommendations, and other factors, influence their use (Davis & Taylor-Vaisey, 1997; Sox, 1994). The existence of conflicting CPGs with differing recommendations regarding the same intervention or population, such as those that have recently been reported for several types of cancer screening, probably undermine their use. Characteristics of the healthcare professional also influence the use of CPGs. For example, personal involvement in CPG development, awareness of as well as agreement and familiarity with CPGs may influence their use (Cabana et al., 1999; Davis & Taylor-Vaisey, 1997; Haynes, 1993). Vetting by and support from professional nursing organizations is important to the successful implementation of nursing care guidelines (Davies, Edwards, Ploeg, & Virani, 2008; Ploeg, Davies, Edwards, Gifford, & Miller, 2007). Healthcare providers who perceive CPGs as "cookbook medicine" or as a threat to practitioner autonomy are not likely to follow a CPG. Patient-related factors, such as patient age or the presence of multiple comorbid conditions, influence the practitioner's use of CPGs (Francke, Smit, de Veer, & Mistiaen, 2008; Sox, 1994). Characteristics of the practice setting, such as availability of time and personnel, work pressures, and even costs to the practice related to the implementation of a CPG, influence its use (Francke et al., 2008). An emerging issue that will affect provider use of CPGs, or at least the explanations of their application with patients, is consumers' understanding of and attitudes toward CPGs (Carman et al., 2010; Francke et al., 2008). Recent evidence reveals that patients do not understand that EBP and CPGs are meant to improve their health and the quality of healthcare delivered without increasing patient costs (Carman et al., 2010). Instead, they believe that care, at least provided by their own physician, is optimal, and that use of a CPG will restrict their access to desired care. Some also believe CPGs are used only to protect physicians from malpractice claims. These patient attitudes and beliefs could have a significant effect on their acceptance of CPG recommendations.

Qualitative and quantitative methods and one meta-review have examined the perceptions of administrators, nurses, and a variety of other healthcare providers regarding the factors that support and hinder guideline implementation in practice. (Davies et al., 2008; Dogherty, Harrison, Graham, Vandyk, & Keeping-Burke, 2013; Francke et al., 2008; Ploeg et al., 2007). One new model specifically focuses on successful implementation of guidelines in nursing (Matther-Maich, Ploeg, Dobbins, & Jack, 2013).

Two publications sum up knowledge regarding the impact of major factors on CPG implementation. Francke et al. (2008) completed a systematic meta-review of evidence regarding factors that impact guideline implementation and strategies used to support implementation. They summarized their findings by characterizing evidence that impacts the implementation of guidelines into one of four categories: the guideline itself, the professionals involved, the patients involved, and the practice environment. They found that guidelines that are "easy to understand" and grounded in evidence are more likely to be successfully implemented. There was inadequate data to determine the relative impact of individual implementation strategies, though most projects used two or more strategies and those that were integrated into care processes by the individual healthcare provider were the most successful. Lack of knowledge about and agreement with the guideline among healthcare providers were identified as major impediments to implementation. Patients who did not understand the value in following a guideline or provider concerns regarding the presence of multiple comorbid conditions in a patient hindered guideline implementation. Finally, negative staff or leadership attitudes and lack of time and resources were the environmental factors impeding the implementation of guidelines.

Dogherty et al. (2013) completed a thematic analysis of critical incident technique data from nurse leaders involved in guideline implementation. Their analysis emphasized factors to support successful implementation. They found that focus on a high-priority problem and use of evidence that is not only relevant to the practice, but also easy to access and apply are critical. They also cited the importance of a strong cohesive team (multidisciplinary engagement of stakeholders who share responsibility), "strategic choreography" (planning, providing resources, anticipating and navigating through challenges, etc.), and enlisting a skilled leader to facilitate the implementation (p. 133).

A recent systematic review examined the factors influencing physician implementation of CPG-based, computer-based clinical decision support systems (CDSSs; Kilsdonk, Peute, & Jaspers, 2017). They used the human, organizational, and technology-fit (HOT-fit) model to review CPG CDSS implementation drivers and barriers in 35 studies (20 qualitative and 12 quantitative). They identified 127 human, 61 organizational, and 210 technology-related factors and another 23 factors related to net benefits from CPG CDSS implementation. Factors found to impede implementation included physician concerns that CPG CDSS interferes with physician autonomy and authority and patient communications and relationships, interrupts workflow, and increases time expenditure to complete their work. Factors found to facilitate implementation included confidence in the quality of evidence underlying the CPG and its development, hands-on training before the system "goes live" and access to post "go live" training as well as easily accessible technical support, easy access to high-speed computers with software that streamlines integration of real-time CDSS into electronic health record/provider order entry documentation workflow, and inclusion of recommendations regarding complementary medicine. Environmental factors that would facilitate implementation of CPG CDSS included support of the CPG CDSS by colleagues, access to adequate numbers of high-quality computers, hands-on training, and technology support. The authors included a list of specific recommendations for those involved in the implementation of CPG CDSS systems (Box 1, p. 61, in Kilsdonk et al., 2017).

The federal government and some private payers are devising or using payment initiatives related to the use of CPGs. Although the evidence to support these plans is at best controversial, Medicare has implemented incentive programs to reward providers, hospitals, nursing homes, and home health agencies that demonstrate application of EBP as well as patient outcomes monitoring (Tanenbaum, 2009). These programs reflect a desire to improve patient care and control costs through the use of patient outcome monitoring combined with the application of research to practice. The CMS PQRI, also known as *pay for performance* (P4P), began in 2007. It allows providers (including NPs), who report satisfactory patient outcome data related to covered professional services to qualify to earn additional payments. Under the CMS Inpatient Prospective Payment System, hospitals report inpatient care process (including discharge instructions, evaluation of left ventricular function, prescription of an angiotensin-converting enzyme [ACE] inhibitor or an angiotensin II receptor blocker [ARB], and provision of smoking-cessation information to heart failure patients, and antibiotic selection and timing, collection of blood cultures, and administration of influenza vaccine for patients with pneumonia) and patient outcome data (including mortality, safety of care, readmission, patient experience, effectiveness of care, timeliness of care, and efficient use of medical imaging; CMS, 2011). The Value-Based Purchasing Program of the Affordable Care Act provides hospitals with financial incentives for not only reporting these quality data, but also for meeting established standards and demonstrating quality improvements. These data are also posted publicly by CMS on the Hospital Compare website (www.medicare.gov/hospitalcompare/about/what-is-hos.html; CMS, 2011; Easter & Tamburri, 2018).

Concerns have been expressed regarding the potential unexpected consequence of P4P systems, in that the need to meet patient outcomes' benchmarks could cause the provider to avoid patients with comorbid or difficult-to-treat problems ("cherry picking"), which might dilute the provider's ability to show improved patient outcomes (Dennison & Hughes, 2009). Penalties for poor patient outcomes have also been adopted by Medicare. Since 2009, hospitals have not been reimbursed for services provided to treat nosocomial infections and other preventable conditions (e.g., catheter-related urinary tract infections, CLABSI, decubitus ulcers, air emboli), prompting improved documentation of these conditions at or prior to admission. It has also driven agencies to examine their patient outcomes and to search out and apply evidence-based solutions, often in the form of CPGs, to prevent these adverse patient outcomes and associated revenue losses.

CPG use has also migrated into the healthcare regulatory arena, most notably via accreditation requirements of The Joint Commission. CPGs have also been used by groups responsible for provider credentialing and competency assessment (Anderson, 1993). In addition, Medicare, through its quality performance rating, publicly posts data regarding hospital performance on compliance with some CPGs. For example, hospital performance on recommendations, such as appropriate care for patients with sepsis and timely administration of aspirin to patients with a myocardial infarction, are posted at the Hospital Compare website (www.medicare.gov/hospitalcompare/search.html; Dennison & Hughes, 2009).

Little has been written regarding the legal implications to use of CPGs (see also Chapter 18, Legal Issues in Translation). The IOM's vision in 1992 was for CPGs to improve care rather than establish a legal standard of care (Ruhl & Siegal, 2017). It is important to remember that CPGs are designed to apply evidence to the care of populations of patients. In some circumstances, patient preferences and honoring a patient's informed consent preclude strict adherence to a CPG. In other situations, some components of a CPG could be contraindicated in individual patients. Principles of EBP include consideration of patient preferences and unique needs. However, some practice guidelines have been used, along with expert testimony, to establish standards of care in medical malpractice claims (Mittman & Siu, 1992; Ruhl & Siegal, 2017). In those cases, if followed, the CPGs may be used to demonstrate that the care provided by a healthcare practitioner met the accepted standards. Also, because negligence requires that the provider take an action that is not consistent with what a reasonable person would do under similar circumstances, if the provider does not follow the relevant CPG because of a contraindication or patient preference, a resulting injury to the patient would not necessarily be the result of negligence (Oza, El-Dika, & Adams, 2016).

■ EVALUATING CPGs

The development and expanded use of CPGs to facilitate the integration of evidence into practice is associated with several challenges. First, the development and use of CPGs encourage a critical scrutiny of the research literature. Optimally, recommendations included for the CPG should be supported by up-to-date systematic reviews and meta-analyses. However, this is not always possible because of the limitations in the availability of adequate depth, breadth, and quality of research, including availability of systematic reviews and meta-analyses. This would logically lead to a fuller discussion regarding the quality and meaning of evidence that should be considered in the development of a CPG. For example, if research evidence is not available, is there other empiric, experiential, or practice-based data, such as big data, that can be used to support recommendations? Questions also arise regarding whether CPGs developed in Western countries are useful and relevant to resource-poor, less-developed countries. In addition, because of the evolving nature of knowledge and practice, the knowledge and evidence basis for CPGs, and as a consequence the CPGs themselves, become out of date over time. In addition, as new research is completed, CPGs need to be updated or replaced.

It is important to understand the validity, quality, ease of use, and other characteristics of a CPG when deciding whether to apply it in practice (Kingston et al., 2000). Qualities of CPGs, including ease of use, complexity, clear scientific basis, a strong link between evidence and recommendations, and other factors, influence their use (Davis & Taylor-Vaisey, 1997; Sox, 1994).

The Appraisal of Guidelines for Research and Evaluation (AGREE) Collaboration is an international group of researchers who have worked together to create instruments (AGREE, AGREE II) that use theoretically derived criteria to evaluate the quality and applicability of CPGs (AGREE Collaboration, 2001; Brouwers et al., 2010a, 2010b, 2010c). The AGREE instrument was revised in 2010, with one item deleted, one item added, and minor changes made in numbering of items and language used in several items (#18–21, and #23). Item #7 from AGREE, "The guideline has been piloted among end users," was deleted. Item #9 in AGREE II is new and reads, "The strengths and limitations of the body of guideline are clearly described." An example of the minor language changes made includes item #18 in AGREE, "The guideline is supported with tools for application." Whereas in the AGREE II instrument, the corresponding item (renumbered #19) is the guideline that provides advice and/or tools on how the recommendations can be put into practice. The AGREE II instrument and manual (2017) can be accessed at no charge (www.agreetrust.org/wp-content/uploads/2017/12/AGREE-II-Users-Manual-and-23-item-Instrument-2009-Update-2017.pdf).

The AGREE II instrument is meant to be used by developers of CPG, healthcare providers using CPG, educators who prepare future healthcare providers, and policy makers who are considering and recommending the adoption of a CPG. It poses 23 questions related to six topical areas related to the guideline, including scope and purpose, stakeholder involvement, rigor of development, clarity of presentation, applicability, and editorial independence (Table 4.1). Each question is rated on a continuum from *strongly agree* to *strongly disagree,* with a corresponding score of 1 (*strongly disagree*) to 7 (*strongly agree*). Domain scores can be obtained and standardized by comparing the obtained scores to maximum possible scores. Typically, more than one individual uses the instrument to rate the CPG on each question. Results of the assessment of each of the domains are then used to make an overall assessment and recommendation regarding the use of the guideline in practice.

The AGREE and AGREE II instruments have been used by clinicians and organizations in more than seven different countries to evaluate CPGs related to diabetes, hypertension, headaches, fever in children, and cancer, and disorders of the neurologic, psychiatric, cardiovascular, pulmonary, gastrointestinal, hematologic,

TABLE 4.1 AGREE II Instrument Items for Evaluating Clinical Practice Guidelines

AGREE Domain	Domain Items
Scope and purpose	The overall objective of the guideline is specifically described.
	The health question(s) covered by the guideline is (are) specifically described.
	The population (patients, public, etc.) to whom the guideline is meant to apply is specifically described.
Stakeholder involvement	The guideline development group includes individuals from all the relevant professional groups.
	The views and preferences of the target population (patients, public, etc.) have been sought.
	The target users of the guideline are clearly defined.
Rigor of development	Systematic methods were used to search for evidence.
	The criteria for selecting the evidence are clearly described.
	The strengths and limitations of the body of evidence are clearly described.
	The methods used for formulating the recommendations are clearly described.
	The health benefits, side effects, and risks have been considered in formulating the recommendations.
	There is an explicit link between the recommendations and the supporting evidence.
	The guideline has been externally reviewed by experts prior to its publication.
	A procedure for updating the guideline is provided.

(*continued*)

TABLE 4.1 AGREE II Instrument Items for Evaluating Clinical Practice Guidelines (*continued*)

AGREE Domain	Domain Items
Clarity and presentation	The recommendations are specific and unambiguous.
	The different options for management of the condition or health issue are clearly presented.
	Key recommendations are easily identifiable.
	The guideline provides advice and/or tools on how the recommendations can be put into practice.
Applicability	The guideline describes facilitators and barriers to its application.
	The potential resource implications of applying the recommendations have been considered.
	The guideline presents monitoring and/or auditing criteria.
Editorial independence	The views of the funding body have not influenced the content of the guideline.
	Competing interests of guideline development group members have been recorded and addressed.

Note: Users should refer to the manual for the AGREE II item criteria and instructions on how to score the items.

AGREE, Appraisal of Guidelines for Research and Evaluation.

Sources: From Brouwers, M. C., Kho, M. E., Browman, G. P., Burgers, J. S., Cluzeau, F., Feder, G., . . . Littlejohns, P. (2010). AGREE II: Advancing guideline development, reporting and evaluation in health care. *Canadian Medical Association Journal, 182*(18), E839–E842. AGREE Next Steps Consortium (2009). The AGREE II instrument [Electronic version]. Retrieved from http://www.agreetrust.org

immunologic, renal, reproductive, musculoskeletal, and skin systems. They have also been used to evaluate complementary medicine, traditional Chinese medicine, and survivorship CPGs, as well as CPGs for dental, pharmacologic, and critical care.

To determine the use of the AGREE and AGREE II instruments, investigators used the two instruments to evaluate 68 CPGs published in 2011 to 2012 and found that the results for items and domains in both versions of the instrument correlated highly.

It is my hope that more clinicians will use the AGREE LL instrument to determine the quality and applicability of existing CPGs, as well as to develop future CPGs.

■ METHODS TO SUPPORT THE IMPLEMENTATION OF CPGs

Translation science is developing and disseminating evidence-based strategies to facilitate successful implementation of CPGs. Factors that should be considered in developing an implementation plan have been identified. Effective implementation methods and those that improve provider adherence with CPGs have also been reported. Evidence comes from individual studies as well as numerous systematic reviews of research and meta-analyses. In fact, the Cochrane group has published a series of reviews related to knowledge translation methods, any of which could be used to support the implementation of practice guidelines.

Strategies reported to support physician adoption of guidelines included educational programs that actively engage the learner and leverage peer influence, embedding guideline components and reminder systems in the medical record, and visible administrative support of guideline adoption (Davis & Taylor-Vaisey, 1997; Grimshaw et al., 2004; Wensing, van der Weijden, & Grol, 1998). Although similar approaches facilitate implementation of practice guidelines among nurses, nurses' adoption is also influenced by official support of the CPG by their professional association and working and collaborating as a team (Davies et al., 2008; Ploeg et al., 2007). Barriers to successful implementation among nurses include negative attitudes and beliefs among staff, lack of time or resources, and failure to integrate guideline components across care structures and processes at the individual and organizational levels.

Most commonly evaluated strategies used to improve provider adherence to care recommendations and guidelines include provider education, audit and feedback, clinician reminder or alert systems, and computerized CDSS. A growing area for application of CPGs is mobile health (mHealth) applications (apps), which can be used by healthcare providers or patients.

Clinician Education

Several systematic reviews and meta-analyses have examined the impact of education on changes in clinician adherence to practice recommendations (Forsetlund et al., 2009; Giguère et al., 2012; Scott et al., 2012). In the first review, printed educational materials, whether delivered alone or in addition to other interventions, were found to have a small impact on provider practices (Giguère et al., 2012). Another found that educational interventions were the most common strategy used to support the implementation of a standardized care process, protocol, or guideline. Isolated educational meetings or materials or a combination of both with or without reminders, a clinical advocate (champions), or audit and feedback were examined. The systematic review reported that education alone produced mixed results, and concluded it had little impact on practice and was not adequate to support adoption of the practice change (Scott et al., 2012). A meta-analysis examined the impact of education compared to no intervention and reported that a 6% to 10% change in clinician adherence to recommended practice could be attributed to an educational meeting (Forsetlund et al., 2009). The meta-analysis also found that programs that included both didactic as well as active learner engagement and focused on content regarding serious rather than less-serious patient outcomes had a larger impact, but that education alone was not likely to have a large impact on complex behavior change.

Audit and Feedback

Audit and feedback consists of a process in which data on the performance of healthcare professionals are provided to an individual provider or provider group to allow them to compare their performance to a known benchmark. The goal of this process is to allow individuals and groups to recognize gaps in performance and modify their practice in order to achieve better performance related to the benchmark. Several systematic reviews and meta-analyses of audit and feedback have found that this method produces small improvements in provider adherence to standard practices (Hysong, 2009; Ivers et al., 2012; Jamtvedt, Young, Kristoffersen, O'Brien, & Oxman, 2006; Jamtvedt, Young, Kristoffersen, Thomson O'Brien, & Oxman, 2003). They also reported that the greatest improvement in performance was associated with low baseline compliance with the standard, feedback delivered verbally or in writing by a supervisor or colleague, and provision of information regarding the expected performance and actions to improve performance (Hysong, 2009; Ivers et al., 2012; Jamtvedt et al., 2003, 2006). Since methods used in audit and feedback may influence its impact, the use of guiding principles for the same is recommended (Foy et al., 2005).

Clinician Reminder and Alert Systems

Clinical reminders are notices provided to a practitioner at the time of care that improve care by alerting the practitioner to document needed information, complete a task, or follow up on a previous action. Several systematic reviews (Arditi, Rège-Walther, Wyatt, Durieux, & Burnand, 2012; Dexheimer, Talbot, Sanders, Rosenbloom, & Aronsky, 2008; Shojania et al., 2009) and one overview of systematic reviews (Cheung et al., 2012) examined the evidence regarding the use of reminders in improving provider adherence to practice recommendations and guidelines. Originally, these reminders were simply notes attached to a patient's chart, but more recently, with the implementation of electronic health records and computerized provider ordering systems, they have evolved into automatic email messages, screen pop-ups, and other types of notices. Some require a provider response or acknowledgment. Although the data are mixed, these notices have been found to have a moderate impact on provider behavior (Arditi et al., 2012; Cheung et al., 2012; Dexheimer et al., 2008; Shojania et al., 2009).

Computerized Clinical Decision Support

For more than 30 years, healthcare systems of all sizes have been immersed in the development, implementation, evaluation, and refining of electronic health records and computerized provider order entry systems (CPOEs). These systems typically include features that support clinical decision-making. They help providers to ensure that patients receive the most appropriate and timely care. CDSSs help the provider to make decisions regarding the diagnosis, disease management, or medication therapy for an individual patient. Some CPOEs include robust CDSSs and others do not (Almutairi, Alseghayyir, Al-Alshikh, Arafah, & Househ, 2012). When best practice recommendations are integrated into CPOE-based CDSSs, guideline implementation is facilitated. CPGs tailored to fit into care-flow processes and that integrate patient data to produce timely patient-specific care guidance are called *computer-interpretable guidelines* (*CIG*; Peleg, 2013). In the future, more CIG systems need to be developed to support patient-centered care. In addition to integrating patient data to develop patient-specific guidance, an effective method needs to be developed to address the needs of individuals with multiple comorbid conditions. Currently, providers struggle to integrate sometimes conflicting care recommendations derived from multiple CPGs (Abidi, 2017; Wilk et al., 2017).

Systematic reviews have examined the impact of CDSSs on provider performance and patient outcomes. Systems that include advice on drug dosing improved a number of measures of drug therapy effectiveness, including patient outcomes (Gillaizeau et al., 2013; Okelo et al., 2013). Two systematic reviews have examined the use of CDSSs on practitioner behavior (Garg et al., 2005; Kawamoto, Houlihan, Balas, & Lobach, 2005). Garg et al. (2005) found that CDSSs that use an automatically activated provider cue were associated with improved provider performance, whereas systems that required the provider to select to use the CDSS were not associated with improved performance. In addition to automatic activation, other features of CDSSs that were found to be predictive of improved provider performance were support at the time and location of decision-making and provision of specific care recommendations (Kawamoto et al., 2005).

■ MOBILE TECHNOLOGY

Over the last two decades, use of mobile technology has grown dramatically, giving rise to the development of health- and healthcare-related software (mHealth). These technologies provide opportunities to access, retrieve, collect, display, share, analyze, and transmit healthcare information and data. mHealth can support clinical decision-making, rapid communication and consultation with experts, and reduce delays and errors in diagnosis and treatment (Edlin & Deshpande, 2013). Today, it is estimated that more than 75% of people worldwide have access to smartphones, and that more than 165,000 mHealth apps are available (Lalloo et al., 2017). Early mHealth apps focused on provider education, providing access to textbooks, journals, diagnostic and treatment reference materials (e.g., ISABELL, Up-to-Date, medical calculators (e.g., medcalc, Mediquations), prescribing guides (e.g., Epocrates, Johns Hopkins Antibiotic Guide), and instructional videos (Edlin & Deshpande, 2013). But today, many mHealth apps are designed for use by consumers. It is unknown how many consumer- or provider-focused mHealth apps are founded in CPG or other evidence.

A number of research publications related to mHealth apps were reviewed to provide insights into the current state of CPG and evidence integration and to identify future opportunities in this area. One examined the integration of patient/provider-linked mHealth that allowed patients to monitor their conditions, follow self-monitoring prompts, and receive medical management when needed (Peleg et al., 2017). A small number of patients with atrial fibrillation (AF) and gestational diabetes (GDM) piloted the app, which kept them safe while leading a normal daily life. Patient compliance with monitoring was very high in the GDM group (82%–98%) and higher than expected in the AF group (65%–75%). Providers intervened to start insulin in two out of 19 patients with GDM and to change the diagnosis and treatment for two out of 10 patients with AF. Although no specific CPGs were identified, the authors characterized the system as a CIG, in which CPG and patient data are integrated to produce patient-specific care guidance. This report exemplified the highest level of integration and sophistication found in the mHealth app literature. It is an outstanding model for the development of future mHealth apps.

A simpler app used the CAIDE Dementia Risk Screening Tool, a valid and reliable instrument, to allow consumers or providers to calculate the future risk of cognitive decline (Sindi et al., 2015). After calculating the individual's risk, the app displays a color-coded interpretation aid, and then, based on the score, offers educational materials regarding risk reduction (e.g., cognitive stimulation and exercise, BP and cholesterol control, provider referral recommendations as needed). The app records and retains data, so that subsequent assessments can be compared over time. Although the CAIDE Tool provides valid and reliable risk estimation, the authors did not describe the evidence basis for the risk reduction recommendations.

The "Brush DJ" mHealth app was created to support adherence to good oral hygiene (Underwood, Birdsail, & Kay, 2015). It includes several CPG-based prompts, alerts, preventive health information displays and external links. Its most notable feature is a "brushing timer" that plays user-selected music and cues the individual to maintain brushing for the recommended 2 minutes. Adults, children, and parents brushing small children's teeth can use the device. The app was introduced in the United Kingdom in 2011 and by 2015 had been downloaded more than 155,000 times in 182 countries. Of note, mHealth apps such as this are submitted to the UK National Health Services Health Apps Library and must demonstrate an evidence basis and clinical safety, as well as meet data-protection regulations. Individuals who use the app have reported that they are motivated to brush longer (88%), so that their teeth feel cleaner (70%), and their gums bleed less (39%).

Two studies report using scales to evaluate the quality of evidence on which mHealth Apps are based (Guo et al., 2017; Machado et al., 2016). Marchado et al. did a systematic review of low-back pain (LBP) self-management apps that included use of the Mobile App Rating Scale (MARS; Stoyanov et al., 2015). They assessed the LBP apps' compliance with 2016 National Institute for Health and Care Excellence (NICE) LBP guidelines. The MARS includes 23 items within five categories (engagement, functionality, esthetics, information quality [two items], and overall quality). Each item is rated between 1 and 5. The scale has demonstrated internal consistency and inter-rater reliability. Marchado et al. found that out of 63 LBP apps, only 10% used strategies consistent with the NICE LBP CPG. None of the apps had been tested with patients, and the overall app MARS scores (reported as a mean of the summed item scores) ranged from 1.83 to 3.94, with low (2.5) information quality scores due to the absence of an evidence basis. Guo et al. reported on the development of a scale to rate the quality of exercise program apps based on the CPG established by the American College of Sports Medicine (ACSM). Their 27-item instrument was used to evaluate compliance of 28 apps with the ACSM CPG recommendations. The instrument demonstrated inter- and intra-rater reliability as well as criterion validity. No app scored higher than 35 out of 70, indicating poor compliance with the CPG. The use of both of these mHealth app scoring techniques demonstrated the lack of evidence that underlies many mHealth apps.

Several scoping reviews, systematic reviews, and meta-analyses examined the evidence basis for recommendations found in mHealth apps for headaches, stress management, treatment of speech disorders in children, and anxiety (Coulon, Monroe, & West, 2016; Firth et al., 2017; Furlong, Morris, Serry, & Erickson, 2018; Mosadeghi-Nik, Askari, & Fatehi, 2016). Furlong et al. used the MARS to evaluate speech apps and identified four that were excellent and 25 that were good, but found the remaining 107 apps scored average to poor. Coulon et al. (2016), Firth et al. (2017), and Mosadeghi-Nik et al. (2016) found very few mHealth apps that even met criteria for inclusion in their analyses, and that most of the mHealth apps they examined failed to base their features or recommendations on evidence or CPGs.

The growth in use of mHealth apps by consumers and healthcare practitioners indicates that this technology should be harnessed to disseminate EBP and CPG. Providers should work with information technology experts and other stakeholders to develop effective evidence-based mHealth apps (Machado et al., 2016). Apps must be evaluated to show their therapeutic benefits (Coulon et al., 2016). mHealth Apps have been found to be very difficult to identify and locate, and so a logical and accessible cataloguing method needs to be developed so that both consumers and healthcare practitioners can access high-quality systems (Furlong et al., 2018).

■ ASSESSING THE IMPACT ON OUTCOMES IN THE APPLICATION OF CPGs

The work is not done even if the CPG is found to be of high quality and applicable to practice. It is important to carefully implement the CPG in a real practice setting and to subsequently evaluate its effects on the final product, the outcome, through outcome assessment. Typically, outcome assessment, such as development of CPGs or implementation of a practice improvement project, is conducted by a team. Resources and support for the assessment (e.g., personnel, funds, or access to databases) may come from inside as well as outside the practice site. Researchers or statisticians (e.g., university faculty) within the community can help in planning and carrying out the assessment process.

When assessing the effect of the application of evidence to practice, outcomes to be assessed should be chosen based on four criteria: salience, objectivity, reality, and common currency (Minnick, 2009). "Salience is the quality of being related to the phenomenon of interest. Objectivity is the ability of the outcome to be measured without bias" (p. 110). Reality is "the extent to which the outcome definition . . . is true to life" (Minnick, 2009, p. 110). Consultation with stakeholders can improve the likelihood that the outcome of interest meets these three criteria. *Common currency* refers to whether the way the outcome is defined and measured is standardized across settings. Familiarity with literature related to the outcome as well as consultation with others who work with the outcome of interest will help in the identification of any generally accepted definition and method of measurement.

Another quality that may be important is temporality. This is important when the project has a limited implementation period. For example, if a project will be implemented for 3 months, it is important to know whether it is possible to change the outcome over that period or whether it would be better to use another indicator. To overcome these challenges, one needs to be sure that the definition of outcomes used on the PICO are consistent across the project and aims and are consistent with the evidence.

The link between the evidence-based improvement intervention (e.g., the application of the CPG) and the outcome to be assessed needs to be clear. Even with clear linkages, at least seven challenges have been identified that interfere in one's ability to trace a direct relationship between the cause (application of an evidence-based intervention) and its effect (effect on the outcome of interest; Minnick, 2009). They include patient adherence to the treatment, inability to control multiple comorbidities, nonclinical (e.g., demographic) differences among participating patients, passage of time between intervention and measurement of the outcome, lack of availability of baseline data, involvement of many providers in the setting or in the patient's care, and general complexity inherent in today's healthcare delivery settings. It is important to recognize these challenges and to try to incorporate ways to mitigate these issues in designing the assessment (e.g., use repeated-measures methods, collect information on participating patient's demographics and comorbidities from medical records for use as covariates in analysis, compare outcomes that occurred during the same months of the year for both the "before" and "after" groups). A "broad knowledge of patients, providers, and systems variables" (Minnick, 2009, p. 113) as well as substantive support from the practice or institution (time of key stakeholders, financial resources, information technology expertise, staff personnel, etc.) is important for the success of this process.

Data analysis is an important component of outcome assessment (see Chapter 14, Information Technology: A Foundation for Translation, on evaluation for more detail). Data linked to the intended outcomes must be collected and analyzed to fully understand the effect of the translated evidence on outcomes. It is likely that any project will require consideration of data related not only to patients but also to the context of the care environment (staffing, census, organizational processes, etc.). It is important to enlist expert assistance during the planning phase, so that relevant data are included during data collection. This is another reason to consider including individuals with knowledge of research and statistical analysis methods on the assessment team. All projects should evaluate, at a minimum, descriptive statistics related to the setting, the project, and its outcomes. Some projects (e.g., those that use the typical quality improvement in pretest and posttest design) might use chi-square or *t*-test to characterize the differences found between the two times or two groups, and other projects could allow the use of correlation techniques to understand the results of the project.

■ FUTURE USE OF CPGs TO IMPROVE PATIENT OUTCOMES

Although data support the effect of guidelines on the processes of care (Cason, Tyner, Saunders, & Broome, 2007; Grimshaw & Russell, 1993; Kornbluth et al., 2006) and methods that can be used to support their implementation, their effect on outcomes is just beginning to be documented (Smith & Hillner, 2001; Worrall, Chaulk, & Freake, 1997). Does the implementation of guidelines really promote improved outcomes? How can CPGs be best implemented and how can their use be sustained? How can patient outcomes derived from the application of CPGs be assessed, analyzed, and integrated to further improve the CPG and overall care? Additional research is needed, and providers' experiences and insights regarding the use of CPGs need to be reported. What is certain is that healthcare professionals and institutions will continue to be called on to use all available methods to improve the quality and safety of healthcare delivered, so that the most important outcome, patient health, is optimized.

■ REFERENCES

Abidi, S. (2017) A knowledge-modeling approach to integrate multiple clinical guidelines to provide evidence-based clinical decision support for managing comorbid conditions. *Journal of Medical Systems, 41*(12), 193. doi:10.1007/s10916-017-0841-1

Ackerman, M. H. (1999). What would Vesalius think? *American Journal of Critical Care, 8*(2), 70–71.

Almutairi, M. S., Alseghayyir, R. M., Al-Alshikh, A. A., Arafah, H. M., & Househ, M. S. (2012). Implementation of computerized physician order entry (CPOE) with clinical decision support (CDS) features in Riyadh hospitals to improve quality of information. *Studies in Health Technology and Informatics, 180*, 776–780.

Anderson, G. (1993). Implementing practice guidelines. *Canadian Medical Association Journal, 148*(5), 753–755.

Appraisal of Guidelines for Research and Evaluation Collaboration. (2001). *Appraisal of Guidelines for Research & Evaluation (AGREE) instrument*. London, UK: Author. Retrived from http://apps.who.int/rhl/agree-instrumentfinal.pdf

Arditi, C., Rège-Walther, M., Wyatt, J. C., Durieux, P., & Burnand, B. (2012). Computer-generated reminders delivered on paper to healthcare professionals: Effects on professional practice and health care outcomes. *Cochrane Database of Systematic Reviews, 2012*(12), CD001175. doi:10.1002/14651858.CD001175.pub3

Brooks, B. A., & Barrett, S. (1998). Core competencies for outcomes management in nursing. *Outcomes Management for Nursing Practice, 2*(2), 87–89.

Brouwers, M. C., Kho, M. E., Browman, G. P., Burgers, J. S., Cluzeau, F., Feder, G., . . . Makarski, J. (2010a). Development of the AGREE II, part 1: Performance, usefulness and areas for improvement. *Canadian Medical Association Journal, 182*(10), 1045–1052. doi:10.1503/cmaj.091714

Brouwers, M. C., Kho, M. E., Browman, G. P., Burgers, J. S., Cluzeau, F., Feder, G., . . . Makarski, J. (2010b). Development of the AGREE II, part 2: Assessment of validity of items and tools to support application. *Canadian Medical Association Journal, 182*(10), E472–E478. doi:10.1503/cmaj.091716

Brouwers, M. C., Kho, M. E., Browman, G. P., Burgers, J. S., Cluzeau, F., Feder, G., . . . Zitzelsberger, L. (2010c). AGREE II: Advancing guideline development, reporting, and evaluation in health care. *Preventive Medicine, 51*(5), 421–424. doi:10.1503/cmaj.090449

Cabana, M. D., Rand, C. S., Powe, N. R., Wu, A. W., Wilson, M. H., Abboud, P. A., & Rubin, H. R. (1999). Why don't physicians follow clinical practice guidelines? A framework for improvement. *Journal of the American Medical Association, 282*(15), 1458–1465. doi:10.1001/jama.282.15.1458

Carman, K. L., Maurer, M., Yegian, J. M., Dardess, P., McGee, J., Evers, M., & Marlo, K. O. (2010). Evidence that consumers are skeptical about evidence-based health care. *Health Affairs, 29*(7), 1400–1406. doi:10.1377/hithaff.2009.0296

Cason, C. L., Tyner, T., Saunders, S., & Broome, L. (2007). Nurses implementation of guidelines for ventilator-associated pneumonia from the Centers for Disease Control and Prevention. *American Journal of Critical Care, 16*(1), 28–38.

Centers for Medicare & Medicaid Services. (2011). Medicare program; hospital inpatient value-based purchasing program. Final rule. *Federal Register, 76*, 26490–26547.

Cheung, A., Weir, M., Mayhew, A., Kozloff, N., Brown, K., & Grimshaw, J. (2012). Overview of systematic reviews of the effectiveness of reminders in improving healthcare professional behavior. *Systematic Reviews, 1*(36), 1–8. doi:10.1186/2046-4053-1-36

Coulon, S. M., Monroe, C. M., West, D. S. (2016). A systematic, multi-domain review of mobile smartphone apps for evidence-based stress management. *American Journal of Preventive Medicine, 51*(1), 95–105.

Damiani, E., Donati, A., Serafini, G., Rinaldi, L., Adrario, E., Pelaia, P., . . . Girardis, M. (2015). Effect of performance improvement programs on compliance with sepsis bundles and mortality: A systematic review and meta-analysis of observational studies. *PLoS One, 10*(5), e0125827. doi:10.1371/journal.pone.0125827

Davies, B., Edwards, N., Ploeg, J., & Virani, T. (2008). Insights about the process and impact of implementing nursing guidelines on delivery of care in hospitals and community settings. *BMC Health Services Research, 8*(29), 1–15. doi:10.1186/1472-6963-8-29

Davis, D. A., & Taylor-Vaisey, A. (1997). Translating guidelines into practice: A systematic review of theoretic concepts, practical experience and research evidence in the adoption of clinical practice guidelines. *Canadian Medical Association Journal, 157*(4), 408–416.

Deaton, C. (2001). Outcomes measurement and evidence-based nursing practice. *Journal of Cardiovascular Nursing, 15*(2), 83–86. doi:10.1097/00005082-200101000-00009

Dennison, C. R., & Hughes, S. (2009). Reforming cardiovascular care: Quality measurement and improvement, and pay-for-performance. *Journal of Cardiovascular Nursing, 24*(5), 341–343. doi:10.1097/JCN.0b013e3181b4346e

Dexheimer, J. W., Talbot, T. R., Sanders, D. L., Rosenbloom, S. T., & Aronsky, D. (2008). Prompting clinicians about preventive care measures: A systematic review of randomized controlled trials. *Journal of the American Medical Informatics Association, 15*(3), 311–320. doi:10.1197/jamia.M2555

Dogherty, E., Harrison, M., Graham, I., Vandyk, A., & Keeping-Burke, L. (2013). Turning knowledge into action at the point-of-care: The collective experience of nurses facilitating the implementation of evidence-based practice. *Worldviews on Evidence-Based Nursing 10*(3), 129–139. doi:10.1111/wvn.12009

Donabedian, A. (1985). Explorations in quality assessment and monitoring. In *The methods and findings of quality assessment and monitoring: An illustrated analysis* (Vol. 3). Ann Arbor, MI: Health Administration Press.

Donabedian, A. (2005). Evaluating the quality of medical care. *Millbank Quarterly, 83*(4), 691–729. doi:10.1111/j.1468-0009.2005.00397.x

Easter, K., & Tamburri, L. M. (2018). Understanding patient safety and quality outcome data. *Critical Care Nurse, 38*(6), 58–66. doi:10.4037/ccn2018979

Edlin, J., & Deshpande, R. (2013). Caveats of smartphone applications for the cardiothoracic trainee. *Journal of Thoracic and Cardiovascular Surgery, 146*(6), 1321–1326. doi:10.1016/j.jtcvs.2013.08.033

Firth, J., Torous, J., Nicholas, J., Carney, R., Rosenbaum, S., & Sarris J. (2017). Can smartphone mental health interventions reduce symptoms of anxiety? A meta-analysis of randomized controlled trials. *Journal of Affective Disorders, 218*, 15–22. doi:10.1016/j.jad.2017.04.046

Forsetlund, L., Bjørndal, A., Rashidian, A., Jamtvedt, G., O'Brien, M. A., Wolf, F., . . . Oxman, A. D. (2009). Continuing education meetings and workshops: Effects on professional practice and health care outcomes. *Cochrane Database of Systematic Reviews, 2009*(2), CD003030. doi:10.1002/14651858.CD003030.pub2

Foster, R. L. (2001). Who is responsible for measuring nursing outcomes? *Journal of the Society of Pediatric Nurses, 6*(3), 107–108. doi:10.1111/j.1744-6155.2001.tb00131.x

Foy, R., Eccles, M. P., Jamtvedt, G., Young, J., Grimshaw, J. M., & Baker, R. (2005). What do we know about how to do audit and feedback? Pitfalls in applying evidence from a systematic review. *BMC Health Services Research, 5*(50), 1–7. doi:10.1186/1472-6963-5-50

Francke, A., Smit, M., de Veer, A., & Mistiaen, P. (2008). Factors influencing the implementation of clinical guidelines for health care professionals: A systematic meta-review. *BMC Medical Informatics and Decision Making, 8*(38), 1–11. doi:10.1186/1472-6947-8-38

Furlong, L., Morris, M., Serry, T., & Erickson, S. (2018). Mobile apps for treatment of speech disorders in children: An evidence-based analysis of quality and efficacy. *PLoS One, 13*(8), e0201513. doi:10.1371/journal.pone.0201513

Garg, A. X., Adhikari, N. K., McDonald, H., Rosas-Arellano, M. P., Devereaux, P. J., Beyene, J., . . . Haynes, R. B. (2005). Effects of computerized clinical decision support systems on practitioner performance and patient outcomes: A systematic review. *Journal of the American Medical Association, 293*(10), 1223–1238. doi:10.1001/jama.293.10.1223

Giguère, A., Légaré, F., Grimshaw, J., Turcotte, S., Fiander, M., Grudniewicz, A., . . . Gagnon, M. (2012). Printed educational materials: Effects on professional practice and healthcare outcomes. *Cochrane Database of Systematic Reviews, 2012*(10), CD004398. doi:10.1002/14651858.CD004398.pub3

Gillaizeau, F., Chan, E., Trinquart, L., Colombet, I., Walton, R. T., Rège-Walther, M., . . . Durieux, P. (2013). Computerized advice on drug dosage to improve prescribing practice. *Cochrane Database of Systematic Reviews, 2013*(11), CD002894. doi:10.1002/14651858.CD002894.pub3

Green, L. W. (2006). Public health asks of systems science: To advance our evidence-based practice, can you help us get more practice-based evidence? *American Journal of Public Health, 96*(3), 406–409. doi:10.2105/AJPH.2005.066035

Grimshaw, J. M., & Russell, I. T. (1993). Effect of clinical guidelines on medical practice: A systematic review of rigorous evaluations. *Lancet, 342*(8883), 1317–1322. doi:10.1016/0140-6736(93)92244-n

Grimshaw, J. M., Thomas, R., MacLennan, G., Fraser, C., Ramsay, C., Vale, L., . . . Donaldson, C. (2004). Effectiveness and efficiency of guideline dissemination and implementation strategies. *Health Technology Assessment, 8*(6), 1–72.

Guo, Y., Bian. J., Leavitt, T., Vincent, H K.,Vander Zalm, L., Teurlings, T. L., . . . Modave F. (2017). Assessing the quality of mobile exercise apps based on the american college of sports medicine guidelines: A reliable and valid scoring instrument. *Journal of Medical Internet Research, 19*(3), e67. doi:10.2196/jmir.6976

Hammermeister, K., Shroyer, A., Sethi, G., & Grover, F. (1995). Why it is important to demonstrate linkages between outcomes of care and processes and structures of care. *Medical Care, 33*(10), OS5–OS16. doi:10.1097/00005650-199510001-00002

Haynes, R. B. (1993). Some problems in applying evidence in clinical practice. *Annals of the New York Academy of Sciences, 703*, 210–225. doi:10.1111/j.1749-6632.1993.tb26350.x

Heater, B. S., Becker, A. M., & Olson, R. K. (1988). Nursing interventions and patient outcomes: A meta-analysis of studies. *Nursing Research, 37*(5), 303–307. doi:10.1097/00006199-198809000-00008

Heslop, L., & Lu, S. (2014). Nursing-sensitive indicators: A concept analysis. *Journal of Advanced Nursing, 70*(11), 2469–2482. doi:10.1111/jan.12503

Hughes, R. G. (2008). Tools and strategies for quality improvement and patient safety. In R. G. Hughes (Ed.), *Patient safety and quality: An evidence-based handbook for nurses* . Rockville, MD: Agency for Healthcare Research and Quality. Retrieved from http://www.ncbi.nlm.nih.gov/books/NBK2682

Hysong, S. J. (2009). Meta-analysis: Audit and feedback features impact effectiveness on care quality. *Medical Care, 47*(3), 356–363. doi:10.1097/MLR.0b013e3181893f6b

Institute of Medicine. (1990). Health, health care, and quality of care. In K. N. Lohr (Ed.), *Medicare: A strategy for quality assurance* (pp. 19–44). Washington, DC: National Academies Press.

Institute of Medicine. (2001). *Crossing the quality chasm: A new health care system for the 21st century*. Washington, DC: National Academies Press.

Ivers, N., Jamtvedt, G., Flottorp, S., Young, J. M., Odgaard-Jensen, J., French, S. D., . . . Oxman, A. D. (2012). Audit and feedback: Effects on professional practice and healthcare outcomes. *Cochrane Database of Systematic Reviews, 2012*(6), CD000259. doi:10.1002/14651858.CD000259.pub3

Jamtvedt, G., Young, J. M., Kristoffersen, D. T., O'Brien, M. A., & Oxman, A. D. (2006). Audit and feedback: Effects on professional practice and health care outcomes. *Cochrane Database of Systematic Reviews, 2006*(2), CD000259.

Jamtvedt, G., Young, J. M., Kristoffersen, D. T., Thomson O'Brien, M. A., & Oxman, A. D. (2003). Audit and feedback: Effects on professional practice and health care outcomes. *Cochrane Database of Systematic Reviews, 2003*(3), CD000259.

Joseph, A. M. (2007). The impact of nursing on patient and organizational outcomes. *Nursing Economic, 25*(1), 30–34.

Kawamoto, K., Houlihan, C. A., Balas, E. A., & Lobach, D. F. (2005). Improving clinical practice using clinical decision support systems: A systematic review of trials to identify features critical to success. *British Medical Journal, 330*(7494), 1–8. doi:10.1136/bmj.38398.500764.8F

Kilsdonk, E., Peute, L. W., & Jaspers, M. W. (2017). Factors influencing implementation success of guideline-based clinical decision support systems: A systematic review and gaps analysis. *International Journal of Medical Informatics, 98*, 56–64. doi:10.1016/j.ijmedinf.2016.12.001

Kingston, M. E., Krumberger, J. M., & Peruzzi, W. T. (2000). Enhancing outcomes: Guidelines, standards, and protocols. *AACN Clinical Issues, 11*(3), 363–374. doi:10.1097/00044067-200008000-00004

Kornbluth, A., Hayes, M., Feldman, S., Hunt, M., Fried-Boxt, E., Lichtiger, S., . . . Young, J. (2006). Do guidelines matter? Implementation of the ACG and AGA osteoporosis screening guidelines in inflammatory bowel disease (IBD) patients who meet the guidelines criteria. *American Journal of Gastroenterology, 101*(7), 1546–1550. doi:10.1111/j.1572-0241.2006.00571.x

Kurtzman, E. T., & Corrigan, J. M. (2007). Measuring the contribution of nursing to quality, patient safety and health care outcomes. *Policy, Politics & Nursing Practice, 8*(1), 20–36. doi:10.1177/1527154407302115

Lalloo, C., Shah, U., Davies-Chalmers, C., Rivera, J., Stinson, J., & Campbell, F. (2017). Commercially available Smartphone apps to support postoperative pain self-management: Scoping review. *JMIR Mhealth and Uhealth, 5*(10), e162. doi:10.2196/mhealth.8230

Lavallée, J. F., Gray, T. A., Dumville, J., Russell, W., & Cullum, N. (2017). The effects of care bundles on patient outcomes: A systematic review and meta-analysis. *Implementation Science, 12*(1), 142. doi:10.1186/s13012-017-0670-0

Lohr, K. N. (1988). Outcome measurement: Concepts and questions. *Inquiry, 25*(1), 37–50. doi:10.1177/1527154407302115

Lohr, K. N., & Field, M. J. (1992). A provisional instrument for assessing clinical practice guidelines. In M. J. Field & K. N. Lohr (Eds.), *Guidelines for clinical practice: From development to use*. Washington, DC: Institute of Medicine, National Academies Press.

Machado, G. C., Pinheiro, M. B., Lee, H., Ahmed, O. H., Hendrick, P., Williams, C., & Kamper, S. J. (2016). Smartphone apps for the self-management of low back pain: A systematic review. *Best Practice and Research in Clinical Rheumatology, 30*(6):1098–1109. doi:10.1016/j.berh.2017.04.002

Marek, K. D. (1997). Measuring the effectiveness of nursing care. *Outcomes Management for Nursing Practice, 1*(1), 8–12.

Matther-Maich, N., Ploeg, J., Dobbins, M., & Jack, S. (2013). Supporting the uptake of nursing guidelines: What you really need to know to move guidelines into practice. *Worldviews on Evidence-Based Nursing, 10*(2), 104–115. doi:10.1111/j.1741-6787.2012.00259.x

McGlynn, E. A., Asch, S. M., Adams, J., Keesey, J., Hicks, J., DeCristofaro, A., & Kerr, E. A. (2003). The quality of health care delivered to adults in the United States. *New England Journal of Medicine, 348*(26), 2635–2645. doi:10.1056/NEJMsa022615

Minnick, A. F. (2009). General design and implementation challenges in outcomes assessment. In R. M. Kleinpell (Ed.), *Outcome assessment in advanced practice nursing* (2nd ed., pp. 107–118). New York, NY: Springer Publishing Company.

Mitchell, P. H. (2008). Defining patient safety and quality care. In R. G. Hughes (Ed.), *Patient safety and quality: An evidence-based handbook for nurses*. Rockville, MD: Agency for Healthcare Research and Quality. Retrieved from http://www.ncbi.nlm.nih.gov/books/NBK2681

Mittman, B. S., & Siu, A. L. (1992). Changing provider behavior: Applying research on outcomes and effectiveness in health care. In S. M. Shortell & U. E. Reinhardt (Eds.), *Improving health policy and management*. Ann Arbor, MI: Health Administration Press.

Mosadeghi-Nik, M., Askari, M. S., & Fatehi, F. (2016). Mobile health (mHealth) for headache disorders: A review of the evidence base. *Journal of Telemedicine and Telecare, 22*(8), 472–477. doi:10.1177/1357633X16673275

Mullins, C. D., Baldwin, R., & Perfetto, E. M. (1996). What are outcomes? *Journal of the American Pharmacists Association, NS36*(1), 39–49.

National Database of Nursing Quality Indicators. (2010). NDNQI: Transforming data into quality care [Brochure]. Retrieved from http://public.qualityforum.org/actionregistry/Lists/List%20of%20Actions/Attachments/141/NDNQIBrochure.pdf?Mobile=1

Newhouse, R., & Poe, S. (2005). *Measuring patient safety*. Sudbury, MA: Jones & Bartlett.

Oermann, M. H., & Floyd, J. A. (2002). Outcomes research: An essential component of the advanced practice nurse role. *Clinical Nurse Specialist, 16*(3), 140–144. doi:10.1097/00002800-200205000-00007

Okelo, S. O., Butz, A. M., Sharma, R., Diette, G. B., Pitts, S. I., King, T. M., . . . Robinson, K. A. (2013). Interventions to modify health care provider adherence to asthma guidelines: A systematic review. *Pediatrics, 132*(3), 517–534. doi:10.1542/peds.2013-0779

Ospina, M. B., Mrklas, K., Deucchar, L., Rowe, B. H., Keigh, R., Bhutani, M., & Stickland, M. K. (2017). A systematicc review of the effectiveness of discharge care bundles for patients with COPD. *Thorax, 72*(1), 31–39. doi:10.1136/thoraxjnl-2016-208820

Oza, V. M., El-Dika, S., & Adams, M. A. (2016). Reaching safe harbor: Legal implications of clinical practice guidelines. *Clinical Gastroenterology & Hepatology, 14*(2), 172–174. doi:10.1016/j.cgh.2015.10.003

Parse, R. R. (2006). Outcomes: Saying what you mean. *Nursing Science Quarterly, 19*(3), 189. doi:10.1177/0894318406289432

Peleg, M. (2013). Computer-interpretable clinical guidelines: A methodological review. *Journal of Biomedical Informatics, 46*(4), 744–763. doi:10.1016/j.jbi.2013.06.009

Peleg, M., Shahar, Y., Quaglini, S., Broens, T., Budasu, R., Fung, N., . . . van Schooten, B. (2017). Assessment of personalized and distributed patient guidance system. *International Journal of Medical Informatics, 101*, 108–130. doi:10.1016/j.ijmedinf.2017.02.010

Ploeg, J., Davies, B., Edwards, N., Gifford, W., & Miller, P. (2007). Factors influencing best-practice guideline implementation: Lessons learned from administrators, nursing staff and project leaders. *Worldviews on Evidence-Based Nursing, 4*(4), 210–219. doi:10.1111/j.1741-6787.2007.00106.x

Resar, R., Griffin, F., Haraden, C., & Nolan, T. (2012). Using care bundles to improve health care quality. IHI innovation series white paper. Cambridge, MA: Institute for Healthcare Improvement.

Resar, R., Pronovost, P., Haraden, C., Simmonds, T., Rainey, T., & Nolan, T. (2005). Using a bundle approach to improve ventilator care processes and reduce ventilator-associated pneumonia. *The Joint Commission Journal on Quality and Patient Safety, 31*(5), 243–248.

Rotter, T., Kinsman, L., James, E., Machotta, A., Gothe, H., Willis, J., . . . Kugler, J. (2009). Clinical pathways: Effects on professional practice, patient outcomes, length of stay and hospital costs. *Cochrane Database of Systematic Reviews, 2009*(3), CD006632. doi:10.1002/14651858.CD006632.pub2

Ruhl, D. S., & Siegal, G. (2017). Medical malpractice implications of clinical practice guidelines. *Otolaryngology—Head and Neck Surgery, 157*(2), 175–177. doi:10.1177/0194599817707943

Sadeghi-Bazargani, H., Tabrizi, J. S., & Azami-Aghdash, S. (2014). Barriers to evidence-based medicine: A systematic review. *Journal of Evaluation in Clinical Practice, 20*(6), 793–802. doi:10.1111/jep.12222

Scott, S., Albrecht, L., O'Leary, K., Ball, G., Hartling, L., Hofmeyer, A., . . . Dryden, D. (2012). Systematic review of knowledge translation strategies in the allied health professions. *Implementation Science, 7*(70), 1–17. doi:10.1186/1748-5908-7-70

Shojania, K. G., Jennings, A., Mayhew, A., Ramsay, C. R., Eccles, M. P., & Grimshaw, J. (2009). The effects of on-screen, point of care computer reminders on processes and outcomes of care. *Cochrane Database of Systematic Reviews, 2009*(3), CD001096. doi:10.1002/14651858.CD001096.pub2

Sindi, S., Calov, E., Fokkens, J., Ngandu, T., Soininen, H., Tuomilehto, J., & Kivipelto, M. (2015). The CAIDE Dementia Risk Score App: The development of an evidence-based mobile application to predict the risk of dementia. *Alzheimer's & Dementia (Amst), 1*(3), 328–333. doi:10.1016/j.dadm.2015.06.005

Smith, T. J., & Hillner, B. E. (2001). Ensuring quality cancer care by the use of clinical practice guidelines and critical pathways. *Journal of Clinical Oncology, 19*(11), 2886–2897. doi:10.1200/JCO.2001.19.11.2886

Sox, H. C. (1994). Practice guidelines: 1994. *American Journal of Medicine, 97*(3), 205–207. doi:10.1016/0002-9343(94)90001-9

Stoyanov, S. R., Hides, L., Kavanagh, D. J., Zelenko, O., Tjondronegoro, D., & Mani, M. (2015). Mobile app rating scale: A new tool for assessing the quality of health mobile apps. *JMIR mHealth and uHealth, 3*(1), e27–e36. doi:10.2196/mhealth.3422

Tablan, O. C., Anderson, L. J., Besser, R., Bridges, C., Hajjeh, R., Centers for Disease Control and Prevention, & Healthcare Infection Control Practices Advisory Committee. (2004). Guidelines for preventing health-care-associated pneumonia, 2003: Recommendations of CDC and Healthcare Infection Control Practices Advisory Committee. *Morbidity and Mortality Weekly Report. Recommendations and Reports/Centers for Disease Control, 53*(RR–3), 1–36.

Tanenbaum, S. J. (2009). Pay for performance in Medicare: Evidentiary irony and the politics of value. *Journal of Health Politics, Policy and Law, 34*(5), 717–746. doi:10.1215/03616878-2009-023

The Joint Commission. (2008). Using evidence-based practice and outcomes management to improve care. *The Joint Commission Benchmark, 10*(3), 9–10.

Underwood, B., Birdsall, J., & Kay, E. (2015). The use of a mobile app to motivate evidence-based oral hygiene behavior. *British Dental Journal, 219*(4), E2. doi:10.1038/sj.bdj.2015.660

Van Driel, M. L., De Sutter, A. I., Christiaens, T. C., & De Maeseneer, J. M. (2005). Quality of care: The need for medical, contextual, and policy evidence in primary care. *Journal of Evaluation in Clinical Practice, 11*(5), 417–429. doi:10.1111/j.1365-2753.2005.00549.x

Wensing, M., van der Weijden, T., & Grol, R. (1998). Implementing guidelines and innovations in general practice: Which interventions are effective? *British Journal of General Practice, 48*(427), 991–997.

Wilk, S., Michalowski, M., Michalowski, W., Rosu, D., Carrier, M., & Kezadri-Hamaiz, M. (2017). Comprehensive mitigation framework for concurrent application of multiple clinical practice guidelines. *Biomedical Informatics, 66*, 52–71. doi:10.1016/j.jbi.2016.12.002

Worrall, G., Chaulk, P., & Freake, D. (1997). The effects of clinical practice guidelines on patient outcomes in primary care: A systematic review. *Canadian Medical Association Journal, 156*(12), 1705–1712.

CHAPTER FIVE

Translation of Evidence for Improving Safety and Quality

Kathleen M. White

There is a right thing to do with regard to quality of care: improve it. If that takes courage, so be it.
—DON BERWICK

THE QUALITY OF CARE IN U.S. HOSPITALS is a cause of widespread concern (Murray & Frenk, 2010). This is particularly disquieting because there has been a dramatic increase in quality and patient safety-related activities during the past decade (Leape, 2010). When the Health and Medicine Division of the National Academies of Sciences, Engineering, and Medicine released the seminal reports, *To Err Is Human* in 1999 and *Crossing the Quality Chasm* in 2001, the assertions that between 44,000 and 98,000 preventable deaths occur annually in U.S. hospitals were both startling and riveting. The Health and Medicine Division's minimum goal of a 50% reduction in errors over 5 years seemed aggressive, but plausible (Institute of Medicine [IOM], 1999, 2001). A RAND research and development report suggested that U.S. hospitalized patients receive, on average, half the therapies that evidence suggests they should (McGlynn et al., 2003) and fueled the urgency for improvement created by the Health and Medicine Division reports. Subsequent national surveys suggested that patient safety was a top priority for hospital leaders, including boards of trustees (Barry, 2005; Callendar, Hastings, Hemsley, Morris, & Peregrine, 2007; Goeschel, Wachter, & Prnovost, 2010; Jiang, Lockee, Bass, & Fraser, 2008). High expectations prevailed; yet, years after the Health and Medicine Division reports were released, health services researchers have voiced concerns over the slow pace of progress (Agency for Healthcare Research and Quality [AHRQ], 2009; Auerbach, Landefeld, & Shojania, 2007; Clancy, 2009; Leape et al., 2009; Wachter, 2010).

Two recent studies have introduced additional dimensions into the continuing concern for quality and safety in healthcare. Weissman et al. (2008) compared adverse events reported by patients in postdischarge interviews to adverse events found in medical record audits. The study found that 23% of patients identified an adverse event that affected their care, compared with a rate of 11% using medical record audit procedures. In fact, in the interviews, patients identified 21 serious and preventable adverse events that were not found in the medical record (Weissman et al., 2008). Patient engagement in their healthcare is a strategy that needs more attention.

In 2013, John James reported a current and sometimes controversial estimate of medical errors in healthcare today. He updated the estimate from 1999 by reviewing studies from 2008 to 2011. The review included four studies, and the author stated:

> [It is] our opinion that none of the 4 studies alone can provide a defensible estimate for hospitals across the United States; however, by combining the studies, an evidence-based estimate of the number of lethal post-antibiotic effects (PAEs) across the country can be developed.

That estimate, combining the four studies, concluded that there are at least 210,000 preventable adverse events per year that contribute to the death of hospitalized patients, based on evidence found in hospital medical records using the Global Trigger Tool. James also discussed the possibility that this number could reach 400,000 if omissions, failure to make diagnosis, and undetected diagnostic errors are also added into the preventable adverse event formula.

Further research continues to attempt to determine the magnitude of the problem and raises additional questions. A British study by Hogan et al. (2015) found that only 3.6% of inpatient deaths were potentially avoidable, which translates to approximately 26,000 preventable deaths each year in the United States. However, Makary and Daniel (2016) analyzed medical death rate data over an 8-year period and calculated that more than 250,000 deaths per year are due to medical error in the United States. This figure puts death from medical error behind heart disease and cancer, but ahead of respiratory disease.

Now, 20 years after the landmark report from the Health and Medicine Division, *To Err Is Human,* was released, this ongoing debate on the number of deaths per year—98,000, 210,000, or more—attributed to preventable adverse events, the state of quality, and safety in healthcare continues to demand our attention. There is broad agreement that healthcare is more complex, methods to improve healthcare are more challenging, and progress is more elusive than anyone imagined. The problem of preventable harm in healthcare continues to be high on the agenda, and the generation of new evidence to improve the system is critical.

Consumer research and front-page news reveal that public frustrations are growing because of the lack of information on quality of care and blatant examples of healthcare dangers (Consumers Union, 2009; M. Graham et al., 2004; Weingart et al., 2010). Health disparities research suggests that there is uneven distribution of improvements in quality of care, and a decline in performance on many measures, when assessed against minority status (AHRQ, 2009). Patient safety and quality of care research suggests that progress is slow, new problems are emerging, and on many national performance measures, either the quality of care stayed the same or got worse during the past decade (Bates & Singh, 2018; Bogdanich, 2010; The Commonwealth Fund Commission on a High Performance Health System, 2008). Health policy research validates that the costs of poor quality of care are rising, regulatory interests are intensifying, and policy approaches to clinical problems are increasing (Leape, 2010; Woodward et al., 2010). Clearly, accountability for the translation of current and emerging evidence into healthcare practice is one important avenue that all clinicians must espouse.

Why has improvement not gone as expected? The authors of *To Err Is Human* recommended four key strategies to improve the quality of care and safety of patients in the United States:

1. Establish a national focus to create leadership, research, tools, and protocols to increase the knowledge base (science) about safety.
2. Develop a nationwide public mandatory incident reporting system like those used in aviation and other risk-reporting industries, and encourage healthcare organizations and practitioners to develop and participate in voluntary reporting systems to identify and learn from errors.
3. Raise performance standards and expectations for improvements in safety through the actions of oversight organizations, professional groups, and group purchasers of healthcare.
4. Implement safety systems in healthcare organizations to ensure safe practices at the delivery level.

The second Health and Medicine Division report, *Crossing the Quality Chasm*, which assessed the nation's healthcare delivery system falling short in its ability to translate knowledge into practice and apply new technology safely and appropriately, recommended six aims for improvement: that healthcare be safe, timely, effective, efficient, equitable, and patient centered and suggested 10 simple principles to inform efforts to redesign the health system and provide consistent, high-quality healthcare:

1. Care should be based on a continuous healing relationship.
2. Care should be customized according to patient needs and values.
3. The patient is the source of control.
4. Knowledge should be shared and information should flow freely.
5. Decision-making should be evidence based.
6. Safety is a system property.
7. Transparency is necessary.
8. Needs should be anticipated.
9. Waste should be continuously decreased.
10. Cooperation among clinicians must be a priority.

Interest in meeting the recommendations from these landmark reports to provide evidence-based, cost-effective, and accountable care has never been higher, and the stakes have never been greater. Unfortunately, a central, coordinated, national infrastructure to implement quality and safety strategies still does not exist. Clinician safety and quality experts, administrators, and policy makers continue to design strategies to address the Health and Medicine Division's strategies. Institutional and system infrastructure to support their efforts has emerged; yet, the complexity of where and how to approach this challenge can stifle even the most courageous innovator.

Over the past 20 years, national programs have emerged to address safety and quality improvement. The Joint Commission (TJC) established the National Patient Safety Goals (NPSG) program in 2002 to help accredited organizations identify and address areas of concern for patient safety, such as patient safety standards and processes, how to meet performance measures, and how to analyze and learn from sentinel events. The NPSG offers evidence-based quality and safety strategies that focus on identifying patients correctly, improving staff communication, using medications safely, using alarms safely, preventing infection, identifying patient safety risks, and preventing mistakes in surgery (https://www.jointcommission.org/standards_information/npsgs.aspx).

The focus on quality in healthcare has provided the opportunity for many national organizations to develop strategies and measures for healthcare quality. However, as discussed before, there is no one central infrastructure overseeing quality measurement. Evidence-based quality measures are regularly proposed and mandated by both public and private organizations, such as TJC, Centers for Medicare & Medicaid Services (CMS), National Quality Forum (NQF), the AHRQ, and National Committee on Quality Assurance (NCQA), to name a few. Websites with report cards on quality measures abound, and healthcare organizations have developed complex internal infrastructures for data collection and reporting of these measures.

If evidence-based practice is clinical decision-making that integrates the best available scientific evidence with the best available experiential (patient and practitioner) evidence, and considers internal and external influences on practice (Newhouse, Poe, Dearholt, Pugh, & White, 2005), what should be the accountability standard when evidence is scant, clinical expertise is diverse, the system of care delivery is evolving, and patients' needs vary widely? Research to answer these questions is flourishing. The study of the diffusion of innovations in healthcare is increasing exponentially (Greenhalgh, Robert, Macfarlane, Bate, & Kyriakidou, 2004; Rogers, 1995), research on knowledge translation is adding clarity to the phases of moving research evidence into clinical practice, and emerging health services research exploring knowledge-to-action (KTA) translation is gaining attention by practitioners, policy makers, patients, purchasers, and the public (I. D. Graham et al., 2006). Nurses have a pivotal role in keeping patients safe and in narrowing the gap between evidence-based practice and common practice. As administrators, educators, researchers, and bedside clinicians, the mandate for nurses to lead patient safety and quality efforts is here and now.

Thus, in full recognition of the nascent nature of the science, this chapter focuses evidence for improving safety and quality within the context of the Health and Medicine Division's four strategic recommendations and offers practical insights and tools for nurse leaders at all levels of practice. This chapter discusses (a) the national momentum that is moving healthcare from awareness and acknowledgment of quality and patient safety deficits to accountability for quality of care and patient safety outcomes; (b) the importance of viewing healthcare delivery as a science to discover and translate evidence to improve quality and safety; (c) the role of high-reliability organizations in quality and safety improvement efforts; (d) an example of a practical organizing framework used for quality and safety translation initiatives; and (e) several successful innovative patient safety and quality initiatives that have translated evidence into practice for healthcare improvement.

■ QUALITY AND SAFETY MOVEMENT

Analogous to the "perfect storm," it seems that although conditions are finally right for patient safety and quality to actually improve, we are still battling the storm. A critical mass of industry leaders is clearly committed to improving patient safety, is willing to learn from their own mistakes, and, in an unprecedented fashion, is willing to work together to support patient safety research, implementation research, and dissemination research, all with an unwavering focus on improved healthcare delivery. Hope is on the horizon.

The Patient Safety and Quality Improvement Act of 2005 (https://www.hhs.gov/hipaa/for-professionals/patient-safety/statute-and-rule/index.html) was passed after years of debate and revision. The goal was a national law to make it easier for providers to report and learn from medical errors. It took 3 years for the AHRQ to issue the first proposed rules to implement that legislation (February 2008), and the law took effect in 2009. The rules authorized the creation of patient safety organizations (PSOs), which bring groups together to improve patient safety learning by sharing data from voluntary reporting under privacy and confidentiality protections provided in the law (Bates & Singh, 2018). Another national initiative, the Partnership for Patients, coordinated through the CMS is also focusing on preventable harm through its Hospital Improvement Innovation Network.

Public reporting of hospital quality and safety data is increasing in both the United States and abroad. As data are reported, there are new challenges regarding what to report and how to use reported data. Scientific and policy discussions focus on the strength of the evidence for what is reported, whether the reported data are sound and equally important, and whether the reported data are useful to stimulate improvement activity (Battles & Stevens, 2009; Benn et al., 2009; Jha, Orav, & Epstein, 2009; Pham et al., 2010; Rosenthal & Riley, 2001; Rothberg, Morsi, Benjamin, Pekow, & Lindenauer, 2008).

Accrediting bodies developed standards highlighting the importance of and delineating accountability for quality and safety within hospitals (NQF, 2005). TJC reports that although compliance with its safety goals and standards is high, there has been limited change in the safety outcomes that it monitors (https://www.jointcommission.org/standards_information/npsgs.aspx). However, it continues to refine standards and safety goals, align them with emerging evidence, and enlist the support of scientific partners and professional societies in a model of collaborative effort that is novel and promising (Farrell, 2009; TJC, 2008).

The NQF's mission is to improve the quality of American healthcare. It uses a consensus development process to bring together stakeholders around specific areas of practice and to develop and endorse standards that can be used to measure and publicly report healthcare quality. This set of endorsed measures focuses on healthcare processes, outcomes, patient perceptions, and organizational structure and/or systems that are associated with the ability to provide high-quality healthcare. It currently has over 600 consensus standards that are updated every 2 years and new ones proposed (www.qualityforum.org/Measuring_Performance/Measuring_Performance.aspx).

Industry quality leaders, such as the Institute for Healthcare Improvement (IHI), continue to shine a light on pressing quality and safety issues (Batalden & Davidoff, 2007; Berwick, 2009; Conway, 2008), encourage providers to become more efficient and effective (Berwick, 2003), and provide a forum for quality improvement, patient safety education, and training at all levels within healthcare, from board members to frontline staff. Business groups such as Leapfrog (www.leapfroggroup.org) are aligning their standards for hospital performance with industry efforts such as reducing central line-associated bloodstream infection (CLABSI). Perhaps most important, health policy leaders are also on board, and the recent health policy reform legislation has specific language and provisions to expedite improvement. The Patient-Centered Outcomes Research Act of 2009 sets the stage for consideration of health delivery as a science.

Finally, the most significant development in the national momentum for patient safety and quality is the U.S. Department of Health and Human Services's (HHS) National Quality Strategy. The National Quality Strategy, led by the AHRQ, was mandated by the Affordable Care Act and is a major step toward a national quality and safety infrastructure (AHRQ, 2015a; www.ahrq.gov/workingforquality/about.htm#aims). The National Quality Strategy pursues three broad aims, referred to as the *Triple Aim*:

1. Better care: Improve the overall quality by making healthcare more patient centered, reliable, accessible, and safe.
2. Healthy people/healthy communities: Improve the health of the U.S. population by supporting proven interventions to address behavioral, social, and environmental determinants of health in addition to delivering higher quality care.
3. Affordable care: Reduce the cost of quality healthcare for individuals, families, employers, and government.

The National Quality Strategy focuses on six priorities: (a) making care safer by reducing harm caused in the delivery of care; (b) ensuring that each person and family is engaged as partners in their care; (c) promoting effective communication and coordination of care; (d) promoting the most effective prevention and treatment practices for the leading causes of mortality, starting with cardiovascular disease; (e) working with communities to promote wide use of best practices to enable healthy living; and (f) making quality care more affordable for individuals, families, employers, and governments by developing and spreading new healthcare delivery models. The CMS (2015), as a part of the National Quality Strategy, has developed a CMS Quality Strategy that uses quality initiatives to mandate public reporting, pay for reporting, and quality improvement. The CMS and the NQF work collaboratively on quality measures.

The efforts are aligning, the momentum is building, and the potential is real. There is a significant opportunity for nurses to be involved in these efforts to lead the transformation, or it is doomed to falter. No other discipline is closer to the core work, regardless of the setting, the patient population, and the delivery model.

HEALTHCARE DELIVERY AS A SCIENCE

Patient safety and quality practices are mired in traditional and often archaic systems of healthcare delivery. Until recently, funding for U.S. healthcare research focused almost entirely on discovering disease mechanisms and identifying new therapies with minimal investments in analyzing how to get those discoveries disseminated and translated safely and effectively into the healthcare of our patients. Correcting this failure requires viewing healthcare delivery as a science. This involves conducting rigorous scientific research on methods to improve healthcare delivery that produces hard evidence for improvement, with clear and measurable results. Only then will it be possible to summarize this evidence into clear recommendations for evidence-based healthcare practices; develop measures; monitor performance with valid, reliable data; hold clinicians and administrators accountable for the outcomes; and set explicit national improvement targets. Until now, even when research revealed effective methods to improve patient safety and quality of care, the lack of a national infrastructure to disseminate the knowledge broadly, study its uptake and translation, and evaluate its generalizability through rigorous measurement was an almost insurmountable barrier to progress.

As discussed previously, a major challenge to improvement in quality and safety of healthcare is the measurement of that improvement. The healthcare system's capacity to monitor progress in quality and safety efforts is growing and improving, but there is still limited capacity to inform the public or clinicians about the success of our efforts to make patient care safer. The attributes of quality measures are generally well accepted; they need to be valid, important, usable, and feasible.

Validity

Validity refers to whether a study is able to answer the questions it scientifically intends to answer. There are many types of validity, and they warrant deep understanding and discussion as standards and measures take shape (Berenholtz et al., 2007). For the purposes of evidence for quality and patient safety, it is most important to understand that, without a scientific approach to quality and safety improvements, the risk is that erroneous conclusions may be drawn from projects, providers may think improvements have occurred when they have not, unintended consequences may occur, and consumers will have no legitimate way to *choose quality* (Pronovost, Goeschel, & Wachter, 2008; Pronovost, Miller, & Wachter, 2007).

Data Quality Control

Regardless of the type of performance measure, data quality control has received relatively little attention. The limited literature examining data quality control in quality and patient safety studies raises substantial concern. Policy makers, hospital leaders, and clinicians make important decisions based on the assumption that quality-improvement project results are accurate. Quality-control methods are critical to help ensure the accuracy of any effort to collect, analyze, and report data (Needham et al., 2009).

Prioritizing Quality-Improvement Targets

Problems in healthcare are immense and resources are limited. It is crucial to prioritize what we measure and what resources we commit to measuring both clinical performance and patient outcomes. The number of measures for mandated reporting is growing exponentially with seemingly little consideration of what is important. Although there are attempts to prioritize quality-improvement targets (the NQF Quality Partners is one strategy), much more needs to be done in this regard. Systematic ways to prioritize national quality measurement incorporating both prediction models of disease burden and risk mitigation models need to be developed. Tools and methods that are successful in other industries, such as aviation, may be applicable.

Usable Measures

The current method of providing national measures of performance that is a high-level surrogate for actual performance is viewed critically by many clinicians, who favor quality metrics that are collected locally and have local face validity. National surrogate measures do not allow the public to evaluate local quality, and unique local measures do not allow consumers to make an informed choice about their provider and to *comparison shop*. Ideally, measures should be scalable, and the ultimate unit of measure should be the patient, clinician, or patient care area. Once these measures are developed and implemented, they may be aggregated to provide hospital, health system, state, and national information.

Feasibility

Once measures are developed, there are undeniable challenges to the feasibility of collecting data to monitor progress. There are strong trade-offs between manual-based data collection and the opposite extreme of using discharge data collection that, although feasible, suffers from lack of validity. New data-mining strategies using advanced information technologies offer huge potential to close this gap. Quality and patient safety scientists will need to consider how to achieve standardized definitions of preventable harms and ways to incorporate the data elements into electronic medical records, easing the burden of manual data collection without forfeiting the validity of the measures used to monitor progress. Such solutions will present both operational and policy challenges. For example, this will likely require joint documentation between nurses and physicians, one of many changes in historical practice patterns that nurse and physician leaders will need to embrace to enhance patient safety. In addition, organizations will need to pay for the investment of clinical time into development of information technologies. Without that investment, there is a potential that hospitals may "automate" ineffective paper and delivery system processes.

The healthcare industry is moving forward and there are many successes to be celebrated. However, the challenges to showing improvements in healthcare quality and safety remain. The translation of evidence-based practices into the routines of healthcare providers and organizations must continue to evolve. Not all harm is preventable, so it is crucial that patient safety and quality efforts focus on the use of evidence-based interventions and systems of care that are designed to prevent harm. There is growing recognition that healthcare leaders must be accountable for the patient safety and quality of care; however, basic standards, common taxonomy, and uniform quality and safety reporting requirements are needed.

■ HIGH-RELIABILITY ORGANIZATIONS

High-reliability organizations are organizations that operate in complex, high-hazard domains for extended periods of time without serious accidents or catastrophic failures (AHRQ, 2015b; https://psnet.ahrq.gov/primers/primer/31/high-reliability). A classic example of high reliability is seen in the military aircraft carrier: despite significant production pressures (aircrafts take off and land every 48–60 seconds), constantly changing conditions, and a hierarchical organizational structure, all personnel associated with the aircraft carrier consistently prioritize safety and have both the authority and the responsibility to make real-time operational adjustments to always maintain safe operations as the top priority. The concept of high reliability has been receiving increasing attention in healthcare because of the complexity of healthcare operations and the risk for significant catastrophic consequences when failures occur. The frequency and severity of failures in healthcare stand in sharp contrast to the safety successes that industries outside healthcare have achieved and sustained. Commercial air travel, nuclear power, and even amusement parks are other examples (Chassin & Loeb, 2013; Weick & Sutcliffe, 2007). Applying the principles and lessons learned from other high-reliability organizations and industries may enable hospitals and the healthcare industry to improve their record on quality and safety.

High reliability is best described as a condition of persistent mindfulness of relentless prioritization of safety and quality over other performance measures (Weick & Sutcliffe, 2007). High-reliability organizations have five characteristic ways of thinking: preoccupation with failure; reluctance to simplify explanations for operations, successes, and failures; sensitivity to operations (situation awareness); deference to frontline expertise; and commitment to resilience (Weick & Sutcliffe, 2007).

Chassin and Loeb (2013) synthesized the literature on high reliability and proposed a framework that involves three key domains for hospitals to focus on to achieve high reliability: leadership engagement, development of a robust safety culture, and use of effective process-improvement tools.

■ AN INNOVATIVE FRAMEWORK FOR PATIENT QUALITY AND SAFETY IMPROVEMENT

Systematic processes used to translate evidence to improve quality and safety in healthcare are needed. One way to approach implementation and dissemination of evidence is through the use of frameworks or models for translation. Several models that have been developed specifically for quality and safety improvements are discussed.

The Comprehensive Unit-Based Safety Program

The Comprehensive Unit-Based Safety Program (CUSP) uses an iterative approach to improve a unit's teamwork and safety culture. Root-cause analyses of medical-error events identify the lack of teamwork as a contributing factor, and TJC (2015) sentinel events reports cite poor communication. The CUSP has been associated with teamwork and safety culture improvements (Timmel et al., 2010). The CUSP empowers frontline staff to identify and focus their efforts to improve safety problems in their local work environments and also provides a structure to improve safety throughout a hospital.

The CUSP involves five steps (AHRQ, 2015c; www.ahrq.gov/professionals/education/curriculum-tools/cusptoolkit/modules/learn/index.html):

1. Educate on the science of safety.
2. Identify defects in care.
3. Assign executive leaders to a unit-level CUSP team.
4. Learn from one defect per month.
5. Implement tools, such as teamwork and communication, to improve safety in the work environment and develop a safety culture.

Step 1 aims to educate about the science of safety through a short training video and group discussions. The learning objectives of the science of safety are to (a) accept that safety is part of the work system, (b) appreciate the basic attributes of safe design (standardize work, develop independent checks for important processes, and learn from mistakes) and recognize that these attributes apply to technical work and adaptive work, and (c) understand that interdisciplinary teams make wiser decisions because they have diverse and independent input.

Step 2 invites staff to identify "how the next patient will be harmed." It is important to introduce this after most staff members have completed the science of safety training. Generally, the nurse manager or the CUSP team leader facilitates the process, which includes all unit staff, as well as physicians and support staff members who frequent the unit (not just nurses). The two-question survey (How is the next patient likely to be harmed on our unit? and What ideas do you have that might reduce this risk?) is distributed at a staff meeting or placed in mailboxes, and a survey dropbox is provided for this activity, so that the responses may be candid and anonymous. The team leader compiles the results and shares them at a CUSP team meeting. The team decides which safety hazards pose the greatest threat and develops a plan to work on those hazards first.

Step 3 requires the CEO to assign a senior hospital leader as a member of each unit-level CUSP project team. The senior leader meets monthly with the team, reviews hazards identified in step 2, participates in the process to select improvement priorities, helps secure the resources and institutional support needed so that the team can proceed with its plan, and then holds the team accountable for following through on the plan (Pronovost et al., 2004).

Step 4 teaches the teams to learn, not merely recover, from mistakes. Using a simple, structured tool, the teams investigate defects in care (Pronovost et al., 2006). The tool prompts users to answer what happened, why it happened, what they did to reduce the risk, and whether their actions actually reduced this risk. The completed one-page written summary of the investigation is shared widely. This helps focus opportunities. For example, some teams discovered that stocking of the central-line cart was erratic and needed a defined protocol and audit process. Other teams identified that staff did not always follow central- line maintenance procedures. These lessons prompted other teams to check their local practice.

Step 5 encourages teams to try tools to improve communication and teamwork. The daily-goals checklist is one of the first tools many teams try because it is clearly patient safety focused (Holzmueller, Timmel, Kent, Schulick, & Pronovost, 2009; Schwartz, Nelson, Saliski, Hunt, & Pronovost, 2008). The checklist starts and finishes with a patient focus rather than a nursing or medical focus. It asks: What patient safety risks does this patient face? How can we mitigate them? and What do we (the caregiver team) need to do today to move this patient to the next level of care? Completed during interdisciplinary rounds, the team creates the daily-goals form collectively, so that all staff members (including nurses, doctors, therapists) understand the plan and their discipline-specific responsibility to implement the plan (AHRQ, 2015c; www.ahrq.gov/professionals/education/curriculum-tools/cusptoolkit/toolkit/index.html; www.hopkinsmedicine.org/innovation_quality_patient_care/areas_expertise/improve_patient_safety/cusp).

Learning Collaboratives

In 1995, the IHI developed a model to achieve what they called "breakthrough improvement" (IHI, 2003) and has continued to improve healthcare while containing or reducing costs through the Breakthrough Collaborative Series (2013). The vision of the Breakthrough Series is that sound science exists to improve the costs and outcomes of current healthcare practices; but unfortunately, there is a gap between what we know and what we do. The Breakthrough Series seeks to help organizations create structures to learn from each other and recognizes experts in topic areas where improvements are needed.

The collaborative strategy for improvement has become a common model for supporting quality- improvement efforts by bringing people together to work collaboratively on a shared improvement goal. The collaborative model uses human factor engineering techniques and other behavioral approaches to improve translation of evidence into practice. A *collaborative* is a group of practitioners from different sites who meet periodically to learn change ideas and quality methods and to exchange their experiences in making changes (Ovreitveit, 2002).

The core components of a collaborative approach are a shared and agreed-upon important problem; an evidence-based and proven solution; support from executive leadership; and interprofessional teams of workers who are brought together to learn, share, and implement the change. Ovreitveit (2002) reviewed the collaborative experiences of the United States, the United Kingdom, and the Nordic countries and suggested 10 tips on how to run an effective collaborative, which are still applicable today:

1. Choose a subject for which the specific methods, if implemented, can be effective.
2. Define and agree on the purpose of the collaborative prior to implementation, so that those interested can decide whether to participate.
3. Agree on the roles and expectations of participants, including time, resources, and efforts that would need to be devoted to implementing the change.
4. Agree on challenging but achievable and clear targets that are easily and objectively measureable.
5. Prepare to hit the ground running at the first meeting by sending out materials and checklists ahead of time to allow the participants to prepare for the first meeting. This will allow for teams to consider how the change can be adapted to their local setting and also understand the requirements of participating.
6. Organize and run meetings effectively and provide for carefully designed communication between the meetings.
7. Agree on the data to be collected, use existing data whenever possible, and develop skills to plan and carry out the appropriate data collection and analysis.
8. Focus the team on developing change-management skills in order to be successful.
9. Sustain the changes to survive the individual's learning, which is the foundation of continuous improvement.
10. Learn skills and share quality methods and change ideas. This can be done by both structured opportunities for exchanging ideas and facilitating informal communication among collaborative members.

Collaboratives, if run well, can be a cost-effective method for improvement and implementing a large-scale and agreed-upon practice change. The interaction to achieve mutual learning that occurs with the collaborative and the support and motivation from experts has been shown to have a tremendous impact on healthcare providers and on developing stakeholder buy-in to translate evidence and best practices into the healthcare setting (Clancy, Margolis, & Miller, 2013). A few examples of current and successful learning collaboratives are discussed in the next section.

■ TRANSLATION EXEMPLARS OF EVIDENCE TO PRACTICE FOR QUALITY AND SAFETY IN HEALTHCARE

Stop BSI: A National and International Exemplar for Patient Safety and Quality Improvement

Infections that patients develop while receiving care in a healthcare setting for another condition are termed *healthcare-associated infections (HAIs)*. HAIs occur in healthcare settings everywhere throughout the world, affecting hundreds of millions of patients each year and are generally considered preventable. HAI prevention is one of the 20 "priority areas" identified in the Health and Medicine Division's 2003 report *Transforming Health Care Quality*. CLABSIs are one type of HAI. CLABSI is a primary laboratory-confirmed bloodstream infection in a patient with a central line at the time of or within 48 hours prior to the onset of symptoms and the infection is not related to an infection from another site. Umscheid et al. (2011) estimated that as many as 65% to 70% of CLABSIs may be preventable with the implementation of evidence-based strategies. Over the past 15 years, many countries, regions, organizations, and professional groups throughout the world have developed evidence-based clinical practice guidelines (CPGs) pertaining to the prevention of CLABSIs. There is high-level evidence to translate into practice to prevent these central-line infections to improve quality of care.

In the United States, a program aimed to reduce CLABSIs using a unit-based method that implemented an evidence-based care strategy was developed by the Johns Hopkins University Quality and Safety Research Group (QSRG). This translation of evidence to practice had significant results in eliminating CLABSIs. After success at the Johns Hopkins Hospital (JHH), a statewide initiative of more than 100 ICU teams in Michigan used the model and achieved a 66% reduction in CLABSI and a median CLABSI rate of 0 (Pronovost et al., 2006). The mandate to spread the "On the CUSP: Stop BSI" program that the research demonstrated was effective at JHH and in more than 100 ICUs in Michigan, was stimulated by public pressure (Faber, Bosch, Wollersheim, Leatherman, & Grol, 2009), political pressure, and private pressure via philanthropic donations specifically earmarked to replicate the work in other states. Thus far, the teams have sustained these improvements for more than 4 years (Pronovost et al., 2010). Together, those pressures contributed to a national improvement target issued by the HHS and an AHRQ-funded national collaborative. The collaborative aimed to have all hospitals in every state in the country, the District of Columbia, and Puerto Rico reduce CLABSIs to the levels achieved in Michigan and to have sound data to demonstrate the improvement. The progress in the United States and worldwide has been significant in reducing CLABSIs and points to their preventability, translating evidence-based strategies into daily routines of patient care. The World Health Organization (WHO) is working with the JHH team to implement the program throughout England and Spain. The Spanish project, called the *Bacteremia Zero Project*, was successful in reducing the incidence of CLABSIs by approximately 50% in 192 ICUs in Spain between 2008 and 2010.

Statewide Collaborative to Reduce Environmental Surface Contamination in Healthcare Settings

Over the past decade, a growing body of evidence suggests that contamination of environmental surfaces throughout healthcare facilities plays an important role in the transmission of key healthcare-associated pathogens, including methicillin-resistant *Staphylococcus aureus* (MRSA), vancomycin-resistant *Enterococcus* (VRE), *Clostridium difficile* (C. diff.), *Acinetobacter*, and norovirus. Evidence suggests that environmental contamination contributes to HAIs through a variety of pathways, including contamination of hands and transfer of pathogens from patients, visitors, and healthcare workers. The Centers for Disease Control and Prevention (CDC) has recommended that all healthcare facilities develop programs to optimize the thoroughness of high-touch surface cleaning and use a monitoring system to ensure that healthcare facilities are being cleaned to standards and policies set forth by the management.

The Maryland Patient Safety Center convened Maryland hospitals, long-term care facilities, and ambulatory care centers to develop the Clean Collaborative, an initiative to improve facility cleanliness as a means of reducing HAIs. The goal of the Clean Collaborative was to identify best management practices (BMPs) for cleaning and disinfecting surface areas; to educate and promote BMPs via webinars, factsheets, and a scholarly dissemination; improve cleanliness of the facility; and reduce the incidence of facility-acquired MRSA, VRE and C. diff. (www.marylandpatientsafety.org/CleanCollaborative.aspx). The collaborative selected an adenosine triphosphate (ATP) monitoring validation technology system to measure cleaning effectiveness and created a web-based portal for inputting participant data. It developed a list of sampling locations and protocols for collecting samples in patient rooms and public areas based on industry guidelines and trained participants (Solomon et al., 2018).

The results of this statewide evidence-based collaborative were significant. Twenty-one of the 24 participating facilities (88%) achieved a 10% reduction in relative light units (RLUs) from the baseline. Even more impressive was that 75% of the facilities exceeded this goal by reducing the RLUs by more than 50%. In addition, the facilities participating in the Clean Collaborative achieved a 14.2% decrease in C. diff. rates compared to only a 5.9% decrease during the same time period among nonparticipating facilities (Solomon et al, 2018).

Surviving Sepsis: A National and International Campaign to Improve Quality Care

The Surviving Sepsis Campaign (SSC), a joint collaboration of the Society of Critical Care Medicine and the European Society of Intensive Care Medicine, began in 2002 with the stated goal of reducing mortality worldwide from severe sepsis and septic shock by 25% in 5 years using a seven-point evidence-based agenda, including:

1. Building awareness of sepsis
2. Improving diagnosis
3. Increasing the use of appropriate treatment
4. Educating healthcare professionals
5. Improving post-ICU care
6. Developing guidelines of care
7. Implementing a performance improvement program (Surviving Sepsis Campaign: International, 2015)

The campaign has launched a quality-improvement initiative to increase early recognition and treatment of sepsis in patients on hospital medical, surgical, and telemetry units worldwide. *Septicemia*, commonly referred to as *sepsis*, is a serious blood infection that triggers a cascading, whole-body inflammatory response that, if left untreated, can rapidly lead to progressive organ failure, shock, and death. Most often caused by bacteria or bacterial toxins in the bloodstream (bacteremia with sepsis), more than 1 million cases of septicemia are reported in the United States each year. Costs of septicemia treatment are high, with total hospital costs estimated to be more than $24 billion in 2007. Despite resources incurred in treatment, an estimated 25% to 50% of patients succumb to this condition, making septicemia the 10th leading cause of death in the United States (Sutton & Friedman, 2013). It is one of the most common healthcare-associated complications, which is potentially preventable by implementing evidence-based guidelines for care (Dellinger et al., 2013; Figure 5.1).

Patient Engagement:An Evidence-Based Approach to Enhancing Health Quality and Safety

There is a growing body of evidence that supports the belief that patients who are actively involved in their healthcare experience better health outcomes and lower costs of healthcare, which are surrogate measures of healthcare quality and two of the aims of the triple aim of the CMS for quality healthcare. Patient engagement has publicly been referred to as one way to meet the triple aim: to improve health outcomes, to provide better patient care, and to lower costs. Consequently, many healthcare organizations are currently involved in developing and implementing evidence-based strategies to increase patient engagement in healthcare. "Patient activation" refers to a patient's knowledge, skills, ability, and willingness to manage his or her own health and care, but what is this new concept of patient engagement? Patient engagement is a broader term that combines patients' willingness to be involved with specific interventions that increase their positive health behaviors. The American Institute for Research proposed a framework to translate evidence – the use of evidence-based interventions – to increase patient engagement (Carman et al., 2013; see Exhibit 1 in www.healthaffairs.org/doi/10.1377/hlthaff.2012.1133).

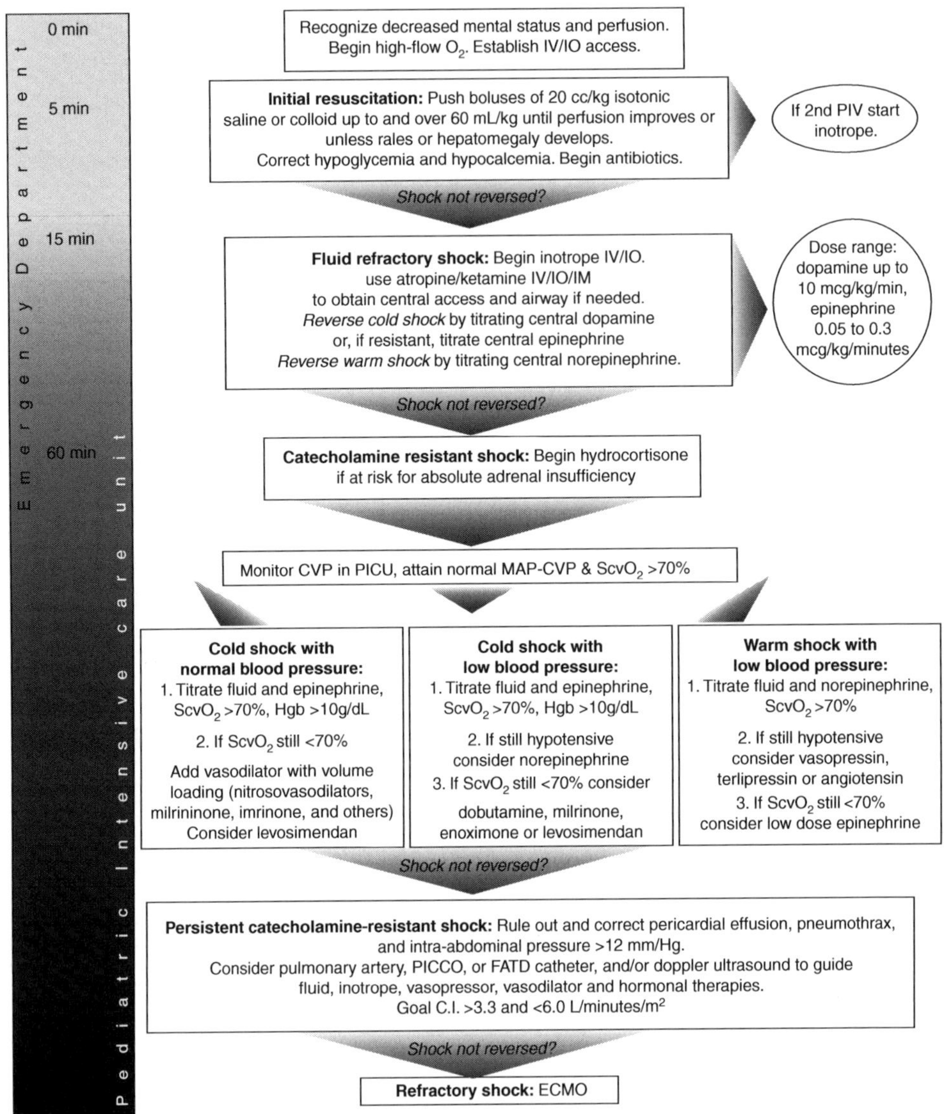

FIGURE 5.1 Evidence-based guidelines for care in the prevention of septicemia.

CI, confidence interval; CVP, central venous pressure; ECMO, extracorporeal membrane oxygenation; FATD, femoral artery thermodilution; Hgb, hemoglobin; IM, intramuscular; IO, intraosseous; IV, intravenous; MAP, mean arterial pressure; PICCO, pulse contour cardiac output; PICU, pediatric intensive care unit; PIV, peripheral intravenous line; $Scvo_2$, central venous oxygen saturation.

Source: Reproduced from Brierley, J., Carcillo, J., Choong, K., Cornell, T., Decaen, A., Deymann, A., . . . Zuckerberg, A. (2009). Clinical practice parameters for hemodynamic support of pediatric and neonatal septic shock: 2007 update from the American College of Critical Care Medicine. *Critical Care Medicine*, *37*, 666–688.

The first level of the framework deals with direct patient care. It suggests that patients should receive information about their healthcare problems and freely discuss healthcare choices and preferences with their providers. As is clearly seen from this level of interaction, patients are able to combine this access to current available evidence with their healthcare preferences to increase the quality of and their satisfaction with the provider's clinical judgment and plan of care. Evidence-based interventions used for these interactions include patient portals, email, social media, and electronic tracking for both health and wellness. This level of interaction and engagement by patients with their providers is a major goal of many healthcare reform initiatives, such as meaningful use, the patient-centered medical home, and accountable care organizations. Patient engagement strategies make good business sense. Patients want access to their medical records, appointment scheduling, prescription refills, and after-hours messaging with their providers.

In the second level of the framework, patient engagement is enhanced by organizational design and evidence-based administrative practices. Healthcare organizations reach out to patients to "engage" them to offer input concerning their healthcare needs and preferences. This is aimed at increasing satisfaction with the response to needs and provision of care and services that are desired but occur at the organizational level. Again, use of certain evidence-based strategies makes good business sense by improving efficiency, lowering costs, and increasing consumer satisfaction with the healthcare organization in a very competitive healthcare industry.

As consumers' responsibilities for their healthcare and its costs continue to increase, they will demand more transparency, access to quality and safety data, and increased satisfaction and convenience. A recent survey of 2,339 U.S. residents by PricewaterhouseCoopers Health Research Institute (HRI) found that:

- More than a quarter of respondents said they would prefer to interact with their provider digitally rather than in person or by telephone.
- Younger consumers found price to be a more important factor in healthcare choices than older consumers, but also valued "trusted advice" more than cost alone.
- Half of the younger consumers said they would choose a lower ranked hospital if it looked modern.
- Forty percent said they would trust a large retailer, such as Target or Wal-Mart, with their healthcare, and nearly as many said they would trust digitally enabled companies such as online retailers.
- Two thirds said they were happy with their core benefits, but only about half were satisfied with their overall healthcare experience.

The report concluded that these data show that the one-size-fits-all service offerings and brand-positioning strategies of healthcare providers and organizations are over. The report went on to say that value propositions throughout healthcare must be tailored to the consumer, and patient engagement strategies are a promising avenue.

The last level of the framework aims the responsibility for patient engagement strategies at the policy- making level. At this level, consumer input is once again sought, but to meet community and population health needs and to guide funding decisions and representation on policy-making groups and committees that advise resource allocation decisions. The policy makers at this level of the framework may be involved in the organizations, systems of care, governmental agencies, and/or broader societal regulation.

■ CONCLUSIONS

This chapter has discussed translation of evidence for safety and quality in healthcare, including the underwhelming state of progress made since *To Err Is Human* was published and the challenges we currently face, and has provided innovative exemplars of translation efforts to improve healthcare. There are many other examples, and the focus on patient safety and quality demands continued attention from the healthcare team. Nurses, who are integral point-of-care providers and members of that healthcare team, are charged with improving our healthcare system. At this early stage of bringing the science of quality and safety to healthcare delivery, it is critical that above all else, nurses understand the importance of their voice, keep patients as their "North Star," and remember that their efforts to generate new evidence, translate new evidence into practice, and to disseminate these efforts broadly are a commitment to be part of leading the evolutionary process. At this juncture, we are still developing new ways to translate emerging evidence into practice most effectively. We must learn together: nurses, doctors, patients, administrators, and regulators. Every paradigm we have in healthcare came from an age when scientific discovery was slow, the data were patient specific, and we considered many of the most distressing outcomes inevitable. All of that has changed and we must change as well. The future is ours, and although it may seem murky, chaotic, and uncertain, it is rich with the potential for breathtaking progress.

■ REFERENCES

Agency for Healthcare Research and Quality. (2009). *National healthcare disparities report*. Rockville, MD: Author.

Agency for Healthcare Research and Quality. (2010). *Patient safety organizations*. Retrieved from https://pso.ahrq.gov

Agency for Healthcare Research and Quality. (2015a). *National quality strategy*. Retrieved from http://www.ahrq.gov/workingforquality/about.htm#aims

Agency for Healthcare Research and Quality. (2015b). *High reliability*. Retrieved from https://psnet.ahrq.gov/primers/primer/31/high-reliability

Agency for Healthcare Research and Quality. (2015c). *Learn about CUSP*. Rockville, MD: Author. Retrieved from http://www.ahrq.gov/professionals/education/curriculum-tools/cusptoolkit/modules/learn/index.html

Auerbach, A. D., Landefeld, C. S., & Shojania, K. G. (2007). The tension between needing to improve care and knowing how to do it. *New England Journal of Medicine*, *357*(6), 608–613. doi:10.1056/nejmsb070738

Barry, D. R. (2005). Governance: Critical issues for hospital CEOs and boards. *Frontiers of Health Services Management*, *21*(3), 25–29. doi:10.1097/01974520-200501000-00004

Batalden, P. B., & Davidoff, F. (2007). What is "quality improvement" and how can it transform healthcare? *Quality and Safety in Health Care*, *16*(1), 2–3. doi:10.1136/qshc.2006.022046

Bates, D. W., & Singh, H. (2018). Two decades since to err is human: An assessment of progress and emerging priorities in patient safety. *Health Affairs*, *37*(11), 1736–1743. doi:10.1377/hlthaff.2018.0738

Battles, J. B., & Stevens, D. P. (2009). Adverse event reporting systems and safer healthcare. *Quality and Safety in Health Care*, *18*(1), 2. doi:10.1136/qshc.2008.031997

Benn, J., Koutantji, M., Wallace, L., Spurgeon, P., Rejman, M., Healey, A., & Vincent, C. (2009). Feedback from incident reporting: Information and action to improve patient safety. *Quality and Safety in Health Care, 18*(1), 11–21. doi:10.1136/qshc.2007.024166

Berenholtz, S. M., Pronovost, P. J., Ngo, K., Barie, P. S., Hitt, J., Kuti, J. L., . . . Dorman, T. (2007). Developing quality measures for sepsis care in the ICU. *The Joint Commission Journal on Quality and Patient Safety, 33*(9), 559–568. doi:10.1016/s1553-7250(07)33060-2

Berwick, D. M. (2003). Disseminating innovations in health care. *Journal of the American Medical Association, 289*(15), 1969. doi:10.1001/jama.289.15.1969

Berwick, D. M. (2009). What "patient-centered" should mean: Confessions of an extremist. *Health Affairs, 28*(4), w555–w565. doi:10.1377/hlthaff.28.4.w555

Bogdanich, W. (2010, January 23). Radiation offers new cures, and ways to do harm. *The New York Times*. Retrieved from www.nytimes.com/2010/01/24/health/24radiation.html

Brierley, J., Carcillo, J., Choong, K., Cornell, T., Decaen, A., Deymann, A., . . . Zuckerberg, A. (2009). Clinical practice parameters for hemodynamic support of pediatric and neonatal septic shock: 2007 update from the American College of Critical Care Medicine. *Critical Care Medicine, 37*, 666–688.

Callendar, A. N., Hastings, D. A., Hemsley, M. C., Morris, L., & Peregrine, M. W. (2007). *Corporate responsibility and health care quality: A resource for health care boards of directors*. Washington, DC: U.S. Department of Health and Human Services, American Health Lawyers Association.

Carman, K. L., Dardess, P., Maurer, M., Sofaer, S., Adams, K., Bechtel, C., & Sweeney, J. (2013). Patient and family engagement: A framework for understanding the elements and developing interventions and policies. *Health Affairs, 32*(2), 223–231. doi:10.1377/hlthaff.2012.1133

Centers for Medicare & Medicaid Services. (2015). *Quality measures*. Retrieved from https://www.cms.gov/Medicare/Quality-Initiatives-Patient-Assessment-Instruments/QualityMeasures/index.html?redirect=/QUALITYMEASURES

Chassin, M. R., & Loeb, J. M. (2013). High-reliability health care: Getting there from here. *Milbank Quarterly, 92(3)*, 459–490. doi:10.1111/1468-0009.12023

Clancy, C. M. (2009). Ten years after to err is human. *American Journal of Medical Quality, 24*(6), 525–528. doi:10.1177/1062860609349728

Clancy, C. M., Margolis, P. A., & Miller, M. (2013). Collaborative networks for both improvement and research. *Pediatrics, 131*(Suppl.), S210–S214. doi:10.1542/peds.2012-3786h

Commonwealth Fund Commission on a High Performance Health System. (2008). *Why not the best? Results from the national scorecard on U.S. health system performance*. New York, NY: Author.

Consumers Union. (2009). *Healthcare experience and concerns*. Retrieved from http//consumersunion.org/research/healthcare-experience-and-concerns-september-2009

Conway, J. (2008). Getting boards on board: Engaging governing boards in quality and safety. *The Joint Commission Journal on Quality and Patient Safety, 34*(4), 214–220. doi:10.1016/s1553-7250(08)34028-8

Dellinger, R. P., Levy, M. M., Rhodes, A., Annane, D., Gerlach, H., Opal, S. M., . . . Surviving Sepsis Campaign Guidelines Committee including the Pediatric Subgroup. (2013). Surviving sepsis campaign: International guidelines for management of severe sepsis and septic shock: 2012. *Critical Care Medicine, 41*(2), 296–327. doi:10.1097/CCM.0b013e31827e83af

Faber, M., Bosch, M., Wollersheim, H., Leatherman, S., & Grol, R. (2009). Public reporting in health care: How do consumers use quality-of-care information? A systematic review. *Medical Care, 47*(1), 1–8.

Farrell, R. P. (2009). *National patient safety goals for 2009—Universal protocol*. Oakbrook Terrace, IL: Joint Commission Resources.

Goeschel, C. A., Wachter, R. M., & Pronovost, P. J. (2010). Responsibility for quality improvement and patient safety: Hospital board and medical staff leadership challenges. *Chest, 138*(1), 171–178. doi:10.1378/chest.09-2051

Graham, I. D., Logan, J., Harrison, M. B., Straus, S. E., Tetroe, J., Caswell, W., & Robinson, N. (2006). Lost in knowledge translation: Time for a map? *Journal of Continuing Education in the Health Professions, 26*(1), 13–24. doi:10.1002/chp.47

Graham, M., Kubose, T., Jordan, D., Zhang, J., Johnson, T., & Patel, V. (2004). Heuristic evaluation of infusion pumps: Implications for patient safety in intensive care units. *International Journal of Medical Informatics, 73*(11–12), 771–779. doi:10.1016/j.ijmedinf.2004.08.002

Greenhalgh, T., Robert, G., Macfarlane, F., Bate, P., & Kyriakidou, O. (2004). Diffusion of innovations in service organizations: Systematic review and recommendations. *Milbank Quarterly, 82*(4), 581–629. doi:10.1111/j.0887-378x.2004.00325.x

Hogan, H., Zipfel, R., Neuburger, J., Hutchings, A., Darzi, A., & Black, N. (2015). Avoidability of hospital deaths and association with hospital-wide mortality ratios: Retrospective case record review and regression analysis. *British Medical Journal, 351, h3239.*

Holzmueller, C. G., Timmel, J., Kent, P. S., Schulick, R. D., & Pronovost, P. J. (2009). Implementing a team-based daily goals sheet in a non-ICU setting. *The Joint Commission Journal on Quality and Patient Safety, 35*(7), 384–388. doi:10.1016/s1553-7250(09)35054-0

Institute for Healthcare Improvement. (2003). *The breakthrough series: IHI's collaborative model for achieving breakthrough improvement.* Retrieved from http://www.ihi.org/resources/pages/ihiwhitepapers/thebreakthroughseriesihiscollaborativemodelforachievingbreakthroughimprovement.aspx

Institute of Medicine. (1999). In L. T. Kohn, J. M. Corrigan, & M. S. Donaldson (Eds.), *To err is human: Building a safer health system*. Washington, DC: National Academies Press.

Institute of Medicine. (2001). *Crossing the quality chasm: A new health system for the 21st century*. Washington, DC: National Academies Press.

Jha, A. K., Orav, E. J., & Epstein, A. M. (2009). Public reporting of discharge planning and rates of readmissions. *New England Journal of Medicine, 361*(27), 2637–2645. doi:10.1056/nejmsa0904859

Jiang, H. J., Lockee, C., Bass, K., & Fraser, I. (2008). Board engagement in quality: Findings of a survey of hospital and system leaders. *Journal of Healthcare Management, 53*(2), 121–134. doi:10.1097/00115514-200803000-00009

Leape, L., Berwick, D., Clancy, C., Conway, J., Gluck, P., Guest, J., . . . Isaac, T. (2009). Transforming healthcare: A safety imperative. *Quality and Safety in Health Care, 18*(6), 424–428. doi:10.1136/qshc.2009.036954

Leape, L. L. (2010). *Transparency and public reporting are essential for a safe health care system*. The Commonwealth Fund. Retrieved from http://www.commonwealthfund.org/publications/perspectives-on-health-reform-briefs/2010/mar/transparency-and-public-reporting-are-essential-for-a-safe-health-care-system

Makary, M. A., & Daniel, M. (2016). Medical error—The third leading cause of death in the US. *British Medical Journal*, 353, i2139.

McGlynn, E. A., Asch, S. M., Addams, J., Keesey, J., Hicks, J., DeCristofaro, A., & Kerr, E. (2003). The quality of health care delivered to adults in the United States. *New England Journal of Medicine, 348*(26), 2635–2645. doi:10.1056/nejmsa022615

Murray, C. J., & Frenk, J. (2010). Ranking 37th—Measuring the performance of the U.S. health care system. *New England Journal of Medicine, 362*(2), 98–99. doi:10.1056/nejmp0910064

National Quality Forum (NQF). (2005). Hospital governing board and quality of care: A call to responsibility. *Trustee: The Journal for Hospital Governing Boards, 58*(3), 15–18.

Needham, D. M., Sinopoli, D. J., Dinglas, V. D., Berenholtz, S. M., Korupolu, R., Watson, S. R., . . . Pronovost, P. J. (2009). Improving data quality control in quality improvement projects. *International Journal for Quality in Health Care, 21*(2), 145–150. doi:10.1093/intqhc/mzp005

Newhouse, R., Dearholt, S., Poe, S., Pugh, L., & White, K. (2005). Evidence-based practice: A practical approach to implementation. *Journal of Nursing Administration, 35*(1), 35–40. doi:10.1097/00005110-200501000-00013

Ovreitveit, J. (2002). How to run an effective improvement collaborative. *International Journal of Health Care Quality Assurance, 15*(5), 192–196. doi:10.1108/09526860210437403

Patient Safety and Quality Improvement Act of 2005. Retrieved from https://www.hhs.gov/hipaa/for-professionals/patient-safety/statute-and-rule/index.html

Pham, J. C., Colantuoni, E., Dominici, F., Shore, A., Macrae, C., Scobie, S., . . . Pronovost, P. J. (2010). The harm susceptibility model: A method to prioritise risks identified in patient safety reporting systems. *Quality and Safety in Health Care, 19*(5), 440–445.

Pronovost, P. J., Berenholtz, S. M., Goeschel, C. A., Needham, D. M., Sexton, J. B., Thompson, D. A., . . . Hunt, E. (2006). Creating high reliability in healthcare organizations. *Health Services Research, 41*(4 Pt 2), 1599–1617. doi:10.1111/j.1475-6773.2006.00567.x

Pronovost, P. J., Goeschel, C. A., Colantuoni, E., Watson, S., Lubomski, L. H., Berenholtz, S. M., . . . Needham, D. (2010). Sustaining reductions in catheterrelated bloodstream infections in Michigan intensive care units: Observational study. *British Medical Journal, 340*(feb041), c309. doi:10.1136/bmj.c309

Pronovost, P. J., Goeschel, C. A., & Wachter, R. M. (2008). The wisdom and justice of not paying for "preventable complications." *Journal of the American Medical Association, 299*(18), 2197–2199.

Pronovost, P. J., Holzmueller, C. G., Martinez, E., Cafeo, C. L., Hunt, D., Dickson, C., . . . Makary, M. A. (2006). A practical tool to learn from defects in patient care. *The Joint Commission Journal on Quality and Safety, 32*(2), 102–108. doi:10.1016/s1553-7250(06)32014-4

Pronovost, P. J., Miller, M., & Wachter, R. M. (2007). The GAAP in quality measurement and reporting. *Journal of the American Medical Association*, *298*(15), 1800–1802.

Pronovost, P. J., Weast, B., Bishop, K., Paine, L., Griffith, R., Rosenstein, B. J., . . . Davis, R. (2004). Senior executive adopt-a-work unit: A model for safety improvement. *The Joint Commission Journal on Quality and Safety*, *30*(2), 59–68. doi:10.1016/s1549-3741(04)30007-9

Rogers, E. (Ed.). (1995). *Diffusion of innovations* (4th ed.). New York, NY: Free Press.

Rosenthal, J., & Riley, T. (2001). *Patient safety and medical errors: A roadmap for state action*. Portland, ME: National Academy for State Health Policy.

Rothberg, M. B., Morsi, E., Benjamin, E. M., Pekow, P. S., & Lindenauer, P. K. (2008). Choosing the best hospital: The limitations of public quality reporting. *Health Affairs*, *27*(6), 1680–1687. doi:10.1377/hlthaff.27.6.1680

Schwartz, J. M., Nelson, K. L., Saliski, M., Hunt, E. A., & Pronovost, P. J. (2008). The daily goals communication sheet: A simple and novel tool for improved communication and care. *The Joint Commission Journal on Quality and Patient Safety*, *34*(10), 608–613. doi:10.1016/s1553-7250(08)34076-8

Solomon, S. L., Plisko, J. D., Wittig, S. M., Edwards, L. V., Imhoff, R. H., DiPietro, B., & Plisko M. J. (2018). Reducing environmental surface contamination in healthcare settings: A statewide collaborative. *American Journal of Infection Control, 46*(8), e71–e73. doi:10.1016/j.ajic.2018.03.016

Surviving Sepsis Campaign: International. (2015). *About the surviving sepsis campaign*. Retrieved from http://www.survivingsepsis.org/About-SSC/Pages/default.aspx

Sutton, J., & Friedman, B. (2013). *Healthcare cost and utilization project (HCUP), trends in septicemia hospitalizations and readmissions in selected HCUP states, 2005 and 2010* (HCUP Statistical Brief #161). Rockville, MD: Agency for Healthcare Research and Quality. Retrieved from http://www.hcup-us.ahrq.gov/reports/statbriefs/sb161.pdf

The Joint Commission. (2008). *NPSG 02.05.01 standardized approach to hand-offs*. Retrieved from http://www.jointcommission.org/sentinel_event_statistics_quarterly

The Joint Commission. (2015). Sentinel event data: Root causes by event type. Retrieved from http://www.jointcommission.org/sentinel_event.aspx

The Joint Commission. (2019). Retrieved from https://www.jointcommission.org/standards_information/npsgs.aspx).

Timmel, J., Kent, P. S., Holzmueller, C. G., Paine, L. A., Schulick, R. D., & Pronovost, P. J. (2010). Impact of the Comprehensive Unit-based Safety Program (CUSP) on safety culture in a surgical inpatient unit. *The Joint Commission Journal on Quality and Patient Safety*, *36*(6), 252–260. doi:10.1016/s1553-7250(10)36040-5

Umscheid, C. A., Mitchell, M. D., Doshi, J. A., Agarwal, R., Willilams, K., & Brenna, P. J. (2011). Estimating the proportion of healthcare-associated infections that are reasonably preventable and the related mortality and costs. *Infection Control and Hospital Epidemiology*, *32*(2), 101–114. doi:10.1086/657912

Wachter, R. M. (2010). Patient safety at ten: Unmistakable progress, troubling gaps. *Health Affairs, 29*(1), 165–173. doi: 10.1377/hlthaff.2009.0785

Weick, K. E., & Sutcliffe, K. M. (2007). *Managing the unexpected* (2nd ed.). San Francisco, CA: Jossey-Bass.

Weingart, S. N., Toro, J., Spencer, J., Duncombe, D., Gross, A., Bartel, S., . . . Connor, M. (2010). Medication errors involving oral chemotherapy. *Cancer, 116*(10), 2455–2464.

Weissman, J. S., Schneider, E. C., Weingart, S. N., Epstein, A. M., David-Kasdan, J., Feibelmann, S., . . . Gatsonis, C. (2008). Comparing patient-reported hospital adverse events with medical records reviews: Do patients know something that hospitals do not? *Annals of Internal Medicine*, *149(2)*, 100–108. doi:10.7326/0003-4819-149-2-200807150-00006.

Woodward, H. I., Mytton, O. T., Lemer, C., Yardley, I. E., Ellis, B. M., Rutter, P. D., . . . Wu, A. W. (2010). What have we learned about interventions to reduce medical errors? *Annual Review of Public Health*, *31(1)*, 479–497. doi:10.1146/annurev.publhealth.012809.103544

CHAPTER SIX

Translation of Evidence for Leadership

Mary F. Terhaar

Be the fire. Wish for the wind.
—NASEEM TALEB

MUCH HAS CHANGED SINCE THE FIRST AND SECOND EDITIONS of this book were published: The demand for translation is far more pressing and the impact for leadership is more profound. The Triple Aim that challenged healthcare providers and systems to deliver favorable patient outcomes, experience, and value has been expanded to include a fourth aim that emphasizes the vital importance of the quality of life and work experience for the clinicians and staff who provide care (Berwick, Nolan, & Whittington, 2008; Bodenheimer & Sinsky, 2014). The Institute of Medicine's (IOM) charge for professionals to achieve timely translation of evidence; dissolve specialty-based silos; and embrace patient-centered, goal-directed teamwork remains relevant (Institute of Medicine [IOM], 2009; National Academy of Science [NAS], 2017, 2018). More recently, movement toward accountable care has placed the work of healthcare, those who work in the field, and the results achieved under a high-resolution microscope. Together, these conditions create unprecedented opportunity for innovation and leadership, which demands new knowledge, behavior, and effectiveness.

There is urgency to these demands because fee-for-service care is quickly coming to an end. No longer can hospitals and providers receive payment for care delivered to manage consequences of error and treat avoidable sequelae. No longer can hospital days drive revenue. No longer can tertiary treatment by specialists hold as the core of healthcare. The system of healthcare, as we have known it, is an oil rig on fire and it is time to jump from the platform (Robert Wood Johnson Foundation [RWJF], 2013). Jumping from that burning platform requires courage. Some say that the jump will be triggered by fear. It will require a grasp of the conditions that mandate action. For individual clinicians to make the jump, an understanding of the changing reality will be required. For the entire team to jump, strong leadership will be the key.

Accountable leaders rise to the challenges of reducing error (IOM, 2000), achieving true quality (IOM, 2001), and transforming the workplace (IOM, 2004). *To Err Is Human: Building a Safer Health System* (IOM, 2000) directs healthcare as an industry to reduce error in meaningful ways that significantly improve health. *Crossing the Quality Chasm: A New Health System for the 21st Century* (IOM, 2001) calls clinicians, leaders, and administrators to keep patients in the center of and in control of their own care. The same document challenges the professions to deliver on America's investment in research by developing ways to accomplish timely application that improves outcomes. *Keeping Patients Safe: Transforming the Work Environment of Nurses* (IOM, 2004) calls for resolution of the root causes of error and poor quality. With respect to each challenge, evidence can inform the targets set, strategies selected, routine operations, execution of innovations, and evaluation of performance. Leaders need evidence for their practice. For the discipline to act on that evidence, an infrastructure to support such action, and teams that share a commitment to deliver on the Triple Aim of care, quality, and value, are needed (Berwick, 2008). The scholarship that was produced and disseminated to support evidence-based practice and leadership has expanded and penetrated practice settings. More is known about approaches and methods that help gain traction when bringing evidence to inform action (Sandstrom, Borglin, Nilsson, & Willman, 2011; Shea, 2011).

The purpose of this chapter is to present a body of knowledge about leadership that applies to the work of translation. Because culture and environment are addressed in other chapters, the focus here is on the strategies and practices of leaders whose teams engage in translation to achieve the Quadruple Aim, attain professional success, ensure practice excellence, and abandon the burning platform of healthcare as we have known it.

Upon completion of this chapter, the reader will have an understanding of:

1. The most impactful and broadly adopted leadership theories that can be practiced to support translation.
2. A set of evidence-based practices adopted by effective nurse leaders engaged in translation and innovation.

Clinical knowledge generation, transformation, and application have been identified by the NAS as integral to improving health in the United States. The group identified six points as critical for success: data structured for priority action, context-applicable findings, workflow-friendly continuous learning and improvement, strategies for integrating knowledge generation into the business proposition, innovation that enhances efficiency, and patient- and provider-resonant research returns (NAS, 2017). NAS leaders further identified challenges related to finances, infrastructure, moral stress, compassion fatigue, and power and hierarchy among professionals as inflection points for their efforts to improve. Effective leadership is essential to effectively addressing every one of these points across every aspect of healthcare, nursing practice, and successful improvement. Without effective leadership safety is compromised, quality care is unattainable due to plummeting patient satisfaction, costs rise, and talented staff depart for better opportunities (Aiken, Clarke, Sloane, Sochalski, & Silber, 2002).

Because evidence presented throughout this book makes the case for the work of translation and because the leader creates the environment in which translation and innovation can take place, it is important to describe the evidence base for effective leadership practice. Such practice is necessary to create both a culture and a context that will promote and sustain impactful translation and innovation.

Earlier chapters have addressed each of the concerns identified by the NAS. This chapter shifts the focus to understanding the evidence available to inform leadership and support its critical role in translation. This chapter presents the most effective theories to guide leadership and the practices used by leaders to produce positive outcomes. Four such practices are supported by evidence and included as criteria for Magnet Recognition (American Nursing Credentialing Center [ANCC], 2018). These include transformational leadership (previously introduced as a leadership theory); structural empowerment; exemplary professional practice; and knowledge generation, innovation, and improvement.

■ IMPACTFUL AND BROADLY ADOPTED LEADERSHIP THEORIES

Theories serve to describe, explain, and predict. Across all disciplines, they position the user to anticipate, understand, and manage challenges. Among the many leadership theories available, four theories are most commonly practiced and most important to understand. They include transactional, transformational, authentic, and resonant leadership. An overview of these four dominant theories of leadership is presented.

Transactional Leadership

This first theory is included, not because it is effective or evidence based, but because it is common and will form a useful contrast with the theories to follow. One who practices *transactional leadership* operates with a high degree of command and control. This leader provides rules and directions for employees to follow and tolerates little deviation. This constitutes the command function. The transactional leader rewards and punishes followers according to the degree to which they adhere to the rules and directions. This constitutes control. The approach is hierarchal and centralized. It relies on monitoring as well as on specific rewards and sanctions to achieve outcomes (Bass, 1985; Weber, 1947). The transactional leader works with three strategies: contingent reward, active management by exception, and passive management by exception, with each calibrated to employee performance. Power is centralized, rules and contingencies vary, and contingencies are often negatively perceived.

Once the dominant leadership approach *transactional leadership* is recognized as a management theory more precisely than a leadership theory and is receding in its application for many reasons. First, although arguably well suited to mechanistic structures and operations, the approach is becoming increasingly rare. Second, its focus on exchanges that satisfy basic needs on a case-by-case basis is not responsive to the motivations of a knowledge-based workforce. Third, the approach is not consistent with the healthcare environment where a brisk pace of innovation spans all work (Kuhnert & Lewis, 1987). Once considered well suited to industrial work and the military, where consistency was considered the most effective approach to reduce error and cost, transactional leadership had the unintended consequence of suppressing the real-time problem-solving that is essential in today's complex work environments. Finally, transactional leadership is less hospitable to rapid cycle improvement or integration of science into practice on a broad scale.

> *Evidence supports discontinuing transactional leadership, particularly management by exception practices.*
>
> (Cummings et al., 2009)

Transformational Leadership

Transformational leadership is the first of two relational leadership theories that focuses on the follower. It is defined as *the meaningful and creative exchange between leaders and followers to induce vision-driven change in followers* (Bass, 1985). It differs from transactional leadership in important and substantive ways. Transformational leadership is characterized by reciprocal respect and trust, which replaces the rewards and sanctions of transactional leadership. The intent is to make ambitious and transformative accomplishment possible (Bass, 1985).

Transformational leaders demonstrate four dimensions of behavior: inspirational motivation, idealized influence, individualized consideration, and intellectual stimulation. Transformational leaders create the following:

- A sense of confidence and a shared purpose among followers; this is called *inspirational motivation*
- A desire among followers to emulate their approach; this charismatic quality is called *idealized influence*
- A feeling that one's goals and aspirations are important and connected to the leader's mission and purpose; this inclusive and personal leadership feature is called *individualized consideration*
- A value for autonomy and innovation among individual team members, which creates a sense of challenge and personal success; this feature is called *intellectual stimulation*

Transformational leaders model positive behaviors that followers emulate and connect individuals to the overarching mission of the organization and its underlying values (Nguyen et al., 2017). Regardless of the organization in which they lead, transformational leaders inspire and motivate, encourage critical thinking and risk taking, connect personal and organizational values, and strive to satisfy needs of individual followers (Judge & Piccolo, 2004). Being big-picture thinkers with grand visions, transformational leaders are recognized for their charisma and for their impact on both the energy and the creativity of their teams (Mhatre & Riggio, 2014).

The currency of the transformational leader is the connection to followers and work with personal values and purpose. The result is improved outcomes on many levels and in many contexts (Deinert et al., 2015). In the context of extreme stress, as in military deployment, transformational leadership contributes to a sense of embeddedness and commitment, which has been associated with reduced intent to leave (Eberly, Bluhm, Guarana, Avoliod, & Hannahe, 2017). This same sense of embeddedness, belonging, and commitment is significant for followers in other contexts considered to be extreme, such as fire-fighting and nursing, where transformational leadership contributes to retention, engagement, and problem solving (Fairholm, 2001; Niessen, Mädera, Strideb, & Jimmieson, 2017).

Transformational leadership emphasizes relationships over tasks (Cummings et al., 2010). It has more ambitious goals that include satisfaction, career development, collaboration, and well-being. Transformational leadership focuses on the apex rather than the base of Maslow's hierarchy (Groff-Paris & Terhaar, 2011). It focuses on self-actualization of the profession and in those who practice it.

The outcomes of such leadership are many and meaningful. It has been found to impact patients and staff alike. With respect to patients, transformational leadership has been correlated to quality of care and satisfaction (Casida & Pinto-Zipp, 2008) and to reduced adverse events and satisfaction (Wong & Cummings, 2007) and has been linked to the effective management of knowledge (Gowin, Henagan, & McFadden, 2009). With respect to nurses, transformational leadership has been associated with increased satisfaction and retention, engagement and empowerment, commitment, and self-efficacy (Failla & Stichler, 2008; Weberg, 2010). Nurses whose leaders practice using a transformational approach report greater autonomy and performance, satisfaction with leadership, recognition of extra effort in their work, and a sense of availability and presence (Anthony et al., 2005; Cowden, Cummings, & Profetto-McGrath, 2011; Gentry, Weber, & Sadri, 2008; Laschinger, Finegan, & Wilk, 2009; Rosengren, Athlin, & Segesten, 2007; Sellgren, Ekval, & Tomson, 2006).

Evidence supports the practice of transformational leadership, including four key leader behaviors:

1. *inspirational motivation*
2. *idealized influence*
3. *individualized consideration*
4. *intellectual stimulation*

(Bass, 1985)

Authentic Leadership

Authentic leadership is a theory that developed at "the intersection of the leadership, ethics, and positive organizational behavior and scholarship literatures" (Walumbwa, Avolio, Gardner, Wersning, & Peterson, 2008, p. 92).

Authentic leaders are self-aware, have an internalized moral compass, process information in a balanced way, and act with transparency in their relationships (Banks, Davis McCauley, Gardner, & Guler, 2016). Because they are open to close relationships with others, including followers, authentic leaders are experienced by their followers as behaving in ways that are consistent with their personal beliefs and values. Followers report feeling greater connection with their own values, motives, and goals (Luthans & Aviolo, 2003; Walumbwa et al., 2008).

In the workplace, creating consistency and transparency between what one communicates and what actions one takes contributes to a positive environment in which individuals are successful, productive, and satisfied. These are the strengths of the authentic leader (Walumbwa et al., 2008). These core practices of transparency, authenticity, and consistency are essential to follower productivity and satisfaction. Less likely than transformational leaders to be charismatic, authentic leaders connect with individuals with a focus on strengths and the result is reciprocity in relationships and talent development that adds value for the individual and the mission (K. S. Cameron, Dutton, Quinn, & Wrzensniewski, 2003; Cooper & Nelson, 2006).

The practice of authentic leadership has been associated with important outcomes, including followers' satisfaction with both their job and their leader, improved job performance, increased organizational citizenship, higher group performance, and favorable evaluation of leader effectiveness (Banks et al., 2016).

Resonant Leadership

Resonant leaders are self-aware and emotionally intelligent. They care for themselves, which strengthens their capacity to lead others. They consistently practice with mindfulness, hope, and compassion for themselves and their followers (Boyatzis & McKee, 2005). These practices increase the potential and capacity of individual followers and the team as a whole.

The resonant leader is *mindful*. This leader is aware of her or his own values and motivations and equally aware of the values and motivations of the members of her or his team. This mindfulness helps to create connections between individuals and the work. It is also useful to monitor the energy of the team and to balance demands with resources.

The resonant leader is *hopeful*. This leader creates an optimistic environment in which positivity is contagious and yields results for the individuals, the team, and the organization.

The resonant leader is *compassionate*. There is a focus on service to and support of each individual member of the team. Just as the leader attends to his or her own balance and personal resources, this leader attends in the same mindful way to the needs and resources of the individual members of his or her team.

The significant demands of leadership, which increasingly focus on service as well as on productivity, can, in the absence of the counterbalance of self-care, lead to discouraged, ineffective, depleted leadership. Such depleted leadership compromises the culture and climate as well as the success of followers and overall achievement of the mission. A leader may lean in to the work, invest long hours, apply dramatic effort, and expect followers to do the same. Although this pattern of behavior can produce favorable results in the short term, it is unsustainable over the long term and yields diminishing returns across multiple challenges in rapid sequence. Such a downward spiral has been labeled *sacrifice syndrome*. Unchecked, it results in dissonance and diminution, which permeate the entire work unit and organization (Boyatzis & McKee, 2005).

Alternatively, these same leadership demands can be counteracted by a *cycle of renewal*. Renewal involves self-care practices, which are key to leadership success. The leader's practice of renewal models the practice for followers. More important, its effectiveness is evident in the leader's performance and buoys the performance of the entire group.

> Effective leaders attend to their own physical, mental, and emotional renewal by consistently practicing the following:
>
> 1. Mindfulness
> 2. Hope
> 3. Compassion
>
> (Boyatzis & McKee, 2005)

Context for Application of Leadership Theory

One might expect that relational leadership approaches (transformational and authentic leadership) would require stability in team membership to allow development of trusting relationships over time. In practice, this does not prove to be true. Relational approaches have significant positive impacts on project work even when conducted by transient teams and even those within larger organizations (Ding, Li, Zhang, Sheng, & Wang, 2017). For example, in high-stress deployment situations, relational approaches can be established and have been demonstrated to yield results that outperform transactional approaches that were originally intended for command-and-control situations (Niessen et al., 2017). This finding has relevance for healthcare and for translation because the work commonly brings together individuals from disparate work groups who undertake a shared effort to achieve a predetermined goal (often a pressing one) with limited time, structure, and resources (Shenhar & Dvir, 2007).

Academic leadership is no different as transformational leadership contributes to development of wisdom in faculty (Pesut & Thompson, 2018). In the context of great change and disruption in universities, colleges, and across higher education, transformational leadership is increasingly the practice of those in positions of responsibility (Giddens & Morton, 2018; Thompson & Miller, 2018). Leadership of professional organizations reinforces the impact of transformational leadership on a broader scale (Sebastian et al., 2018).

EVIDENCE-BASED LEADERSHIP PRACTICES

For decades, nursing as a discipline has focused on leadership, both in research and in practice. Evidence supports broad adoption of several practices that include structural empowerment, job sculpting, workforce engagement, and lifelong learning (Gifford et al., 2018).

Structural Empowerment

Leaders who ensure members of their team have access to information, support, resources, and opportunities that promote success engage in a practice called *structural empowerment* (Kanter, 1993; Laschinger, Finegan, Shamian, & Wilk, 2004). These leaders configure their organizations and work units to promote robust and informed decision-making and development of individuals within their teams and work units. These leaders ensure that organizational structures follow Kanter's theory of structural engagement (Clavelle, Porter O'Grady, & Drenkard, 2013). Structural empowerment, more than leadership behavior or other characteristics of the workforce, is associated with job satisfaction among nurses (Dahinten, Lee, & MacPhee, 2016).

Across industry, workgroups that experience structural empowerment report higher satisfaction and their organizations benefit from greater workforce stability and productivity (Orgambídez-Ramos & Borrego-Alés, 2014). Nurses who practice in structurally empowered environments report higher levels of control over their practice (Laschinger & Leiter, 2006), greater satisfaction with work (Laschinger, Finegan, Shamian, & Wilk, 2004), more engagement (Boamah, Spence, Laschinger, Wong, & Clarke, 2018), and greater trust (Laschinger, Shamian, & Thomson, 2001). Conversely, absence of structural empowerment has been associated with unfavorable patient outcomes, including medication errors, pressure ulcers, pneumonia, failure to rescue, and increased mortality (Laschinger, 2008; Laschinger & Leiter, 2006). Closely aligned with the essential characteristics of Magnet facilities, structural empowerment is associated with favorable nursing performance, patient outcomes, and interprofessional collaboration (Boamah et al., 2018).

Shared governance (SG) is one approach to achieving structural empowerment that comingles many best practices for leadership. It has been broadly embraced because it yields unparalleled results for patients, nurses, and organizations (Kretzschmer et al., 2017). Positive outcomes associated with SG include increased perceptions of nursing autonomy, staff satisfaction, improved patient satisfaction, increased retention of nursing staff, and reduced errors (Newmann, 2011).

For these reasons, SG has been broadly adopted across Magnet organizations as a means to promote structural empowerment. It provides a structure to engage nurses in decisions about practice (Clavelle et al., 2013; Stimpfel, Rosen, & McHugh, 2015).

SG has been associated with favorable outcomes for patients, staff, and the institutions where it is practiced. Despite having high impact on variables of concern to individual nurses and the profession as a whole, SG is broadly perceived as an administrative structure that allows staff input rather than a structure actually belonging to and arising from the nursing staff (Clavelle et al., 2013).

Workforce Engagement

Workforce engagement is a desired target across any enterprise. Personal resources, job-related resources, and the nature of the work itself combine to influence engagement of individuals and groups and overall organizational outcomes (Bakker & Demarouti, 2007). Engagement is "a positive, fulfilling, work related state of mind that is characterized by vigor, dedication, and absorption" (Schaufeli & Bakker, 2004, p. 295).

Optimism, self-efficiency, resilience, and self-esteem comprise personal resources. Social support, performance feedback, skill development, and fit combine with opportunities to function with autonomy and opportunities to learn (Aiken et al., 2003). Together, these comprise job resources; they combine to promote engagement and positive outcomes (Bakker & Demerouti, 2008).

Engagement in the nursing workforce refers to a state in which nurses inform and participate in organizational decisions that influence their practice, collaborate with colleagues both within nursing and other disciplines, and benefit from meaningful and diverse opportunities for professional development. Engagement is influenced by a host of conditions, including the setting in which nurses practice, staffing patterns, and nurse–patient ratios (Aiken et al., 2008a, 2008b, 2011; Carthon et al., 2019; Garcia-Sierra, Fernandez-Castro, Martinez-Zaragoza, 2016; McHugh et al., 2016).

In nursing, engagement is associated with improved outcomes for the nurses themselves, the patients they serve, and the organization in which they practice. For example, hospitals in which staff demonstrate low levels of engagement see measurable improvement in outcomes with even small increases in engagement (Carthon et al., 2019). High engagement is associated with favorable patient outcomes, including reduced mortality,

Job Sculpting

Although connection between skills and job requirements contributes to productivity, it does not equate to satisfaction or retention. Effective leaders recognize this and seek opportunities to present challenges that connect the efforts and productivity of individual followers to deeply held values and aspirations using a practice called *job sculpting* (Butler & Waldrop, 2009). Although some individuals have a high interest in technology and analytics, interests of others may focus more precisely on creativity, conceptual or theoretical work, coaching and mentoring, managing relationships, control of the enterprise, or communications (Wang, Demerouti, & Le Blanc, 2017). Such diversity of interests among followers can contribute to the success of a project as well as that of the team, while at the same time, increasing satisfaction and retention. Translation is an excellent vehicle to make these connections to individual followers' deeply held values, to kindle engagement, and to improve mission critical outcomes.

Lifelong Learning

Lessons From Magnet Hospitals

The superiority of outcomes achieved by *Magnet hospitals* is well and broadly documented. Infrastructure and perceptions of a supportive work environment are central to the body of work related to Magnet hospitals. Magnet hospitals are those that are able to present evidence of the presence of the Forces of Magnetism. They share a climate, culture, and environment in which nursing thrives and produces significant constructive outcomes for patients, the institution, practicing nurses, other professionals, and the community (Smith, Tallman, & Kelly, 2006). As a result of significant investment in practice, these hospitals report perceptions among the nurses who practice in them that the culture and the climate support excellence (Schmalenberg & Kramer, 2008).

Healthcare lagged behind other high-stakes industries with respect to reducing error, was slow to heighten awareness of risk, recognize potential for failure, focus on adaptability, create readiness for the unexpected, emphasize knowledge and expertise above title and credential, encourage a big-picture perspective, and develop flexibility to flatten any structure as needed. These process improvements are widely recognized as effective in other industries (Weick & Sutcliffe, 2001). As with other industries beginning the work of consistently producing error-free outcomes, healthcare has relied heavily on technology. More recent strategies have emphasized knowledge workers and well-engineered systems based on a growing body of knowledge about effective leadership practices capable of reducing error and risk (Frankel, Leonard, & Denham, 2006). A solid base of evidence supports the involvement of nurses in decisions that impact practice, including work design, workflow, and work process. Such involvement contributes to satisfaction and retention of nurses (Lacey et al., 2007; Laschinger et al., 2004; Moore & Hutchison, 2007) and at the same time improves clinical, quality, operational, and financial outcomes (Porter-O'Grady, 2000, 2001, 2004, 2009).

The IOM report *Keeping Patients Safe: Transforming the Work Environment of Nurses* (IOM, 2004) summarized the evidence and made five recommendations for nurses and nurse leaders to improve the quality and safety of the nursing work environment:

1. Participate in *decision-making* at all levels, including redesign of work and workflow.
2. Promote *evidence-based management practices.*
3. Maximize the *workforce capabilities of RNs* and identify the need of RN staffing for each patient care unit per shift.
   a. It is recommended that nursing homes have at least one RN on duty at all times.
   b. It is recommended that staffing levels increase as the number of patients increases.
4. Redesign both the *work* and the *workspace* to prevent and mitigate errors.
   a. It is recommended that nursing shifts be limited to 12 hours in any 24-hour period, and no more than 60 hours in a 7-day stretch.
5. Create and sustain a *culture of safety* (IOM, 2004).

Collaborative Care

In response to demands to place the patient at the center and in control, many different, new models for care have evolved and all depend on strong, inclusive leadership. Some models have implemented comprehensive approaches to care that begin on admission and extend through discharge planning, follow-up, and home visits. Disease management, coaching, education, peer support, tele-health, and intensive primary care are all value-added components of care. All rely on engaged, supported staff with the knowledge and resources they need to successfully meet the needs of challenging patients (Naylor & Keating, 2008; Naylor et al., 2011).

Fair and Just Culture

Change in any organization has the potential to stimulate resistance, which ranks high among the reasons that innovations fail. People whose work is impacted by any innovation need to trust that the new approach is safe and valid, need confidence in the leadership driving change, and need to believe that outcomes will be maintained or improved. A practice environment characterized by justice in expectations and treatment across members (distributive justice) and as a base for policy (procedural justice) is referred to as a *fair and just culture*. Such a culture is associated with improved retention, satisfaction, performance, and quality (St-Pierre & Holmes, 2010).

A. Cameron and Masterson (2000) identified this significant aspect of the change process as the *leader–member exchange* (LMX). LMX has been noted to affect perceived fairness in interpersonal interaction and policy (Piccolo, Bardes, Mayer, & Judge, 2008). Although evidence suggests that leaders create this sense of fairness and justice in the workplace, achieving financial performance and productivity targets conspire to decrease the number of managers and leaders available to accomplish this important work. The increased requirements placed on managers as they take on relatively more responsibility have been characterized as distributive injustice on the managers themselves (Thorpe & Loo, 2003). This extends to the entire staff inasmuch as it threatens to keep leaders from the important work of creating a fair and just culture for all (St-Pierre & Holmes, 2010).

Nurse leaders can create an environment in which every team member feels a responsibility and is accountable for ensuring that the value of keeping patients safe is upheld. Moving toward a just culture requires that nurse leaders hold themselves and staff accountable as errors are disclosed. This accountability includes understanding why errors occur and identifying what systems, processes, and conditions are at fault. Nurse leaders are also accountable to manage staff so that at-risk behaviors are identified and managed to reduce the risk of error.

The following characteristics indicate an organization at risk according to the three-behavior model developed by Marx (2001):

- Honest human errors made in the context of error-prone systems
- At-risk behavior (failure to recognize)
- Reckless behavior (conscious disregard), including intentional rule violations

Evidence-based leadership will discriminate among these three classes and respond in a way that is effective to manage the behavior. The effective leader will recognize human error and focus on solutions rather than blame, monitor for and mitigate risky behaviors, and manage and eliminate recklessness.

Executive Rounds

Collaborative-walk rounds by leaders and providers have been demonstrated to provide a counterbalance to the pressures of the market to place financial outcomes above quality. Such rounds can increase engagement and accountability and improve outcomes (Frankel et al., 2003; Frankel, Leonard, & Denham, 2006). They help to establish a strategic and tactical focus on safety, service, and operations (Gawande, 2009; Pronovost et al., 2002, 2006, 2010; Pronovost, Berenholtz, & Needham, 2008). In one study, 48 sets of rounds were conducted monthly on 47 different patient care units. Executive leaders, nurses, and others who engaged in direct patient care addressed near misses and operational failures with the goal of identifying and mitigating the cause. Data were entered into a log-enabling meta-level analysis of the sources of errors across the organization (Frankel et al., 2003). From a quality-improvement perspective, the data from the log indicated that all parties participating in the rounds found them to be productive. From a leadership perspective, executives engaged in discussions about direct patient care are better informed because they approach decisions that affect that care and the individuals who provide it.

Including executives in clinical rounds ensures that high-level decisions about resources and environment are informed by real challenges faced by both clinicians and patients. Such rounds enable leadership to put a practical and personal face on the data shared in dashboards and reports (Denham, 2005, 2006, 2010; Denham et al., 2005). Potentially uncomfortable for the executive, exposure to the point of service translates to informed decisions and improved outcomes. Successful industries have long been aware of the risk of failure, which is useful in planning to avoid such risk. Leaders who participate in walk rounds can have a more vivid understanding of both the risk and the implications of failure, and this can translate into an environment more conducive to practice (Frankel et al., 2006).

Interprofessional Collaboration

In a recent Cochrane Review, five randomized controlled trials were found to focus on strategies to enhance interprofessional collaboration. All five trials were found to have design flaws or methodological weaknesses. Sample sizes were small and interventions were different (walking rounds, videoconferencing, audioconferencing, case studies, and team meetings). Some measured length of stay (LOS) and others measured charge per case. Improvement was not consistently reported (Zwarenstein, Goldman, & Reeves, 2009). As a result, further study with larger samples and consistent methods and interventions is needed to support evidence-based collaborative practice.

Rounds are a means to strengthen collaboration. Executive rounds, referred to earlier as *walk rounds*, achieve context and impact for decisions made in boardrooms.

But daily rounds made by physicians, nurses, and all disciplines engaged in care and leadership facilitate clear and direct communication and problem-solving along with education and decision support. These rounds decrease mortality, sequelae, and error (Pronovost et al., 1999, 2006). Effective, regular, and respectful communication reduces frustration among members of the healthcare team, which is one of the root causes of many avoidable errors (Manojlovich & DeCicco, 2007; Manojlovich, Sidani, Covell, & Antonakos, 2011).

Team Training

Training for teams to enhance functioning and communication has been proven to be effective in multiple studies (Cooper & Gaba, 2002; Helmreich & Musson, 2000; Leonard, Graham, & Bonacum, 2004). The IOM (2004) built on this work in its third report titled *Keeping Patients Safe: Transforming the Work Environment of Nurses*. The document provides a road map for nurse leaders with detailed recommendations for staffing, skillsets, work, workspace, shifts, culture, and structure.

Developing the ability of physicians, nurses, and others engaged in patient care to work effectively as teams is one strategy with the potential to improve collaboration, quality of care, and the work environment. In one elective, medical students were introduced to nonphysician caregivers with the goals of developing understanding, improving communication, introducing the possibilities for collaboration, demonstrating how services offered by other professionals complement the work of the physicians, and improving the students' skills in communicating with nonphysicians. At the close of the 2-week-long rotation with a nonphysician professional, students reported a sense of empowerment as a result of their new skills and understanding (Pathak, Holzmueller, Haller, & Pronovost, 2010).

Training for teams is not effective without a culture that values and supports the behaviors on a day-to-day basis. So the "team" must be situated within a culture and permeate all work. It is also true that teamwork is learned. Accommodation is needed in the education for caregiving professionals. Traditionally proved in the silos of nursing schools apart from medical schools, social work schools, and other professional schools, effective education for healthcare professionals needs to incorporate scenarios and team activities in which the realities of practice and the interdependence of work come into clear focus and, in doing so, become more effective (Frankel et al., 2006).

Performance Envelope

For any strategy to take root, leadership is required. The work of quality needs to be visible, compelling, and pervasive across the organization and needs a champion with the visibility, authority, tenacity, data, and credibility to take the team through many waves of change (Denham, 2005, 2006). The notion of the performance development proposes that it is possible to reverse a late-adopter position commonly adopted by executive and financial officers, by engaging this level of leadership in systems design. This approach promotes safety and at the same time eliminates conditions that inhibit initiative and capability of people from all disciplines on the frontline and in support positions (Denham, 2010). The performance envelopment is the safe zone of performance within system-design limits and includes recognizing the capabilities of people. Success begins and ends with leadership (Denham, 2010).

Sustained Improvement Based on Evidence

Pronovost et al. (2008) determined that bloodstream infections per 1,000 catheter days could be reduced and improved performance sustained in critical care units across the state of Michigan. The team implemented five recommendations from the Centers for Disease Control and Prevention, including (a) washing hands before catheter insertion, (b) using full-barrier precautions, (c) preparing the skin with chlorhexidine before insertion, (d) using the femoral site only when use of another site is impossible, and (e) removing catheters as soon as the patient's condition permits. Eighty-seven percent of the 103 ICUs originally participating in the project reported a total of 1,532 ICU months of data, comprising 300 to 310 catheter days as part of a second study focused on sustainability. Catheter-related bloodstream infection rates reported as mean scores decreased from 7.7 at baseline to 1.3 at 16 to 18 months and 1.1 at 34 to 36 months following implementation. During the same period, bloodstream infection rates were unchanged. The intervention designed to reduce catheter-related infections was considered to be specific and effective and produced sustained improvement in the target measure (Hyzy et al., 2010).

Operations

Operations of the work environment are significant for practice. In a systematic review of the literature, including 9,000 titles and abstracts focused on the practice environment, Schalk, Bijl, Halfens, Hollands, and Cummings (2010) identified strategies documented as effective to improve the environment. These strategies included very basic items: primary nursing, education tools, individualized care, supervision, and violence prevention. Each of these strategies was supported as effective in only one or two quality studies. So, although these strategies have face value and empirical evidence to support application, they lack a strong and deep empirical base.

■ ROLE OF ORGANIZATION IN TRANSLATION

Leaders strategically develop capacities that drive innovation critical to the successful translation of evidence into meaningful performance improvement. These include will, ideas, and execution. Will takes the form of clearly developed aims communicated and embraced across the enterprise. Ideas come from a workforce and leadership constantly engaged in achieving excellence (Reinertsen, Bisognano, & Pugh, 2008). Execution requires having the discipline to manage performance to attain targets, to use data to evaluate progress, and to refine plans of action to achieve aims.

Transforming Care at the Bedside

The Transforming Care at the Bedside (TCAB) initiative, a national program of the RWJF and Institute for Healthcare Improvement (IHI), began in July 2003 and concluded in August 2008. Because of the intensity and complexity of care, which is routinely being delivered in hospital medical–surgical units, and as a result of projections that as many as 35% to 40% of unexpected hospital deaths will occur on such units, the RWJF and the IHI created an initiative called *TCAB*. Its intent was to improve care on medical–surgical units and to increase the amount of time nurses spend caring for patients at the bedside. The initiative was built around improvements in four main categories (Figure 6.1): (a) safe and reliable care, (b) vitality and teamwork, (c) patient-centered care, and (d) value-added care processes (IHI, 2008). TCAB started with 10 hospitals, but it has been so successful that more than five hospitals have joined the TCAB Learning and Innovation Community, and 68 hospitals are participating in the American Organization of Nurse Executives TCAB Collaborative. The key to this success is leadership support for and implementation of evidence-based management practices such as communication models that support consistent and clear communication among caregivers, professional support programs such as preceptorships and educational opportunities, and redesigned workspaces that enhance efficiency and reduce waste (Rutherford, Lee, & Greiner, 2004; Viney, Batcheller, Houston, & Belcik, 2006).

Microsystems

Recent work in clinical microsystems promises to provide a framework for leaders and teams intending to improve systems and outcomes (Reis, Scott, & Rempel, 2009). Leadership, at the level of the microsystem, focuses on day-to-day challenges of infrastructure and operations.

> Clinical microsystems are the small, functional, front-line units that provide most healthcare to most people. They are the essential building blocks of larger organizations and of the health system. They are the place where patients and providers meet. The quality and value of care produced by a large health system can be no better than the services generated by the small systems of which it is composed. (Nelson et al., 2002, p. 473)

The microsystems approach is inclusive and democratic, with results informed by processes in the hands of those who execute the work (Batalden, Nelson, Edwards, Godfrey, & Mohr, 2003). In nursing and healthcare, clinical microsystems engage clinicians who provide direct services in ongoing work to improve quality. As a result, larger numbers of caregivers are informed in detail about the work. They grow competent and confident to identify potential practice issues. In doing so, they improve quality and performance. They develop skills and confidence to address problems in real time and decrease their tolerance of recalcitrant practice problems (Williams, Dickinson, Robinson, & Allen, 2009).

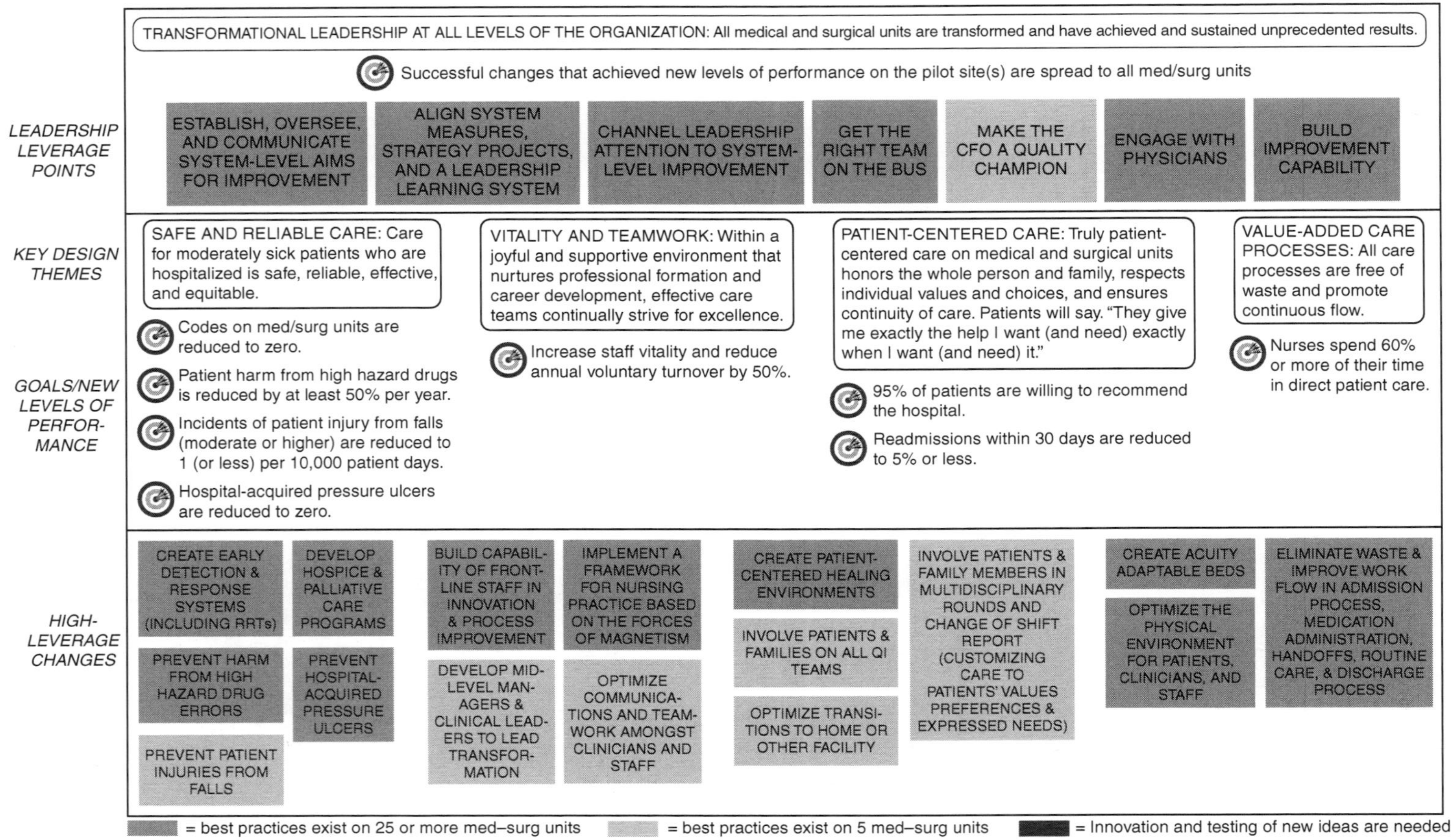

TRANSFORMATIONAL LEADERSHIP AT ALL LEVELS OF THE ORGANIZATION: All medical and surgical units are transformed and have achieved and sustained unprecedented results.

Successful changes that achieved new levels of performance on the pilot site(s) are spread to all med/surg units

LEADERSHIP LEVERAGE POINTS

ESTABLISH, OVERSEE, AND COMMUNICATE SYSTEM-LEVEL AIMS FOR IMPROVEMENT

ALIGN SYSTEM MEASURES, STRATEGY PROJECTS, AND A LEADERSHIP LEARNING SYSTEM

CHANNEL LEADERSHIP ATTENTION TO SYSTEM-LEVEL IMPROVEMENT

GET THE RIGHT TEAM ON THE BUS

MAKE THE CFO A QUALITY CHAMPION

ENGAGE WITH PHYSICIANS

BUILD IMPROVEMENT CAPABILITY

KEY DESIGN THEMES

SAFE AND RELIABLE CARE: Care for moderately sick patients who are hospitalized is safe, reliable, effective, and equitable.

VITALITY AND TEAMWORK: Within a joyful and supportive environment that nurtures professional formation and career development, effective care teams continually strive for excellence.

PATIENT-CENTERED CARE: Truly patient-centered care on medical and surgical units honors the whole person and family, respects individual values and choices, and ensures continuity of care. Patients will say. "They give me exactly the help I want (and need) exactly when I want (and need) it."

VALUE-ADDED CARE PROCESSES: All care processes are free of waste and promote continuous flow.

GOALS/NEW LEVELS OF PERFORMANCE

Codes on med/surg units are reduced to zero.

Patient harm from high hazard drugs is reduced by at least 50% per year.

Incidents of patient injury from falls (moderate or higher) are reduced to 1 (or less) per 10,000 patient days.

Hospital-acquired pressure ulcers are reduced to zero.

Increase staff vitality and reduce annual voluntary turnover by 50%.

95% of patients are willing to recommend the hospital.

Readmissions within 30 days are reduced to 5% or less.

Nurses spend 60% or more of their time in direct patient care.

HIGH-LEVERAGE CHANGES

CREATE EARLY DETECTION & RESPONSE SYSTEMS (INCLUDING RRTs)

DEVELOP HOSPICE & PALLIATIVE CARE PROGRAMS

PREVENT HARM FROM HIGH HAZARD DRUG ERRORS

PREVENT HOSPITAL-ACQUIRED PRESSURE ULCERS

PREVENT PATIENT INJURIES FROM FALLS

BUILD CAPABILITY OF FRONT-LINE STAFF IN INNOVATION & PROCESS IMPROVEMENT

IMPLEMENT A FRAMEWORK FOR NURSING PRACTICE BASED ON THE FORCES OF MAGNETISM

DEVELOP MID-LEVEL MANAGERS & CLINICAL LEADERS TO LEAD TRANSFORMATION

OPTIMIZE COMMUNICATIONS AND TEAMWORK AMONGST CLINICIANS AND STAFF

CREATE PATIENT-CENTERED HEALING ENVIRONMENTS

INVOLVE PATIENTS & FAMILIES ON ALL QI TEAMS

OPTIMIZE TRANSITIONS TO HOME OR OTHER FACILITY

INVOLVE PATIENTS & FAMILY MEMBERS IN MULTIDISCIPLINARY ROUNDS AND CHANGE OF SHIFT REPORT (CUSTOMIZING CARE TO PATIENTS' VALUES PREFERENCES & EXPRESSED NEEDS)

CREATE ACUITY ADAPTABLE BEDS

OPTIMIZE THE PHYSICAL ENVIRONMENT FOR PATIENTS, CLINICIANS, AND STAFF

ELIMINATE WASTE & IMPROVE WORK FLOW IN ADMISSION PROCESS, MEDICATION ADMINISTRATION, HANDOFFS, ROUTINE CARE, & DISCHARGE PROCESS

= best practices exist on 25 or more med–surg units

= best practices exist on 5 med–surg units

= Innovation and testing of new ideas are needed

FIGURE 6.1 TCAB model.

CFO, chief financial officer; QI, quality improvement; RRT, rapid response team.

Source: Reprinted from www.IHI.org with permission of the Institute for Healthcare Improvement, ©2019.

A microsystems approach is based on the body of evidence that draws a clear connection between the nurses' work environment and the quality of care (Ulrich et al., 2007). Investment in the practice environment and the work of nursing yields improved outcomes. This is the basis for microsystems, the platform for nurse leaders to achieve meaningful, sustained process and quality improvements, and the process to be used to connect people with purpose.

■ CONCLUSIONS

In my graduate education, I had a wise faculty member who liked to quote A. A. Milne (1928):

> Here is Edward Bear, coming downstairs now, bump, bump, bump on the back of his head . . . sometimes he thinks there really is another way if only he could stop bumping a minute and think about it.

Translation offers a means to stop bumping on the back of our heads: to terminate the cycle of habitual practice and to substitute evidence for opinion. Leaders who would support and advance translation can do so by themselves, translating evidence into their leadership practice. They can be transparent in doing so the same way a capable clinical instructor accomplishes his or her work, by decoding his or her thoughts and actions and emphasizing the intent and evidence base for the decisions he or she makes, the actions he or she takes, and the practices he or she adopts.

Leading by example necessitates that managers, administrators, and executives evaluate evidence and apply strong and valid findings through innovation focused on carefully selected, well-crafted quality targets. Nurse leaders will be well served by modeling a spirit of inquiry, speaking the language of evidence-based practice and translation, and developing the organization's capacity to accomplish significant and measurable performance improvement. Doing so would enable these leaders to connect people with purpose, facilitate organizational learning, and position their enterprise to thrive in the face of the many and diverse challenges to come. Nothing less will suffice to move nurses, our profession, and our interprofessional teams to jump from the burning platform of care, as we have known it, to care informed by evidence.

■ REFERENCES

Aiken, L. H., Cimiotti, J. P., Sloane, D. M., Smith, H. L., Flynn, L., & Neff. D. F. (2011). Effects of nurse staffing and nurse education on patient deaths in hospitals with different nurse work environments. *Medical Care*, *49*(12), 1047–1053. doi:10.1097/mlr.0b013e3182330b6e

Aiken, L. H., Clarke, S. P., Cheung, R. B., Sloane, D. M., & Silber, J. H. (2003). Educational levels of hospital nurses and surgical patient mortality. *Journal of the American Medical Association*, *290*(12), 1607–1623. doi:10.1001/jama.290.12.1617

Aiken, L. H., Clarke, S. P., Sloane, D. M., Lake, E. T., & Cheney, T. (2008a). Effects of hospital care environment on patient mortality and nurse outcomes. *Journal of Nursing Administration*, *38*(5), 223–229. doi:10.1097/01.nna.0000312773.42352.d7

Aiken, L. H., Clarke, S. P., Sloane, D. M., Lake, E. T., & Cheney, T. (2008b). Effects of hospital care environment on patient mortality and nurse outcomes. *Journal of Nursing Administration*, *39*(7/8), S45–S51. doi:10.1097/nna.0b013e3181aeb4cf

Aiken, L. H., Clarke, S. P., Sloane, D. M., Lake, E. T., & Cheney, T. (2009). Effects of hospital care environment on patient mortality and nurse outcomes. *Journal of Nursing Administration*, *39*(Suppl. 7–8), S45–S51. doi:10.1097/nna.0b013e3181aeb4cf

Aiken, L. H., Clarke, S. P., Sloane, D. M., Sochalski, J. A., Busse, R., Silber J. H., . . . Shamian, J. (2001). Nurses' reports on hospital care in five countries. *Health Affairs*, *20*(3), 43–53. doi:10.1377/hlthaff.20.3.43

Aiken, L. H., Clarke, S. P., Sloane, D. M., Sochalski, J., & Silber, J. H. (2002). Hospital staffing and patient mortality, nurse burnout, and job dissatisfaction. *Journal of the American Medical Association*, *288*(16), 1987–1993. doi:10.1001/jama.288.16.1987

Aiken, L. H., Clarke, S. P., Sloane, D. M., Sochalski, J. A., & Silber, J. H. (2010). Hospital nurse staffing and patient mortality, nurse burnout, and job dissatisfaction. *Journal of the American Medical Association*, *288*(16), 1987–1993. doi:10.1001/jama.288.16.1987

Aiken, L. H., Havens, D. S., & Sloane, D. M. (2009). The Magnet nursing services recognition program. *American Journal of Nursing*, *100*(3), 26–36. doi:10.1097/00000446-200003000-00040

American Nursing Credentialing Center. (2018). *ANCC Magnet Recognition program*. Retrieved from https://www.nursingworld.org/organizational-programs/magnet

Anthony, M. K., Standing, T. S., Glick, J., Duffy, M., Paschall, F., Sauer, M. R., . . . Dumpe M. L. (2005). Leadership and nurse retention: The pivotal role of nurse managers. *Journal of Nursing Administration*, 35(3), 146–155. doi:10.1097/00005110-200503000-00008

Avolio, B. J., & Bass, B. M. (2004). *Multifactoral leadership questionnaire*. Mind Garden Inc. Retrieved from www.mindgarden.com/16-multifactor-leadership-questionnaire

Bakker, A. B., & Demerouti, E. (2007). The Job Demands Resources model: State of the art. *Journal of Managerial Psychology, 22*(3), 309–328.

Bakker, A. B., & Demerouti, E. (2008). Towards a model of work engagement. *Career Development International, 13*(3), 209–223.

Banks, G. C., Davis McCauley, K., Gardner, W. L., & Guler, C. E. (2016). A meta-analytic review of authentic and transformational leadership: A test for redundancy. *Leadership Quarterly,* 27(4), 634–652. doi:10.1016/j.leaqua.2016.02.006

Bass, B. M. (1985). *Leadership and performance beyond expectations*. New York, NY: Free Press.

Batalden, P. B., Nelson, E. C., Edwards, W. H., Godfrey, M. M., & Mohr, J. J. (2003). Microsystems in health care: Part 9. Developing small clinical units to attain peak performance. The *Joint Commission Journal on Quality and Patient Safety*, *29*(11), 575–585. doi:10.1016/s1549-3741(03)29068-7

Berwick, D. M. (2008). The science of improvement. *Journal of the American Medical Association*, *299*(10), 1182–1184. doi:10.1001/jama.299.10.1182

Berwick, D. M., Nolan, T. W., & Whittington, J. (2008). The Triple Aim: Care, health, and cost. *Health Affairs*, 27(3), 759–769. doi:10.1377/hlthaff.27.3.759

Boamah, S. A., Spence Laschinger, H. K., Wong, C., & Clarke, S. (2018). Effect of transformational leadership on job satisfaction and patient safety outcomes. *Nursing Outlook,* 66(2), 180–189. doi:10.1016/j.outlook.2017.10.004

Bodenheimer, T., & Sinsky, C. (2014). From triple to quadruple aim: Care of the patient requires care of the provider. *Annals of Family Medicine*, *12*(6), 573–576. doi: 10.1370/afm.1713

Boyatzis, R., & McKee, A. (2005). *Renewing yourself and connecting with others through mindfulness, hope and compassion*. Brighton, MA: Harvard Business School Press.

Butler, T., & Waldrup, J. (2009). Job sculpting: The art of retaining your best people. *Harvard Business Review,* 77(5).

Cameron, A., & Masterson, A. (2000). Managing the unmanageable? Nurse executive directors and new role developments in nursing. *Journal of Advanced Nursing*, *31*(5), 1081–1088. doi:10.1046/j.1365-2648.2000.01384.x

Cameron, K. S., Dutton, J. E., Quinn, R. E., & Wrzensneiwski, A. (2003). *Positive organizational scholarship: Foundations of a new discipline*. San Francisco, CA. Berrett-Koehler.

Carthon, B. J., Hatfield, L., Plover, C., Dierkes, A., Davis, L., Hedgeland, T., . . . Aiken, L (2019). Association of Nurse engagement and nurse staffing on patient safety. *Journal of Nursing Care Quality*, *34*(1), 40–46. doi:10.1097/ncq.0000000000000334

Casida, J., & Pinto-Zipp, G. (2008). Leadership-organizational culture relationships in nursing units of acute care hospitals. *Nursing Economic$*, *26*(1), 7–15.

Clavelle, J. T., Porter O'Grady, T., & Drenkard, K. (2013). Structural empowerment and the nursing practice environment in Magnet® organizations. *Journal of Nursing Administration,* 43(11), 566–573. doi:10.1097/01.nna.0000434512.81997.3f

Cooper, J. B., & Gaba, D. (2002). No myth: Anesthesia is a model for addressing patient safety. *Anesthesiology, 97*(6), 1335–1337. doi:10.1097/00000542-200212000-00003

Cowden, T., Cummings, G., & Profetto-McGrath, J. (2011). Leadership practices and staff nurses' intent to stay: A systematic review. *Journal of Nursing Management, 19*(4), 461–477. doi:10.1111/j.1365-2834.2011.01209.x

Cummings, G. G., MacGregor, T., Davey, M., Lee, H., Wong, C. A., Lo, E., . . . Stafford, E. (2010). Leadership styles and outcome patterns for the nursing workforce and work environment: A systematic review. *International Journal of Nursing Studies, 47*(3), 363–385. doi:10.1016/j.ijnurstu.2009.08.006

Dahinten, V. S., Lee, S. E., & MacPhee, M. (2016). Disentangling the relationships between staff nurses" workplace empowerment and job satisfaction. *Journal of Nursing Management, 24*(8), 1060–1070. doi:10.1111/jonm.12407

Deinert, A., Homan, A. C., Boer, D., Voelpel, S. V., & Gutermann, D. (2015). Transformational leadership sub-dimensions and their link to leaders' personality and performance. *Leadership Quarterly, 26*(6), 1095–1120. doi:10.1016/j.leaqua.2015.08.001

Denham, C., Bagian, J., Daley, J., Edgman-Levitan, S., Gelinas, L., O'Leary, D., . . . Wachter, R. (2005). No excuses: The reality that demands action. *Journal of Patient Safety, 1*(3), 154–169. doi:10.1097/01.jps.0000183854.29928.4d

Denham, C. R. (2005). Patient safety practices: Leaders can turn barriers into accelerators. *Journal of Patient Safety, 1*(1), 41–55. doi:10.1097/01209203-200503000-00009

Denham, C. R. (2006). Leaders need dashboards, dashboards need leaders. *Journal of Patient Safety, 2*(2), 45–53.

Denham, C. R. (2010). Greenlight issues for the CFO: Investing in patient safety. *Journal of Patient Safety, 6*(1), 52–56. doi:10.1097/pts.0b013e3181c72c9e

Ding, X., Li, Q., Zhang, H., Sheng, Z., & Wang, Z. (2017). Linking transformational leadership and work outcomes in temporary organizations: A social identity approach. *International Journal of Project Management, 35*(4), 543–556. doi: 10.1016/j.ijproman.2017.02.005

Eberly, M. B., Bluhmb, D. J., Guaranac, C., Avoliod, B. J., & Hannahe, S.T. (2017). Staying after the storm: How transformational leadership relates to follower turnover intentions in extreme contexts. *Journal of Vocational Behavior, 102*, 72–85. doi:10.1016/j.jvb.2017.07.004

Failla, K. R., & Stichler, J. F. (2008). Manager and staff perceptions of the manager's leadership style. *Journal of Nursing Administration, 38*(11), 480–487. doi:10.1097/01.nna.0000339472.19725.31

Fairholm, M. R. (2001). *The themes and theory of leadership: James MacGregor Burns and the philosophy of leadership*. Washington, DC: The George Washington University.

Frankel, A., Graydon-Baker, E., Neppl, C., Simmonds, T., Gustafson, M., & Gandhi, T. K. (2003). Patient safety leadership WalkRounds. *The Joint Commission Journal of Quality and Safety, 29*(1), 16–26. doi:10.1016/s1549-3741(03)29003-1

Frankel, A. S., Leonard, M. W., & Denham, C. R. (2006). Fair and just culture, team behavior, and leadership engagement: The tools to achieve high reliability. *Health Services Research, 41*(4 Pt. 2), 1690–1709. doi:10.1111/j.1475-6773.2006.00572.x

Garcia-Sierra, R., Fernandez-Castro, J., Martinez-Zaragoza, F., (2016). Work engagement in nursing: an integrative review of the literature. *Journal of Nursing Management, 24*(2), E101–E111. doi:10.1111/jonm.12312

Gawande, A. (2009). *The checklist manifesto: How to get things right*. New York, NY: Metropolitan Books.

Gentry, W. A., Weber, T. J., & Sadri, G. (2008). Examining career-related mentoring and managerial performance across cultures: A multilevel analysis. *Journal of Vocational Behavior, 72*(2), 241–253. doi:10.1016/j.jvb.2007.10.1014

Giddens, J. (2018). Transformational leadership: What every nursing dean should know. *Journal of Professional Nursing, 34*(2), 117–121. doi:10.1016/j.profnurs.2017.10.004

Giddens, J. & Morton, P. (2018). Pearls of Wisdom for chief academic nursing leaders. *Journal of Professional Nursing, 34*(2), 75–81. doi:10.1016/j.profnurs.2017.10.002

Gifford, W. A., Squires, J. E., Angus, D. E., Ashley, L. A., Brosseau, L., Craik, J. M., . . . Graham, I. D. (2018). Managerial leadership for research use in nursing and allied health care professions: a systematic review. *Implementation Science, 13*(1), 127. doi:10.1186/s13012-018-0817-7

Gowin, C. R., Henagan, S. C., & McFadden, K. L. (2009). Knowledge management as a mediator for efficacy of transformational leadership and quality management initiatives in US healthcare. *Health Care Management Review, 34*(2), 129–140. doi:10.1097/hmr.0b013e31819e9169

Groff-Paris, L. M., & Terhaar, M. F. (2011). Using Maslow's pyramid and the National Database of Nursing Quality Indicators to attain a healthier work environment. *Online Journal of Issues in Nursing, 16*(1). doi:10.3912/OJIN.Vol16No01PPT05

Helmreich, R. L., & Musson, D. M. (2000). Surgery as team endeavor. *Canadian Journal of Anesthesia, 47*(5), 391–392. doi:10.1007/bf03018965

Hyzy, R. C., Flanders, S. A., Pronovost, P. J., Berenholtz, S. M., Watson, S., George, C., . . . Auerbach, A. D. (2010). Characteristics of intensive care units in Michigan: Not an open and closed case. *Journal of Hospital Medicine, 5*(1), 4–9. doi:10.1002/jhm.567

Institute for Healthcare Improvement & Robert Wood Johnson Foundation. (2008). *Transforming care at the bedside. How-to guide: Engaging front-line staff in innovation and quality improvement.* Retrieved from http://www.ihi.org/education/IHIOpenSchool/Courses/Documents/CourseraDocuments/12_TCABHowtoGuideEngagingFrontLineStaffSep08.pdf

Institute of Medicine. (2000). *To err is human: Building a safer health system.* Washington, DC: National Academies Press.

Institute of Medicine. (2001). *Crossing the quality chasm: A new health system for the 21st century.* Washington, DC: National Academies Press.

Institute of Medicine. (2004). *Keeping patients safe: Transforming the work environment of nurses.* Washington, DC: National Academies Press.

Institute of Medicine. (2009). *Initial national priorities for comparative effectiveness research.* Washington, DC: National Academies Press.

Judge, T. A., & Piccolo, R. F. (2004). Transformational and transactional leadership: A meta-analytic test of their relative validity. *Journal of Applied Psychology, 89*(5), 755–768. doi:10.1037/0021-9010.89.5.755

Kanter, R. M. (1993). *Men and women of the corporation* (2nd ed.). New York, NY: Basic Books.

Kretzschmer, S., Walker, M., Myers, J., Vogt, K., Massouda, J., Gottbrath, D., . . . Logsdon, M. C. (2017). Nursing empowerment, workplace environment, and job satisfaction in nurses employed in an academic health science center. *Journal for Nurses in Professional Development, 33*(4), 196–202. doi:10.1097/nnd.0000000000000363

Kuhnert, K. W., & Lewis, P. (1987). Transactional and transformational leadership: A constructive/developmental analysis. *Academy of Management Review, 12*(4), 648–657. doi:10.5465/amr.1987.4306717

Lacey, S. R., Cox, K. S., Lorfing, K. C., Teasley, S. L., Carroll, C. A., & Sexton, K. (2007). Nursing support, workload, and intent to stay in magnet, magnet-aspiring, and non-magnet hospitals. *Journal of Nursing Administration, 37*(4), 199–205. doi:10.1097/01.nna.0000266839.61931.b6

Laschinger, H. K. S. (2008). Effect of empowerment on professional practice environments, work satisfaction, and patient care quality: Further testing the Nursing Worklife Model. *Journal of Nursing Care Quality, 23*(4), 322–330.

Laschinger, H. K. S. (2010). Positive working relationships matter for better nurse and patient outcomes. *Journal of Nursing Management, 18*(8), 875–877. doi:10.1111/j.1365-2834.2010.01206.x

Laschinger, H. K. S., Finegan, J., & Wilk, P. (2009). The impact of unit leadership and empowerment on nurses' organizational commitment. *Journal of Nursing Administration, 39*(5), 228–235. doi:10.1097/nna.0b013e3181a23d2b

Laschinger, H. K. S., Finegan, J. E., Shamian, J., & Wilk, P. (2004). A longitudinal analysis of the impact of workplace empowerment on work satisfaction. *Journal of Organizational Behavior, 25*(4), 527–545. doi:10.1002/job.256

Laschinger, H. K. S., & Leiter, M. P. (2006). The impact of nursing work environments on patient safety outcomes: The mediating role of burnout/engagement. *Journal of Nursing Administration, 36*(5), 259–267. doi:10.1097/00005110-200605000-00019

Laschinger, H. K. S., Shamian, J., & Thomson, D. (2001). Impact of magnet hospital characteristics on nurses' perceptions of trust, burnout, quality of care, and work satisfaction. *Nursing Economic$, 19*(5), 209–219.

Laschinger, H. K. S., Wong, C. A., Cummings, G. C., & Grau, A. L. (2014). Resonant leadership and workplace empowerment: The value of positive organizational cultures in reducing workplace incivility. *Nursing Economic$, 32*(1), 1–16.

Leonard, M., Graham, S., & Bonacum, D. (2004). The human factor: The critical importance of effective teamwork and communication providing safe care. *Quality and Safety in Healthcare, 13*(Suppl. 1), i85–i90.

Luthans, F., & Avolio, B. J. (2003). Authentic leadership development. In K. S. Cameron, J. E. Dutton, & R. E. Quinn (Eds.), *Positive organizational scholarship* (pp. 241–258). San Francisco, CA: Berrett-Koehler.

Manojlovich, M., & DeCicco, B. (2007). Healthy work environments, nurse–physician communication, and patients' outcomes. *American Journal of Critical Care, 16*(6), 536–543.

Manojlovich, M., Sidani, S., Covell, C. L., & Antonakos, C. L. (2011). Nursing dose: Linking staffing variables to adverse patient outcomes. *Nursing Research, 60*(4), 214–220. doi:10.1097/nnr.0b013e31822228dc

Marx, D. (2001). *Patient safety and the "just culture": A primer for health care executives*. New York, NY: Columbia University. Retrieved from http://psnet.ahrq.gov/resource.aspx?resourceID=1582

McHugh, M. D., Rochman, M. F., Sloane. D. M., Berg, R. A., Mancini, M. E., Nadkarni, V. M., . . . Aiken L. H (2016). Better nurse staffing and nurse work environments associated with increased survival of in-hospital cardiac arrest patients. *Medical Care, 54*(1), 74–80. doi:10.1097/mlr.0000000000000456

Mhatre, K. H., & Riggio, R. E. (2014). Charismatic and transformational leadership: Past, present, and future. In D. V. Day (Ed.), *Oxford library of psychology. The Oxford handbook of leadership and organizations* (pp. 221–240). New York, NY: Oxford University Press.

Milne, A. A. (1928). *The house at pooh corner*. New York, NY: Dutton Children's Books.

Moore, S. C., & Hutchison, S. A. (2007). Developing leaders at every level: Accountability and empowerment actualized through shared governance. *Journal of Nursing Administration, 37*(12), 564–568. doi:10.1097/01.nna.0000302386.76119.22

National Academy of Science. (2017). Accelerating medical evidence generation: Summary. Retrieved from https://nam.edu/wp-content/uploads/2017/06/SUMMARY-Accelerating-Medical-Evidence-Generation.pdf

National Academy of Science. (2018). A design thinking, systems approach to well-being within education and practice: Proceedings of a workshop. Retrieved from https://www.nap.edu/download/25151

Naylor, M., & Keating, S. A. (2008). Transitional care: Moving patients from one care setting to another. *American Journal of Nursing, 108*(Suppl. 9), 58–63. doi:10.1097/01.naj.0000336420.34946.3a

Naylor, M. D., Aiken, L. H., Kurtzman, E. T., Olds, D. M., & Hirschman, K. B. (2011). The importance of transitional care in achieving health reform. *Health Affairs, 30*(4), 746–754. doi:10.1377/hlthaff.2011.0041

Nelson, E. C., Batalden, P. B., Huber, T. P., Mohr, J. J., Godfrey, M. M., Headrick, L. A., & Wasson, J. H. (2002). Microsystems in health care: Part 1. Learning from high performing front-line clinical units. *The Joint Commission Journal of Quality Improvement, 28*(9), 472–493. doi:10.1016/s1070-3241(02)28051-7

Newmann, K. P. (2011). Transforming organizational culture through nursing shared governance. *Nursing Clinics of North America, 46*(1), 45–48. doi:10.1016/j.cnur.2010.10.002

Nguyen, T. T., Mia, L., Winata, L., & Chong, V. K. (2017). Effect of transformational-leadership style and management control system on managerial performance. *Journal of Business Research, 70*, 202–213. doi:10.1016/j.jbusres.2016.08.018

Niessen, C., Mädera, I., Strideb, C., & Jimmieson, N. L. (2017). Thriving when exhausted: The role of perceived transformational leadership. *Journal of Vocational Behavior, 103*(Part B), 41–51. doi:10.1016/j.jvb.2017.07.012

Orgambídez-Ramos, A., & Borrego-Alés, Y. (2014). Empowering employees: Structural empowerment as antecedent of job satisfaction in university settings. *Psychological Thought, 7*(1), 28–36. doi:10.5964/psyct.v7i1.88

Pathak, S., Holzmueller, C. G., Haller, K. B., & Pronovost, P. J. (2010). A mile in their shoes: Interdisciplinary education at the Johns Hopkins University School of Medicine. *American Journal of Medical Quality, 25*(6), 462–467. doi:10.1177/1062860610366591

Pesut, D. J., & Thompson, S. A. (2018). Nursing leadership in academic nursing: The wisdom of development and the development of wisdom. *Journal of Professional Nursing, 34*(2), 122–127. doi:10.1016/j.profnurs.2017.11.004

Piccolo, R. F., Bardes, M., Mayer, D. M., & Judge T. A. (2008). Does high quality leader–member exchange accentuate the effects of organizational justice? *European Journal of Work and Organizational Psychology, 17*(2), 273–298. doi:10.1080/13594320701743517

Porter-O'Grady, T. (2000). Governance at the crossroads. Post-millennium trustees face difficult decisions in a new age of health care. *Health Progress, 81*(6), 38–41, 55.

Porter-O'Grady, T. (2001). Is shared governance still relevant? *Journal of Nursing Administration, 31*(10), 468–473.

Porter-O'Grady, T. (2004). Overview: Shared governance: Is it a model for nurses to gain control over their practice? *Online Journal of Issues in Nursing, 9*(1). Retrieved from http://ojin.nursingworld.org/MainMenuCategories/ANAMarketplace/ANAPeriodicals/OJIN/TableofContents/Volume92004/No1Jan04/Overview.html

Porter-O'Grady, T. (2009). Creating a context for excellence and innovation: Comparing chief nurse executive leadership practices in magnet and non-magnet hospitals. *Nursing Administration Quarterly, 33*(3), 198–204. doi:10.1097/naq.0b013e3181acca44

Pronovost, P., Needham, D., Berenholtz, S., Sinopoli, D., Chu, H., Sexton, B., . . . Goeschel, C. (2006). An intervention to decrease catheter-related bloodstream infections in the ICU. *New England Journal of Medicine, 355*(26), 2725–2732. doi:10.1056/nejmoa061115

Pronovost, P. J., Angus, D. C., Dorman, T., Robinson, K. A., Dremsizov, T. T., & Young, T. L. (2002). Physician staffing patterns and clinical outcomes in critically ill patients: A systematic review. *Journal of the American Medical Association*, *288*(17), 2151–2162. doi:10.1001/jama.288.17.2151

Pronovost, P. J., Berenholtz, S. M., & Needham, D. M. (2008). Translating evidence into practice: A model for large scale knowledge translation. *British Medical Journal*, *337*, a1714. doi:10.1136/bmj.a1714

Pronovost, P. J., Goeschel, C. A., Colantuoni, E., Watson, S., Lubomski, L. H., Berenholtz, S. M., . . . Needham, D. (2010). Sustaining reductions in catheter-related bloodstream infections in Michigan intensive care units: Observational study. *British Medical Journal*, *340*, c309. doi:10.1136/bmj.c309

Pronovost, P. J., Jenckes, M. W., Dorman, T., Garrett, E., Breslow, M. J., Rosenfeld, B. A., . . . Bass, E. (1999). Organizational characteristics of intensive care units related to outcomes of abdominal aortic surgery. *Journal of the American Medical Association*, *281*(14), 1310–1317.

Reinertsen, J. L., Bisognano, M., & Pugh, M. D. (2008). *Seven leadership leverage points for organization-level improvement in health care* (2nd ed.). Cambridge, MA: Institute for Healthcare Improvement.

Reis, M. D., Scott, S. D., & Rempel, G. R. (2009). Including parents in the evaluation of clinical microsystems in the neonatal intensive care unit. *Advances in Neonatal Care*, *9*(4), 174–179. doi:10.1097/anc.0b013e3181afab3c

Robert Wood Johnson Foundation. (2013). *A burning platform and trust: Key ingredients for payment reform. Robert Wood Johnson Foundation*. Retrieved from http://www.rwjf.org/content/dam/farm/reports/issue_briefs/2013/rwjf409726

Rosengren, K., Athlin, E., & Segesten, K. (2007). Presence and availability: Staff concepts of nursing leadership on an intensive care unit. *Journal of Nursing Management*, *15*(5), 522–529. doi:10.1111/j.1365-2834.2007.00712.x

Rutherford, P., Lee, B., & Greiner, A. (2004). *Transforming care at the bedside* (IHI Innovation Series white paper). Boston, MA: Institute for Healthcare Improvement. Retrieved from www.IHI.org

Sandstrom, B., Borglin, G., Nilsson, R., & Willman, A. (2011). Promoting the implementation of evidence-based-practice: A literature review focusing on the role of nursing leadership. *Worldviews on Evidence-Based Nursing*, *8*(4), 212–223. doi:10.1111/j.1741-6787.2011.00216.x

Schalk, D. M., Bijl, M. L., Halfens, R. J., Hollands, L., & Cummings, G. G. (2010). Interventions aimed at improving the nursing work environment: A systematic review. *Implementation Science*, *5*(1), 34. doi:10.1186/1748-5908-5-34

Schaufeli, W. B., & Bakker, A. B. (2004). Job demands, job resources, and their relationship with burnout and engagement: a multi-sample study. *Journal of Organizational Behavior*, *25*, 293–315. doi:10.1002/job.248

Schmalenberg, C., & Kramer, M. (2008). Essentials of a productive nurse work environment. *Nursing Research*, *57*(1), 2–13. doi:10.1097/01.nnr.0000280657.04008.2a

Sebastian, J. G., Breslin, E. T., Trautman, D. E., Cary, A. H., Rosseter, R. J., & Vlahov, D. (2018). Leadership by collaboration: Nursing's bold new vision for academic practice partnerships. *Journal of Professional Nursing*, *34*(2), 110–116. doi:10.1016/j.profnurs.2017.11.006

Sellgren, S., Ekval, G., & Tomson, G. (2006). Leadership styles in nursing management: Preferred and perceived. *Journal of Nursing Management*, *14*(5), 348–355. doi:10.1111/j.1365-2934.2006.00624.x

Shea, B. J. (2011). A decade of knowledge translation research—What has changed? *Journal of Clinical Epidemiology*, *64*(1), 3–5. doi:10.1016/j.jclinepi.2010.07.009

Shenhar, A. J., & Dvir, D. (2007). *Re-inventing project management: The diamond approach to successful growth and innovation*. Brighton, MA: Harvard Business School Press.

Smith, H., Tallman, R., & Kelly, K. (2006). Magnet hospital characteristics and northern Canadian nurses' job satisfaction. *Nursing Leadership* , *19*(3), 73–86. doi:10.12927/cjnl.2006.18379

St-Pierre, I., & Holmes, D. (2010). The relationship between organizational justice and workplace aggression. *Journal of Advanced Nursing*, *66*(5), 1169–1182. doi:10.1111/j.1365-2648.2010.05281.x

Stimpfel, A. W., Rosen, J. E., & McHugh, M. D. (2015). Understanding the role of the professional practice environment on quality of care in Magnet and non-magnet hospitals. *The Journal of Nursing Administration*, *45*(10 Suppl.), S52–S58.

Thompson, S. A., & Miller, K. L. (2018). Disruptive trends in higher education: Leadership skills for successful leaders. *Journal of Professional Nursing*, *34*(2), 92–96. doi:10.1016/j.profnurs.2017.11.008

Thorpe, K., & Loo, R. (2003). Balancing professional and personal satisfaction of nurse managers: Current and future perspectives in a changing health care system. *Journal of Nursing Management*, *11*(5), 321–330. doi:10.1046/j.1365-2834.2003.00397.x

Ulrich, B. T., Woods, D., Hart, K. A., Lavandero, R., Leggett, J., & Taylor, D. (2007). Critical care nurses' work environments: Value of excellence in beacon units and magnet organizations. *Critical Care Nurse*, *27*(3), 68–77.

Viney, M., Batcheller, J., Houston, S., & Belcik, K. (2006). Transforming care at the bedside: Designing new care systems in an age of complexity. *Journal of Nursing Care Quality*, *21*(2), 143–150. doi:10.1097/00001786-200604000-00010

Walumbwa, F. O., Avolio, B. J., Gardner, W. L., Wersning, T. S., & Peterson, S. J. (2008). Authentic leadership: Development and validation of a theory-based measure†. *Journal of Management*, *34*(1), 89–126. doi:10.1177/0149206307308913

Wang, H. J., Demerouti, E., & Le Blanc, P. (2017). Transformational leadership, adaptability, and job crafting: The moderating role of organizational identification. *Journal of Vocational Behavior, 100*, 185–195. doi:10.1016/j.jvb.2017.03.009

Weber, M. (1947). *The theory of social and economic organization* (A. M. Henderson & T. Parsons, Trans.) New York, NY: Oxford University Press.

Weberg, D. (2010). Transformational leadership and staff retention: An evidence review with implications for healthcare systems. *Nursing Administration Quarterly*, *34*(3), 246–258. doi:10.1097/naq.0b013e3181e70298

Weick, K. E., & Sutcliffe, K. M. (2001). *Managing the unexpected: Assuring high performance in an age of complexity*. San Francisco, CA: Jossey Bass.

Williams, I., Dickinson, H., Robinson, S., & Allen, C. (2009). Clinical microsystems and the NHS: A sustainable method for improvement? *Healthcare Organization and Management*, *23*(1), 119–132. doi:10.1108/14777260910942597

Wong, C. A., & Cummings, G. G. (2007). The relationship between nursing leadership and patient outcomes: A systematic review. *Journal of Nursing Management*, *15*(5), 508–521. doi:10.1111/j.1365-2834.2007.00723.x

Zwarenstein, M., Goldman, J., & Reeves, S. (2009). Interprofessional collaboration: Effects of practice-based interventions on professional practice and healthcare outcomes. *Cochrane Database of Systematic Reviews*, *2009*(3), CD000072. doi:10.1002/14651858.CD000072.pub2

CHAPTER SEVEN

Translation of Evidence for Health Policy

Kathleen M. White

In order to advocate effectively for lifesaving legislation, advocates must have clear and compelling scientific evidence to provide a basis for policy change.
—Millie Webb, Mothers Against Drunk Driving

Understanding the Policy Process Is Critical to the incorporation of newly generated research evidence into healthcare practice and policy. However, there is a large gap between the research and policy worlds. It is widely recognized that the translation of research evidence into practice and policy is determined as much by the decision-making context and other influences as by the evidence (Oliver, Innvar, Lorenc, Woodman, & Thomas., 2014). Lavis, Ross, and Hurley (2002) paraphrased the title of a journal article to describe the gap between research and policy as "the paradox of health services research: if it is not used, why do we produce so much of it?" Why do we not see consistent translation of new scientific evidence into public policy? How might the interactions between researchers and policy makers become more relevant to real-world problems? What strategies will improve knowledge translation into healthcare policy? Brownson, Royer, Ewing, and McBride (2006) suggested that researchers and policy makers are "travelers in parallel universes"; yet, linking scientific advances to public policy has tremendous promise to advance the health and well-being of the population (Brownson et al., 2006). Brownson, Chriqui, and Stamatakis (2009) discussed the importance of implementing evidence-based policy, citing that the 10 great public health achievements of the 20th century, such as seat belt laws, tobacco control, and injury prevention, were model achievements that occurred because of a policy change. However, they found that only 6.5% of the sponsors of these achievements provided details that showed that the policies or laws were based on scientific information. There are two ways that research findings are communicated: first, by establishing relevance to current issues and, second, by using a local example to frame the effects of a policy impact, which are critical to knowing when and how quickly the research will be considered for use (Armstrong et al., 2013). Effective methods of dissemination and implementation are needed to put evidence into real-world settings, including the policy environment (Brownson & Jones, 2009). Lewis (2011), describing the relationship between research and policy making as "still hazy after all these years," suggests that continued efforts are needed to understand the decision-making processes and enhance the role of research-based evidence in policy.

Because of the difficulty in achieving evidence-based policy, the use of terminology that refers to *evidence-informed* policy is gaining recognition that allows for evidence to consider political realities, change-management practices, and influence provider behaviors and local preferences (Lavis, Oxman, Lewin, & Fretheim, 2009; Kelley & Papa, 2012). The World Health Organization (WHO; n.d.) has created an Evidence-Informed Policy Network, referred to as *EVIPNet*, to promote the use of evidence to improve healthcare practices and policies globally (www.who.int/evidence/en). This chapter discusses evidence and the policy-making process and offers strategies and examples of evidence translated into policy at various public and private levels of policy making.

■ POLICY AND THE POLICY PROCESS

Policy is defined as the choices a society, an organization, or a group makes regarding its goals and priorities and how it will allocate its resources to those priorities. The design of policy involves specifying ends or goals to be pursued and the means for achieving those goals, and reflects the values, beliefs, and attitudes of those designing the policy (Mason, Chaffee, & Leavitt, 2011).

Public policy is defined as any action by local, state, or national government that is created in response to demands of the society to achieve desired goals, values, and practices. Public policy includes laws, regulations, organization/agency guidelines, private sector initiatives, and national or international specialty initiatives.

Health policy specifically addresses how and by whom healthcare is delivered and financed and the environmental influences on health, and it has direct and indirect impact on people's health. The WHO defines *health policy* as an agreement or consensus on the health issues, goals, and objectives to be addressed, the priorities among those objectives, and the main directions for achieving them.

Policy making is a complex, dynamic, and constantly evolving process. Ideally, the policy process, whether for a public policy or a healthcare policy in particular, follows five steps: (a) getting on the public agenda, (b) policy formulation, (c) policy adoption, (d) policy implementation, and (e) policy evaluation (Anderson, 2011). However, the five steps are rarely linear or cyclical. The introduction of research evidence has the ability to influence the policy-making process during any of the steps.

There are several approaches to policy making and the decision-making that ensues as policies are developed. The first is the *rational approach* to policy decision-making. Derived from classic economic theory, this approach is considered to be rational, not only because it has a logical and linear sequence, but also because it assumes full information, comparing all possible alternatives to solve the problem. The limitations to this approach are evident, primarily because an exhaustive analysis of benefits and costs to every possible alternative for dealing with a problem is not practical; it is time-consuming and expensive. The *incremental approach*, also referred to as *incrementalism*, involves small steps to policy change. Many individuals who are involved in the policy process argue against making radical changes and are reluctant to change things too quickly; consequently, policies get tweaked over time rather than dramatically changed all at once. Using this more practical approach, only a few of the many possible alternatives are considered and tend to be the ones that involve only small changes in existing policy rather than radical innovations. Changes are made only "at the margin." Another approach to the policy decision-making is known as the *garbage can approach*. This approach considers that, at any particular time, there is a mix of problems and possible solutions and that this mix of problems and solutions determines the policy outcome.

Kingdon's *multiple streams approach* (2003) to policy decision-making explains three streams (problem, policy, and politics) to implement evidence-based policy and to communicate and package the policy. This approach attempts to explain why some problems and alternatives are recognized and considered for the policy agenda, whereas others are not. The first stream is the *problem*. It is in this stream that problems come to the attention of policy makers, and the decision is made that something must be done about it or it goes away. Problems come to attention through triggering events, feedback, or new knowledge. The *policy* stream is seen when alternatives or solutions are generated by the policy community. During this time in the policy process, new knowledge or ideas must be considered feasible and practical to implement to reach the policy agenda. The *politics* stream includes the current context within which the problem and policy streams are operating, including national mood, organized interests, and current events. When these three streams converge at a given point in time, a problem is recognized, a viable solution is identified, and a change occurs in the political stream. Kingdon (2003) says that a "window of opportunity" opens and a policy change can be enacted.

■ WHY IS TRANSLATION OF RESEARCH TO POLICY DIFFICULT?

An often-cited and important systematic review of evidence from 24 interview studies on facilitators and barriers to the use of research evidence by policy makers yielded weak results (Innvaer, Vist, Trommald, & Oxman, 2002). The use of the evidence was largely descriptive and qualitative and provided limited support for commonly held beliefs. They found that the degree to which evidence is used directly or selectively varies in relation to different types of decision makers and different types of policy questions. In the review of 24 articles, common barriers (and their frequency in parentheses) to the use of research evidence in policy making were identified:

- Absence of personal contact between researchers and policy makers (11/24)
- Lack of timeliness or relevance of research (9/24)
- Mutual mistrust, including perceived political naivety of scientists and scientific naivety of policy makers (8/24)

- Power and budget struggles (7/24)
- Poor quality of research (6/24)
- Political instability or high turnover of policy-making staff (5/24)

The barriers also identified the most common facilitators (and their frequency) of the use of research in policy making from the review:

- Personal contact between researchers and policy makers (13/24)
- Timeliness and relevance of the research (13/24)
- Research that included a summary with clear recommendations (11/24)
- Good-quality research (6/24)
- Research that confirms current policy or endorsed self-interest (6/24)
- Community pressure or client's demand for research (4/24)
- Research that included effectiveness data (3/24).

Finally, the review identified five strategies to increase policy makers' use of research for policy making, focusing on what the researcher should do: (a) have a personal and close two-way communication with the policy maker; (b) ensure that research is perceived as timely, relevant, and of high quality; (c) include effectiveness data; (d) argue that research is relevant to the demands of policy makers and the community; and (e) provide policy recommendation reports, along with the technical research reports.

An update of the Innvaer et al. systematic review was undertaken by Oliver et al. (2014). This systematic review identified 145 new studies, half published after 2010, that showed a much wider range of policy topics, including criminal justice, traffic policy, drug policy, and partnership research. The top five barriers were availability and access to research/improved dissemination, clarity/relevance/reliability of research findings, timing/opportunity, policy maker research skills, and cost. The top five facilitators were availability and access to research/improved dissemination, collaboration, clarity/relevance/reliability of research findings, relationship with policy makers, and relationship with researchers.

Studies by Lavis, Lomas, Hamid, and Sewankambo (2006) and Brownson et al. (2006) identified challenges to translating new research evidence to practice and policy. Brownson et al. (2006) found that the most important challenge is the clash of cultures between the researcher and the policy maker, citing that even with sound scientific data some policies do not get implemented because of lack of public support or competing policy issues. This clash of cultures or "two-communities" view is discussed later in this chapter. Both studies found that timing is a challenge. Lavis (2006) found that research evidence competes with other ideas in the decision-making process, and Brownson et al. (2006) proposed that the generation of new knowledge is not predictable and does not coincide with issues that are on the public agenda. Both studies discussed the frustration that policy makers have with research results and that research evidence is often not easy to use or understand. Policy makers are limited by the amount of information they can process. The effective communication of research findings in a relevant, timely, and compelling manner is necessary to inform the process. Brownson et al. (2006) suggested that policy makers want precise estimates, and researchers often provide confidence intervals that are difficult to sell or project. Finally, these studies also found that the lack of data on relevant new research evidence is a major challenge to translating research to policy. Both studies suggested that the use of case studies or anecdotes to increase relevance and to understand the value of the new evidence is important for researchers when communicating with decision makers.

Later, Brownson and Jones (2009) identified eight specific barriers to implementing effective evidence-based health policy: (a) a lack of value placed on prevention, (b) an insufficient evidence base, (c) mismatched time horizons, (d) the power of vested interests, (e) researchers isolated from the policy process, (f) complex and messy policy-making process, (g) some individuals on the team not understanding the policy-making process, and, (h) practitioners lacking the skills to influence evidence-based policy.

New research evidence is often found in the know–do gap, where the evidence is not translated or acted upon in a timely way (Graham Kothan, McCutcheon, & on behalf of the Integrated Knowledge Translation Research Network Project Leads, 2018). Graham et al. propose moving evidence into practice and policy through integrated knowledge translation, where knowledge users work with researchers throughout the research process, starting with the first research question.

■ THEORY AND ORGANIZING FRAMEWORKS FOR TRANSLATION OF EVIDENCE TO POLICY

Research processes include a question, methods designed specifically to answer the question, data collection, analysis, and interpretation (Lavis, 2006). The public policy-making process is less linear, more unpredictable, and the vicissitudes of debate and politics can cause the issue to languish with uncertain outcome.

The classic literature on technology transfer raised the question about who is responsible for ensuring the application of new technology (Kamien & Schwartz, 1975; Lynch & Gregor, 2003). This responsibility debate, referred to as the *technology push* or the *need or demand pull*, refers to the source and motivation for the innovation. The source is either the scientist who develops the innovation (technology push) or the demand for the innovation based on perceived need (demand pull). According to this *push–pull* theory, an innovation is likely to occur and be applied when a means to develop the innovation and the need for it are simultaneously recognized. This debate has been applied to other disciplines, and more recent discussions in the translation literature have focused on a science–push versus a user–pull debate. The science push is the development of new knowledge driven by science. The user pull is making evidence available when there is demand from policy makers for evidence to drive policy.

Nathan Caplan's two-communities theory (1979) attempted to explain the use or nonuse of research for policy making as a symptom of the cultural or behavioral gap between researchers and policy makers. The theory posits that there are cultural differences between the research and policy-making communities, which have different views of the world, and these are explained as a gap in values, language, reward systems, and professional affiliations. For example, the researcher is concerned mainly with pure science and esoteric issues, whereas the policy maker is more interested in immediate relevance and therefore has an action orientation. This simple dichotomy of use versus nonuse between the two communities must be acknowledged and understood, but researchers and policy makers cannot be complacent or assume that this is the way it has to be. Caplan, Morrison, and Stambaugh (1975) also found that these two groups—the researchers and the policy makers—see themselves and each other differently. The social scientists in the research saw themselves as rational, objective, and open to new ideas, and they saw the policy makers as action and interest oriented and indifferent to evidence and new ideas. The policy makers saw themselves as responsive, action oriented, and pragmatic, and saw the scientists as naïve, jargon ridden, and lacking in practicality. To have an impact on developing and implementing evidence-based policy, the two groups must develop a mutual understanding of the important policy questions and the evidence that is needed to answer them.

Weiss (1979) discusses the three meanings of research as (a) data, (b) ideas, and (c) argumentation and indicates that research is only one of many sources of information used by policy makers. She believes that the goal of research is to clarify and accelerate opinion to contribute to the policy process. Her work adds another dimension to the use–nonuse discussion and suggests that it is not a simple dichotomy of use and nonuse, but that translation of new knowledge is built on a gradual shift in conceptual thinking over time. She posits that the real decision-making is "consideration for use," and she argues that there is an "enlightenment function" of research. She identifies seven models or meanings of research use:

1. Knowledge driven—application of basic research
2. Problem solving—communication of research on agreed-upon problem to the policy maker
3. Enlightenment—education of the policy maker
4. Political—rationalization for previously agreed-upon decision
5. Tactical—requesting additional information to delay action
6. Interactive—competing information sources which implies a search for policy-relevant information
7. Intellectual enterprise—policy research as one of many intellectual pursuits

The challenge for the research community is to improve the use of research findings in policy making. There are numerous frameworks found in the literature that attempt to explain decision-making (or lack of decision-making) and translation (or lack of translation) of new knowledge into the policy process. A significant challenge in the translation of research evidence into practice and policy is that those attempting to translate the findings interpret and apply these frameworks in different ways (Milat & Li, 2017).

Lavis, Robertson, Woodside, McLeod, and Abelson (2003) developed an organizing framework for knowledge transfer into policy and posit that the push–pull tug of knowledge transfer can be loosened by attention to the message and the target audience. The framework has five key elements: (a) the *message,* or how an actionable message should be developed and transferred to decision makers; (b) the *target audience,* or *to whom* the research knowledge should be transferred;, (c) the *messenger,* or *by whom* the research knowledge should be transferred; (d) the *knowledge transfer process,* or how the research knowledge should be transferred; and (e) the *evaluation,* or use of objective performance measures to evaluate the effect of the transfer of the research knowledge. Lavis et al. (2003) suggest that there are four key target audiences to consider: general public, service providers, managerial decision makers, and policy decision makers, and that the message should be crafted individually to each target audience. They also stress the importance of stakeholder involvement in the development of healthcare policy.

There are other models or frameworks for translation of research into policy making worth mentioning. Dobbins, Ciliska, Cockerill, Barnsley, and DiCenso's (2002) *framework for dissemination and utilization of research for health care policy and practice* describes a process for the adoption of research evidence into healthcare decision-making. The framework includes the complex interrelationships among the individual, the organization, the environment, and the innovation. This framework uses Everett Rogers's five stages for the diffusion of innovation to describe the journey of the innovation into practice policy: knowledge, persuasion, decision, implementation, and confirmation. Schmid, Pratt, and Witmer (2006) developed a framework for public policy relevant to physical activity, and Rütten et al. (2003) applied the concept of *logic of events* in a model that is determined by wants, abilities, duties, and opportunities to develop and carry out health policy and evaluate impact.

Gold (2009) proposed a framework that showed 10 pathways through which research may be used in policy making and the factors that mediate the translation of research into messages that are communicated to and used by policy makers. The 10 pathways are divided into:

1. Traditional pathways where meritorious findings drive use (big bang, gradual accumulation and diffusion, and formal synthesis)
2. Intermediaries that help to communicate the research messages (researchers as communicators and experts, formal intermediary-brokered translation, and the mass media)
3. Users who seek to enhance the value of research (commissioned synthesis around policy problems, user-commissioned studies, users that provide input into new research, and researchers as users)

Of course, a single pathway is rarely seen, and a composite of these pathways is more realistic and should be the focus of translation efforts to incorporate new knowledge into policy. The value that this analysis adds is the emphasis on the linkages of the pathways and building bridges between the research and user communities. Gold (2009) emphasizes the importance of a publicly available repository of research findings and synthesis of those findings, not only around important public policy agenda issues, but also in emerging healthcare problems and issues, but also to raise awareness and to stimulate further research on important topics.

Weinick and Shin (2003), as part of work for the Agency for Healthcare Research and Quality, developed a framework for developing data-driven capabilities to support policy decision-making. The framework has four stages and focuses on the importance of stakeholders in making policy decisions. The first stage is *definition and priorities,* which includes articulating a common definition of the policy problem among the stakeholders, clarifying stakeholder concerns and priorities, and understanding what questions need to be answered with evidence. The second stage is *generating data* or determining what data are available to support a policy decision. This stage involves assembling a matrix of all available data sources, including an evaluation of what the data represent and confidence in the data, determining the available measures, identifying the need for new or additional data, and developing an inventory of current and past initiatives. The third stage is *assessment* or explaining what the data say about the current state of the problem, undertaking activities that include analyzing data, clarifying the limitations of current knowledge, and disseminating the findings. The fourth and final stage is *action*. The main activity of the action stage is selecting a policy option that is supported by the data. This includes evaluating the impact of past and current initiatives and any unintended consequences, estimating the short- and long-term effects of the options, and making the policy recommendation. This stage should also include an evaluation of values at issue, anticipation of the outcomes of policy options, and development of a plan for communication of the policy choice.

In 2007, the WHO did a review of the capacity issues underlying different aspects of the relationship between researchers and policy makers (Green & Bennett, 2007). Green and Bennett (2007) used a framework to guide the process to show that there is not a linear relationship between the generation of evidence and policy making and that there are many factors involved in how new knowledge gets translated into policy. The framework first describes four functional processes: (a) priority setting for research, (b) knowledge generation and dissemination, (c) evidence filtering and amplification, and (d) the policy process. As evidence-informed (this framework does not use evidence-based policy) policy making occurs, it is recognized that there are many direct and indirect influences on the policy making, including ideology and values, ability to use the evidence, personal experience and intuition, special interests, and external influences. There are many examples of this filtering and amplification of evidence in the policy arena. Special interests often use this as a way to pick out or *filter* their particular research outputs, translate them into policy messages, and attempt to influence policy makers. The next level of concern for the framework is the various organizations that are carrying out the functions described previously and their interrelationships. They identified these organizations as funding bodies, research institutions, advocacy organizations, the media, think tanks, and government bodies. Finally, the framework includes certain organizational capacities that the organizations must have to carry out the functions, such as leadership and governance, adequate and sustainable resources, and communication and networks. These all operate within a broader national context and wider environment that includes external funders, external research organizations, and external advocacy groups. The added value of this framework to the discussion of translation of research to policy making is the previously recognized important role of the organization in the policy-making process and the help given to researchers and policy makers to understand what works for whom and in what circumstances.

■ STAKEHOLDERS

Knowledge translation for evidence-based policy has been described as a unidirectional flow of information that resulted in a specific policy. If the flow of information was from the researcher to the policy maker, it was called the *science-push* or *knowledge-driven* model (Jacobson, Butterill, & Goering, 2003). Conversely, if the policy maker commissioned the information to address a policy problem, it was referred to as a *demand-pull* or *problem-solving* model.

Jacobson et al. (2003) developed a framework for knowledge translation: understanding user context from a review of literature and its own experience. The framework contains five domains: (a) the user group, (b) the issue, (c) the research, (d) the researcher–user relationship, and (e) the dissemination strategies. Within each domain, the authors pose questions to the researcher that can serve as a way of organizing the translation to the user group.

The first domain is the *user group*. There are many questions posed under this domain, and they focus on the context in which the user group operates; the morphology, politics, and decision-making practices of the user group; how the user group uses information; and its experience with translation (Box 7.1).

The second domain is the *issue* and includes questions about the effect of the issue on the user group, how the user group currently deals with the issue and whether this is changing or not, whether there is uncertainty or conflict surrounding the issue, and what risks are associated with the issue (Jacobson et al., 2003).

The *research* itself is the third domain and encourages the researcher to think about the source, focus, and methodology of the research; the quality, consistency, and ambiguity of the research; the relevance of the research to the user group, such as whether the research has an immediate application, whether it is action oriented, and whether it is compatible with the user-group's expectations or priorities; and, finally, what the implications of the research are for the user group and how politically charged they are (Jacobson et al., 2003).

The fourth domain is the *researcher–user relationship* and focuses the researcher on the linkage between the researcher and the user group, how much trust and rapport exist, whether they have a history of working together, how frequently they have contact with one another, and whether the researcher and the user group have agreed on the outcomes of the translation and about the responsibilities and interactions each will have during knowledge translation (Jacobson et al., 2003).

The final domain deals with how the translation will be organized and the *dissemination strategies* that will be used during the translation, such as the manner of communication, format, the detail needed, use of feedback and reminders, and the

BOX 7.1 User-Group Questions

In what formal or informal structures is the user group embedded?

What is the political climate surrounding the user group?

To whom is the user group accountable?

Are changes expected in any of these?

How big is the user group?

How centralized is the user group?

How institutionalized is the user group?

What are the politics within the user group?

What kinds of decisions does the user group make?

What is the user group's attitude toward decision-making?

What criteria does the user group use to make decisions?

What actions are available to the user group?

What are the stages or phases of the user group's decision-making work?

What is the user group's pace of work?

What sources of information does the user group access and use?

How does the user group process information (i.e., how does it access, disseminate, and apply information internally)?

For what purposes does the user group use information?

Has the user group demonstrated an ability to learn?

What incentives exist for the user group to use research? Is the user group cynical about research and researchers?

How sophisticated is the user-group's knowledge of research methods and terminology?

Does the user group have a history of being involved in knowledge translation?

What knowledge translation structures and processes already exist?

What resources does the user group devote to knowledge translation?

What are the user group's expectations of the researcher? Of the knowledge translation process?

How many user-group members will be involved in the knowledge translation process? Who are they?

Source: From Jacobson, N., Butterill, D., & Goering, P. (2003). Development of a framework for knowledge translation: Understanding user context. *Journal of Health Services Research & Policy*, 8(2), 94–99. doi:10.1258/135581903321466067

extent and the ways in which the researcher should continue to be available to the user group after the conclusion of the knowledge translation (Jacobson et al., 2003).

Attention to these domains by the researcher will improve translation planning and implementation and raise awareness of the information needed by users, which can increase the uptake of the research results. The early involvement of multiple stakeholders with specific vested interests is more likely to develop consensus and yield a user-friendly policy that can be successfully implemented and sustained (Irvin et al., 2007; Nieva et al., 2005).

SELECTED TRANSLATION OF EVIDENCE TO POLICY

Sorian and Baugh recognized the importance of state participation in setting health policy based on evidence. They raised the following questions: (a) How useful is policy research in making policy decisions? (b) Is research information getting to policy makers in a timely and useful manner? (c) How can the needs of researchers and policy makers be better aligned? In an attempt to answer these questions, researchers from Georgetown University's Institute for Health Care Research and Policy and the T. Baugh and Company marketing firm conducted a telephonic survey of state-based health policy makers. They interviewed 97 legislators, 97 legislative staff members, and 87 executive managers of health-related state agencies (Sorian & Baugh, 2002) to identify pathways and factors that could assist communicating health policy research findings to state policy makers. Results of the survey showed that 53% of the respondents only skim materials and that they never get to 35% of the material. They reported that 49% of the information they receive is not relevant, and when probed about what would make it relevant, 67% said that they needed the information to be focused on current debate or 25% on real people. They also identified what made information least useful to them: 36% said when the information is not relevant or focused on real problems; 22% said when it is too long or dense; 20% reported information not to be relevant when it was too theoretical, technical, or used jargon; and 19% were concerned about bias.

Pollack, Samuels, Frattaroli, and Gielen (2010) discussed numerous examples of injury-prevention measures that were proven effective, such as passenger-restraint devices, smoke alarms, residential sprinklers, and use of motorcycle and bicycle helmets. Their experience has shown that personal contact between researchers and policy makers and timely conveyance of easy-to-understand information that is relevant to the policy context facilitates the acceleration of translation of knowledge to action to prevent injury and protect the population. In addition, it is important to include information on the burden of the problem, costs associated with action or inaction, and options for policy formulation (Jilcott, Ammerman, Sommers, & Glasgow, 2007; Pollack et al., 2010).

Tomson et al. (2005) reported on the usefulness of research evidence in implementing a national drug policy in the Lao People's Democratic Republic. Their research concluded that a close interaction between the researchers and the policy makers and attention to broad dissemination of results are important for acceptance of new evidence for drug policies, but that more research is needed to understand the interaction necessary between researchers and decision makers.

In 2005, Congress passed legislation as part of the Deficit Reduction Act that requires the secretary of the Department of Health and Human Services (DHHS) through the Centers for Medicare & Medicaid Services (CMS) to identify healthcare conditions among patients admitted to the hospital that (a) are high cost, high volume, or both; (b) result in the assignment of a case to a diagnosis-related group, which has a higher payment scale when present as a secondary diagnosis; and (c) could reasonably have been prevented through the application of evidence-based guidelines (DHHS, CMS, 2011). The new law was applicable to 3,500 acute care hospitals reimbursed by Medicare. On July 31, 2008, CMS identified 10 categories of conditions that met the three criteria stated previously and were selected for this hospital-acquired condition payment provision in the fiscal year 2009 final rule:

1. Foreign object retained after surgery
2. Air embolism
3. Blood incompatibility
4. Stage III and IV pressure ulcers
5. Falls and trauma, including fractures, dislocations, intracranial injuries, crushing injuries, burns, and electric shock
6. Manifestations of poor glycemic control, such as diabetic ketoacidosis, nonketotic hyperosmolar coma, hypoglycemic coma, secondary diabetes with ketoacidosis, and secondary diabetes with hyperosmolarity
7. Catheter-associated urinary tract infection
8. Vascular catheter-associated infection
9. Surgical site infection following (a) coronary artery bypass graft; (b) bariatric surgeries such as laparoscopic gastric bypass, gastroenterostomy, and laparoscopic gastric restrictive surgery; and (c) orthopedic procedures of the spine, neck, shoulder, and elbow
10. Deep vein thrombosis/pulmonary embolism following total knee or hip replacement

Medicare will no longer pay hospitals at higher rates for the increased costs of care if any of these 10 conditions that have been determined to be reasonably preventable by following generally accepted evidence-based practice guidelines are acquired during the hospitalization.

This policy, using evidence-based practice guidelines based on the translation of research to practice and now to policy, is important for standardizing and improving access to appropriate treatment for patients. The benefits should be significant to healthcare (White, 2008).

The transitional care model (TCM), developed by researchers at the University of Pennsylvania and funded by the National Institutes of Health, is another example of the translation of an evidence-based strategy into a practice delivery model. The model uses advanced practice registered nurses with specialized training to care for older adults with multiple chronic conditions and to support their family caregivers (Naylor et al., 2004, 2009). The TCM has had significant and sustained outcomes, including avoiding hospital readmissions and ED visits for primary and coexisting conditions; improvements in health outcomes after discharge; enhancement in patient and family caregiver satisfaction; and reductions in total healthcare costs (Naylor & Sochalski, 2010). This success of the TCM has positioned it for translation into national healthcare policy. Aetna has adopted the TCM to achieve better outcomes for its older adult enrollees with multiple chronic problems. AARP has recommended expansion of the services of the TCM to its members. The National Quality Forum has endorsed the deployment of evidence-based transitional care, such as the TCM, as one of the 25 national preferred practices for care coordination. Finally, the Patient Protection and Affordable Care Act of 2010, President Obama's healthcare reform legislation, includes support for design, measurement, and payment innovation around evidence-based transitional care.

A final and important clinical example of translation of evidence into policy is attempting to reduce early elective deliveries of newborns. Approximately 10% to 15% of all births in the United States are performed early without any medical reason for the early birth induction. These early births scheduled without a medical reason, also known as *early elective deliveries*, occur between 37 and 39 weeks' of pregnancy. Elective deliveries may occur by either induction or cesarean section (C-section) and are associated with an increased risk of maternal and neonatal morbidity and longer hospital stays for both mothers and newborns, as compared to deliveries occurring between 39 and 40 completed weeks' gestation. These early births have increased the risk of maternal and infant complications. For more than 30 years, the American College of Obstetricians and Gynecologists has promoted a clinical guideline discouraging elective deliveries prior to 39 weeks' gestation without medical or obstetrical need. Over the past several years, organizations, such as the March of Dimes, Childbirth Connections, the LeapFrog Group, and the Association of Women's Health, Obstetric and Neonatal Nurses, have raised concerns about babies being scheduled for birth too soon. In 2012, CMS and state Medicaid programs launched two evidence-based initiatives designed to improve maternal and infant health outcomes by reducing the number of early elective deliveries that lack a medical reason (American College of Obstetricians and Gynecologists, 2009). One initiative, Strong Start for Mothers and Newborns, led by the CMS and Medicaid Innovation working in partnership with the Center for Medicaid and Children's Health Insurance Program (CHIP) Services (CMCS), includes two primary strategies: (a) testing ways to encourage best practices for reducing the number of early elective deliveries that lack medical indication across all payer types and (b) testing three models of enhanced prenatal care for reducing preterm births among women covered by Medicaid/CHIP. The other national initiative, CMS Expert Panel for Improving Maternal and Infant Health Outcomes, is identifying specific opportunities and strategies to provide better care while reducing the cost of care for mothers and infants covered by Medicaid/CHIP (https://www.medicaid.gov/medicaid/quality-of-care/improvement-initiatives/maternal-and-infant-health/index.html).

STRATEGIES TO INCREASE THE UPTAKE OF RESEARCH TO POLICY

The literature abounds with discussion of strategies intended to increase the uptake of evidence into policy or lessons learned from an attempt to translate research into policy. As has been said about moving evidence into practice, there is a similar need to move from knowing to doing (Nutley, Walter, & Davies, 2003). Lavis et al. (2002) conclude that careful attention must be paid to where we look for research use; what we are looking for; the conditions under which the research is used and not used; and, most important, the way in which research is used as well as its use in the context of other competing influences in the policy-making process. Brownson et al. (2006) suggest several actions to bridge the research–policy chasm, but all are aimed at the researcher: Understand the complexity and drivers in decision-making; find a way to understand and be involved in the policy process; communicate information more effectively; make better use of analytic tools; educate staffers on science; develop systems for policy surveillance; conduct policy research; improve training and educational programs for scientists; build appropriate, transdisciplinary teams; and cultivate political champions. Likewise, policy makers have a responsibility to bridge this chasm.

Mercer et al. (2010) wrote a case study examining the lessons learned from translating evidence on the effectiveness of laws to lower the legal blood alcohol limit for drivers. They reported that the successful translation of evidence into policy was related to the following: (a) salience of the health problem and policy intervention, in addition to the compelling relationships among the health problem, policy intervention, and health outcomes; (b) use of systematic review methods to synthesize the full body of evidence; (c) use of a recognized, credible, and impartial process for assessing the evidence; (d) development of evidence-based policy recommendations by an independent, impartial body; (e) ability to capitalize on readiness and teachable moments; (f) active participation of key partners and intended users throughout all stages of the process; (g) use of personalized channels, targeted formats, and compelling graphics to disseminate the evidence; (h) capacity to involve multiple stakeholders in encouraging uptake and adherence; and (i) attention paid to addressing sustainability.

Brownson et al. (2011) developed four types of policy briefs on mammography screening and sent them to three groups of state-level policy makers, legislative staff, legislators, and executive branch administrators, to measure their understandability, credibility, and likelihood to be used and/or shared. They found that the likelihood of using the briefs was highest among the legislators, among women, those older than 52 years with a graduate education, and those who identified themselves as socially liberal. However, they also found that each of the groups of policy makers preferred a different type of brief, data focused versus story focused and state versus local data, so that the "one-size-fits-all" approach when delivering information to policy makers may be less effective than communicating information based on the type of policy maker.

The literature discusses many ways to facilitate the uptake of research to policy, yet it is widely recognized that it is still a difficult challenge (Dickson & Flynn, 2009;

Hinshaw & Grady, 2011). However, experience has taught that there are several key strategies that will increase the likelihood that policy makers will use evidence in their decision-making for policy development. First, and most important, is for the researcher to develop effective two-way communication with the policy maker. This should begin ahead of the policy question reaching the public agenda. An open dialogue between the research community and the policy makers about healthcare issues of concern in real time will increase the likelihood that each communicates the needs in the research and policy-making processes. Second, it is important that researchers take the time to ensure that the research is perceived as timely, relevant, and of high quality.

In today's environment, the inclusion of effectiveness data as evidence is a key to success in informing choices that both clinicians and patients are confronting. New evidence that affects comparative effectiveness should be reviewed and incorporated when relevant and appropriate (Coopey, James, Lawrence, & Clancy, 2008).

Finally, because of the abundance of data and information available to policy makers, strategies that provide a synthesis of the relevant evidence to inform policies are critical for uptake. The Robert Wood Johnson Foundation (RWJF) developed the Synthesis Project (Figure 7.1) to give policy makers access to reliable information, develop insights into complex policy decisions, and produce briefs and reports that synthesize research findings on perennial health policy questions. The project started with a question: Why aren't research results more useful to policy makers (Colby, Quinn, Williams, Bilheimer, & Goodell, 2008)? Policy makers answered and identified three needs for use of research evidence in the development of policy: clear translation, accessible and easy-to-use information, and relevance to the policy context (Colby et al., 2008). They explained that policy makers are besieged with information, but results are not translated for policy decisions; research does not address pressing policy questions; journal articles and research reports are written for researchers, not policy makers; and policy makers have little time to stay abreast of current research (Cohen & Neumann, 2009). The

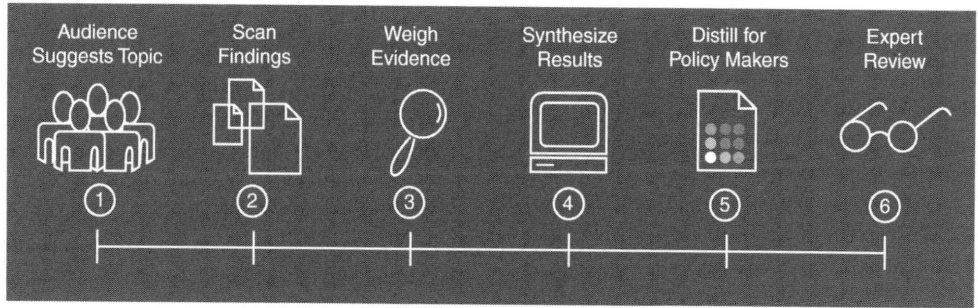

FIGURE 7.1 The Robert Wood Johnson Foundation Synthesis Project framework.

Source: From Cohen, J., & Neumann, P. (2009). *The cost savings and cost-effectiveness of clinical preventive care*. Robert Wood Johnson Foundation Research Synthesis Report No. 18. Retrieved from www.rwjf.org/content/dam/farm/reports/issue_briefs/2009/rwjf46045/subassets/rwjf46045_1

RWJF Synthesis initiative developed products to address policy makers' requests for short, skimmable, and policy-focused information, focusing on the findings, not the methods (Colby et al., 2008). They developed policy briefs, research synthesis reports, and data charts. These project deliverables are structured around policy questions rather than research issues; they distill and weigh the strength of research evidence in a rigorous and objective manner; and they draw out the policy implications of findings (www.rwjf.org/pr/synthesisabout.jsp). Finally, they attempt to tell a "synthesis story" that addresses four questions: (a) Why is this of interest to policy makers? (b) What "story" does the evidence tell? (c) What choices does the evidence suggest would be most effective? (d) What are the implications for policy makers (Colby et al., 2008)?

There are two other valuable techniques that are used to synthesize data and evidence for policy makers. The policy brief, often referred to as the *two pager*, is written by those trying to influence or impact a policy maker or a decision. The purpose of a policy brief is to assist the policy maker to evaluate policy options on a specific issue. Policy briefs offer policy options informed by evidence with rationale and consequences for choosing each option. The brief usually makes a recommendation for a preferred and specific course of action (Box 7.2).

The second technique uses a research approach that systematically reviews the evidence to reduce a large amount of evidence on an issue of concern and reports a synthesis of the evidence that determines the quality, quantity, and consistency of that evidence (Dobbins, 2010; Dobbins, Cockerill, & Barnsley, 2001; Haby et al., 2016, Marquez et al., 2018; Yost et al., 2014). A systematic review applies defined scientific methods to appraise and summarize the evidence. As part of those scientific methods, the systematic review attempts to identify and limit bias and to improve the reliability of any recommendations proposed from the synthesis of the evidence. Murthy et al. (2012) reviewed eight studies evaluating the effectiveness of the use of systematic reviews. The overall synthesized quality of the evidence reviewed was low to moderate. They concluded that a mass mailing of the systematic review evidence can be an effective strategy to get the message out if there is growing awareness of the need for the change. Petkovic et al. (2016) found that evidence summaries are more likely to increase policy makers' understanding of the importance of the new evidence; however, they concluded that the use of systematic reviews of evidence for policy making is unclear. Hence, if the goal is to develop awareness and share new evidence, a multifaceted approach is necessary (Tricco et al., 2016). Marquez et al. (2018) evaluated the best formats for communicating systematic-review findings to increase uptake of the evidence. They found that the most important facilitators were that the content is relevant, resources for implementation have to be available, that there is collaboration between the researcher and decision maker and that the decision is motivated to use the results.

The combination of the information from many studies on a specific issue can increase the strength of the overall evidence more than any one study result could yield, increasing its power (Box 7.3).

BOX 7.2 How to Write a Policy Brief: The Two Pager

Components of a Policy Brief

1. **Executive summary or abstract**—The executive summary or abstract should be a short summary of approximately 150 words, which states clearly and succinctly the purpose of the policy brief and its recommendations.
2. **Statement of the issue/problem**—The statement of the issue is the first section of the policy brief and is a short statement of the problem with a clear description of a definition of the issue. Sometimes the statement of the issue is phrased as a question that requires a decision.
3. **Background section**—The background section describes the background and history of the issue. Be clear, precise, and succinct. This section should include only the essential facts that a decision maker "needs to know" to understand the context of the problem. There are usually reams of information that can be included in this section; however, consider that your job is to filter out all the possible information about this issue and what you think the policy maker really needs to read. For example, discuss any preexisting policies, any policy options that have been considered in the past, or merely describe what has taken place in the past or been done by others for and against this issue. It is important to note that the absence of action in the past may be considered a policy decision.
4. **Statement of your organization's interests in the issue**—The statement of your organization's interest in the issue is important to remind the policy maker or reader why the issue matters for that organization, group, or the country.
5. **Policy options**—The policy-options section of the policy brief delineates the possible courses of action or inaction. Usually the decision maker is given at least three potential courses of action. Those three courses of action include the status quo, maximum change, and some policy option in between no action and maximum change. Sometimes there is more than one choice in between, which then increases the number of policy options and the complexity of decision-making. Include the advantages and disadvantages of each policy option.
6. **Recommendation**—In the recommendation section, state what your recommendation is for action. This is usually done by prioritizing the relative pros and cons of the options presented and then making a recommendation for one option.
7. **Sources or consultations**—Include references, sources of information, and interviews or consultations conducted with experts on the issue.

BOX 7.3 What Is a Systematic Review?

A systematic review is a summary of the literature that uses explicit methods to perform a comprehensive literature search and critical appraisal of individual studies. This critical appraisal reviews for strength, quality, and consistency of the evidence. The review may also use appropriate statistical techniques to combine these valid studies (Straus, Richardson, Glasziou, & Haynes, 2005). A systematic review provides a mechanism to identify studies with strong and weak designs and limit the bias of the weaker designs that might overestimate the effects or benefits of the evidence.

For policy making, the systematic review uses specific and reproducible search strategies to generate evidence to answer a specific policy question. The systematic review provides the strongest type of evidence that is available on the policy issue, both published and unpublished. A review of the strength and quality is conducted on all of the existing evidence on that policy topic/question (Jadad et al., 1996). The review of the evidence is then combined into a single analysis where explicit methods are used to limit bias and to evaluate the quality of the evidence (GRADE* Working Group, 2004).

Websites that house current systematic reviews of evidence include:

www.cochrane.org

www.joannabriggs.edu.au

www.ahrq.gov *or* www.ngc.gov

■ CONCLUSIONS

This chapter has discussed the importance of translating new evidence into practice and policy. For evidence to be translated into policy, the evidence must be communicated in an understandable and accessible manner to policy makers. Lavis, Posada, Haines, and Osei (2004) recommend using systematic reviews to summarize new evidence and answer three simple questions for policy makers: (a) Could it work? (b) What will it take to make it work? and (c) Is the balance of risk and benefit worth it?

However, politics will always have a role in policy making. When it comes to the translation of research into healthcare policy, attention must be directed to recognizing the importance of the current healthcare policy agenda and how problems or issues got on and off the policy agenda. This also means regularly interacting with policy makers to understand what is currently making news, what is of interest to all of the audiences with which they have to contend (consumers, policy makers, and practitioners alike), and finding out what the policy questions are for which they need data to answer. This would create a perfect world where policy is informed by evidence and that policy could be directed to improve health and reduce health inequalities in our healthcare system.

REFERENCES

American College of Obstetricians and Gynecologists. (2009). Committee on Practice Bulletins. ACOG practice bulletin No. 107. Induction of labor. *Obstetrics and Gynecology, 114*, 386–397.

Anderson, J. E. (2011). *Public policymaking: An introduction* (7th ed.). Boston, MA: Wadsworth Cengage Learning.

Armstrong, R., Whaters, E., Dobbins, M., Anderson, L., Moore, L., Petticrew, M., . . . Swinburn, B. (2013). Knowledge translation strategies to improve the use of evidence in public health decision making in local government: Intervention design and implementation plan. *Implementation Science, 8(1)*, 121. doi:10.1186/1748-5908-8-121

Brownson, R. C., Chriqui, J. F., & Stamatakis, K. A. (2009). Understanding evidence-based public health policy. *American Journal of Public Health, 99*(9), 1576–1583. doi:10.2105/ajph.2008.156224

Brownson, R. C., Dodson, E. A., Stamatakis, K. A., Casy, C. M., Eltite, M. B., Luke, D. A., . . . Kreunter, M. W. (2011). Communicating evidence-based information on cancer prevention to state-level policy makers. *Journal National Cancer Institute, 103*(4), 306–316. doi:10.1093/jnci/djq529

Brownson, R. C., & Jones, E. (2009). Bridging the gap: Translating research into policy and practice. *Preventive Medicine, 49*(4), 313–315. doi:10.1016/j.ypmed.2009.06.008

Brownson, R. C., Royer, C., Ewing, R., & McBride, T. D. (2006). Researchers and policymakers: Travelers in parallel universes. *American Journal of Preventive Medicine, 30*(2), 164–172. doi:10.1016/j.amepre.2005.10.004

Caplan, N. (1979). The two-communities theory and knowledge utilization. *American Behavioral Scientist, 22*(3), 459–470. doi:10.1177/000276427902200308

Caplan, N. S., Morrison, A., & Stambaugh, R. J. (1975). *The use of social science knowledge in policy decisions at the national level: A report to respondents*. Ann Arbor, MI: University of Michigan.

Cohen, J., & Neumann, P. (2009). *The cost savings and cost-effectiveness of clinical preventive care*. Robert Wood Johnson Foundation Research Synthesis Report No. 18. Retrieved from https://www.rwjf.org/en/library/research/2009/09/cost-savings-and-cost-effectiveness-of-clinical-preventive-care.html

Colby, D. C., Quinn, B. C., Williams, C. H., Bilheimer, L. T., & Goodell, S. (2008). Research glut and information famine: Making research evidence more useful for policymakers. *Health Affairs, 27*(4), 1177–1182. doi:10.1377/hlthaff.27.4.1177

Coopey, M., James, M. D., Lawrence, W., & Clancy, C. M. (2008). The challenge of comparative effectiveness: Getting the right information to the right people at the right time. *Journal of Nursing Care Quality, 23*(1), 1–5. doi:10.1097/01.ncq.0000303797.76962.9e

Department of Health and Human Services, Center for Medicare and Medicaid Services. (2011). *Hospital-acquired conditions*. Baltimore, MD: Authors. Retrieved from http://www.cms.gov/HospitalAcqCond/06_Hospital-Acquired_Conditions.asp

Dickson, G., & Flynn, L. (2009). *Nursing policy research: Turning evidence-based research into health policy*. New York, NY: Springer Publishing Company.

Dobbins, M. (2010). Dissemination and use of research evidence for policy and practice. In J. Rycroft-Malone & T. Bucknall (Eds.), *Models & frameworks for implementing evidence-based practice*. Chichester, UK: John Wiley & Sons.

Dobbins, M., Ciliska, D., Cockerill, R., Barnsley, J., & DiCenso, A. (2002). A framework for the dissemination and utilization of research for health-care policy and practice. *Online Journal of Knowledge Synthesis for Nursing, E9(1)*, 149–160. doi:10.1111/j.1524-475x.2002.00149.x

Dobbins, M., Cockerill, R., & Barnsley, J. (2001). Factors affecting the utilization of systematic reviews: A study of public health decision makers. *International Journal of Technology Assessment in Health Care, 17*(2), 203–214. doi:10.1017/s0266462300105069

Gold, M. (2009). Pathways to the use of health services research in policy. *Health Services Research, 44*(4), 1111–1136. doi:10.1111/j.1475-6773.2009.00958.x

GRADE* Working Group. (2004). Grading quality of evidence and strength of recommendations. *British Medical Journal, 328*(7454), 1490–1494.

Graham, I. D., Kothan, A., McCutcheon, C., & On behalf of the Integrated Knowledge Translation Research Network Project Leads. (2018). Moving knowledge into action for more effective practice, programmes and policy: Protocol for a research programme on integrated knowledge translation. *Implementation Science, 13*(1), 22. doi:10.1186/s13012-017-0700-y

Green, A., & Bennett, S. (Eds.). (2007). *Sound choices: Enhancing capacity for evidence-informed health policy*. Geneva, Switzerland: World Health Organization.

Haby, M. M., Chapman, E., Clark, R., Barreto, J. Reveiz, L., & Lavis, J. (2016). What are the best methodologies for rapid reviews of the research evidence for evidence-informed decision making in health policy and practice: A rapid review. *Health Research Policy and Systems, 14*(1), 83. doi:10.1186/s12961-016-0155-7

Hinshaw, A. S., & Grady, P. (Eds.). (2011). *Shaping health policy through nursing research*. New York, NY: Springer Publishing Company.

Innvaer, S., Vist, G., Trommald, M., & Oxman, A. (2002). Health policy-makers' perceptions of their use of evidence: A systematic review. *Journal of Health Services Research & Policy*, 7(4), 239–244. doi:10.1258/135581902320432778

Irvin, C. B., Afilalo, M., Sherman, S. C., Stack, S. J., Huckson, S., Kanji, A., & Skin, B. (2007). The use of health care policy to facilitate evidence-based knowledge translation in emergency medicine. *Academic Emergency Medicine*, *14*(11), 1030–1035. doi:10.1197/j.aem.2007.06.022

Jacobson, N., Butterill, D., & Goering, P. (2003). Development of a framework for knowledge translation: Understanding user context. *Journal of Health Services Research & Policy*, *8*(2), 94–99. doi:10.1258/135581903321466067

Jadad, A. R., Moore, R. A., Carroll, D., Jenkinson, C., Reynolds, D. J., Gavaghan, D. J., & Quay, H. J. (1996). Assessing the quality of reports of randomized clinical trials: Is blinding necessary? *Controlled Clinical Trials, 17*(1), 1–12. doi:10.1016/0197-2456(95)00134-4

Jilcott, S., Ammerman, A., Sommers, J., & Glasgow, R. E. (2007). Applying the RE-AIM framework to assess the public health impact of policy change. *Annals of Behavioral Medicine*, *34*(2), 105–114. doi: 10.1007/bf02872666

Kamien, M., & Schwartz, N. (1975). Market structure and innovation: A survey. *Journal of Economic Literature*, *13*, 1–37.

Kelley, B., & Papa, K. (2012). *Academy health research insights: Using HSR to influence policy change and population health improvement*. Washington, DC: Academy Health.

Kingdon, J. W. (2003). *Agendas, alternatives, and public policies* (2nd ed.). New York, NY: Addison-Wesley Educational Publishers.

Lavis, J., Oxman, A., Lewin, S., & Fretheim, A. (2009). SUPPORT Tools for evidence-informed health Policymaking (STP). *Introduction. Health Research Policy and Systems*, 7(Suppl. 1), 478–505. Retrieved from http://www.health-policy-systems.com/content/pdf/1478-4505-7-S1-I1.pdf

Lavis, J. N. (2006). Research, public policymaking, and knowledge-translation processes: Canadian efforts to build bridges. *Journal of Continuing Education in the Health Professions*, *26*(1), 37–45. doi:10.1002/chp.49

Lavis, J. N., Lomas, J., Hamid, M., & Sewankambo, N. K. (2006). Assessing country-level efforts to link research to action. *Bulletin of the World Health Organization*, *84*(8), 620–628.

Lavis, J. N., Posada, F. B., Haines, A., & Osei, E. (2004). Use of research to inform public policymaking. *Lancet*, *364*(9445), 1615–1621. doi:10.1016/s0140-6736(04)17317-0

Lavis, J. N., Robertson, D., Woodside, J. M., McLeod, C. B., & Abelson, J. (2003). How can research organizations more effectively transfer research knowledge to decision makers? *Milbank Quarterly*, *81*(2), 221–248. doi:10.1111/1468-0009.t01-1-00052

Lavis, J. N., Ross, S. E., Hurley, J. E. (2002). Examining the role of health services research in public policymaking. *Milbank Quarterly*, *80*(1), 125–154. doi: 10.1111/1468-0009.00005

Lewis, S. (2011). How research influences policy makers: Still hazy after all these years. *Journal National Cancer Institute, 103*(4), 286–287. doi:10.1093/jnci/djq543

Lynch, T., & Gregor, S. (2003). Technology-push or user-pull? The slow death of the transfer-of-technology approach to intelligent support systems development. In S. Clarke, E. Coaches, M. G. Hunter, & A. Winn (Eds.), *Socio-technical and human cognition elements of information systems*. Hershey, PA: Information Science Publishing.

Marquez, C., Johnson, A. M., Jassemi S., Park, J., Moore, J. E., Blaine, C., . . . Straus, S. E. (2018). Enhancing the uptake of systematic reviews of effects: What is the best format for health care managers and policymakers? A mixed-methods study. *Implementation Science, 13*(1), 84. doi:10.1186/s13012-018-0779-9

Mason, D., Chaffee, M., & Leavitt, J. (2011). *Policy & politics in nursing and health care* (6th ed.). St. Louis, MO: Elsevier Saunders.

Medicaid.gov. (n.d.). *Maternal and infant health care quality*. Retrieved from https://www.medicaid.gov/medicaid/quality-of-care/improvement-initiatives/maternal-and-infant-health/index.html

Mercer, S. L., Sleet, D. A., Elder, R. W., Cole, K. H., Shultz, R. A., & Nichols, J. L. (2010). Translating evidence into policy: Lessons from the case of lowering the legal blood alcohol limit for drivers. *Annals of Epidemiology*, *20*(6), 412–420. doi:10.1016/j.annepidem.2010.03.005

Milat, A. & Li, B. (2017). Narrative review of frameworks for translating research evidence into policy and practice. *Public Health Research & Practice, 27*(1), e2711704. doi:10.17061/phrp2711704

Murthy, L., Shepperd, S., Clarke, M. J., Garner, S. E., Lavis, J. N., Perrier, L., . . . Straus, S. (2012). Interventions to improve the use of systematic reviews in decision-making by health system managers, policy makers and clinicians. *Cochrane Database of Systematic Reviews, 2012*(9), CD009401.

Naylor, M., & Sochalski, J. A. (2010). Scaling up: Bringing the transitional care model into the mainstream. *Commonwealth Fund, 103*, 1–12.

Naylor, M. D., Broken, D. A., Campbell, R. L., Maslin, G., McCauley, K. M., & Schwartz, J. S. (2004). Transitional care of older adults hospitalized with heart failure: A randomized, controlled trial. *Journal of the American Geriatrics Society*, *52*(5), 675–684. doi:10.1111/j.1532-5415.2004.52202.x

Naylor, M. D., Feldman, P. H., Keating, S., Koran, M. J., Kurtzman, E. T., McCoy, M. C., & Krakauer, R. (2009). Translating research into practice: Transitional care for older adults. *Journal of Evaluation in Clinical Practice*, *15*(6), 1164–1170. doi:10.1111/j.1365-2753.2009.01308.x

Nieva, V. F., Murphy, R., Ridley, N., Donaldson, N., Combes, J., Mitchell, P., . . . Carpenter, D. (2005). From science to service: A framework for the transfer of patient safety research into practice. In K. Henriksen, J. Battles, & D. Lewin (Eds.), *Advances in Patient Safety: From research to implementation* (Volume 2: Concepts and Methodology). Rockville, MD: Agency for Healthcare Research and Quality.

Nutley, S., Walter, I., & Davies, H. (2003). Moving from knowing to doing: A framework for understanding the evidence-into-practice agenda. *Evaluation*, *9*(2), 125–148.

Oliver, K., Innvar, S., Lorenc, T., Woodman, J., & Thomas, J. (2014). A systematic review of barriers to and facilitators of the use of evidence by policymakers. *BMC Health Services Research, 14*(1), 2. doi:10.1186/1472-6963-14-2

Petkovic, J., Welch, V., Jacob, M. H., Yoganathan, M., Ayala, A. P., Cunnigham, H., & Tugwell, P. (2016). The effectiveness of evidence summaries on health policymakers and health system managers use of evidence from systematic reviews: A systematic review. *Implementation Science, 11*(1), 162. doi:10.1186/s13012-016-0530-3

Pollack, K. M., Samuels, A., Frattaroli, S., & Gielen, A. C. (2010). The translation imperative: Moving research into policy. *Injury Prevention*, *16*(2), 141–142. doi:10.1136/ip.2010.026740

Rütten, A., Lüschen, G., von Lengerke, T., Abel, T., Kannas, L., Rodríguez Diaz, J. A., . . . van der Zee, J. (2003). Determinants of health policy impact: A theoretical framework for policy analysis. *Sozial- und Präventimedizin*, *48*(5), 293–300. doi:10.1007/s00038-003-2118-3

Schmid, T. L., Pratt, M., & Witmer, L. (2006). A framework for physical activity policy research. *Journal of Physical Activity and Health*, *3*(Suppl. 1), S20–S29. doi:10.1123/jpah.3.s1.s20

Sorian, R., & Baugh, T. (2002). Power of information: Closing the gap between research and policy. *Health Affairs*, *21*(2), 264–273. doi:10.1377/hlthaff.21.2.264

Straus, S. E., Richardson, W., Glasziou, P., & Haynes, R. (2005). *Evidence-based medicine: How to practice and teach evidence-based medicine* (3rd ed.). London, UK: Elsevier.

Tomson, G., Paphassarang, C., Jönsson, K., Houamboun, K., Akkhavong, K., & Wahlström, R. (2005). Decision-makers and the usefulness of research evidence in policy implementation—A case study from Lao PDR. *Social Science & Medicine*, *61*(6), 1291–1299. doi:10.1016/j.socscimed.2005.01.014

Tricco, A. C., Cardoso, R., Thomas, S. M., Motiwala, S., Sullivan, S., Kealey, M. R., . . . Straus, S. E. (2016). Barriers and facilatators to uptake of systematic reviews by policy makers and health care managers: A scoping review. *Implementation Science, 11*(1), 4. doi:10.1186/s13012-016-0370-1

Weinick, R. M., & Shin, P. W. (2003). *Monitoring the health care safety net: Developing data-driven capabilities to support policymaking*. Washington, DC: Agency for Healthcare Research and Quality.

Weiss, C. H. (1979). The many meanings of research utilization. *Public Administration Review*, *39*(5), 426–431. doi:10.2307/3109916

White, K. M. (2008). The new CMS payment system: Too much, too soon? *Nursing Management*, *39*(10), 38–42. doi:10.1097/01.numa.0000338305.87383.57

World Health Organization. (n.d.). *Evidence-informed policy network*. Retrieved from http://www.who.int/evidence/en

Yost, J., Thompson, D., Ganann, R., Aloweni, F., Newman, K., McKibbon, A., . . . Ciliska, D. (2014). Knowledge translation strategies for enhancing nurses' evidence-informed decision making: A scoping review. *Worldviews on Evidence-Based Nursing, 11*(3), 156–167. doi:10.1111/wvn.12043

PART THREE

Methods and Process for Translation

CHAPTER EIGHT

Methods for Translation

Mary F. Terhaar

The role of the musician is to go from concept to full execution. Put another way, it's to go from understanding the content of something to really learning how to communicate it and make sure it's well-received and lives in somebody else.
—Yo-Yo Ma

Improving Health Outcomes Broadly and Significantly Requires the development of reliable ways to translate evidence, including research findings, from the bench to bedside and into the community. Translation helps ensure that the best evidence is applied in one's own practice and that of others. This chapter presents the most common and effective ways to accomplish translation and refers to this set of strategies and approaches as *methods for translation*. Consistently referring to the strategies and approaches used to accomplish translation as methods is useful for four main reasons:

- It will increase clarity in teaching, scholarship, and understanding.
- The *methods* section of a research proposal describes how the study will be conducted. It is useful to create parallel *methods* for translation to precisely and completely describe how, in any given context, evidence will be translated into practice.
- Some translation work will be classified as human-subjects research and will require institutional review board (IRB) review. Because the IRB is familiar with the language of *methods,* referring to the ways the evidence will be translated as *methods* will reduce confusion.
- It is not uncommon to read manuscripts about translation of evidence into practice and find that the intervention itself is a "black box." That is to say, authors do not consistently provide the details to describe the way they accomplished translation. Failure to provide these details prevents replication of the work, interferes with fidelity, and renders impossible any real understanding of the reasons a particular method was or was not effective in a given context.

Providing a clear and complete description of the method used to accomplish translation will promote fidelity to the evidence as well as accountability for the outcomes.

In order to ensure that translation is responsibly planned, adapted, implemented, tended, evaluated, and sustained, it will be useful to develop methods for translation that are effective, to evaluate the results associated with each in particular settings and particular types of practice problems, and to refine these methods for future application. To those ends, this chapter describes 15 methods for translation that are commonly reported in healthcare literature, provides examples of translation projects in which each method has been used, and presents the outcomes associated with each. This approach is consistent with the definition of implementation science as "the scientific study of methods to promote the systematic uptake of research findings and other evidence-based practices into routine practice, and hence, to improve the quality and effectiveness of health services and care" (Eccles & Mittman, 2006, p. 1).

■ FOUNDATION FOR TRANSLATION

There are many ways to get a job done. Therefore, the method needs to be well suited to the nature of the practice change to be accomplished, the context in which the practice change will happen, the individuals responsible to implement the practice change, the experiences and preferences of the team and organization, and the resources available. It is the combination of the method and the project plan that forms the foundation for successful translation.

The methods presented in this chapter can be best understood as serving one of two functions. Some are particularly suited to respond to the needs of large and relatively homogeneous groups of patients, and others are suited to the needs of the outliers and special or uncommon cases. Pathways and guidelines are good examples of methods that perform well for relatively homogeneous groups of patients. On the other hand, academic detailing, decision support, and tool kits may be more effective for the outliers whose needs are less common and less predictable.

Adoption of evidence-based practices is highly variable and the reasons for that are many (Gurses et al., 2008). Regardless of the method used, some clinicians resist. The most robust criticisms posed by resistant clinicians are commonly expressed in one of the following ways:

"I didn't go to school all these years to practice from a cookbook."
"No one approach can meet the needs of every patient."
"These decisions and actions you are restricting are a matter of professional judgment."

Application of these methods is intended to support best practice, but not to interfere with it. They are intended to help clinicians keep pace with the rapid changes in science, to reduce variation in practice that does not improve outcomes, to establish a minimum standard of care below which no patient will fall, and to help clinicians and teams focus on conditions in which special cases require special responses. It is not the pathway or protocol or bundle that improves outcomes, but the thoughtful conversation, evaluation of evidence, and struggle to achieve consensus about best practice that changes the performance of clinicians and improves outcomes for patients, teams, institutions, populations, and communities.

TOP 15 METHODS FOR TRANSLATION

A search of the evidence yields a set of 15 commonly described methods for translation. The list includes academic detailing, audit and feedback (A&F), bundles, clinical pathways, communication-centered methods, decision support, order sets, practice guidelines, process redesign, protocols, quality improvement and rapid cycle performance improvement (RCPI), scorecards and dashboards, teaming, technology-based solutions, and tool kits (practice resources). Each method is defined; its history, genesis, and application are explained. And for each, an example of its application and the results are presented.

1. Academic Detailing

Academic detailing refers to the work of trained consultants who provide unbiased, noncommercial, evidence-based information about medications, interventions, and therapeutic options. Commonly provided to pharmacists, nurse practitioners, physicians, other clinicians, and healthcare system decision makers, academic detailing is used to improve the quality of care and outcomes (Agency for Healthcare Research and Quality [AHRQ], 2013b).

Primary care providers face tremendous pressure to produce. Patients are scheduled tightly, allowing little time to consult the evidence or participate in professional development programs, and yet, the pace of discovery demands clinicians' attention in order to ensure relevance, safety, quality, and efficiency. Pharmaceutical and medical device industries have long understood these conditions and responded by providing continuing medical education in the practice setting. Such programming has helped providers keep current with fast-paced changes in medications, doses, devices, utilization, and treatment options. These offerings, though convenient, were vulnerable to criticisms because of the potential for bias and conflict of interest.

Academic detailing was developed to use the same approach but eliminate potential bias and conflict of interest. Professional detailers are trained to present evidence-based content to help providers keep pace with discovery in order to provide state-of-the-art care. This practice has been established as useful for introducing new medications and new technologies. Significant changes in practice have been documented across 69 separate studies where academic detailing was provided. Conduct of the intervention varied significantly across these studies, which may have contributed to variability in outcomes reported (M. A. O'Brien et al., 2007).

On a broad scale, academic detailing, which is also referred to as *educational outreach visits*, has been used to help providers adopt new clinical guidelines in their practice settings. Both the Canadian health system and Kaiser healthcare system have used detailing to help providers adopt practice guidelines across many diverse practice settings (Brown et al., 2013). Clinicians have increased their adoption and implementation of best practices for prescribing antihypertensives (Bonds et al., 2009; Simon et al., 2007), antibiotics (Coenen, Van Royen, Michiels, & Denekens, 2004), antipsychotics (Benjamin, Swartz, & Forman, 2011; Hermes, Sernyak, & Rosenheck, 2013), and benzodiazepines following academic detailing interventions (Simon et al., 2006; Zwar, Wolk, Gordon, & Sanson-Fisher, 2000). This method has also been effective as an intervention with patients, as in the case of smoking-cessation programs where individual clinicians and patients received academic detailing from a pharmacist (Jin et al., 2014).

The AHRQ recently concluded a 3-year program during which specially trained *detailers* visited practices of more than 1,300 primary care providers to provide information and facilitate evidence-based practice. Here the focus was on adoption of practice guidelines for the management of congestive heart failure, prescribing of antimicrobials and antipsychotics, and management of hypertension (AHRQ, 2013b).

Academic detailing was developed to provide support to individuals and groups practicing in the community as they work to keep abreast of recent developments in science, technology, medications, treatments, and care. Independent providers are the hub of primary care and many find it difficult to take time off from practice to participate in professional development programs. Academic detailing goes one step further than traditional professional development because it allows the content to be tailored to the needs of the provider and the population served. It may focus on medications, technology, or practice guidelines, and the goal is improved patient outcomes and improved population health.

To implement academic detailing, a respected, credentialed expert visits the practice setting and spends time coaching individual clinicians. The goal is to shape practice so that it conforms to guidelines and best practices as supported by strong evidence. The detailer helps the clinician identify and manage or eliminate potential barriers to consistent best practice and outcomes. Educational materials, audits, tracking tools, and practice resources may all be used in the process of detailing.

See Exemplar 19.1: Adherence to Guidelines for Non-High-Density Lipoprotein Screening.

2. Audit and Feedback

"Audit and feedback involves providing a recipient with a summary of their performance over a specified period of time and is a common strategy to promote implementation of evidence-based practices" (Ivers et al., 2014, p. 9). This method, audit and feedback (A&F), for promoting the adoption of best practices is commonly used across healthcare systems, professional organizations, and entities funding research. Based on a logical positivist view, it presupposes that, when provided data about one's performance in relation to a standard adopted by one's profession and peers, individuals seek to conform to the norm or to outperform peers.

A&F extends performance appraisal for individual clinicians a step beyond self-assessment and self-report by providing objective performance data that describe practice in relation to standard expectations. In doing so, A&F facilitates data-informed self-reflection as well as criterion-referenced discussions about practice and outcomes. Although widely used, A&F achieves inconsistent results as reported in two Cochrane Reviews (Ivers et al., 2012; Jamtvedt, Young, Kristofferson, O'Brien, & Oxman, 2006). These reviews establish that A&F performs well under certain conditions. For example, greater improvements were noted when baseline performance was low, when feedback intensity was high, and when reminders or academic detailing were added to A&F. Strong evidence supports the use of A&F in combination with other translation methods. Its use alone, although common, is not supported by the evidence.

To implement A&F, data to be used as outcome or performance measures are selected based on evidence of sensitivity, specificity, reliability, and availability. A process for data collection, analysis, and reporting is developed and implemented. Then, a feedback loop is used to ensure that clinicians are aware of their performance in relation to targets and to the norm of the group. Subsequently, a problem-solving process is activated to help clinicians improve performance to target, and finally the audit is repeated. The goal is to help clinicians evaluate their own practice and promote the best outcomes for groups of patients. Tracking tools, technology, reporting structures, best practice guidelines, analytic support, and coaching may all be used in the process.

See Exemplar 20.1: The Toxigen Initiative.

3. Bundles

A bundle is a structured way of improving the processes of care and patient outcomes: a small, straightforward set of evidence-based practices—generally three to five—that, when performed collectively and reliably, have been proven to improve patient outcomes (Institute for Healthcare Improvement [IHI], 2015).

The concept of the bundle was developed to facilitate faithful translation of evidence into practice when a set of action interventions have been linked to best outcomes. Bundles promote the best possible care for patients undergoing particular treatments with inherent risks (IHI, 2015). Bundles are simply collections of best practices supported by strong evidence, which are adopted by teams of clinicians to improve outcomes (Camporota & Brett, 2011). They may be developed on particular care units (Fulbrook & Mooney, 2003; Gao, Melody, Daniels, Giles, & Fox, 2005), for high-risk populations across multiple facilities (Helder et al., 2013; Robb et al., 2010), across units in a single organization (Carter, 2007), or in specialty organizations (Barochia et al., 2010). Creation of these bundles requires evaluation of the evidence and thoughtful consideration of current practice and the population served.

Bundles have been well received and adhered to in critical care as a means of avoiding complications like ventilator-acquired pneumonias (Lachman & Yuen, 2009; Resar et al., 2005), central-line infections (Helder et al., 2013), and sepsis (Gao et al., 2005; Levy et al., 2004; Masterson, 2009). In the case of sepsis and septic shock, bundles have been associated with improved outcomes in 16 separate investigations. Outcomes have included increased survival (odds ratio, 1.91; 95% confidence interval, 1.49–2.45; p <.0001), decreased time to start, and increased appropriateness of antibiotics (p <.0002) as reported by Barochia et al. (2010).

To implement bundles, clinicians who will use them collaborate in a examination of the evidence. They read, critique, and evaluate the science associated with improved outcomes related to a particular practice problem. Interventions supported as effective by the strongest evidence are gathered into a bundle and the entire set is adopted as the standard of care for a population of patients in a particular practice setting. Bundles target particular outcomes, usually avoid complications, and lend themselves to ongoing monitoring. They are commonly used in combination with A&F.

See Exemplar 20.2: Preventing Catheter-Associated Urinary Tract Infections in Critically Ill Children Using a Bundle Approach.

4. Clinical Pathways

Clinical pathways have been defined as "structured, multidisciplinary care plans used by health services to detail essential steps in the care of patients with a specific clinical problem. They aim to link evidence to practice and optimize clinical outcomes whilst maximizing clinical efficiency" (Rotter et al., 2010, p. 1). Clinical pathways have many names, including *care paths, critical pathways, case management plans,* and *integrated care pathways*. Together, they have been classified as "structured care methodologies," which means they prescribe the approach to care used over time and in doing so, structure care based on evidence, reduce avoidable delay, and support efficiencies in resource management and staffing.

Clinical pathways have been used in healthcare since Zander and Bower first applied them to the care of patients across emergency services, inpatient areas, and home care (Zander, 1985, 1986, 2003). Pathways are commonly seen in practice and the literature and are used to organize and coordinate in detail the assessments, treatments, procedures, medications, diagnostics, patient education, and outcomes expected over the course of care. They have been useful as a method to organize care for individual episodes (surgical procedures) and across continuums (care of women from confirmation of pregnancy through the postpartum period). And they project expected outcomes across an episode or continuum of care enabling the team to track work and performance to target.

Pathways can be used as a method to translate evidence into practice and, in doing so, promote quality, safety, and coordination. However, not all pathways are based on evidence. In fact, the method is borrowed from industry where its focus was on efficiency and prudent resource utilization. Some of the earliest pathways were developed to reduce length of stay and control costs. It is this history that has cast doubt over pathways as a method to promote quality care based on evidence for a set of patients. Because they were introduced as care paths and case management paths, many clinicians associate them with cost control rather than improved outcomes.

Still, when the path is created as a means to translate evidence into practice, it can improve outcomes, quality, and satisfaction and at the same time eliminate cost drivers that do not add value (Terhaar & O'Keefe, 1995).

Pathways have also been used to help detect early signs of complications and initiate treatment without delay. Therefore, they can increase safety, quality, efficiency, coordination, readiness for self-care, and many other target outcomes across diverse practice settings and populations.

Pathways are developed within an organization or health system and as such can and must be fitted to the needs of the population. They have been used to coordinate care for many populations with common needs. Children with supracondylar fractures who received care based on a pathway had favorable results, and both families and surgeons reported high satisfaction with the method (Sung et al., 2013). The same is true for children whose care was coordinated using a pathway for pediatric chronic cough (McCallum, Bailey, Morris, & Chang, 2014), and a reduced incidence of pneumonia was noted for patients on a heart failure pathway (Panella, Marchisio, & Di Stanislao, 2003).

To implement clinical pathways as a method for translation, populations of patients are selected based on similar needs. An inclusive team comprising members of all disciplines involved in the provision of care is assembled. This team considers the evidence and identifies practices supported by strong evidence; this forms the basis for the pathway. Those who build it go on to implement and evaluate the pathway. They gather evidence to monitor progress to target and make revisions as indicated. Taking such a thorough, inclusive, evidence-based, and transparent approach can do much to overcome common concerns. Opponents to this approach assert that pathways lead to cookbook practice and diminish, rather than promote, quality care (Vanhaecht et al., 2012).

See Exemplar 19.2: Screening of Geriatric Behavioral Health Issues in the Emergency Department.

5. Communication-Centered Methods

Communication is defined in business as a crucial process by which participants come to a mutual understanding through the exchange of ideas, emotions, and information, and in doing so both share meaning and create meaning (Communication, n.d.).

In all aspects of practice, communication is key. Miscommunication within a team can lead to poor coordination, which is a common source of error and expense (Greenberg et al., 2007; Leonard, Graham, & Bonacum, 2004; Mills, Neily, & Dunn, 2007). In fact, it is the leading cause of preventable injury and death during hospitalization (The Joint Commission on Accreditation of Healthcare Organizations [JCAHO], 2005), contributes to increased length of stay, and has been identified as one of the most common causes of reduced satisfaction among patients, families, and professional staff (Rice-Simpson, James, & Knox, 2008).

On the other hand, promoting effective communication is a potent antidote to many practice problems. This is the reason that so much emphasis has been placed on communication by the Institute of Medicine (IOM), The Joint Commission, and scholars alike. Whether the concern is with disruptive behavior (Rosenstein & O'Daniel, 2008), collaboration, and communication within a team (Pronovost et al., 2005, 2006) or with flow of information at handoffs in care (Haig, Sutton, & Whittington, 2006), improving communication improves outcomes (Dunn & Murphy, 2008).

At the turn of the millennium, more people in the United States died each year as a result of medical error than from automobile accidents. At the same time, it was predicted that improving the accuracy and civility of communication would go a long way in reducing error and the associated pain, suffering, and expense (IOM, 1999). As a result, many have investigated solutions to communication-related problems. Methods to address it are numerous and varied based on the nature of the communication challenge. *Disruptive communication*, which harms the practice culture and environment, can be improved by raising awareness; developing policies and procedures; reporting processes; and providing education, tools, and forums for discussion (Rosenstein & O'Daniel, 2008). *Incomplete communication*, which leads to errors, can be improved by standardizing communication with approaches like SBAR (situation, background, assessment, recommendation), in which staff structure communication to present the situation, background, assessment, and recommendations for action (Haig et al., 2006). Incomplete communication that results from *failure to communicate* important information can be addressed by using checklists and by implementing a culture where safety is everyone's responsibility. Including staff from all disciplines, management, and executive leadership has been established as effective: The Comprehensive Unit-Based Safety Program (CUSP) model engages the full team, and everyone owns the outcome of safety (Pronovost et al., 2005, 2006). Checklists have also been used as memory aids and to increase the quality of interactions and handoffs, especially in high-stakes or high-pressure situations (Gawande, 2009). Each of these methods was designed to increase the reliability, accessibility, and utility of information to ensure that it is available to those who need it, when they need it, and in ways that promote safety and quality of care.

To implement communication-focused methods for translation, teams identify areas of communication breakdown, select one of the methods suited to resolving the problem, adopt that method in practice, and evaluate the outcome. The goal is to ensure that information flows effectively to promote the best possible outcomes for patients, families, communities, and teams of providers (Frankel, Gardner, Maynard, & Kelly, 2007). Rounds, huddles, communication boards, logs, checklists, various technologies, and resources may all be used in the process of improving communication. Increasing awareness of the risk associated with ineffective, incomplete, or ill-timed communication is key to communication-related improvement (Gold, Helms, & Guterman, 2011).

See Exemplar 21.1: Using Best-Fit Interventions to Improve the Nursing Inter-Shift Handoff Process at a Medical Center in Lebanon.

6. Decision Support

Decision support refers to a set of technology-based strategies designed to put up-to-date evidence in the hands and minds of clinicians facing important decisions about the care of patients and populations. According to HealthIT.gov, "Clinical decision support (CDS) provides clinicians, staff, patients or other individuals with knowledge and person-specific information, intelligently filtered or presented at appropriate times, to enhance health and health care. CDS encompasses a variety of tools to enhance decision-making in the clinical workflow. These tools include computerized alerts and reminders to care providers and patients; clinical guidelines; condition-specific order sets; focused patient data reports and summaries; documentation templates; diagnostic support, and contextually relevant reference information, among other tools" (HealthIT.gov, p. 1, para 1). Decision support is thoroughly presented in Chapter 12, Dissemination of Evidence, and so it is only briefly introduced here.

Computerized alerts, embedded in the electronic health record, can notify providers when routine tests are due, when diagnostic findings fall outside accepted parameters, when potentially dangerous drug interactions with other drugs or foods are possible, or when allergies or concurrent conditions require consideration. Like checklists, alerts reduce error by serving as memory aids and triggers for action.

Automated order sets can be used to decrease variations in practice, facilitate adherence to accepted guidelines, and ensure prescribing practices adhere to an institutional formulary. Order sets can expedite treatment by preauthorizing certain assessments, interventions, and actions, and in doing so, liberate nurses, therapists, technicians, and others to act without delay. Implementing order sets can contain cost of medications, reduce time to treatment, and increase patient satisfaction.

Clinical guidelines can be disseminated via computer or other smart device and accessed by clinicians across practice sites and settings to promote adherence. (More information about guidelines is presented later in this chapter.)

Checklists and other memory aids can be placed in the information system to reduce error, increase adherence to protocols, and ensure a standard of care for all.

Each of these methods for translation is best developed by teams of clinical experts based on strong evidence and then translated into technology-supported applications and functionality that are accessible and useful to other clinicians in practice. (More information is presented in Chapter 13, Education: An Enabler of Translation.)

See Exemplar 19.3: A Systematic Approach Incorporating Family History Improves Identification of Cardiovascular Disease Risk.

7. Order Sets

Order sets are among the first process improvements broadly adopted in healthcare settings. They have the potential to expedite the work of the team, reduce delay in treatment response, and avoid variations in practice that might compromise quality. Establishing standard order sets takes time, but implementing them helps reduce burden on providers associated with basic tasks that require little judgment.

Many studies have established that order sets reduce time to treatment, length of stay, and patient discomfort even as they increase compliance with accepted practice guidelines (Fishbane et al., 2007). Order sets can also decrease provider time spent on order entry and reduce the burden of that work (Chan, Shojania, Easty, & Etchells, 2011). Because order sets rely heavily on information systems, Chapter 13, Education: An Enabler of Translation, will provide a more thorough introduction. They are included here because they need to be recognized and considered as one method to accomplish translation.

See Exemplar 20.3: Preventing Hyperbilirubinemia in Late Preterm Infants Using Evidence-Based Practices.

8. Practice Guidelines

Clinical *practice guidelines* are defined by the IOM as "statements that include recommendations intended to optimize patient care, that are informed by a systematic review of evidence and an assessment of the benefits and harms of alternative care options" (IOM, 2011, p. 15). Guidelines recognized by the National Guideline Clearinghouse of the AHRQ may be promulgated by a professional organization, a medical society, or federal or state agency according to a rigorous set of criteria that require a foundation in strong evidence, disciplined process, and consensus of a broad and inclusive team of clinicians and constituents (AHRQ, 2013a).

Guidelines, in many cases, are themselves the evidence to be translated. Failure to adopt established guidelines is thought to introduce risk for patients and detract from the achievement of best outcomes (Pathman, Konrad, Freed, Freeman, & Koch, 1996). Nonetheless, broad and precise adoption of guidelines continues to challenge many organizations and is the stimulus for translation science and much practice scholarship (Grimshaw & Russell, 1993; Gurses et al., 2008; Gurses, Murphy, Martinez, Berenholtz, & Pronovost, 2009).

Guidelines are well suited to promoting the translation of strong evidence and yet many have no such foundation. In one study that evaluated more than 4,000 practice recommendations, only 14% were found to be based on randomized controlled trials in contrast to 55% that were based on expert opinion or case studies (Lee & Vielemeyer, 2011). This is the concern underlying the assertion that guidelines interfere with professional practice and clinical judgment. In the absence of certainty about the best solution to every problem under any condition, strong evidence can help determine the probability of improved outcomes resulting from certain interventions and this is the basis for practice guidelines (Powers, 2011). When teams of providers determine that strong evidence directs a particular action, then that can be disseminated for use by many other professionals in the form of practice guidelines. Subsequently, outcomes from adoption of guidelines can be monitored to ensure that outcomes are achieved in a particular practice setting and for a particular population of patients.

Guidelines can also be developed within a healthcare organization or system as a method used to translate evidence and improve outcomes. Practice guidelines developed within a service entity are more specific to the population for whom care is provided. These guidelines tend to be practical and applicable within the context for which they were designed. They may be written in the absence of national guidelines or developed to ensure that national guidelines are followed in a particular setting. These homegrown guidelines can always exceed requirements of national guidelines. They cannot set a lesser standard.

Rapidly developing changes in science require clinicians and organizations to be nimble, to be capable of making rapid change in practice when science points to the need to do so (deductively) or when patient need demands it (inductively). The pace at which science advances is commonly uneven: Sometimes it is brisk and at other times sluggish. In the case in which demand for practice change is quicker than the pace of guideline development, the dissonance may result in a need to develop guidelines within the organization. And yet, efforts to develop in-house guidelines before national guidelines have been developed may falter in the face of weak or inconclusive evidence. The key is to have meaningful engagement of professionals who will apply the guidelines across all phases of the work of practice guideline development, implementation, and evaluation (Prior, Guerin, & Grimmer-Somers, 2008).

See Exemplar 19.4: Developing a System of Care for the Transient Ischemic Attack Patient.

9. Process Redesign

The U.S. General Accounting Office (GAO) defined *business process reengineering* or *redesign* as a particularly effective strategy organizations can use to reconsider and retool the approach to the work in order to dramatically improve customer service, cut operational costs, and become world-class competitors (USGAO, 1997).

Reengineering refers to comprehensive and broad sweeping improvements in the way an organization does its work with a focus on improving outcomes and achieving efficiency. *Redesign*, on the other hand, is more focused and modest in its scope with a focus on articulating the components of the work and the interrelationships that produce results. Either way, process redesign and process reengineering focus on improved service, efficiency, and outcomes (Mansar & Reijers, 2007).

For the remainder of this text, *BPR* will refer to *business process redesign*. BPR gives consideration to the customers, products, operations, behaviors, structures, information, technologies, and environment related to services. It focuses on inputs, throughputs, and outputs of a functional unit to emphasize efficiency and service. BPR uses a set of best practices to improve performance. These include task elimination when the work is unnecessary; reconfiguration into aggregates of work to improve performance; use of technology to improve performance; empowerment that minimizes hierarchal structures and situates authority with workers in general and caregivers in healthcare; ordering reassignment, which allows clusters of actions with individuals; resequencing of tasks as appropriate; careful consideration of what is assigned to generalists and specialists; integration that aligns services with customers and providers; taking actions from sequential to parallel execution to reduce cycle time; and reducing the number of functional units of people working on common processes (Mansar & Reijers, 2007).

BPR is used commonly when there is concern about the cycle time of any process or when there is an opportunity to rework all aspects of care. Delays in treatment in general and waiting times in the ED, specifically, are practice problems amenable to BPR (Spaite et al., 2002). Delays in treatment and prolonged cycle times for high-risk populations like those with chest pain, asthmatics, and trauma patients are also good examples. Any situation in which reorganizing and redesigning flow and care processes have the potential to improve outcomes or control cost is a situation where BPR can be useful.

Taking a fresh look at an entire care process enables a group to identify efficiencies, redundancies, and activities that neither add value nor produce results (Shafer et al., 2006). It can reveal outdated practices no longer supported by evidence. Eliminating these types of activities and interventions is the least painful way to save resources, reduce cost, and conserve caregiver effort. These goals are at the core of all microsystems work (Nelson et al., 2002b).

Microsystems thinking has proven to be a useful way to reframe everyday challenges in healthcare practice regardless of the setting or the nature of the problem. "Clinical microsystems are the small, functional, frontline units that provide most healthcare to most people. They are the essential building blocks of larger organizations and of the health system. They are the place where patients and providers meet. The quality and value of care produced by a large health system can be no better than the services generated by the small systems of which it is composed" (Nelson et al., 2002a, p. 472). Concentrating on redesign of microsystem processes has tremendous potential to improve outcomes and deliver on the Triple Aim of improved care, quality, and cost. Translation at this level will be the most nimble, most impactful, and most energizing for providers and patients alike (Barach & Johnson, 2006). Outcomes from redesign using the microsystems approach to redesign include reductions in preventable codes, time to treatment, and overall length of stay in the ED, increase in the number of timely transfers from the ED, and more timely response to call bells (Godfrey, Melin, Meuthing, Batalden, & Nelson, 2008). Other favorable outcomes include reduced noise in intermediate care and reduced days on mechanical ventilation (Batalden, Nelson, Edwards, Godfrey, & Mohr, 2003; Godfrey, Nelson, Wasson, Mohr, & Batalden, 2003).

See Exemplar 19.5: A Nutritional Intervention to Address Metabolic Syndrome in the Navajo.

10. Protocols

The term *protocol* connotes many different meanings. Simply put, a protocol is a set of rules that explain the correct conduct and procedures to be followed in formal situations, a plan for scientific experiment or medical treatment, or a document that describes the details of a treaty or formal agreement between countries.

Soldiers, computer programmers, diplomats, and clinicians, all follow protocols. They are an accepted means of regulating behavior and creating norms for a target group. Clinical protocols are considered to convey more detail than practice guidelines. Yet, both are intended to support effective decision-making in the patient care arena. Protocols usually describe precisely the plan of action for participants in clinical trials. Therefore, in some organizations, the language of the protocol is more familiar and agreeable. A protocol is useful to communicate precise expectations for managing complex patients like those being weaned from the ventilator (Roh et al., 2012), those being sedated in critical care (Tanios, de Wit, Epstein, & Devlin, 2009), or those receiving physiotherapy while in the intensive care unit (ICU; Hanekom, Louw, & Coetzee, 2013). It is also useful to novice clinicians (Prasad, Christie, Bellamy, Rubenfeld, & Kahn, 2010) and to those learning to manage complex patients (Parker & Lawton, 2000). Its utility lies in its specificity and in the extent to which it helps structure caregiver actions and elicits desired patient outcomes.

See Exemplar 20.4: Sedation in the ICU: Changing Traditional Patterns of Practice.

11. Quality Improvement and RCPI

The IOM (1999) report *To Err Is Human: Building a Safer Health System* gave voice to public concerns and sharpened the focus across the United States on healthcare quality, consistency, and error reduction. Quality improvement (QI) is generally the accepted approach to improving outcomes regardless of the nature of the industry, healthcare included (Demming, 1982). It is simply good business to improve outcomes, to consistently deliver quality, and to continually work to reduce error. Many have built careers on efforts to improve quality (Donabedian, 1997). As a result, many different approaches to the work are available along with many examples of these practices and associated outcomes. It is useful to be familiar with the most common QI tools and approaches used across industry in general and in healthcare in particular. These include RCPI, the plan-do-study-act (PDSA) method, Six Sigma, and Lean methodology. Each has different supporters and applications. Each is worth understanding because, coupled with strong evidence, each can support translation and improve outcomes in ways QI alone cannot.

Rapid Cycle Performance Improvement

RCPI makes incremental change, evaluates outcomes, and then repeats the improvement process. The cycle is more predisposed to action than planning, which was its significant contribution when first introduced. Based on the assumption that the team has the knowledge and aptitude it needs to be successful, RCPI then presses team members to make improvements and to carefully tend results (Varkey, Reller, & Resar, 2007). Not designed as a method for translation, RCPI traditionally does not rely on evidence. It is predicated on the innovation of team members who pose and test hypotheses about improved processes (Gold et al., 2011). Still, RCPI easily fits the work of translation when evidence is used to inform the improvement activities. This may hinder the rapidity of change but may well increase its impact. A team steeped in the evidence may find RCPI a very useful approach to translation and improvement.

Plan-Do-Study-Act

The PDSA cycle is among the most familiar and most commonly used RCPI approaches. Accompanied by statistical process control, it was introduced by Shewhart as an approach to continuous, systemic improvement. The process is iterative with a focus on small-scale change executed within rapid cycles that are completed sequentially to accomplish sustainable improvement. PDSA is now used broadly in healthcare because it is a logical cycle for improvement that supports ongoing adjustment and refinement in the plan. When coupled with application of evidence, PDSA supports careful application of evidence and continual refinement based on local data that describe specific patient experiences and responses (Shewhart, 1931; Taylor et al., 2013).

One systematic review of studies that used PDSA cycles to improve performance found considerable variability in the application of the method, sample sizes, number of complete cycles, and reported outcomes. Taylor and colleagues (2013) encourage greater standardization of the method for the purpose of research and note considerable potential for bias in the interpretation of the findings. Research has tested PDSA cycles and provides models for evaluation. The results are positive (Speroff & O'Connor, 2004).

Consider this scenario. When a bundle is implemented, critics assert that it is impossible to evaluate the impact of any one component. RCPI, conversely, would allow the addition of each component of the bundle to be introduced individually and outcomes to be measured over time. Across multiple iterations or steps in improvement, it would then be possible to evaluate the contribution of each component of the bundle and to monitor outcomes without holding progress captive to protracted planning and approval.

An example of the successful application of PDSA as a means to accomplish translation and improve outcomes is reported by Huang et al. (2008). This team used PDSA cycles to introduce improvements that reduced door-to-balloon time for ST-elevation myocardial infarction (STEMI) patients. By focusing on intervals of care, the team progressively reduced postintervention door-to-balloon time by 44 minutes ($p < .001$) to 64 minutes (interquartile range = 56 to 94 minutes) and increased the number of patients whose times satisfied American College of Cardiology/American Heart Association guidelines from 24% to 74% ($p < .001$).

Demming (1982) added sampling, continuous measurement, and applied statistics to the RCPI process with the general mandate that all engaged in QI ought to measure what matters and manage what is measured.

Six Sigma

Six Sigma focuses on reducing defects. Like PDSA, it is not designed as a translation method but is compatible with the work. Evidence can be introduced at many points in the process, most notably when framing the solution. It is at once a management philosophy, a representation of quality, and a method to reduce variation and increase quality.

Six Sigma is one approach to QI. Six Sigma is not six-step approach. It is a process that seeks to reduce variations or deviations in practice that detract from best performance (Schroeder, Linderman, Liedtke, & Choo, 2008). First, the opportunity to improve performance is identified and a team chartered to tackle the work. Then a plan for data gathering and analysis is developed and control charts are built to monitor and manage the improvements and performance. Next, based on the data, the root of the performance defect is identified. Then a solution is proposed and execution planned. And finally, the new level of performance is achieved and monitored for defects (Shewhart, 1931; Varkey et al., 2007).

This methodology of define, measure, analyze, improve, control (DMAIC) transfers easily to improving quality of care. Six Sigma success stories in industry have been told by General Electric, Boeing, Dupont, Toshiba, Kodak, Honeywell, Texas Instruments, and Sony (Kwak & Anbari, 2006). Success stories in healthcare include reducing falls, medication errors, cycle time through radiology, ED waiting times, door-to-bed times, and many others (Chakravorty, 2009; Taner, Sezen, & Antony, 2007).

Lean Methodology

Lean methodology focuses on eliminating waste. It seeks to align resource allocation with the values and benefits to the customer. Any effort or resource that does not improve the customer experience or improve a valued outcome is unnecessary and removed from the process. In healthcare, it might eliminate interventions based on experience and not evidence. Teams using Lean methodology will map the process and eliminate activities that do not add value. This value-stream mapping is comparable to the design work involved in microsystems process mapping. Both drill down to the detail and question the value added by each input.

Lean seeks to reduce waste and not people. It uses a series of steps to describe value, map the value stream, differentiate between activities that add value and those that do not, consider optimal flow, rely on pull (which is readiness downstream in the work process), and pursue perfection. Each of these steps easily applies to healthcare, with pursuit of perfection a fitting overarching goal.

Lean methodology led Toyota Motors to its dominant market position and guided it through challenges in the market related to faulty components and allegations of culpability for customer harm. The idea here is that Lean processes are faster, allow less room for error, and harbor less unnecessary cost.

Lean Six Sigma

Lean Six Sigma is a popular hybrid of the two common methods that focuses on eliminating defects and reducing waste. This blended approach is increasingly common in industry and has been adopted in The Joint Commission Center for Transforming Healthcare.

See Exemplar 21.2: Mitigation of Intravenous Medication Administration Barriers: A Comprehensive Unit-Based Safety Program (CUSP) Initiative.

12. Scorecards and Dashboards

Healthcare scorecards and dashboards have captured the interest of those engaged in QI for decades. The thinking is that such performance trackers will appeal to the competitive nature of individual providers and teams, and, in doing so, focus interest on improving performance and outcomes (Hibbard & Jewett, 1997). The power of this approach is rooted in the selection of metrics that matter; metrics that are reliable, sensitive, and specific; and metrics that represent important differences in quality of care without bias (Dranove, Kessler, McClellan, & Satterthwaite, 2002).

Scorecards and dashboards are the subject of more than 2,000 publications with 65% of those investigations having been conducted in the United States. Many were conducted by professionals or teams of professionals spanning diverse practice disciplines (S. E. O'Brien, Lorenzetti, Lewis, Kennedy, & Ghali, 2010). At the organization level, dashboards can trend performance to targets for reimbursement and compliance (Mukamel & Spector, 2003). In combination with statistical process control, they are useful for communicating performance with consumers, team members, and the community to gain competitive advantage.

Teams and organizations using dashboards and scorecards face several challenges. They must determine the sources to be used for reliable, unbiased data and the plan to display data that will promote understanding by broad groups of readers with different interests and levels of sophistication (Shahian, Silverstein, Lovett, Wolf, & Normand, 2007). These dashboards and scorecards are commonly used in combination with A&F, academic detailing, or some kind of professional development programming like department-wide morbidity and mortality rounds or risk management review. These sets of strategies increase engagement of the clinicians whose practice needs to be informed by and improved as a result of the data.

Dashboards have most commonly been used to improve practice in cardiology and cardiac surgery, primary care, psychological/mental health, nursing homes, and general surgery (M. A. O'Brien et al., 2007). These tools are used by administrators and clinicians alike (Shahian et al., 2007) in acute and subacute care as well as in the community. There are concerns about the purposes to which such data could be used and emphasis is placed on the protection of disadvantaged and underserved populations whose outcomes may differ from the norm for the community as a whole (Davies, Washington, & Bindman, 2002).

See Exemplar 21.3: Rapid Access to Tertiary Care: Mitigating Barriers Impacting Clinical, Financial, and Operational Outcomes.

13. Teaming

The IOM charged healthcare professionals with placing patients in the center of healthcare and with situating control with them as well (IOM, 2002). To accomplish this requires a more collaborative approach than ever before seen in practice (World Health Organization [WHO], 2008).

Teams are a part of human society spanning gender, race, and culture. Metaphors for *team* are commonly available, span boundaries, and are easily understood. For these reasons, the language of teaming has penetrated healthcare (Naylor et al., 2010). *Team-based care* has been defined as

> the provision of comprehensive health services to individuals, families, and/or their communities by at least two health professionals who work

> collaboratively along with patients, family caregivers, and community service providers on shared goals within and across settings. (Mitchell, Wynia, et al., 2012, p. 13)

Transforming teams is key to their success (Sevin, Moore, Sheppard, Jacobs, & Hupke, 2009). There are many examples of effective teamwork and its impact on healthcare and outcomes (Langley, Nolan, Nolan, Norman, & Provost, 1996; Leonard et al., 2004; Markova, Mateo, & Roth, 2012). The work of Catchpole et al. (2007) is a good example. Teaming strategies from Formula 1 racing were combined with strategies from aviation to structure handoff from the operating suite to the postanesthesia care unit (PACU) and critical care. The approach was originally built for highly specialized teams whose effective collaboration is essential in high-stakes, high-pressure situations. The result was a reduction in technical errors from 5.42 (95% CI ± 1.24) to 3.15 (95% CI ± 0.71), a reduction in handover omissions from 2.09 (95% CI ± 1.14) to 1.07 (95% CI ± 0.55), and a decreased cycle time from 10.8 minutes (95% CI ± 1.6) to 9.4 minutes (95% CI ± 1.29). Moreover, 39% of the patients in the baseline group had more than one error in the handoff as compared to 11.5% in the treatment group. Catchpole and colleagues (2007) determined that this new team approach improved performance and outcomes.

Huddles, rounds, collaborative practice models, and many other methods are used to increase the quality of teamwork and patient care. The best approach to introducing teamwork and collaboration remains unclear (Salas et al., 2009). Approaches like TeamSTEPPS (Team Strategies and Tools to Enhance Performance and Patient Safety) have been incorporated in entry-to-practice education to prepare students from all disciplines for the collaboration that professional practice will require. Such approaches have the potential to promote safety and retention on a broad scale (Robertson et al., 2010). Because of the breadth and significance of this content, Chapter 13, Education: An Enabler of Translation, presents it fully. Nonetheless, it is important to identify here in this compendium that teaming methods are numerous and essential to translation.

See Exemplar 21.4: Improving Effective Communication Within the Neonatal Interdisciplinary Team.

14. Technology-Based Solutions

In *Crossing the Quality Chasm: A New Health System for the 21st Century* (IOM, 2002), the IOM transformed "patient information" from the core substance of a medical record used to drive reimbursement to the knowledge and information essential to ensure safe, effective care (Berwick, 2008). The focus shifted from generating documents to driving solutions, and this shift demanded new and more effective ways to share and disseminate vital information. New technologies are at the center of this transformation (Blumenthal, 2009).

Just as technology can disseminate data, it can support and accelerate translation. Technology has been used to automate order sets, facilitate compliance with practice guidelines, remind clinicians of small steps in high-stakes processes, facilitate communication, and standardize the flow of information. Chapter 12, Dissemination of Evidence, addresses fully the use of technology in translation.

See Exemplar 21.5: Use of Pagers With an Alarm Escalation System to Reduce Cardiac Monitor Alarm Signals.

15. Tool Kits (Practice Resources)

Driving innovation into the market requires deep understanding of conditions in that market and the context in which the particular innovation will be introduced. This step places demands on time and resources of those who develop the innovation. One solution in industry to achieving this handoff is to prepare tool kits that help the users make modifications and adaptations to the innovation themselves. This expedites adoption and frees the innovator to continue to make more solutions (Von Hippel, 2001; Von Hippel & Katz, 2002). This way of thinking and working is particularly useful in the healthcare market where the innovation is research and the challenge is translation.

The AHRQ identifies the use of tool kits as a useful strategy to promote translation of evidence into action or policy. The agency defines them as follows (2013b):

- A "tool kit" is an action-oriented compilation of related information, resources, or tools that together can guide users to develop a plan or organize efforts to conform to evidence-based recommendations or meet evidence-based specific practice standards.
- A "tool" is an instrument (e.g., survey, guidelines, or checklist) that helps users accomplish a specific task that contributes to meeting a specific evidence-based recommendation or practice standard.

Tool kits and practice resources are designed for the purpose of facilitating the use of knowledge in practice to improve outcomes. They may be memory aids, decision-support tools, or collections of materials needed in particular high-risk or challenging situations. The priority is to facilitate safe, effective practice and favorable outcomes. The code cart is a tool kit broadly adopted across healthcare settings. These carts are standardized, make available all the resources one would need to provide safe care in a high-risk setting, and often contain decision-support or memory aids to assist clinicians in stressful conditions in which performance is essential. The utility of these practice resources goes without question.

The model can be useful in other pressured situations as well and under conditions in which clinicians could be expected to be challenged. The key is to assemble resources, materials, information, and processes to facilitate a favorable outcome.

Consider this example: A facility participates in the National Database of Nursing Quality Indicators (NDNQI) survey and uses the data to inform strategy at the macrosystem level. Leadership at the mesosystem level believes that these data can be used to improve work conditions at the microsystem level. Therefore, a clinical nurse educator gains access to the data and then develops a set of tools that can be used by staff to analyze, interpret, and apply the data to develop solutions to problems he or she faces in the patient care area. In order for the staff to understand the data and apply them to solve problems, the educator develops a set of tools. Staff use these to interpret the data, evaluate the problem, identify potential solutions, implement those strategies, and evaluate the outcome. The educator has prepared a tool kit and has helped the staff participate in an inductive solution to a recalcitrant problem. The staff feel empowered and prepared to repeat the performance improvement cycle. This is the utility of the toolkit (Groff-Paris & Terhaar, 2010).

See Exemplar 20.7: Improving the Pain Experience for Hospitalized Patients With Cancer; and 21.6: Improving the Practice Environment of the Bedside Nurse Using Maslow's Hierarchy of Human Need, NDNQI Data, and a Tool Kit for Change.

■ CONCLUSIONS

It is quite common to read in the discussion section at the close of a translation manuscript that the methods were not fully described and, as a result, replication will be challenging if not impossible. Similarly, authors of systematic reviews commonly emphasize the difficulty they faced in assembling findings related to particular methods because of the variability and inconsistency in the way those methods were presented. For this reason, it will advance the practice of translation and the successful adoption of science in direct care if there is a new level of rigor and discipline brought to the work of translation.

Students in traditional research-focused doctoral programs follow a well-established approach that ensures compliance with scientific process so the knowledge generated is reliable, valid, and generalizable. PhD students prepare a proposal, defend it, and then faithfully complete a dissertation and disseminate the findings. This time-tested approach ensures adherence to the scientific process, focuses precisely on the research question, and controls for the influence of confounding variables. It is characterized by precision, control, and rigor. It is the standard for scholarship accepted globally. The dissertation results in the development of new knowledge that can be applied broadly. Universities are familiar with the processes and the products of this approach because faculty were themselves educated using the same approach. The product is traditionally presented in five chapters: the problem, the background, the methods, the findings, and the conclusions. This template is also the norm for scholarly publications. Adherence to the standard is essential to ensure that knowledge generated and disseminated is valid and trustworthy. It is also necessary for the researcher who wishes to advance professionally.

Given that nursing is a practice discipline, it becomes necessary to establish a complementary language and process for the application of evidence. Translation is younger, by far, than research. Those who practice translation would benefit from the adoption of a consistent, tested, and effective approach and tools that support both implementation and evaluation just as researchers have benefited from the use of consistent methods, models, and frameworks in their work.

Translation science promises to develop tools and methods to increase the effectiveness of efforts to bridge the gap between discovery and application. As that new science develops, those who practice it will need to keep abreast of advancements and contribute to the conversation. The methods presented in this chapter offer a preliminary toolbox for those who seek to improve practice through translation. It will be useful to ply each method as it fits the practice problem and to gather outcomes and test the performance of each.

■ REFERENCES

Agency for Healthcare Research and Quality. (2013a). National Guideline Clearinghouse. *Inclusion criteria*. Retrieved from http://www.guideline.gov/about/inclusion-criteria.aspx

Agency for Healthcare Research and Quality. (2013b). Toolkit guidance. In Calico, F. W., Dillard, C. D., Moscovice, I., & Wakefield, M. K. (2003). A framework and action agenda for quality improvement in rural health care. *Journal of Rural Health, 19*(3), 226–232.

Agency for Healthcare Research and Quality. (2014). *About the academic detailing project*. Retrieved from http://effectivehealthcare.ahrq.gov/index.cfm/who-is-involved-in-the-effective-health-care-program1/about-the-academic-detailing-project

Barach, P., & Johnson, J. K. (2006). Understanding the complexity of redesigning care around the clinical microsystem. *Quality and Safety in Healthcare, 15*(Suppl. 1), i10–i16. doi:10.1136/qshc.2005.015859

Barochia, A. V., Cui, X., Vitberg, D., Suffredini, A. F., O'Grady, N. P., Banks, S. M., . . . Eichacker, P. Q. (2010). Bundled care for septic shock: An analysis of clinical trials. *Critical Care Medicine, 38*(2), 668–678. doi:10.1097/ccm.0b013e3181cb0ddf

Batalden, P. B., Nelson, E. C., Edwards, W. H., Godfrey, M. M., & Mohr, J. J. (2003). Microsystems in health-care: Part 9. Developing small clinical units to attain peak performance. *Journal of Quality Improvement, 29*(11), 575–585. doi:10.1016/s1549-3741(03)29068-7

Benjamin, D., Swartz, M., & Forman, L. (2011). The impact of evidence-based education on prescribing in psychiatry residency. *Journal of Psychiatric Practice, 17*(2), 110–117. doi:10.1097/01.pra.0000396062.12893.5b

Berwick, D. M. (2008). The science of improvement. *Journal of the American Medical Association, 299*(10), 1182–1184. doi:10.1001/jama.299.10.1182

Blumenthal, D. (2009). Stimulating the adoption of health information technology. *New England Journal of Medicine, 360*(15), 1477–1479. doi:10.1056/nejmp0901592

Bonds, D. E., Hogan, P. E., Bertoni, A. G., Chen, H., Clinch, C. R., Hoitt, A. E., . . . Goff, D. C. (2009). A multifaceted intervention to improve blood pressure control: The guideline adherence for heart health (GLAD) study. *American Heart Journal, 157*(2), 278–284. Retrieved from http://www.sciencedirect.com/science/article/pii/S0002870308008272

Brown, D. P., Fenelon, L., Holmes, A., Ramsey, C. R., Wiffen, P. J., & Wilcox, M. (2013). Interventions to improve antibiotic prescribing practices for hospital inpatients. *The Cochraine Library, 2013*(4). Retrieved from http://onlinelibrary.wiley.com/doi/10.1002/14651858.CD003543.pub3/epdf/standard

Camporota, L., & Brett, S. (2011). Care bundles: Implementing evidence or common sense. *Critical Care, 15*(3), 159. doi:10.1186/cc10232

Carter, C. (2007). Implementing the severe sepsis care bundles outside the ICU by outreach. *Nursing in Critical Care, 12*(5), 225–230. doi:10.1111/j.1478-5153.2007.00242.x

Catchpole, K. R., DeLeval, M. R., McEwan, A., Pigott, N., Elliott, M. J., McQuillan, A., . . . Goldman, A. J. (2007). Patient handover from surgery to intensive care: Using Formula 1 pit-stop and aviation models to improve safety and quality. *Pediatric Anesthesia, 17*(5), 470–478. doi:10.1111/j.1460-9592.2006.02239.x

Chakravorty, S. S. (2009). Six sigma programs: An implementation model. *International Journal of Production Economics, 119*(1), 1–16. doi:10.1016/j.ijpe.2009.01.003

Chan, J., Shojania, K. G., Easty, A. C., & Etchells, E. E. (2011). Does user-centered design affect the efficiency, usability, and safety of CPOE order sets? *Journal of the American Medical Informatics Association, 18*(3), 276–281. doi:10.1136/amiajnl-2010-000026

Coenen, S., Van Royen, P., Michiels, B., & Denekens, J. (2004). Optimizing antibiotic prescribing for acute cough in general practice: A cluster-randomized controlled trial. *Journal of Antimicrobiology & Chemotherapy, 54*(3), 661–672. Retrieved from http://www.ncbi.nlm.nih.gov/pubmed/15282232

Communication. (n.d.). In *BusinessDictionary.com*. Retrieved from http://www.businessdictionary.com/definition/communication.html

Davies, H. T. O., Washington, A. E., & Bindman, A. B. (2002). Healthcare report cards: Implications for vulnerable patient groups and the organizations providing care for them. *Journal of Health Politics, Policy and Law*, *27*(3), 379–400. doi:10.1215/03616878-27-3-379

Demming, E. W. (1982). *Out of crisis*. Cambridge, MA: Massachusetts Institute of Technology, Center for Advanced Engineering Study.

Donabedian, A. (1997). The quality of care: How can it be assessed? *Archives of Pathology and Laboratory Medicine*, *121*(11), 1145–1150.

Dranove, D., Kessler, D., McClellan, M., & Satterthwaite, M. (2002). *Is more information better? The effects of "report cards" on health care providers* (NBER Working Paper Series w8697). Cambridge, MA: National Bureau of Economic Research. Retrieved from http://www.nber.org/papers/w8697.pdf

Dunn, W., & Murphy, J. G. (2008). The patient handoff: Medicine's Formula 1 moment. *Chest*, *134*(1), 9–12. doi:10.1378/chest.08-0998

Eccles, M. P., & Mittman, B. S. (2006). Welcome to implementation science. *Implementation Science*, *1*(1), 1–3.

Fishbane, S., Niederman, M. S., Daly, C., Magin, A., Kawabata, M., deCorla-Souza, A., . . . Parker, S. (2007). The impact of standardized order sets and intensive clinical case management on outcomes in community-acquired pneumonia. *Archives in Internal Medicine*, *167*(15), 1664–1669.

Frankel, A., Gardner, R., Maynard, L., & Kelly, A. (2007). Using communication and teamwork skills (CATS) assessment to measure healthcare team performance. *The Joint Commission Journal on Quality and Safety*, *33*(9), 549–558. doi:10.1016/s1553-7250(07)33059-6

Fulbrook, P., & Mooney, S. (2003). Care bundles in critical care: A practical approach to evidence-based practice. *Nursing Critical Care*, *8*(6), 249–255. doi:10.1111/j.1362-1017.2003.00039.x

Gao, F., Melody, T., Daniels, D. F., Giles, S., & Fox, S. (2005). The impact of compliance with 6-hour and 24-hour sepsis bundles on hospital mortality in patients with severe sepsis: A prospective observational study. *Critical Care Forum*, *9*(6), R764–R770.

Gawande, A. (2009). *The checklist manifesto: How to get things done right*. New York, NY: Metropolitan Books.

Godfrey, M. M., Melin, C. N., Meuthing, S. E., Batalden, P. B., & Nelson, E. C. (2008). Microsystems in healthcare: Part 3. Transformation of two hospitals using microsystem, mesosystem, and macrosystem strategies. *Journal on Quality Improvement*, *34*(10), 591–603. doi:10.1016/s1553-7250(08)34074-4

Godfrey, M. M., Nelson, E. C., Wasson, J. H., Mohr, J. J., & Batalden, P. B. (2003). Microsystems in health care: Part 3: Planning patient-centered services. *Joint Commission Journal on Quality and Safety*, *29*(4), 159–170.

Gold, M., Helms, D., & Guterman, S. (2011). Identifying, monitoring, and assessing promising innovations: Using evaluation to support rapid cycle change. *Commonwealth Fund*, *12*, 1–12.

Greenberg, C. C., Regenbogen, S. E., Studdert, D. M., Lipsitz, S. R., Rogers, S. O., Zinner, M. J., & Gawande, A. A. (2007). Patterns of communication breakdowns resulting in injury to surgical patients. *Journal of the American College of Surgeons*, *204*(4), 533–540. Retrieved from http://www.sciencedirect.com/science/article/pii/S107275150700061O#

Grimshaw, J. M., & Russell, I. T. (1993). Effect of clinical guidelines on medical practice: A systematic review of rigorous evaluation. *Lancet*, *342*(8883), 1317–1322.

Groff-Paris, L., & Terhaar, M. (2010). Using Maslow's pyramid and the national database of nursing quality indicators(R) to attain a healthier work environment. *Online Journal of Issues in Nursing*, *16*(1), 6. doi: 10.3912/OJIN.Vol16No01PPT05

Gurses, A. P., Murphy, D. J., Martinez, E. A., Berenholtz, S. M., & Pronovost, P. J. (2009). A practical tool to identify and eliminate barriers to compliance with evidence-based guidelines. *The Joint Commission Journal on Quality and Safety*, *35*(10), 526–532. doi:10.1016/s1553-7250(09)35072-2

Gurses, A. P., Seidl, K. L., Vaidya, V., Bochicchiio, G., Harris, A. D., Hebden, J., & Xiao, Y. (2008). Systems ambiguity and guideline compliance: A qualitative study of how intensive care units follow evidence-based guidelines to reduce healthcare-associated infections. *Quality and Safety in Healthcare*, *17*(5), 351–359. Retrieved from http://qualitysafety.bmj.com/content/17/5/351.long

Haig, K. M., Sutton, S., & Whittington, J. (2006). SBAR: A shared mental model for improving communication between clinicians. *The Joint Commission Journal on Quality and Safety*, *32*(3), 167–175.

Hanekom, S., Louw, Q. A., & Coetzee, A. R. (2013). Implementation of protocol facilitates evidence-based physiotherapy practice in intensive care units. *Physiotherapy*, *99*(2), 139–145. doi:10.1016/j.physio.2012.05.005

HealthIT.gov. (2018). Clinical decision support. Retrieved from https://www.healthit.gov/topic/safety/clinical-decision-support

Helder, O., Kornelisse, R., van der Starre, C., Tibboel, D., Looman, C., Wijnen, R., . . . Ista, E. (2013). Implementation of a children's hospital-wide central venous catheter insertion and maintenance bundle. *BMC Health Services Research, 13*, 417. Retrieved from http://www.ncbi.nlm.nih.gov/pmc/articles/PMC3853717/pdf/1472-6963-13-417.pdf

Hermes, E. D., Sernyak, M. J., & Rosenheck, R. A. (2013). Prescription of second-generation antipsychotics: Responding to treatment risk in real-world practice. *Psychiatric Services, 64*(3), 238–244. Retrieved from http://www.ncbi.nlm.nih.gov/pubmed/23241613

Hibbard, J. H., & Jewett, J. J. (1997). Will quality report cards help consumers? *Health Affairs, 16*(3), 218–228. doi:10.1377/hlthaff.16.3.218

Huang, R. L., Donelli, A., Byrd, J., Mickiewicz, M. A., Slovis, C., Roumie, C., . . . Zhao, D. (2008). Using quality improvement methods to improve door-to-balloon time at an academic medical center. *Journal of Invasive Cardiology*, 20(20), 46–52.

Institute for Healthcare Improvement. (2015). *Improvement stories: What is a bundle?* Retrieved from http://www.ihi.org/resources/Pages/ImprovementStories/WhatIsaBundle.aspx

Institute of Medicine. (1999). *To err is human: Building a safer health system*. Washington, DC: National Academies Press.

Institute of Medicine. (2002). *Crossing the quality chasm: A new health system for the 21st century*. Washington, DC: National Academies Press.

Institute of Medicine. (2011). In R. Graham, M. Mancher, D. M. Wolman, S. Greenfield, & E. Steinberg (Eds.), *Clinical practice guidelines we can trust*. Washington, DC: National Academies Press.

Ivers, N., Jamtvedt, G., Flottorp, S., Young, J. M., Odgaard-Jensen, J., French, S. D., . . . Oxman, A. D. (2012). Audit and feedback: Effects on professional practice and healthcare outcomes (review). *Cochrane Library, 2012*(6), CD000259.

Ivers, N. M., Sales, A., Colquhoun, H., Michie, S., Foy, R., Francis, J., & Grinshaw, J. M. (2014). No more 'business as usual' with audit and feedback interventions: Towards an agenda for reinvigorated intervention. *Implementation Science, 9(1),* 14. doi:10.1186/1748-5908-9-14

Jamtvedt, G., Young, J. M., Kristofferson, D. T., O'Brien, M. A., & Oxman, A. D. (2006). Audit and feedback: Effects on professional practice and healthcare outcomes. *Cochrane Library, 2006*(2), CD000259. doi:10.1002/14651858.cd000259.pub2

Jin, M., Gagnon, A., Levine, M., Thabane, L., Rodriguez, C., & Dolovich, L. (2014). Patient-specific academic detailing for smoking cessation. *Canadian Family Physician, 60*(1), e16–e23. Retrieved from http://www.ncbi.nlm.nih.gov/pmc/articles/PMC3994822

Kwak, Y. H., & Anbari, F. T. (2006). Benefits, obstacles, and future of six-sigma approach. *Technovation, 26*(5–6), 708–715. doi:10.1016/j.technovation.2004.10.003

Lachman, P., & Yuen, S. (2009). Using care bundles to prevent infection in neonatal and paediatric ICUs. *Current Opinion in Infectious Disease*, 22(3), 224–228. doi:10.1097/qco.0b013e3283297b68

Langley, G. J., Nolan, K. M., Nolan, T. W., Norman, C. L., & Provost, L. P. (1996). *The improvement guide*. San Francisco, CA: Jossey-Bass.

Lee, D. H., & Vielemeyer, O. (2011). Analysis of overall level of evidence behind Infectious Disease Society of America practice guidelines. *Archives of Internal Medicine, 171*(1), 18–22. doi:10.1001/archinternmed.2010.482

Leonard, M., Graham, S., & Bonacum, D. (2004). The human factor: The critical importance of effective teamwork and communication in providing safe care. *Quality and Safety in Healthcare, 13*(Suppl. 1), i85–i90.

Levy, M. M., Pronovost, P. J., Dellinger, R. P., Townsend, S., Resar, R. K., Clemmer, T. P., & Ramsay, G. (2004). Sepsis change bundles: Converting guidelines to meaningful change in behavior and clinical outcome. *Critical Care Medicine*, 32(11), S595–S597. doi:10.1097/01.ccm.0000147016.53607.c4

Mansar, S. L., & Reijers, H. A. (2007). Best practices in business process redesign: Use and impact. *Business Process Management Journal, 13*(2), 192–213. doi:10.1108/14637150710740455

Markova, T., Mateo, M., & Roth, L. M. (2012). Implementing teams in a patient-centered medical home residency practice: Lessons learned. *Journal of the American Board of Family Medicine*, 25(2), 224–231. doi:10.3122/jabfm.2012.02.110181

Masterson, R. G. (2009). Sepsis care bundles and clinicians. *Intensive Care Medicine, 35*(7), 1149–1151. doi:10.1007/s00134-009-1462-z

McCallum, G. B., Bailey, E. J., Morris, P. S., & Chang, A. B. (2014). Clinical pathways for chronic cough in children. *Cochrane Collaboration, 2014*(9), CD006595. doi:10.1002/14651858.cd006595.pub3

Mills, P., Neily, J., & Dunn, E. (2007). Teamwork and communication in surgical teams: Implications for patient safety. *Journal of American College of Surgeons, 206*, 107–112.

Mitchell, P., Hall, L., & Gaines, M. (2012). A social compact for advancing team-based high-value health care. *Health Affairs Blog*. Retrieved from http://healthaffairs.org/blog/2012/05/04/a-social-compact-for-advancing-team-based-high-value-health-care

Mitchell, P., Wynia, M., Golden, R., McNellis, B., Okun, S., Webb, C.E., . . . Von Kohorn, I. (2012). Core principles and values of effective team-based health care. *IOM Roundtable on value and science-driven health care* [Discussion Paper]. Washington, DC: Institute of Medicine.

Mukamel, D. B., & Spector, W. D. (2003). Quality report cards and nursing home quality. *The Gerontologist, 43*(2), 58–66. doi:10.1093/geront/43.suppl_2.58

Naylor, M. D., Coburn, K. D., Kurtzman, E. T., Prvu Bettger, J. A., Buck, H., Van Cleave, J., . . . Cott, C. (2010). *Team-based primary care for chronically ill adults: State of the science. Advancing team-based care.* Philadelphia, PA: American Board of Internal Medicine Foundation.

Nelson, E. C., Batalden, P. B., Homa, K., Huber, T. P., Godfrey, M. M., Campbell, C., . . . Wasson, J. H. (2002a). Microsystems in healthcare: Part 2. Creating a rich information environment. *Journal of Quality Improvement, 29*(1), 5–15. doi:10.1016/s1549-3741(03)29002-x

Nelson, E. C., Batalden, P. B., Huber, T. P., Mohr, J. J., Godfrey, M. M., Headrick, L. A., & Wasson, J. H. (2002b). Microsystems in healthcare: Part 1. Learning from high-performing front-line clinical units. *Journal of Quality Improvement, 28*(9), 472–493. doi:10.1016/s1070-3241(02)28051-7

O'Brien, M. A., Rogers, S., Jamtvedt, G., Odgaard-Jensen, J., Iristoffersen, D. T., Forsetlund, L., . . . Harvey, E. L. (2009). Educational outreach visits: Effects on professional practice and health care outcomes. *Cochrane Database of Systematic Reviews, 2007*(4), CD000409.

O'Brien, M. A., Rogers, S., Jamtvedt, G., Oxman, A. D., Odgaard-Jensen, J., Kristoffersen, D. T., . . . Harvey, E. L. (2007, October 17). Educational outreach visits: Effects on professional practice and health outcomes. *Cochrane Database of Systematic Review, 2007*(4), CD000409. Retrieved from http://www.ncbi.nlm.nih.gov/pubmed/17943742

O'Brien, S. E., Lorenzetti, D. L., Lewis, S., Kennedy, J., & Ghali, W. A. (2010). Overview of a formal scoping review on health system report cards. *Implementation Science, 5*(2), 1–12.

Panella, M., Marchisio, S., & Di Stanislao, F. (2003). Reducing clinical variations with clinical pathways: Do pathways work? *International Journal of Quality in Healthcare, 15*(6), 509–521.

Parker, D., & Lawron, R. (2000). Judging the use of clinical protocols by fellow professionals. *Social Science and Medicine, 51*(5), 669–677. doi:10.1016/s0277-9536(00)00013-7

Pathman, D. E., Konrad, T. R., Freed, G. L., Freeman, V. A., & Koch, G. G. (1996). The awareness-to-adherence model of steps to clinical practice guideline compliance: The case of pediatric vaccine recommendations. *Medical Care, 34*(9), 873–889. doi:10.1097/00005650-199609000-00002

Powers, J. H. (2011). Practice guidelines: Belief, criticism, and probability. *Archives of Internal Medicine, 171*(1), 15–17. doi:10.1001/archinternmed.2010.453

Prasad, M., Christie, J. D., Bellamy, S. L., Rubenfeld, G. D., & Kahn, J. M. (2010). The availability of clinical protocols in U.S. teaching intensive care units. *Journal of Critical Care, 25(4)*, 610–619. doi:10.1016/j.jcrc.2010.02.014

Prior, M., Guerin, M., & Grimmer-Somers, K. (2008). The effectiveness of clinical guideline implementation strategies: A synthesis of systematic review findings. *Journal of Evaluation in Clinical Practice, 14*(5), 888–897. doi:10.1111/j.1365-2753.2008.01014.x

Pronovost, P., Weast, B., Rosenstein, B., Sexton, B. J., Holzmueller, C. G., Paine, L., . . . Rubin, H. R. (2005). Implementing and validating a comprehensive unit-based safety program. *Journal of Patient Safety, 1*(1), 33–40. doi:10.1097/01209203-200503000-00008

Pronovost, P. J., King, J., Holzmueller, C. G., Sawyer, M., Bivens, S., Michael, M., . . . Miller, M. (2006). A web-based tool for the comprehensive unit-based safety program. *The Joint Commission Journal on Quality and Safety, 32*(3), 119–129. Retrieved from http://docserver.ingentaconnect.com/deliver/connect/jcaho/15537250/v32n3/s1.pdf?expires=1422047897&id=80564087&titleid=11231&accname=Welch+Medical+Library&checksum=9EE3A790B801CA0582CE1D69E1279EDE

Resar, R., Pronovost, P., Haraden, C., Simmonds, T., Rainey, T., & Nolan, T. (2005). Using a bundle approach to improve ventilator care processes and reduce ventilator-associated pneumonia. *The Joint Commission Journal on Quality and Patient Safety,* 31(5), 243–248. Retrieved from http://docserver.ingentaconnect.com/deliver/connect/jcaho/15537250/v31n5/s1.pdf?expires=1421688935&id=80509706&titleid=11231&accname=Welch+Medical+Library&checksum=70599A0821E4163E70572EB6DD49560F

Rice-Simpson, K., James, D. C., & Knox, E. (2008). Nurse-physician communication during labor and birth: Implications for patient safety. *Journal of Obstetric, Gynecologic, and Neonatal Nursing, 35*(4), 547–556. Retrieved from http://onlinelibrary.wiley.com/doi/10.1111/j.1552-6909.2006.00075.x/pdf

Robb, E., Jarman, B., Suntharalingam, G., Higgens, C., Tennant, R., & Elcock, K. (2010). Using care bundles to reduce in-hospital mortality: Quantitative survey. *British Medical Journal, 340*, c1234. doi:10.1136/bmj.c1234

Robertson, B., Kaplan, B., Hany, A., Higgins, M., Lewitt, M. J., & Ander, D. S. (2010). The use of simulation and modified TeamSTEPPS curriculum for medical and nursing student teams training. *Simulation in Healthcare: Journal of Society for Simulation in Healthcare, 5*(6), 332–337. doi:10.1097/sih.0b013e3181f008ad

Roh, J. H., Synn, A., Lim, C. M., Suh, H. J., Hong, S. B., Huh, J. W., & Koh, Y. (2012). A weaning protocol administered by critical care nurses for the weaning of patients from mechanical ventilation. *Journal of Critical Care, 27*(6), 549–555. doi:10.1016/j.jcrc.2011.11.008

Rosenstein, A. H., & O'Daniel, M. (2008). A survey of the impact of disruptive behaviors and communication defects on patient safety. *Journal of the Commission on Quality and Patient Safety, 43*(8), 464–471. Retrieved from http://docserver.ingentaconnect.com/deliver/connect/jcaho/15537250/v34n8/s5.pdf?expires=1422044975&id=80563666&titleid=11231&accname=Welch+Medical+Library&checksum=C11DC41442A5803D097109AA6B6529E2

Rotter, T., Kinsman, L., James, E. L., Machotta, A., Gothe, H., Willins, J., . . . Kugler, J. (2010). Clinical pathways: Effects on professional practice, patient outcomes, length of stay, and hospital costs. *Cochrane Collaboration, 2010*(3), CD006632. Retrieved from http://onlinelibrary.wiley.com/doi/10.1002/14651858.CD006632.pub2/pdf

Salas, E., Almeida, S. A., Salisbury, M., King, H., Lazzara, E. H., Lyons, R., . . . McQuillan, R. (2009). What are the critical success factors for team training in health care? *The Joint Commission Journal on Quality and Patient Safety, 35*(8), 398–405. Retrieved from http://docserver.ingentaconnect.com/deliver/connect/jcaho/15537250/v35n8/s2.pdf?expires=1422056908&id=80565018&titleid=11231&accname=Welch+Medical+Library&checksum=6EDD104B15B9A39DB55B27829E998756

Schroeder, R. G., Linderman, K., Liedtke, C. & Choo, A. S. (2008). Six sigma: Definition and underlying theory. *Journal of Operations Management, 26(4)*, 536–554. doi:10.1016/j.jom.2007.06.007

Sevin, C., Moore, G., Sheppard, J., Jacobs, T., & Hupke, C. (2009). Transforming care teams to provide the best possible patient-centered, collaborative care. *Journal of Ambulatory Care Management, 32*(1), 24–31. doi:10.1097/01.JAC.0000343121.07844.e0

Shafer, T. J., Wagner, D., Chessare, J., Zampiello, F. A., McBride, V., & Perdue, J. (2006). Organ donation breakthrough collaborative: Increasing organ donation through system redesign. *Critical Care Nurse, 26*(2), 33–48.

Shahian, D. M., Silverstein, T., Lovett, A. F., Wolf, R. E., & Normand, S. L. T. (2007). Comparison of clinical and administrative data sources for hospital coronary artery bypass graft surgery report cards. *Circulation, 115*(12), 1518–1527. doi:10.1161/circulationaha.106.633008

Shewhart, W. A. (1931). *Economic control of quality of manufactured product*. New York, NY: Van Nostrand Company.

Simon, S. R., Rodriguez, H. P., Majumdar, S. R., Kleinman, K., Warner, C., Salem-Schatz, S., & Prosser, L. A. (2007). Economic analysis of a randomized trial of academic detailing interventions to improve use of antihypertensive medications. *Journal of Clinical Hypertension, 9*(1), 15–20. Retrieved from http://onlinelibrary.wiley.com/doi/10.1111/j.1524-6175.2006.05684.x/abstract

Simon, S. R., Smith, D. H., Feldstein, A. C., Perrin, N., Yang, X., Zhou, Y., . . . Soumerai, S. B. (2006). Computerized prescribing alerts and group academic detailing to reduce potentially inappropriate medications in older people. *Journal of American Geriatrics Society, 54*(6), 963–968. Retrieved from http://onlinelibrary.wiley.com/doi/10.1111/j.1532-5415.2006.00734.x/pdf

Spaite, D. W., Bartholomeaux, F., Guisto, J., Lindberg, E., Hull, B., Eyherabide, A., . . . Conroy, C. (2002). Rapid process redesign in a university-based emergency department: Decreasing waiting time intervals and improving patient satisfaction. *Annals of Emergency Medicine, 39*(2), 168–177. doi:10.1067/mem.2002.121215

Speroff, T., & O'Connor, G. F. T. (2004). Study designs for PDSA quality improvement research. *Quality Management in Health Care, 13*(1), 17–32. doi:10.1097/00019514-200401000-00002

Sung, K. H., Chung, C. Y., Lee, K. M., Lee, S. Y., Ahn, S., Park, S., . . . Park, M. S. (2013). Application of clinical pathway using electronic medical record system in pediatric patients with supracondylar fracture of the humerus: A before and after comparative study. *British Medical Informatics & Decision Making, 13*(87). Retrieved from http://www.biomedcentral.com/1472-6947/13/87

Taner, M. T., Sezen, B., & Antony, J. (2007). An overview of six sigma applications in healthcare industry. *International Journal of Healthcare Quality Assurance*, *20*(4), 329–340. doi:10.1108/09526860710754398

Tanios, M. A., de Wit, M., Epstein, S. K., & Devlin, J. W. (2009). Perceived barriers to the use of sedation protocols and daily sedation disruption: A multidisciplinary survey. *Journal of Critical Care*, *24(1)*, 66–73. doi:10.1016/j.jcrc.2008.03.037

Taylor, M. J., McNicholas, C., Nicolay, C., Darzi, A., Bell, D., & Reed, J. E. (2013). Systematic review of the application of the plan-do-study-act method to improve quality in healthcare. *BMJ Safety & Quality,* 23(4), 290–298. doi:10.1136/bmjqs-2013-001862

Terhaar, M. F., & O'Keefe, S. (1995). A new advanced practice role focused on outcomes management. *Journal of Perinatal and Neonatal Nursing, 9*(3), 10–21.

The Joint Commission on Accreditation of Healthcare Organizations. (2005). *Sentinel event statistics*. Oak Brook, IL: Author.

U.S. General Accounting Office Accounting and Information Management Division. (1997). *Business process reengineering assessment guide*. Washington, DC: Author.

Vanhaecht, K., Ovretveit, J., Elliott, M. J., Sermeus, W., Ellershaw, J., & Massimiliano, P. (2012). Have we drawn the wrong conclusions about the value of care pathways? Is a Cochraine review appropriate? *Evaluation and Health Professions*, *35*(1), 28–42. Retrieved from http://ehp.sagepub.com/content/35/1/28.full.pdf+html

Varkey, P., Reller, K., & Resar, R. K. (2007). Basics of quality improvement in health care. *Mayo Clinic Proceedings*, *82*(6), 735–739. doi:10.1016/s0025-6196(11)61194-4

Von Hippel, E. (2001). Perspective: User tool kits for innovation. *Journal of Project Innovation Management*, *18*(4), 247–257. doi:10.1016/s0737-6782(01)00090-x

Von Hippel, E., & Katz, R. (2002). Shifting innovation to users via toolkits. *Management Science*, *48*(7), 821–833. doi:10.1287/mnsc.48.7.821.2817

World Health Organization. (2008). *The World Health Report 2008: Primary health care (now more than ever)*. New York, NY: Author.

Zander, K. (1985). Managed care within acute care settings: Design and implementation via nursing case management. *Health Care Supervisor*, *6*(2), 27–43.

Zander, K. (1986). Case management: Cost, processes, and quality outcomes. *Definition*, *1*(2), 1–4.

Zander, K. (2003). Integrated care pathways: Eleven international trends. *Journal of Integrated Care Pathways*, *6*(3), 101–107. doi:10.1177/147322970200600302

Zwar, N. A., Wolk, J., Gordon, J. J., & Sanson-Fisher, R. W. (2000). Benzodiazepine prescribing by GP registrars: A clinical trial of educational outreach. *Australian Family Physician*, *29*(11), 1104–1107.

CHAPTER NINE

Project Management for Translation

Mary F. Terhaar, Rachael Crickman, and Deborah S. Finnell

Plans are nothing; planning is everything.
—DWIGHT D. EISENHOWER

TRANSLATION IS COMPLEX WORK: NONLINEAR, ADAPTIVE, AND influenced by context that includes the people, resources, and history of the organization that is moving through change. Because of this complexity, those who engage in translation will benefit from a structured approach based on a translation framework that applies one or more translation methods presented a priori in a well-crafted plan of action. Much like the tripod used by a photographer to stabilize the camera in order to capture the best image, the tripod proposed here supports the most effective and faithful translation of evidence.

Scholars have worked to dissemble the process of translation to help others negotiate it. Resultant frameworks guide teams as they move through the process. These frameworks, which are presented in Chapters 2 and 3, constitute the first leg of the tripod.

In much the same way that research methods direct the activities of all who participate in a study and all who would replicate it, translation methods promote fidelity to the findings of strong evidence by directing the activities of all who participate in translation and all who would replicate it. Methods, which are described in Chapter 8, constitute the second leg of the tripod.

The project plan is commonly considered to be less scholarly than the framework or methods because it is less theoretical and more practical, less abstract and more tactical. A well-constructed plan reflects collaboration and consensus of many individuals with specialized expertise. It helps to sequence and coordinate efforts, resources, and activities of many team members, all with different expertise, different concerns, and different information needs. The project plan is one key to successful translation and constitutes the third leg of the tripod.

The planning phase for any project is like the portion of the iceberg beneath the surface of the water because it is so large and so often goes unrecognized. However, lack of attention to planning is dangerous because it has the potential to end any endeavor, even an important one. Reasonable effort invested in a thoughtful project plan supports allocation of time and resources to a project with a high probability of success and potential for gain.

■ TRANSLATION AS PROCESS OR PROJECT TO BE MANAGED

It is useful to think of translation as a kind of project. Well-known projects include landing a man on the moon or a vehicle on a comet or on Mars. Both of these are examples of high-stakes efforts that consume impressive time and resources. They require sustained commitment and real-time problem-solving. All invite scrutiny. All promise important gains for stakeholders if successful and all threaten significant disappointment if they fail.

Approaching any complex project requires tremendous attention to detail, clear communication, effective collaboration among many individuals with highly specialized, frequently discrete knowledge and expertise. Proper sequencing of work, precise timing of activities, and a detailed resource plan contribute to success. Complex projects also require quality controls to minimize or mitigate unintended outcomes and thoughtful contingency planning to ensure the achievement of critical activities and outcomes. Complex projects require a clear statement of the purpose, aims, and target outcomes toward which all effort is directed. They require clarity in scope to describe work to be included in the project and work not to be included. This is called the *project plan*.

Translation is intended to improve outcomes (Institute of Medicine [IOM], 2001, 2003; Mohide & Coker, 2005; Titler, 2002; Titler et al., 2003). It can move an organization or a team toward achievement of the Triple Aim by improving quality of care, patient experience, and cost or value (Berwick, Nolan, & Whittington, 2008). Nurses and colleagues from other practice disciplines engaged in translation can reduce the cycle time from knowledge generation to its application in practice to realize the improved outcomes promised in original research (Foxcroft & Cole, 2003; Titler et al., 2003).

Nurses and teams engaged in this work can face challenges gaining organizational support, achieving intervention fidelity, documenting outcomes, maintaining momentum for change, shifting organizational culture, and finding effective clinical leadership (Bradley et al., 2004). Project management techniques can help to identify potential obstacles and orchestrate strategies to navigate around or over such challenges with minimal disruption to the plan or disturbance to important stakeholders. In this way, project management and planning mitigate each of the previously mentioned threats to the success of the project.

Researchers use scientific process to ensure rigor and control across efforts to develop new knowledge. This process is incorporated in education from middle school onward. It is familiar, effective, and clearly articulated. PhD students, in traditional research-focused doctoral programs, follow a well-established and consistent approach designed to promote optimal compliance with scientific process. They prepare a proposal, defend it, and execute dissertation work using a time-tested approach that ensures fidelity to the scientific process and a consistent level of scholarship. The result is the development of new knowledge following a rigorous, well-vetted process. Universities are familiar with both the processes and the products of this approach because the faculty themselves practiced it during their education. The product, called a *dissertation*, was traditionally presented as five topics: the problem, the background, the methods, the findings, and the conclusions. Each was reported in a separate chapter and combined to create the dissertation document. More recently, many programs and universities are accepting a set of manuscripts in substitution for the five chapters as the evidence of having met expectations for authentic and rigorous scholarship. Currently, many programs are accepting one to three manuscripts, derived from the research or the project as the final scholarly workproducts required to complete the program of study and offer evidence of mastery of the curriculum. This approach results in evidence of scholarship and facilitates dissemination at the same time.

DNPs have had no parallel and broadly accepted process to ensure the rigor and effectiveness of translation. The project plan can serve this function. It can organize and standardize the approach to translation, provide a structure to ensure thorough consideration and planning for complex change, and be used to generate documents that will promote fidelity to the evidence and collaboration within the team engaged in or affected by the change.

Project management is a process employed by many disciplines and enterprises engaged in high-stakes, complex work. Less well-known outside industry, its purposes are to increase the probability of achieving target outcomes, fidelity to a plan, on-time completion of work, and overall success within the budget (Project Management Institute [PMI], 2014). Not intended for knowledge development, project management is a great fit for the challenges of knowledge translation and practice innovation when combined with the frameworks and methods used for evidence-based practice (EBP) described earlier in this book.

Gawande (2010) proposed that healthcare today needs new leadership that looks more like a "pit crew" than a "cowboy": Healthcare needs leadership provided by engaged teams rather than by single physician leaders, as was common in the old paradigm. Because of this need for new leadership, new patterns of behavior and new tools are required. Project management offers tools and strategies that can help these newly created pit crews with the work of translation and innovation. DNPs can lead and facilitate these crews and these innovative translation projects. More important, the work products of DNP scholarship and the scholarship of clinical teams can be strengthened by following the project management process.

The purpose of this chapter is to introduce the phases of project management together with a set of tools and processes that can be used to enhance both the strength of success and the probability of its attainment by teams and team leaders engaged in the work of translation. Project management has demonstrated value for teams charged with completing complex work. It is a strategy with great potential to facilitate translation science. This chapter uses an unfolding case study based on a project designed to reduce exposure to hazardous medication. This case approach will help to illustrate the project-planning process and provide examples of the way the various tools can be used for planning, communicating with stakeholders, and achieving fidelity to the evidence (Crickman & Finnell, 2015).

■ PROJECT MANAGEMENT

The PMI (2014, p. 5) defines a *project* as "a temporary endeavor undertaken to create a unique product, service, or result." Several attributes of projects (Shenhar & Dvir, 2007) are worthy of emphasis with respect to translation.

- Projects are temporary. A team is formed for a purpose. The process is completed and the team disbands.
- Projects are special activities, not the day-to-day operations that routinely constitute one's work. Projects have a particular focus and may be only tangentially related to one's primary work.
- Projects have a beginning and an end and generate a specific, valued outcome.
- Projects can help any enterprise to innovate and adapt to changing customer requirements and market conditions.
- Projects can be used to help migrate knowledge into effective operations.
- Projects can help the organization develop new capabilities, learn, and gain competitive advantage.

Nurses and colleagues from other healthcare disciplines are commonly required to engage in projects because these activities are well suited to accomplishing diverse strategic goals.

Within any enterprise, many priorities compete for time and energy. Translation of specific evidence into practice is one strategy that cuts across many compelling priorities. The goal of improving outcomes through the application of evidence spans boundaries and disciplines. As a result, it provides common ground for managing change processes.

Within healthcare, the delay between knowledge generation and its effective application in practice is far too long: in fact, 7 to 11 years (Foxcroft & Cole, 2003; Funk, Tornquist, & Champagne, 1995). As a result, nursing and other disciplines have invested significant intellectual capital in the EBP process as a means to abbreviate that delay. Overlaying EBP processes with project management practices can help to secure the gains of research and EBP at an accelerated pace in ways that promote adaptability and sustainability within a particular context.

Translation projects, like other complex projects, progress through five phases: initiating, planning, executing, monitoring and controlling, and closing. Each phase focuses on a set of activities and each benefits from the use of particular tools. Managing these phases and applying the respective tools can be of tremendous help to clinicians translating evidence into practice (PMI, 2014). Figure 9.1 depicts the phases of project management as a base for translation. Because this chapter focuses on

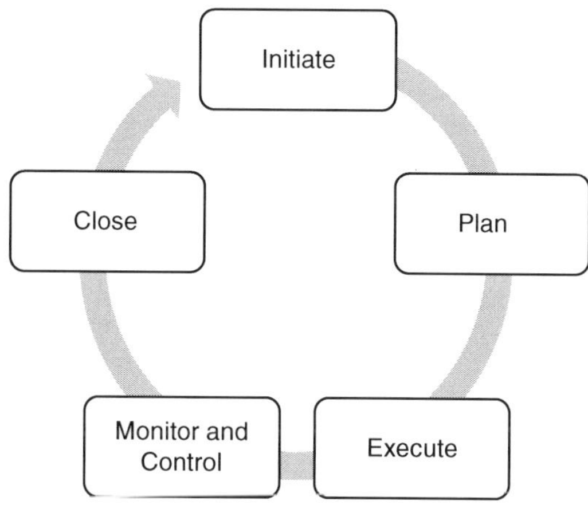

FIGURE 9.1 Phases of project management.

planning for translation, only the first two of the five phases will be addressed here. Execution will be addressed in Chapters 19 to 21. Monitoring and control will be addressed in Chapter 17 and closing out the project will be addressed in Chapters 19 to 21 as well.

The remainder of the chapter is organized around the phases of a project. Each phase is named in the order in which it is conducted. Then the work involved in completing that phase is described. Finally, an evolving case is presented so that each phase of that single project is used as an example of each phase of project management. The unfolding case describes process improvement in a hazardous drug-control program.

Phase 1: Initiating the Translation Project

The first phase of a project is called *initiation*. Merriam-Webster's defines *initiation* as *causing something to begin*. In the case of translation, initiation includes several processes: identifying and clearly stating the problem, examining the evidence, articulating the purpose of the project, setting specific aims to be achieved, and securing approvals and support.

The Problem Statement

Identifying the practice problem is the first step in the initiation of translation. It is the first piece of the project plan. The team must be open to recognizing opportunities to improve performance. Once opportunity is recognized, the practice problem is stated in such a way that it describes the opportunity to improve outcomes, which commonly corresponds to achieving the Triple Aim. Problems may relate to quality of care, patient experience, or the value of services (Berwick et al., 2008). Such problems may involve inconsistencies in practice, failure to adopt best practices, or lack of compliance with accepted guidelines or recent scientific development with potential to improve outcomes for a population served, or they may be associated with achieving competitive advantage in the market.

An example of a problem statement follows. This crisp text briefly describes the problem addressed in the Unfolding Case of the Hazardous Drug-Control Program.

> Health care workers across multiple settings are at risk for adverse health consequences from hazardous drug exposure because of their involvement in the transport, handling, preparation, administration, or disposal of certain medications. (Crickman & Finnell, 2015, p. 73)

Once identified, the problem is stated precisely using local data to establish both scope and magnitude. The data required to articulate the problem are commonly found in quality improvement, risk management, morbidity and mortality, billing, admissions, or discharge data. The source may be one of many departments or disciplines within the organization, or data may come from payers, staff, faculty, or community groups. Once the local data have been used to describe the problem in situ, regional or national data are used to establish context and to understand the performance to target.

The PICO format, which standardizes the statement of the problem in the context of EBP, requires a statement of the **p**roblem, the proposed **i**ntervention, the **c**omparison or **c**urrent practice, and the desired **o**utcome (Newhouse, 2007). This convention is counterproductive in translation because it requires forecasting of the intervention before prosecution of the evidence. So, for translation projects, the PICO is not used. Rather the problem within the organization is stated along with the background and significance in a particular setting. Together, these components of the problem statement will be useful to guide the search and prosecution of the evidence as well as development of the remainder of the project plan. An example of a complete problem statement for the project presented in the Unfolding Case of the Hazardous Drug-Control Program follows.

> Polovich and Clark (2012) examined factors that affect nurses' PPE use, which included barriers to adherence, workplace safety climate, and patient/ nurse ratios. The study revealed that institutional practices and personal behaviors affect occupational exposure. PPE is considered the last line of defense in protecting nurses and other healthcare workers who handle hazardous drugs. Addressing knowledge deficits is essential but may not be sufficient to protect healthcare workers. Knowledge alone does not consistently lead to behavior change; however, acknowledging poor safe handling behavior is critical for reducing exposure (Geer, Curbow, Anna, Lees, & Buckley, 2006).
>
> Compliance with PPE standards for handling chemotherapy remains poor and insufficient to prevent occupational exposure despite the growing body of evidence of PPE efficacy (Gambrell & Moore, 2006; Martin & Larson, 2003; McDiarmid, Oliver, Roth, Rogers, & Escalante, 2010; Polovich & Clark, 2012). (Crickman & Finnell, 2015, p. 75)

Prosecution of the Evidence

Rigorous prosecution of the evidence is essential to translation. Conducted by one individual alone, this is a time-consuming process. Conducted by a team, it can be accomplished efficiently. The team approach helps develop a strong sense of confidence in the solution and shared ownership in the project, which grows through the work during the initiation phase. Prosecution of the evidence, like prosecution of a witness, seeks the truth. It tests veracity of assertions and requires clinicians to suspend judgment until a thorough understanding of the evidence is complete. Translation requires teams to be open to what the evidence teaches. In the end, the translation team will draw reliable conclusions from strong evidence and will be invested in the solution because they will have vetted the evidence thoroughly, using the same set of tools established as reliable and useful in the EBP process.

A search is conducted. Evidence is gathered, reviewed, critiqued, and summarized. Then trustworthy, robust research findings are synthesized and presented for consideration by the team. The solution flows from the prosecution, directs the translation, and is presented in the project plan.

During initiation, an idea is refined and vetted. The problem is clearly defined and data are gathered to establish the scope, significance, and impact of that problem on the organization, the individuals it serves, and the community. After the prosecution of the evidence is complete, the findings are captured in a report so the full team and all stakeholders can interact with the findings, pose questions, and contribute to understanding the fit with the population served, the facility, and the context into which the change will be introduced. A template used at the Johns Hopkins University School of Nursing to outline the purpose and aims of a translation project is presented in Exhibit 9.1 (Dearholt & Dang, 2012).

In the end, the prosecution of the evidence answers a simple question: What does strong evidence direct the team to do in order to address the problem? Anthropomorphism aside, the reason to prosecute the evidence is to find answers based on science that will transform care and, in doing so, improve outcomes for a particular population under particular conditions. This is the core of translation; it is the power in the work; and the plan is central to ensuring that research findings do in fact improve care, quality, and cost. The team and its leader(s) face the challenge of

EXHIBIT 9.1 Summary of the Evidence Table

#	1st Author	Year	Level of Research (or Nonresearch) Evidence	Sample Composition and Size	Results/ Recommendations	Limitations	RATING Strength / Quality

locating, critiquing, understanding, and synthesizing the evidence. The next challenge is to tell the story of the science, capture the confidence and commitment of the healthcare team, and deliver impactful and sustainable improvement. An example of a high-level summary of the evidence from the Unfolding Case of the Hazardous Drug-Control Program follows.

> Five methods to reduce occupational exposure were identified: (a) the development of engineering controls, (b) personal protective equipment (PPE) use, (c) medical and environmental monitoring for common antineoplastic drugs, (d) hazard identification, and (e) a comprehensive hazardous drug control program that provides education and training for healthcare workers. (Crickman & Finnell, 2015, p. 75)

Support and Approval

The executive in any healthcare organization, serving any population in need, has a large set of initiatives in the "inbox," all seeking support. Many of these proposed activities promise to improve care, reduce risk, control cost, or conserve precious human capital. From that universe of possibilities, the executive selects the critical few projects judged to have the highest probability of success and greatest congruence with the mission. A clear and compelling problem statement is key here.

The better the fit between the outcome to be achieved and the mission, vision, values, and resources of the entity, the stronger will be the support for the project. The DNP can provide significant leadership during this phase.

To position a project for favorable preliminary review, it is helpful to present a high-level summary that describes the purpose of the project, the specific aims of the work, and the measurable outcomes to be achieved (clinical, operational, financial, or quality). A tool used for this purpose at the Johns Hopkins University School of Nursing is presented in Exhibit 9.2.

EXHIBIT 9.2 Cover Page and Approvals

Project Title	
Project Leader	
Advisor	
Mentor	
Team Members	
Site	
Purpose	
Background	
Project Aims	
Team Leader's Signature	
Approval Signature	

Project Title

The project title should be a simple statement of the work. It needs to appeal to stakeholders from different disciplines and departments, capture interest, and stimulate readers to read on. It should use compelling language and avoid jargon and acronyms. Imagine that a philanthropist is considering funding the project. If written for that reader, the title will likely satisfy the executive as well. The title for the project presented in the Unfolding Case of the Hazardous Drug-Control Program is "Implementing a Hazardous Drug-Control Program" (Crickman & Finnell, 2015).

Purpose

The purpose statement needs to be clear and compelling. It should describe the intent of the project, command the interest of stakeholders, and recruit the support of those in the position to select the vital few projects that will be supported in a given cycle. The purpose should be specific and its scope should be appropriate to the problem or opportunity at the core of the project. It is a high-level summary of what the project is about.

Think of this statement as the elevator speech for the project. Tight statements that use crisp language and convey an important intention will be most effective. An example of a purpose statement for the Unfolding Case of the Hazardous Drug-Control Program follows.

> The goal of the current study was to implement an evidence-based program that focused on improving the safe handling practices of and reducing the occupational exposure of nurses to hazardous drugs. (Crickman & Finnell, 2015, p. 76)

Aims

Aims are statements of what will be accomplished; what will be better as a result of the translation project. Aims should be singular in focus and precise so they can be evaluated. They should explain the expected direction of change: Will there be an increase or a decrease in something about which there is concern? It is impossible to evaluate compound aims, those that present more than one improvement. So aims are not written that way. Finally, aims need to be specific and inclusive in order to form the basis for the evaluation plan.

An example of a set of aims for the Unfolding Case of the Hazardous Drug-Control Program follows.

The project has two aims:

1. To increase compliance with personal protective equipment among inpatient oncology nurses administering hazardous drugs
2. To reduce environmental contamination with cyclophosphamide in the inpatient oncology nursing unit (Crickman & Finnell, 2015).

These aims will guide all project work. Stating the aims explicitly allows reviewers to critique the project, clarify its focus and scope, and expand or restrict the group's efforts.

The institutional review board (IRB) is familiar with the language of aims. Adopting this convention facilitates the IRB review process for those projects that may be considered human-subjects research.

Background. The background provides a high-level summary of the prosecution of the evidence and explains what the strong evidence directs clinicians and team members to do to resolve the problem. This will become the work of the proposed project. An effective background text establishes the project as a priority and creates confidence in the team as sufficiently prepared and informed to accomplish the aims as stated. Citing strong evidence and connecting the project to the strategic intent and goals of the organization help to create the support required to move the project forward.

Charge or Charter. The work of translation may be charged to a practice council, research committee, or other established group; or it may be conducted by a team that forms itself expressly for the purpose of conducting a single translation project. Regardless, the leadership team benefits from a charge that establishes the authority needed to complete the work. The charge needs to clearly identify the reason behind assembling the team, the problem to be solved, the time frame for the work to be done, the members of the team, and the individual(s) named as the leader(s). The charge may be to improve quality, improve process, reduce rework, reduce cycle time, decrease waste, or increase satisfaction. The clearer and more specific the charge, the greater the probability it will be attained. In translation projects, targets for time, resources, and outcomes are commonly included in the charge.

Leadership. An individual or a group of individuals may be assigned responsibility for the project. These leaders are responsible for achieving the stated purpose as presented in the charge or charter. A coach can be provided to facilitate the work of leaders and team members as well. Because they are likely to be engaged in patient care at the same time that they are asked to fill a leadership role, project leaders may struggle to find the time required to manage a translation project of significant scope. Leaders may be consulted with respect to team formation or charged with actual assembly of the project team themselves. Chapter 6, Translation of Evidence for Leadership, summarizes evidence for effective leadership.

Team. The team of individuals who will play key roles in the project is selected and charged as the project team. This group is most effective when composed of individuals who together possess the necessary knowledge, skill, and authority to accomplish legitimate and sustainable change. A team that lacks any of the requisite knowledge, expertise, or skill can be expanded; can subcontract pieces of the work; or can be provided with education, coaching, or consultation to compensate for a deficit. The stronger and more inclusive the team is, the greater its likelihood of success. Including team members with diverse perspectives will increase the probability of success because potential problems that are identified early are amenable to careful planning and thoughtful solutions.

Team Members Add Diversity and Expertise. Faculty members from schools of nursing, medicine, engineering, pharmacy, public health, or business may be able to provide support for projects and may prove to be good coaches for teams. These individuals may be able to help with measurement plans, data analysis, and interpretation of findings. Faculty may also be able to help obtain IRB approval or extramural funding.

Students from schools of nursing can also be helpful. Students value the opportunity to engage in meaningful work. They bring a strong set of skills that will prove helpful throughout the translation process. They are able to help with reviews of literature and evaluation of evidence. They can review charts, collect and enter data, and help with project management. Later, in the implementation phase, students can collect data, monitor processes, and maintain records and data.

The initiation phase focuses on establishing a good fit between the organization at a given time (including resources, commitments, and strategic intent) and the opportunities and requirements presented by a particular project. It involves two key factors: identifying opportunity or need and establishing readiness and preparation for action. Establishing readiness involves both situational and stakeholder analysis.

Phase 2: Planning the Translation Project

The second phase in project management is developing the plan of action. During this phase the team develops a very granular, very prescriptive approach that ensures faithful translation of the evidence to achieve the purpose and aims stated in phase 1. Several documents, not commonly encountered in the provision of care, will be used during this phase. They include a work breakdown structure (WBS), Gantt chart, situational assessment (strengths, weaknesses, opportunities, threats [SWOT]), stakeholder assessment, communication plan, risk management plan, and assorted supplemental documents. All are used to ensure that providers, clinicians, and colleagues can adhere to the recommendations from strong evidence.

The WBS and the Gantt chart help communicate deep detail so that all engaged in the provision of care can faithfully translate evidence into practice. These two documents are essential to achieving the project aims. Project planners in industry commonly use both tools. However, clinicians may find them a bit redundant and, as a result, selection of the one that best suits a project and facility is recommended.

Work Breakdown Structure

A WBS is central to the success of complex projects. It deconstructs the work of the project into manageable chunks that are called *packages of work*. This deconstruction helps team members and those charged with executing the plan to understand the interrelated nature of the work of many individuals and teams and the sequencing of these interrelated contributions. The WBS is constructed as a hierarchical and visual representation of the work. When executed as originally designed by engineers, the WBS is organized by tasks and each is further broken down into the activities required to accomplish it. By design, all tasks assembled together produce the goal of the project.

The WBS is much like a concept map for the project. The document itself looks simple, but creating this representation of all project work takes considerable thought and attention to detail. Moving a group from a statement of a problem to a consensus

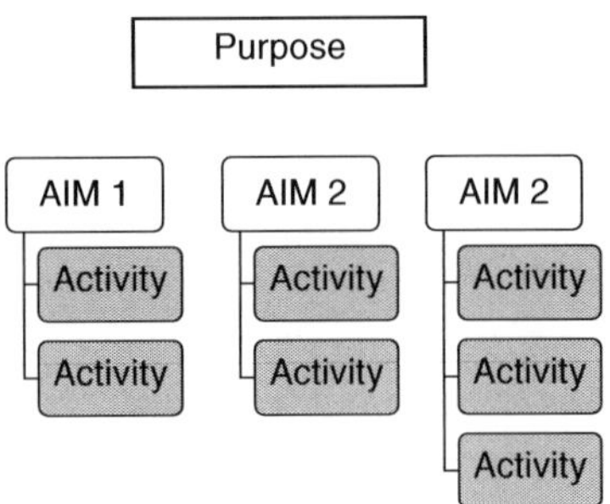

FIGURE 9.2 Work breakdown structure.

about all the activities and efforts required to resolve it takes considerable effort. Fortunately, in the work of translation, evidence can point the way. In translation, strong evidence is the key to establishing consensus. For this reason, the group will consult the evidence tables throughout the development of the WBS and will remind itself to ask repeatedly: What does the strong evidence direct the team to do to address and solve the problem?

In any project, it is useful to begin with the end in mind (Covey, 1989). A clear statement of the target to be achieved in the end and the overall purpose of the project is useful to set and maintain focus. Then, work backward to determine what is necessary to accomplish that end based on the evidence. In translation, use the aims to organize the work and then deconstruct each to identify the actions within the WBS. From each aim, drill deeper to describe all actions and activities required. Continue to drill deeper until the plan is clear and complete. This strategy will help you develop your WBS.

Figure 9.2 contains a template for the WBS. It can help you to create a visual representation of the work. For large or complex projects, a list may be more practical and, as a result, more helpful than a visual model.

In the end, the WBS is comparable to the methods section of a dissertation or research paper. It should contain sufficient detail to allow any reader to replicate the work and, in doing so, recreate the outcomes. Creating the WBS is a challenge that requires those engaged in its development to describe a process or processes in minute detail. Benner (1984) reports that even experts have a difficult time breaking down what they do to basic components. Ask the expert nurse how he or she recognized that a specific patient was in trouble, and that nurse will often share some high-level, integrated thoughts that would not lead a novice to successfully manage the same clinical challenge and would not lead to the same resolution of the problem. An example of a set of a WBS for the Unfolding Case of the Hazardous Drug-Control Program is provided in Exhibit 9.3.

Asking clinical experts to help create the WBS is asking them to break down integrative, high-level thinking into basic steps (Benner, 1984). It is asking those who operate in a quick-thinking and quick-acting paradigm to slow down and linger in the details so others can follow (Kahneman, 2011). It can be tedious work for the expert and yet, failure to complete this work is certainly planning for project failure.

EXHIBIT 9.3 WBS for the Unfolding Case of the Hazardous Drug Control Program

AIM 1: Increase compliance with use of PPE among inpatient oncology nurses administering hazardous drugs.				AIM 2: Reduce environmental contamination of cyclophosphamide in the inpatient oncology nursing unit.				
Education Plan	**Identify Hazardous Drugs**	**Design Assessment Tool**	**Standardize PPE**	**Select Lab**	**Communicate**	**Secure Funds**	**Measure**	**Remeasure**
Develop instructional design.	Determine which drugs merit observation of PPE.	Deconstruct steps for PPE use.	Communicate idea to stakeholders.	Develop product specifications.	Identify those who need to know.	Obtain cost estimate.	Recruit testing assistant (pre).	Obtain baseline measures (post).
Set learning objectives.		Create tool for observations.	Select vendor to provide gowns.	ID all labs able to run swipe analysis.	Determine effective communication.	Explore internal funds.	Train assistant.	Repeat initial measure.
Develop content.	Plan timeline for observations.	Calculate sample size.	Obtain cost estimate.			Explore external funds.	Obtain baseline.	
Create online module.		Determine whether IRB review is required.	Secure gowns.	Invite bids.			Select testing sites.	
Update tools for PPE use.		Obtain baseline.	Use PDSA cycle with gowns.	Review quality.		Seek funding.		
		Repeat observation.	Calculate ROI.	Review cost.		Pay lab.	Gather data.	

ID, identify; IRB, institutional review board; PDSA, plan-do-study-act; PPE, personal protective equipment; ROI, return on investment; WBS, work breakdown structure.

Source: From Crickman, R., & Finnell, D. S. (2015). Systematic review of control measures to reduce hazardous drug exposure for health care workers. *Journal of Nursing Care Quality*, *31*(1), 9–12.

There are many ways to represent the work, but the detail must be included for the project to be successful and for clinicians to accomplish fidelity to strong evidence. The challenge to the team leader is to hold the experts' full engagement in discussions about details and dialogue that takes time away from direct care.

It may be easier to see the value of the WBS using content less familiar to the clinical expert. Consider changing a tire. How does one go about the work? What resources are needed? How does one avoid the risk? What can be learned from experience? What can be learned from the user's manual? Exhibit 9.4 presents a WBS for changing a flat tire. As translation work, this is a poor example because the sources are anecdotal or industry-sponsored driver's manuals. On the other hand, as detailed work developed to help the user, it is illustrative. Because the aims drive the work, explicitly including safety in the aim requires the addition of steps that might otherwise not have been recognized as important.

Gantt Chart

The Gantt chart is a second type of document that can be used to plan and communicate in detail the work of the project. Like the WBS, the Gantt deconstructs the work of translation to provide in-depth detail that describes exactly how the evidence will be translated and what clinicians will do to improve outcomes and achieve the project aims. This chart is one of the most popular and broadly used among all project management tools.

In a Gantt chart, the sets of activities and a very granular representation of the work of the project are listed down the vertical axis of the document. These activities can be organized in sets that correspond to the aim they are intended to accomplish, which is much like the design of the WBS. The Gantt differs from the WBS because it adds columns across the horizontal axes that represent units of time. Bars are created across the units of time for each activity to show the distribution of work over the life cycle of the project. This approach helps forecast, sequence, and distribute effort over time; helps identify when the burden of work is heavy; and emphasizes opportunities more to evenly distribute effort or add resources to accommodate it.

The Gantt is particularly useful as a means to anticipate and organize the work of a project. Beyond planning, it is a great approach that is used during execution to track progress, to evaluate attainment of intermediate goals and deliverables, and to determine achievement of more inclusive aims. The Gantt helps identify when a project is tracking along as planned, which is reassuring. It also helps to identify when the work is behind schedule, which is useful in contingency planning. There are many tools available online to help with generating Gantt charts for any project. An example is presented in Exhibit 9.5.

In the end, the Gantt chart presents a very detailed summary of the work of a project. It promotes organization of work contributed by many individuals and diverse team members to a complex process in service of achieving a set of specific and measurable aims. An example of a set of a Gantt chart for the Unfolding Case of the Hazardous Drug-Control Program is provided in Exhibit 9.6.

Developing the WBS or Gantt. Developing the project plan, either in the form of a WBS or Gantt, is a useful way of representing the work. It helps to ensure that the

EXHIBIT 9.4 WBS for Changing a Flat Tire

Get Safe	Get Equipment	Loosen Tire	Raise the Car	Remove Tire	Replace Tire	Lower the Car	Return to Driving
Grip wheel	Driver's manual	Remove hub cap	Apply the jack per instructions	Place lug nuts in hub cap	Lift spare tyre til openings allign with bolts on wheel	Use jack to lower car	Turn on car
Turn on blinker	Tire	Loosen each lug nut partially (turn left)	Raise car just high enough to clear the ground	Remove tire	Shimmy new tire into place	Place full weight of car on the ground before removing the jack	Disengage parking break
Pull over	Jack	Repeat		Place flat away from traffic	Replace each lug nut	Remove jack	Turn off flashers
Find a level space	Blanket or tarp	Repeat til all are completely loose			Turn each lug nut a few times (turn right)	Replace equipment and tire into the trunk	Turn on blinker
Get out of traffic					Repeat til all are secure		Check for oncoming traffic
Turn off engine							Allow time to merge
Turn on flashers							Return to traffic
Engage parking break							Drive to service station to have tire checked
Call for help							

WBS, work breakdown structure.

EXHIBIT 9.5 Gantt Chart Template

AIM 1										
Activity	1	2	3	4	5	6	7	8	9	10
AIM 2										
Activity	1	2	3	4	5	6	7	8	9	10

project can be fully understood by all members of the team and evaluated for potential effect on work units in the organization, key stakeholders, finances, and resources. This detailed summary of the project helps to establish the work of translation as important, well considered, feasible, resource conserving, and inclusive. The project plan helps create a reasonable expectation that the project will be successful, will produce important results that contribute to the success of the mission, will be completed on time and within budget, and will have a strong return on investment (PMI, 2014).

Sticky Note Process for Developing the WBS. Some people find it helpful to create the WBS by writing "to do" items on sticky notes and then placing them on the wall. This approach requires that team members help to state all the activities required to

EXHIBIT 9.6 Gantt Chart for the Unfolding Case of the Hazardous Drug-Control Program

Project Activity	Person Responsible	Start	End	January	February	March	April	May	June	July	Aug	Sept
AIM 1: Increase compliance with use of PPE among inpatient oncology nurses administering hazardous drugs.												
1. Develop education plan.	RC	03/10/14	06/02/14									
Meet instructional designer.	RC & JS	05/01/14	08/20/14									
Develop instructional design.	RC & JS	05/01/14	08/20/14									
Set learning objectives.	RC & DK		02/28/14									
Align design and objectives.	RC & DK		03/19/14									
Develop content.	RC	05/10/14	07/02/14									
Create online module.	RC & DK	06/20/14	07/02/14									
Update tools for PPE use.												
Create assessments.	RC											
Review content with stakeholders.	RC											
Seek approval from stakeholders.	RC, DK, & KB	05/05/14	06/02/14									
Seek approval from IRB.	RC	06/02/14	07/01/14									
2. Identify hazardous drugs.												

(continued)

EXHIBIT 9.6 Gantt Chart for the Unfolding Case of the Hazardous Drug-Control Program (*continued*)

Project Activity	Person Responsible	Start	End	January	February	March	April	May	June	July	Aug	Sept
Determine which drugs merit observation of PPE.												
Plan timeline for observations.												
3. Design assessment tool.												
Deconstruct steps for PPE use.												
Create tool for observations.												
Calculate sample size.												
Determine whether IRB review is required.												
Obtain baseline.												
4. Standardize PPE.												
Communicate idea with stakeholders.												
Select vendor to provide gowns.												
Obtain cost estimate.												
Secure gowns.												
Calculate ROI.												

IRB, institutional board review; PPE, personal protective equipment; ROI, return on investment.

achieve an aim. Members then brainstorm the ways the aims can be accomplished and post those activities or actions beneath each related aim. Brainstorming continues with a focus on actions and activities required to achieve the aims, and those threads are posted in the subsequent text. This process is repeated until the group has described all activities necessary to achieve the project aims. It is particularly helpful when the team comprises members with different knowledge bases and expertise. It helps to bring the specialty knowledge to the surface and create a shared understanding of a process or processes. In the end, content is recorded and shared by members who work on crafting the final draft of the WBS that is free of redundancies, inconsistencies, or omissions. A common vocabulary can be developed along with a sense of identity and affiliation with other team members and the aims to be achieved.

Situational Assessment: Organizational Readiness for Change

Once the plan has been developed, it is important to formally evaluate readiness of the organization for the intended change. One approach to this situational assessment is to conduct a SWOT analysis that identifies the **s**trengths and **w**eaknesses in the organization with respect to the project, the **o**pportunities inherent in the work of the project, and any potential **t**hreats to project success. The SWOT is most effective when conducted in an open dialogue with key stakeholders and customers.

Strengths refer to key functions the organization does well and the organization's assets. Experienced clinical leaders, a strong financial position, committed customers, dedicated clinicians, an established program of research, and an engaged executive are examples of organizational strengths. Each of these attributes and assets positions an organization or work unit for success. A unit with stable staff, strong leadership, and a good physical plant is favorably positioned to engage in innovation; these are its strengths.

Weaknesses refer to particular areas where the organization identifies need or deficiency. High staff turnover, vacancies in critical roles, knowledge or skill deficits, undesirable payer mix, outdated processes, and old technology are examples of organizational or work-unit weaknesses. These can compromise any organization's position in the market and interfere with its ability to innovate. A unit where staff turnover is high, commitment is low, and staff members are inexperienced will need to address these weaknesses in any plan for innovation.

Opportunities refer to conditions and factors that position an organization for success. Some factors may be external, such as a change in a demographic in the community that has the potential to increase business. Some factors are internal, such as a strong new department head who is ready and eager to take on a challenge. Connecting opportunity to strategic intent supports innovation. Therefore, a pediatric primary care group whose pediatric nurse practitioner (PNP) is earning his or her DNP degree has an opportunity to benefit from hosting that PNP's doctoral project because the DNP student will provide the scholarship to drive meaningful performance improvement.

Threats are factors that can prevent the success of a project. Competing priorities, unforeseen demands on staff and resources, new technology or knowledge, and changes in funding or policy can all threaten a project. It is useful to discriminate between risk and threat. The former, risk, refers to any harm that might be expected to befall participants. It is critical, and in fact an ethical imperative, to identify and manage risk. The latter, threat, refers to harm that could befall the project itself. To the extent that external conditions can be evaluated and identify threat to a project, strategies to reduce their impact can be developed. For example, innovative education for breastfeeding can be threatened when reimbursement is reduced to hold down healthcare costs and when lactation support is on the list of programs to be cut. Anticipating such a threat would point the project team to use cost-effective, high-impact approaches to patient education and support. It would also point the team to calculate return on investment in order to make the business case to sustain the intervention due to its overall value. One tool that may be useful during the situational assessment is presented in Figure 9.3.

The project team uses the SWOT analysis to develop strategies to exploit strengths, compensate for weaknesses, capitalize on opportunities, mitigate threats, and communicate essential information to those affected by the work of the project. Translation will be most effective when its execution is carefully planned with full consideration of the people, resources, culture, and history of the organization into which it is introduced. The SWOT situational assessment for the Unfolding Case of the Hazardous Drug-Control Program is presented in Figure 9.4.

Stakeholder Assessment

Stakeholders are those "individuals or organizations actively involved in the project or those whose interests may be affected by the project execution or project outcome" (PMI, 2014, p. 24). Engaging stakeholders effectively is critical to the success of any project. To do so, it is necessary to establish an understanding of their expectations and requirements so that these can be taken into account when planning and executing the project.

A stakeholder assessment is conducted to identify the extent to which individuals in the organization are affected by the work of the project. It can be used to identify the reasons they are interested or affected and the ways they may become engaged in the work. Time should be taken to map out key individuals, their level of investment, their perspective with respect to the project work and aims, and their importance with respect to the success of the project. Conducting such an assessment can help to surface expectations, identify potential barriers, and discover individuals and conditions that support the project aims. It will also help to plan inclusion strategies, responsibilities, and communication throughout the life cycle of the project. The template for a stakeholder assessment is presented in Exhibit 9.7.

In addition to the stakeholder assessment described in the preceding text, it may be useful to create a visual map of the stakeholders. This approach calls attention to the needs for different levels of engagement in the project. Figure 9.5 contains a visual representation of this map.

- Some individuals have little influence in the organization and are expected to be minimally impacted by the project. The project team will benefit from investigating the concerns, experiences, and ideas of this group. To do so will increase the quality of the project and outcomes.

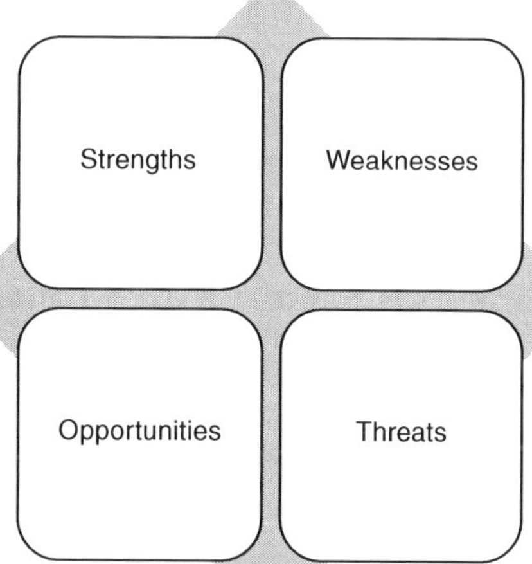

FIGURE 9.3 Situational assessment template.

Strengths

Legislation mandates implementation

Expertise of leadership

It is the right thing to do!

Many strategies and tools in place

Support of key leaders

Passionate and dedicated team leadership

Weaknesses

Hazardous Drug Committee lacking members

Policies and procedures for chemo do not necessarily apply to other hazardous drugs

Limited research evidence for non-chemo hazardous drugs

Insufficient manpower to support execution

Some regulatory requirements not supported by strong evidence

Industry-wide tools not user-friendly

Leadership in ambulatory undetermined

Opportunities

Organization uniquely poised to improve performance across the state

Oncology unit moving to new building (baseline contamination should be zero)

Good potential to connect oncology nurses nationally

High potential to impact national policy

Threats

COST: to upgrade training, personnel, and equipment

FEAR: regarding level of harm, concern for staff, patients, and families

LEGISLATION: delay in implementation

RESISTANCE: among external stakeholders

RAPID: pace of change

CONFUSION: between evidence and legislation

FIGURE 9.4 SWOT for the Unfolding Case of the Hazardous Drug-Control Program.

EXHIBIT 9.7 Stakeholder Assessment Tool

Individual or Team	Stake or Mandate	Potential Involvement	Involvement

- Some individuals are minimally influential in the organization, but their work can be expected to be impacted by the project. In this case, it is prudent to invite consultation so that their perspective can improve the project.
- Some individuals are influential in the organization, but their work is not expected to be impacted by the project. This group should be kept informed of progress.

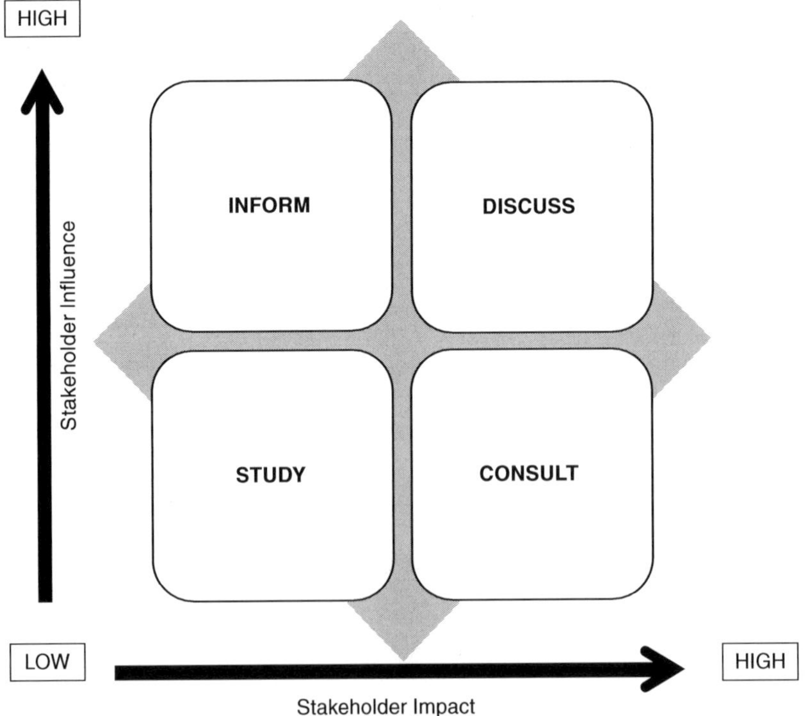

FIGURE 9.5 Stakeholder map.

- And finally, some individuals are influential in the organization and their work has a high probability of being impacted. This group needs to be engaged in ongoing discussion or progress and problem-solving.

Communication Plan

All stakeholders require information about the progress of the project. They need to receive updates on completion of work and attainment of the project aims. Working from the stakeholder analysis and the stakeholder map, and in collaboration with the individuals and teams identified as having legitimate need for information, a plan for communication can be developed. Such a plan will need to identify standing meetings and forums where information can be conveniently and regularly shared. It is also useful to identify vehicles for conveying information that are routinely used by the group and helpful to the stakeholders. An effective communication plan will use these forums and vehicles to keep all stakeholders apprised of progress and informed of any outcomes or unintended consequences that are relevant to their work. It will be useful to engage all stakeholders in development of the plan as well as to seek improvement and approval by the parties involved. Subsequently, faithful execution of the plan is key to high-impact translation of the evidence and resultant improved outcomes.

Shared Responsibility. The work of translation often requires collaboration among many individuals from various disciplines and work units. Coordinating the activities and accountabilities of such a team requires fine-tuning and clear communication. Responsibility charts (R charts) help in situations, for example, when many people are legitimately and necessarily involved in the work. In such a situation, it becomes important that each person understands his or her responsibilities, that those in positions of authority approve work appropriately, and that those who are affected by the work are provided with information they require to perform their own work. The stakeholder analysis and the WBS should be used to facilitate a discussion of responsibilities and to generate a responsibility chart similar to the one presented in Exhibit 9.8.

Risk Management Plan

Any project that involves human subjects requires identification and planning to manage any potential risk to subjects or any individuals involved. As caregivers, nurses advocate that patients be fully informed of any risks inherent in a new treatment or approach to care. The IRB will require full disclosure and a plan to manage any identified risk.

In translation projects, nurses and colleagues also need to be assured that both patients and caregivers are protected against risk. For example, if a translation project requires that caregivers become aware of evidence and apply that evidence in their caregiving, then baseline knowledge will need to be assessed along with knowledge following the intervention. Caregivers deserve assurance that knowledge deficit at baseline will not bring discipline or retaliation. The goal of quality improvement is not to eliminate staff members who would benefit from education but to raise the level of knowledge across the staff in order to raise the quality of care and improve outcomes.

EXHIBIT 9.8 Responsibility Chart for Managing the Integrated Work of Diverse Team Members

Aim										
Activity	Stakeholder 1	Stakeholder 2	Stakeholder 3	Stakeholder 4	Stakeholder 5	Stakeholder 6	Stakeholder 7	Stakeholder 8	Stakeholder 9	Stakeholder 10

Key

A: Needs to provide approval

R: Responsible

R: Co-responsible

C: Consultant

I: Needs to be informed

To protect patients and caregiver participants alike, a risk management plan is prepared. Its purpose is to predict all foreseeable potential risks, to identify the means to identify those who may face risk, and to take appropriate action to mitigate that risk. An example of a risk management plan for the Unfolding Case of the Hazardous Drug-Control Program plan is presented in Exhibit 9.9.

Planning Evaluation

The aims and the WBS provide the infrastructure for the evaluation plan. Each aim is assigned a metric selected for its sensitivity, specificity, and reliability that will be evaluated to determine whether the aim has been achieved. For example, a *fast track* may be implemented in the ED to reduce waiting time. Metrics for this project may include time waiting for intake, time waiting to see the physician, number of people in the waiting room, and patient satisfaction. For the purpose of planning evaluation, the team will identify the measures to be used, determine the source of the data, and plan the statistics to be used to determine the outcome.

EXHIBIT 9.9 **Risk Management Plan for the Unfolding Case of the Hazardous Drug-Control Program**

	Response to Reduce, Avoid, or Manage Risk	Indicator and Threshold	Probability L/M/H	Effect L/M/H	Status
Risk 1: *If a breach of confidentiality occurs*					
1.1	Then the source of the breach will be investigated	Staff commenting on level of compliance or demographic information shared via email	LOW	LOW	
1.2	Then IRB will be notified	Written or verbal	LOW	LOW	
1.3	Then the subjects will be notified	Face to face	LOW	LOW	
1.4	Then measures will be taken to ensure confidentiality	Change passwords, files, etc.	LOW	LOW	
Risk 2: *If a nurse does not don appropriate PPE*					
2.1	Then the observer will provide immediate coaching	Nurse does not don gloves, gown, face mask with eye shield	MOD	LOW	

H, high; IRB, institutional review board; L, low; M, moderate; PPE, personal protective equipment.

A full discussion of the evaluation process is presented in Chapter 17, Best Practices in Translation: Challenges and Barriers to Translation. It is important to note that evaluation must be planned in advance along with all the other work of the project. This is essential to ensure that the necessary data are collected throughout the project to evaluate with a high level of confidence the effectiveness of the innovation derived from the evidence.

Planning to Manage Quality

Translation is commonly framed as quality improvement for two reasons. First, it seeks to apply strong evidence to improve outcomes and, in doing so, has tremendous potential to contribute to the Triple Aim: care, quality, and cost. Second, it is distinguished from research that seeks to discover new knowledge, and often the IRB will articulate a clear and distinct difference.

Teams will find it useful to understand the organization's approach to quality improvement as the context for translation work. To that end, teams will want to understand the answers to several questions.

- How do stakeholders describe and measure quality in this organization or functional unit? Are there a set of metrics that tie to the mission and performance expectations? How were they chosen and who owns the data?
- What quality-improvement activities are underway in the organization or functional unit? Are there competing or complementary priorities? Is there already an investment in this effort? Are there boundaries or contingencies of importance?
- What are the quality goals for the group?
- Has the group been successful in its quality-improvement efforts? What would the group consider to be its significant accomplishments? How were they achieved? What was learned? What was valuable?
- Have there been failures in the work of quality improvement? What was learned? What ought not be repeated?
- What are the baseline measures of quality before the project begins?
- What is the level of quality below which performance must not fall?
- How is benchmarking accomplished?
- Who are the experts? Who are the stakeholders?

It is a best practice to engage others in monitoring the quality and the outcome of the project. It is useful to develop plans to suspend the project or address unintended consequences or problems if there is a negative effect on quality. The success of any project is well served by taking time to describe in detail how a problem is to be reported and addressed, should it occur. The project team will want to discuss the likelihood that this project might compromise quality even though the goal is to improve it and then plan ways to document and communicate quality throughout the life cycle of the project. It is helpful to use graphs, reports, and dashboards, to share information, engage staff in the work of interpreting findings, and establish accountability for quality. A template for a quality-management plan is presented in Exhibit 9.10.

Project Approval and Support

In order to proceed to phases 3 and 4, due diligence is required. A project proposal that presents a thorough problem statement, comprehensive prosecution of the

EXHIBIT 9.10 **Quality Management Plan Template**

Deliverable	Relevant Quality Criteria	Recovery Procedure (If Item Does Not Meet Standard)	Person(s) Responsible

evidence, a compelling purpose, clear and specific aims, a detailed plan of action, assessment of strategic readiness, and stakeholder assessment can be reviewed and presented for formal approval. Such approval may be given directly by the executive, administration, governance body, practice committee, or research committee charged with oversight of translation. In some cases, IRB review will be indicated and in others it will not. Like the original charge or charter, the approval is most effective when it is clear, specific, and detailed.

For the purpose of considering project approval, it is useful to return to the contrast drawn earlier between the PhD and the DNP. The PhD student conducts research called a *dissertation*. Research generates new knowledge. It is rigorous, follows a prescribed process, and is reviewed for quality, rigor, and scholarship. It is also evaluated for its effect on participants known as *human subjects*. The DNP student conducts a translation project or quality-improvement project. Translation applies findings from quality research endeavors to practice, and the authors use a prescribed process known as *project management* to facilitate disciplined implementation and evaluation of the knowledge application.

Entities engaged in the care of patients have in place IRBs responsible for the oversight of all activities that involve research on human subjects with the purpose of generating new, systematically collected knowledge that can be generalized to populations other than the subjects engaged in the study. Depending on the nature of the translation project, review by the IRB may be indicated or required. Because nurses have a privileged relationship with patients, characterized by a high level of trust and a high degree of dependency, a conversation with the IRB is wise at the beginning of any translation project. In many cases, the translation project plan is presented to the IRB for review just like a research project. This ensures that the rights of all participants are protected; data are kept confidential; participants face no unnecessary harm or risk; procedures for recruiting subjects are appropriate; and methods and documents to be used in obtaining consent are clear, complete, and appropriate for the population of concern. Further detail is presented in Figure 9.6.

Organizational Learning

The close of any project, which comprises the fifth and final phase, involves evaluation, dissemination, and organizational learning. Healthcare, like any enterprise, depends on two primary streams of work. The first is the day-to-day operations necessary to accomplish the mission. This is the work of operations and is the focus of traditional management. The second is the work of innovation and growth. This is the work of teams and projects, the work of organizational learning. Both are critical to success. Both are the work of leaders (Shenhar & Dvir, 2007). Consequently, leadership must fully exploit all learning and development achieved in the conduct of projects it supports. At every phase of the project, leaders need to ask: What has been learned? and How can that be applied across the organization? Through engaged and inquisitive leadership, enterprises can achieve their potential as learning organizations whose practices are consistently disciplined by evidence, where the time between knowledge generation and its application is as brief as possible, and as a result business is strong.

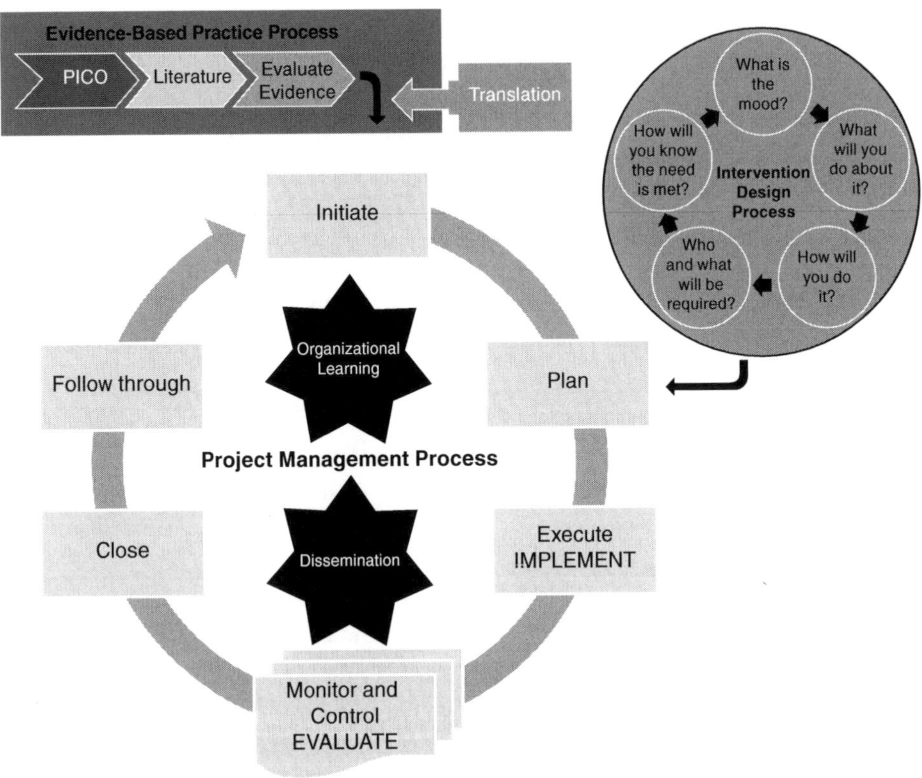

FIGURE 9.6 Organizational learning and dissemination.
PICO, problem, intervention, comparison or current practice, outcome.

A well-managed project is like a story well told. With a good book, the beginning captures the interest of the readers and makes them want to turn the page. The chapters are compelling in and of themselves, and all contribute to the final effect. In the end, the reader judges that a book was worth the time required to read it because he or she knows more, feels something new, or is motivated to change.

A good project plan is much like a good book. The proposal generates interest in the project, which converts to commitment. The plan itself guides the work. In the end, the project is favorably judged when the aims are achieved.

■ CONCLUSIONS

The work of translation is well served by thoughtful, inclusive planning that makes good use of project management tools and strategies. The process begins when clinicians identify an opportunity to improve care, performance, and outcomes. They ask the question, "What is the problem?" Stated clearly, the problem focuses the intent of the team on improvement.

Once there is agreement about the answer to the question, "What is the need?" the team can ask, "What ought to be done?" This question focuses on prosecution of the evidence and guides the team to identify the best approach to the problem.

Next, the team can ask, "How would the thing best be done?" This guides members to identify the components of a solution derived from robust research and scholarship. Next, the team can design a plan to ensure fidelity to the recommendations of strong evidence. This evidence can direct the interventions, the controls, and the monitoring of progress required to ensure safety and quality.

Then the team can ask, "Who and what will be required?" and then plan for those resources. The next question it can ask is, "How will it be determined that the need is met?" and then plan for a rigorous evaluation. The result will be that evidence is translated into practice by clinicians who are best able to judge its efficacy, monitor its outcomes, and refine practice across healthcare.

■ DISSEMINATION

Crickman, R., & Finnell, D. S. (2016). A systematic review of control measures to reduce hazardous drug exposure for health care workers. *Journal of Nursing Care Quality*, *31*(2), 183–190.

Crickman, R., & Finnell, D. S. (2017). Limiting occupational exposure to chemotherapy: Implementation of a hazardous drug control program. *Clinical Journal of Oncology*, *21*(1), 73–78.

■ REFERENCES

Benner, P. (1984). *From novice to expert: Excellence and power in clinical nursing practice*. Menlo Park, CA: Addison-Wesley.

Berwick, D. M., Nolan, T. W., & Whittington, J. (2008). The Triple Aim: Care, health, and cost. *Health Affairs*, *27*(3), 759–769.

Bradley, E. H., Webster, T. R., Baker, D., Schlesinger, M., Inouye, S. K., Barth, M. C., . . . Koran, M. J. (2004). *Translating research into practice: Speeding the adoption of innovative health care programs* (Issue Brief No. 724). New York, NY: Commonwealth Fund.

Covey, S. R. (1989). *The seven habits of highly effective people*. Salt Lake City, UT: Franklin Covey Company.

Crickman, R., & Finnell, D. S. (2015). Systematic review of control measures to reduce hazardous drug exposure for health care workers. *Journal of Nursing Care Quality*, 31(1), 9–12.

Dearholt, S. L., & Dang, D. (2012). *Johns Hopkins Nursing evidence-based practice model and guidelines* (2nd ed.). Indianapolis, IN: Sigma Theta Tau International.

Foxcroft, D. R., & Cole, N. (2003). Organizational infrastructures to promote evidence-based nursing practice. *Cochrane Database of Systematic Reviews*, *2003*(4), CD002212. doi:10.1002/14651858.CD002212

Funk, S. G., Tornquist, E. M., & Champagne, M. T. (1995). Barriers and facilitators of research utilization: An integrative review. *Nursing Clinics of North America*, *30*(3), 395–407.

Gawande, A. (2010). Health care needs a new kind of hero: Interview by Gardiner Morse. *Harvard Business Review*, *88*(4), 60–61.

Institute of Medicine. (2001). *Crossing the quality chasm: A new health system for the 21st century*. Washington, DC: National Academies Press.

Institute of Medicine. (2003). *Priority areas for national action: Transforming health care quality*. Washington, DC: National Academies Press.

Kahneman, D. (2011). *Thinking, fast and slow*. New York, NY: Penguin Books.

Mohide, E. A., & Coker, E. (2005). Toward clinical scholarship: Promoting evidence-based practice in the clinical setting. *Journal of Professional Nursing*, *21*(6), 372–379. doi:10.1016/j.profnurs.2005.10.003

Newhouse, R. P. (2007). Diffusing confusion among evidence-based practice, quality improvement and research. *Journal of Nursing Administration*, *37*(10), 432–435. doi:10.1097/01.nna.0000285156.58903.d3

Project Management Institute. (2014). *Project management body of knowledge* (5th ed.). Newtown Square, PA: ANSI Publications.

Shenhar, A. J., & Dvir, D. (2007). *Reinventing project management: The diamond approach to successful growth and innovation*. Boston, MA: Harvard Business School Press.

Titler, M. G. (2002). Use of research in practice. In G. LoBiondo-Wood & J. Haber (Eds.), *Nursing research methods: Critical appraisal and utilization* (5th ed., pp. 411–444). St. Louis, MO: Mosby.

Titler, M. G., Herr, K., Ardery, G., Brooks, J., Buckwalter, K. C., Clarke, W. R., . . . Xie, X. J. (2003). TRIP intervention saves healthcare dollars and improves quality of care. In *Translating research into practice: What's working? What's missing? What's next?* Washington, DC: Agency for Healthcare Research and Quality.

■ REFERENCES FOR THE UNFOLDING CASE

Crickman, R., & Finnell, D.S. (2016). Systematic review of control measures to reduce hazardous drug exposure for healthcare workers. *Journal of Nursing Care Quality, 31*, 183–190.

Gambrell, J., & Moore, S. (2006). Assessing workplace compliance with handling of antineoplastic agents. *Clinical Journal of Oncology Nursing, 10*, 473–477.

Geer, L. A., Curbow, B. A., Anna, D. H., Lees, P. S., & Buckley, T. J. (2006). Development of a questionnaire to assess worker knowledge, attitudes and perceptions underlying dermal exposure. *Scandinavian Journal of Work, Environment and Health, 32*, 209–218.

Martin, S., & Larson, E. (2003). Chemotherapy-handling practices of outpatient and office-based oncology nurses. *Oncology Nursing Forum, 30*, 575–581.

McDiarmid, M. A., Oliver, M. S., Roth, T. S., Rogers, B., & Escalante, C. (2010). Chromosome 5 and 7 abnormalities in oncology personnel handling anticancer drugs. *Journal of Occupational and Environmental Medicine, 52*, 1028–1034.

Polovich, M., & Clark, P. C. (2012). Factors influencing oncology nurses' use of hazardous drug safe-handling precautions [Online exclusive]. *Oncology Nursing Forum, 39*, E299–E309. doi:10.1188/12.ONF.E299-E309

CHAPTER TEN

Ethical Responsibilities of Translation of Evidence and Evaluation of Outcomes

Mary F. Terhaar

Make a habit of two things: to help; or at least to do no harm.
—Hippocrates

Nursing is Ranked as the Most Trusted Among all Professions for a 17th year in a Row with fully 84% of Americans rating their trust in the honesty and ethics of nurses as high (Brenan, 2018). Such public trust is hard earned. Protecting it is the ongoing responsibility of every nurse, every clinician, researcher, academic, and leader alike. DNPs, such as researchers, have a special responsibility to protect this trust by ensuring the conduct of their scholarly projects and all translation work conducted after graduation follows ethical guidelines established to protect human subjects.

All health professionals seek to follow three core ethical principles outlined in the Belmont Report (U.S. Department of Health and Human Services [HHS], 1974; The National Commission for the Protection of Human Subjects of Biomedical and Behavioral Research, 1979). We seek to practice beneficence (accomplish good for individuals in our care), to practice nonmaleficence (do no harm), and to protect and promote justice (demonstrate respect for the rights of all individuals, and protect the less advantaged and vulnerable from abuse or exclusion from benefits of discovery that are due to all). These core ethical principles guide all health professionals in the conduct of research and are equally relevant to the work of translation.

Expectations for researchers in general and nurse researchers in particular are clearly described and governed by international law, U.S. regulations and professional standards. Because DNPs work to improve quality, value, and outcomes of care, their efforts are no different in this respect. The purpose of this chapter is to offer an overview of the regulations and standards that provide guidance and structure to research, translation, quality improvement, program evaluation, and other practice-based scholarship.

Upon completion of this chapter, the reader will have an understanding of:

1. The distinctions between research and translation, and the relevance of ethical standards
2. The professional standards that guide nurses engaged in translation
3. The international and U.S. regulations relevant to the work of translation
4. The history that creates demand for protection of those who participate in research and some translation activities
5. Protection of human subjects in the work of translation
6. The best practices for working with the institutional review board (IRB), which is charged with responsibility to protect human subjects, investigators, institutions, and society

■ DISTINCTIONS BETWEEN RESEARCH AND TRANSLATION

Research is defined as "a systematic investigation, including research development, testing, and evaluation, designed to develop or contribute to generalizable knowledge" (Protection of Human Subjects, 2018). *Translation*, on the other hand, does not have one precise definition. It has been described as proceeding through four phases across which the details of an intervention achieve its fullest potential, and the controls on its application are relaxed (Westfall, Mold, & Fagnan, 2007). The author proposes defining *translation* as *a range of activities that migrate research findings from the point of discovery (the lab) to the point of consistent and effective application in the provision of patient care (point of care) with precision, caution, confidence, safety, and efficacy.*

Clear distinctions can be drawn between research and translation (National Commission on the Protection of Human Subjects, 1979; Szanton, Taylor & Terhaar, 2013). Understanding this distinction is important for planning the work itself and for interacting effectively with the IRB, its staff, and its membership. The distinction between research and translation can be understood in relation to several important points. These include the intent of the work, the potential for risk to participants, the promise of benefits to those same participants, and expectations that findings will be published or disseminated. These points of contrast are described here and summarized in Table 10.1.

Intent

Research is intended, designed, and conducted to answer previously unanswered questions in order to produce new, reliable, and generalizable knowledge. The goal of research is to advance science and benefit society as a whole. Benefit to individual participants is neither the primary nor proximate goal.

TABLE 10.1 Distinctions Between Research and Translation

	Research	Translation
Intent	Generate new knowledge	Apply strong evidence to improve outcomes
Risk	Risk may be present	Little risk because solutions come from science
Benefit	Participants may or may not be expected to benefit	Participants are expected to benefit
Generalizability	Produce generalizable findings	Evaluate impact of science on target population
Dissemination	Primary goal	Secondary gain
	Expectation	Not routinely expected

Translation is intended, designed, and conducted in order to directly benefit the participants. In this context, generalizable findings would be secondary gains of the work. Benefit to individual participants is the primary and immediate goal.

Risk

Research creates new knowledge and, because it exists at the boundaries of what is known, it may have associated risks. It is the responsibility of every researcher to minimize risk. Still, it may be impossible to do so. It may even be impossible to precisely forecast and disclose the nature of the risk inherent in an investigation. As a result of this uncertainty, society has implemented regulations, procedures, and structures to ensure that participants are properly informed of any potential risk associated with their participation in an investigation. Individuals who participate in research have the right to be made aware of any risks and to consent or decline to participate. This is a central tenet of ethical conduct and the basis for the practice of seeking informed consent.

Translation seeks to apply only strong evidence to the care of individuals and populations and as a result can be expected to introduce only low to minimal risk. Clinicians engaged in translation have a responsibility to test the efficacy and impact of solutions using rigorous evaluation methods. In cases in which translation is expected to carry some risk, nurses and teams engaged in the work share a responsibility to contravene and mitigate risk as well as a responsibility to disclose that risk and honor each individual patient's rights to consent or decline to participate.

Benefit

Another key difference between research and translation relates to the benefits individuals can expect as a result of participation in the investigation. Human subjects who participate in research have no assurance that they themselves will benefit as a result of participation. Researchers have a responsibility to disclose this and ensure that participants understand the situation accurately.

Conversely, translation activities seek to apply solutions based on strong evidence in order to solve problems and improve outcomes. Activities are conducted for the explicit purpose of achieving positive outcomes for participants in a specific setting. These activities are commonly classified as quality initiatives and informed consent may or may not be required based on the decision of the IRB.

As healthcare disciplines move science from the bench to the bedside, the intent becomes increasingly focused on the individual. Risks are reduced and benefits become more predictable and reliable. In the end, the goal is to ensure that science consistently and effectively informs practice and improves outcomes.

Generalizability

Research is conducted to yield "generalizable" results. The researcher seeks solutions that can be applied beyond the particular, well-controlled setting and population where the study was conducted. In order to yield generalizable findings, the researcher must control extraneous variables that increase confidence in the findings. They must achieve a sample size that allows statistical power and supports generalizability of the findings (Protection of Human Subjects, 2017).

Translation differs with respect to generalizability. Activities are conducted with the explicit purpose of improving outcomes for the participants, for members of a specific population, in a specific the setting. The intervention being evaluated is commonly classified as quality improvement, translation, or program evaluation.

Dissemination

The results of research are routinely disseminated consistent with the intent to discover and add to the body of knowledge. For the researcher, publication is expected. Conversely, the intent of translation is to improve outcomes for a particular population in a particular setting. As a result, findings may or may not be disseminated outside the setting where the work is conducted. Publication of translation may result, but that is less common than is the case with research.

■ PROFESSIONAL STANDARDS THAT GUIDE RESEARCH AND TRANSLATION

Nurses engaged in research and translation are guided by a code of ethics and a social contract. Both the code of ethics and social contract between society and members of the nursing profession mandate that nurses' efforts, regardless of role, setting, or academic preparation, all seek to advance the health, well-being, safety, wholeness, integrity, values, and agency of individuals in our care and that we demonstrate respect for the dignity, worth, and rights of every person. The complete American Nurses Association (ANA) *Code of Ethics* is available through ANA's Nursing World website (https://www.nursingworld.org/practice-policy/nursing-excellence/ethics).

GUIDANCE AND REGULATIONS

Because there have been numerous instances throughout history when researchers have failed to protect the rights of human subjects in the conduct of investigations and because there have been activities that were conducted in the name of research that failed to meet basic scientific and ethical standards, numerous position papers and white papers are available to provide guidance to investigators and protect participants from harm. These include the Belmont Report, the Common Rule, and several additional landmark documents that are described in the text that follows. below.

The Belmont Report

The National Commission for the Protection of Human Subjects of Biomedical and Behavioral Research released the Belmont Report in 1977. This report provides guidance to researchers by outlining three essential ethical principles that should undergird all research: respect for persons, beneficence, and justice.

Respect for persons derives from our social contract as professionals. Nurses engaged in both research and translation are bound to respect the autonomy and self-determination of all participants, especially those with diminished capacity who are in need of protection. Demonstrating respect for persons demands that participants in research be volunteers, be informed fully and clearly about the study, and what might be expected as a result of participation.

Beneficence is the professional expectation that nurses act to benefit others, that nurses will "do good." It obliges researchers to accomplish maximum benefit and minimum harm and relies on their experience, scholarship, best judgement, care, and expertise to do so.

Justice demands a fair distribution of benefits and burdens in society. Justice is a direct correlate to respect in that it requires no population be disadvantaged, unfairly burdened, or removed from the benefits of research.

Each of the principles outlined in the Belmont Report applies to translation equally well as it applies to research and needs to inform every step of the process of translation. Respect for persons requires that individuals have the right to consent or to decline to consent to participate in research. Under conditions deemed appropriate by the IRB, individuals who participate in translation may be required to give informed consent for participation.

The Common Rule

Code of Federal Regulations, Title 45, part 46 (45 CFR 46; Protection of Human Subjects), often referred to as the *Common Rule*, stipulates requirements and procedures for organizations that address assurances, IRB operations, informed consent, and proper ethical conduct of research. It describes protections for vulnerable populations, including pregnant women, fetuses, and neonates (subpart B); prisoners (subpart C); and children (subpart D). Vulnerable populations include individuals who may lack capacity to understand information necessary to make informed decisions, may lack agency to advocate for themselves, or may be vulnerable to coercion or influence. As a result, society bears the responsibility to protect their best interests: Researchers and clinicians do as well.

The Common Rule was initially promulgated in 1991, and amended in 2005. We refer to this version of the Common Rule as the *pre-2018 Requirements*. The Common Rule was substantially revised in 2017 and has been amended twice to delay the date that regulated entities must comply with the revised version of the rule. We refer to this version as the *revised Common Rule*, the *2018 Requirements*, or the *2018 Rule*.

The 2018 Rule provides direction to investigators regarding informed consent documents and processes, review of lower risk investigations, and other IRB administrative responsibilities. Specifically, 49 CFR 11 provides important new definitions for human subjects, research, and public health surveillance.

Human subject includes any living individual about whom an investigator (whether professional or student) is conducting research and includes any activities that involve:

- Obtaining information or biospecimens through intervention or interaction with the individual, and using, studying, or analyzing information or biospecimens
- Obtaining, using, studying, analyzing, or generating identifiable private information or identifiable biospecimens

The 2018 Rule further provides direction to investigators regarding which activities are considered to be *research* and which are not. To be specific, the revised rule excludes the following activities from the category of research:

1. Certain scholarly and journalistic activities
2. Certain public health surveillance activities
3. Collection and analysis of information, specimens, or records, by or for a criminal justice agency for certain criminal justice or investigative purposes
4. Certain authorized operational activities for national security purposes

The 2018 Rule defines *public health surveillance* as "the collection and testing of information or biospecimens, conducted, supported, requested, ordered, required, or authorized by a public health authority." Such activities are to be conducted for the purpose of informing public policy and/or preparing effective responses to threats to the public health. The 2018 Rule further stipulates that the IRB must review and approve all public health surveillance activities. In addition, the 2018 Rule supports immediate implementation of *three burden-reducing provisions* during the interim before compliance of the revised version is required.

■ HISTORY THAT CREATES DEMAND FOR PROTECTIONS

Throughout history, scientists have accomplished great gains in knowledge. Unfortunately, at times these discoveries have come at great expense for individuals in society, especially the vulnerable and disenfranchised, and have resulted in great suffering (Ferrari, 2014). Professionals need to recall these instances and understand the lessons they teach in order to prevent further harm. A few examples of misguided efforts and failed professional ethics are provided here.

Nuremberg War Crimes

Many investigations were conducted in the internment camps of the Third Reich by individuals who called their work *science* (U.S. Government Printing Office, 1949a, 1949b). At the hands of these German scientists millions of unwilling participants were exposed to great hardships and suffering for the purpose of generating new knowledge. Prisoners were exposed to conditions of extreme hypothermia, pathogens were introduced, and drug trials were conducted (Roelcke, 2014). Unknown active agents were injected beyond the fourth month of pregnancy as abortives and sterilization procedures were performed (Czarnowski, 2014). Subjects were first exposed to typhus and malaria and then to experimental treatments and management (Czarnowski, 2014). Because researchers demonstrated abject disregard for the value of human life, great conflict about the validity of the work and the utility of the findings persists today (Caplan, 2014).

These prisoners-turned-subjects for malicious research during the Holocaust were treated as though they had no rights. They were provided no information about what was happening to them, had no opportunity to consent or decline to consent, and in fact had their rights stripped from them by more powerful individuals. They routinely faced coercion and punishment, and none could hope for benefit from the experiments conducted on them. The research methods used were weak and flawed. The findings lack value or impact. No community engaged in constructive oversight and no one intervened on behalf of the participants to relieve suffering (Rubenfeld, 2014).

> You, the scientists of the world, must remember that the research is done for the sake of mankind and not for the sake of science; you must never detach yourselves from the subjects you serve.
>
> I hope with all my heart that our sad stories will in some way impel the international community to devise laws and rules to govern human experimentation. The dignity of all human beings must be respected, preserved, and protected at all costs. Life without it is a mere existence.
>
> I experienced such loss of dignity every day as a guinea pig in Dr. Mengele's laboratory. These same doctors had taken an oath to help and to save human life.
>
> **E. M. Kor**

Some believe the grave and expansive violations of human rights that occurred during the Holocaust had their roots in benevolence gone wrong. Misguided beliefs about achieving good ends for society by conducting research on its imperfect members led to a catalog of violations, a miasma of suffering, and a broad range of experiments without value or application that have been vilified by peer review. The greatest enduring contribution of these atrocities is an international system of rules and expectations for accountability that sanction scientists and clinicians who would repeat any aspect of that misadventure (Ferrari, 2014).

Tuskegee Syphilis Study

In the more recent past, between 1932 and 1972, researchers made observations and gathered data from 625 research subjects, 425 of whom were syphilitic. All subjects were impoverished, Black men from Tuskegee, Alabama. All received heavy metals as treatment for the disease and not penicillin, which was available and documented as effective treatment for the disease in the early 1940s. Participants were treated as controls, were never informed that they suffered from the illness, and were never offered standard treatment. Investigators in this study observed the participants and described the long-term presentation and outcomes of untreated disease in the name of science.

By the study was shut down, 276 participants had died. Autopsies conducted on 160 bodies of participants revealed syphilis as the primary cause of death (Centers for Disease Control and Prevention [CDC], 2013). Participants had not been properly informed about the risks inherent in the study, did not give proper consent, were denied benefit of effective treatment and known science, and suffered for the discovery of new knowledge that would benefit others in society but not themselves.

Willowbrook School

In the early 1950s, researchers exposed children with intellectual disabilities who received care in a residential facility (institution) to hepatitis A with the intent to study its progression and management. Children did not give their permission (assent) and neither were they deemed to have the capacity to do so. As a result of this exposure, participants contracted the chronic illness, were not afforded standard treatment, and suffered at the hands of researchers to create new knowledge and science from which they themselves could not reasonably be expected to benefit (Goldby, Krugman, Pappworth, & Edsall, 1971). The issues of injustice raised by the community led to reforms in the care of institutionalized children and to guidelines regarding the rights of children to protection as a vulnerable population (Fansiwala, 2016).

Jewish Chronic Disease Hospital Study

Abuse of human subjects and failure to advocate for populations is not a problem of the past. It is a problem that presented in the New York Jewish Chronic Disease Hospital in the late 1950s where 22 senior citizens being treated for malignancies were, without their consent, injected with cancer cells to test their ability to fight the disease. Having previously been refused permission to conduct this research at another reputable institution, the investigator moved to a new site that abdicated responsibility to protect a cohort of elders. This vulnerable elder population was already ill, was not informed of the experimental injections they were given, did not have the opportunity to become informed, was unable to decline participation, and had no reasonable expectation of benefit from participation. On many levels, the investigation violated the principles of justice, beneficence, and nonmaleficence (Ratzan, 1981).

Publications in Reputable Professional Journals

Beecher (1966) described a set of investigations published in reputable, peer-reviewed journals in which research presented real and significant risk of harm to subjects without their having been informed or having consented to that risk. This finding raised discomfort and concern in the scientific community. Perhaps distracted by aspirations to eliminate disease and suffering on a grand scale, some researchers have caused or at least tolerated infliction of great harm on individual subjects with their work. Having done so is an unacceptable violation of basic human rights. The lessons taught by these cases set clear expectations for all who would engage in activities that involve human subjects.

Henrietta Lacks

Henrietta Lacks had an aggressive cancer in the early 1950s. During a treatment procedure, cells were obtained from her and subsequently used for diagnostics and experimentation. Hers is the first cell line propagated in the lab: HeLa cells. These HeLa cells have enabled remarkable discoveries and advancement in the treatment of cancer. Still, Ms. Lacks did not give her consent for their use and neither she nor her family benefit-ed from the cell line or the discoveries they made possible. So HeLa cells raise concerns about informed consent and justice in healthcare and research (Beskow, 2016).

This case has great relevance for research. It clarified expectations for handling of samples and use of cells beyond the initial investigation. With respect to translation, the case of Ms. Lacks and her family emphasizes the vital importance of using clear and simple language during the process of consent to ensure participants understand their rights and are in no way coerced into participation.

■ WORKING WITH THE IRB

IRBs have been charged with the responsibility of protecting the rights and safety of individuals who might choose to participate in research. Independent review of proposals is required for all studies seeking funding from the National Institutes of Health (NIH). Such a review is also a common practice in hospitals and healthcare entities across the United States as a means to prevent conflict of interest, injustice, exploitation, violation of basic human rights, and conduct of research lacking scientific or social merit (Grady, 2015).

Composition of the IRB

According to the Common Rule, IRBs have at least five members, including at a minimum one health professional, one member representing the sciences, one member from outside the sciences, and one member from the community who is not associated with the enterprise (45 CFR 46.107; 21 CFR 56.107). The board must have representation from both sexes and also from different races or ethnic groups in the community. This diversity in composition is essential to ensure diversity of thought as well as thorough and careful attention to the full impact of a proposal. Members are expected to recuse themselves if they identify any conflict of interest or commitment. Inclusion of ad hoc content experts can help one to ensure that the group is sufficiently informed to determine whether a study satisfies the full requirements of the board and can be approved (45 CFR 46.108; 21 CFR 56.107).

The Role of the IRB

Each IRB establishes its own procedures and operations in agreement with the common rule. These procedures provide for initial review, continuing review, auditing and reporting processes, conditions for a quorum, and noncompliance (45C FR 46.108; 21 CFR 56.108). A majority vote is required for decisions, including approval, modification, and disapproval, as well as changes or amendments to the study plan or team (45 CFR 46.109; 21 CFR 56.109). The IRB also has authority to approve, require modifications, disapprove research, require informed consent and documentation, approve a waiver, and investigators are to receive such notification in writing (45 CFR 46.108; 21 CFR 56.108). Continuing review follows the criteria for the Common Rule (45 CFR 46.111; 21 CFR 56.111).

Each IRB is responsible to ensure that risks have been minimized and are reasonable with respect to both potential benefits and the knowledge to be generated. IRBs are responsible to ensure that subject selection is equitable and fair for the vulnerable population. They ensure that participants will have the opportunity for informed consent and that their decisions will be documented. The IRB is also responsible to ensure adequate monitoring, protection of confidentiality, and safeguards for potentially vulnerable populations from coercion or undue influence (45 CFR 46.113; 21 CFR 56.113). Institutional officials cannot override IRB decisions (45 CFR 46), and the IRB has authority to suspend or terminate any research to prevent serious harm or noncompliance.

Requirements for IRB Review

The IRB will require the full research plan for review. The plan needs to explain the purpose and background of the work; describe any potential risks or benefits; explain the process used to obtain informed consent and include the documents to be used; explain the process for assent if indicated; describe the population to be recruited and the procedures to be followed; explain how confidentiality and anonymity will be safeguarded; describe the plan for data management, handling, and protection; explain the research design and methods; and address any additional concerns for the IRB or study participants. Details as described in the Collaborative Institutional Training Initiative (CITI) are outlined in Table 10.2.

The proposal may be submitted using a standard form or an online program. The written proposal should be complete, scholarly, detailed, logical, and clear. Cite important sources. Check for errors and correct them. Provide all tools and instruments to be used for recruitment, data collection, and patient education.

Students should coordinate all document preparation with faculty advisors and on-site collaborators. Communication with IRB staff should be coordinated, organized, and demonstrate respect for the time and resources of the IRB.

Levels of IRB Review

The IRB has three different levels of review: full review, expedited review, and exempt. These are explained here and summarized in Table 10.3.

Full review is required when study participants can be expected to face greater than minimal risk. Many IRBs require full review when the intent is to create generalizable findings with the intent to publish and add to the body of science.

Expedited review is appropriate when minimal risk is involved as is the case with secondary analysis of data. This level of review is appropriate when identification of the subjects and/or their responses would not reasonably be expected to place participants at risk of criminal, civil, financial, reputational harm or stigma; or when research does not involve human subjects. IRB criteria are used to identify appropriateness for expedited review

Exemption is appropriate when no more than minimal risk and/or when secondary data analysis is involved, as in educational or survey research. IRB criteria are used to identify appropriateness for exemption.

It is within the purview of the IRB to develop tools and processes that facilitate their work and guide researchers seeking review. Decision-support tools may be available from the IRB or the academic institution. An example of such a tool is presented in Figure 10.1.

Recent revised federal regulations distinguish between research and quality-improvement activities, and other scholarly activities, including oral histories, public health surveillance, criminal investigations activities, and other activities related to intelligence, homeland security, and national defense (Protection of Human Subjects, 2017). Still, it is essential that researchers and those engaged in translation do not themselves make the determination that their work be considered expedited or exempt. This decision is best made by the IRB chair or staff in collaboration with the investigator. Documentation of the decision becomes an important requirement for future scholarship, publication, and other collaborations (HHS, Office for Human Research Protections [OHRP], 1998).

TABLE 10.2 Minimum Information on an IRB Application for IRB Assessment

Topic	Details
Risk/anticipated benefit analysis	Identification and assessment of risks and anticipated benefits
	Determination that risks are minimized
	Determination that risks are reasonable in relation to potential benefits
Informed consent	Informed consent process and procedures
	Documentation of informed consent (form)
Assent	The affirmative agreement of a minor or decisionally impaired individual to participate in research
	Assent process
	Documentation of assent
Selection of subjects	Equitable selection in terms of gender, race, and ethnicity
	Benefits are distributed fairly among the community's populations
	Additional safeguards are provided for vulnerable populations susceptible to pressure to participate (for example, prisoners, individuals with impaired decision-making capacity, or economically or educationally disadvantaged persons).
Privacy and confidentiality	Ensure that subject recruitment does not invade individual privacy and that procedures are in place to ensure that the confidentiality of the information collected during the research is maintained
Research plan for collection, storage, and analysis of data	Clinical research studies often include data safety-monitoring plans and/or data safety-monitoring boards/committees (DSMBs/DSMCs); IRBs will review the plans to ensure they are adequate to ensure the safety of subjects
	Researchers are qualified to collect, handle, and analyze the data responsibly and have a plan for analyzing the data in a meaningful fashion
Research design/ methods	Are appropriate and scientifically valid, and therefore do not unnecessarily expose subjects to risk
Additional Information	About identification, recruitment, and safeguards if the research involves special populations
Additional Items IRBs Must Review	Qualifications of the principal investigator and scientific collaborators
	Complete description of the proposed research
	Provisions for the adequate protection of rights and welfare of subjects
	Compliance with pertinent federal and state laws/regulations, and organizational policies
	Investigator's brochure/investigator protocols (for U.S. Food and Drug Administration-regulated research)

IRB, institutional review board.

Source: Data from Collaborative Institutional Training Initiative. (2019). CITI Program. Retrieved from https://about.citiprogram.org/en/homepage

TABLE 10.3 Levels of IRB Review

Level of Review	Details
Convened	Greater than minimal risk to participants
	Vulnerable populations involved
Expedited	Judged by IRB to introduce minimal risk (as published in federal regulations)
Exempt	Some research conducted in established educational settings
(DHHS criteria)	Research involving educational tests and surveys
	Research involving benign behavioral interventions (brief, painless, harmless, non-invasive, not likely to have lasting negative impact) is not offensive, not embarrassing
	Secondary use of data for which regulatory criteria are satisfied
	Federally supported demonstration projects for the public benefit that involve study and/or evaluation
	Taste and food-quality studies
	Storage and maintenance of data for secondary analysis
	Secondary analysis of data for which broad consent is required
Quality improvement	Focus on knowledge implementation
	Emphasis on process or program improvement
	Intent to deliver quality care and adopt accepted standards

DHHS, U.S. Department of Health and Human Services; IRB, institutional review board.

Source: U. S. Department of Health and Human Services. (2019). *Common Rule 2019: Federal policy for the protection of human subjects*. Rockville, MD: Office of Human Research Protections.

■ CONCLUSIONS

All nurses are ethically obliged to prevent harm, promote human dignity, support the right to self-determination, and protect privacy and confidentiality (ANA, 2015). These obligations are as binding for the new nurse as they are for the experienced nurse. They are binding for the nurse engaged in translation just as they are for the nurse conducting research.

Because the work of translation is relatively young in contrast to the work of research, there is relatively more variability and less experience with its practice. As a result, it is essential that individuals and teams engaged in translation follow the established practices designed to protect patients from harm and institutions from risk. Ongoing communication with the IRB and careful adherence to its procedures and policies are critical to fulfilling our obligations to protect individuals in our care, communities, and our profession throughout the work of translation.

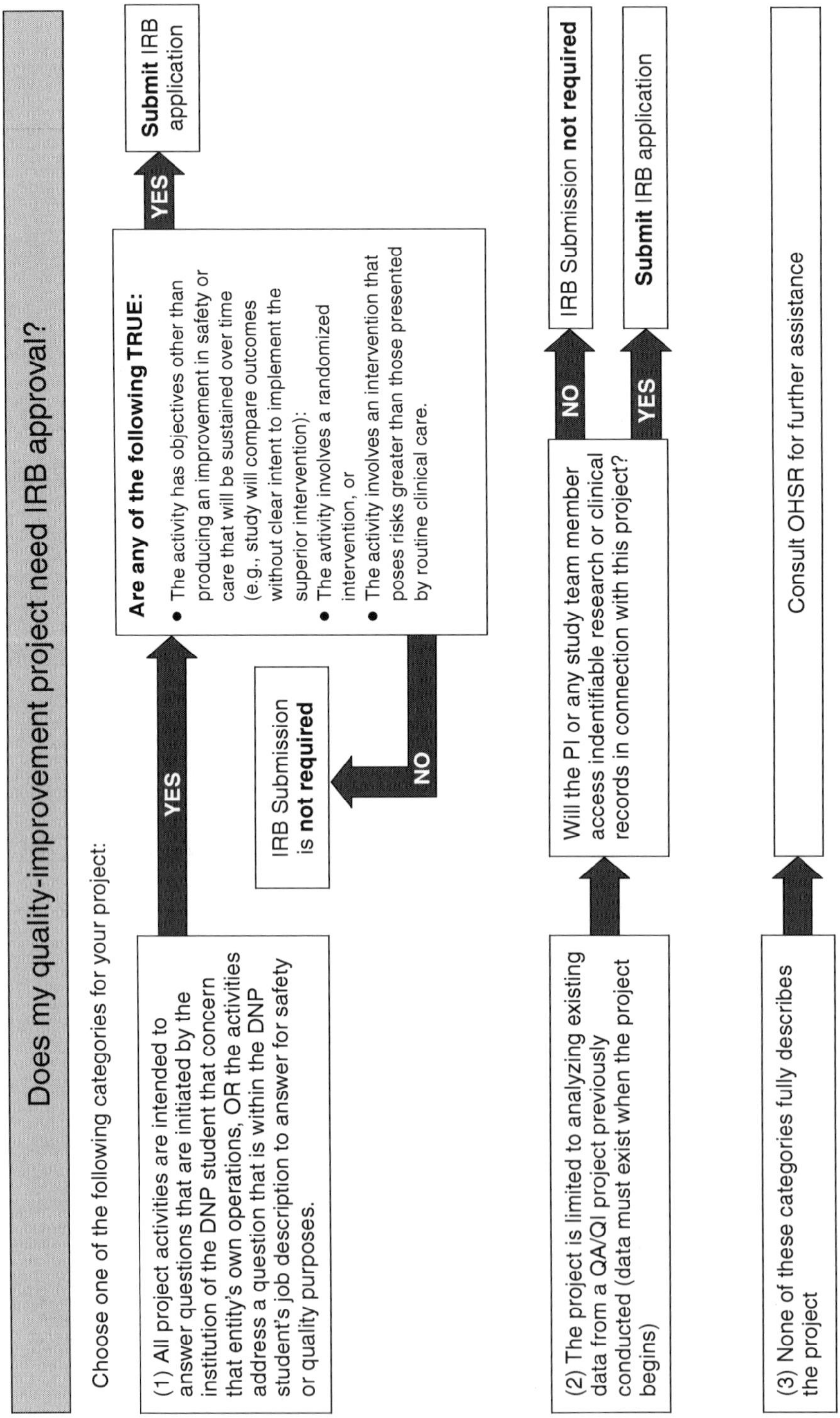

FIGURE 10.1 Decision-support tool for seeking IRB review.

IRB, institutional review board; OHSR, Office of Human Subjects Research; PI, principal investigator; QA/QI, quality assurance/quality improvement.

Source: From Szanton, S. L., Taylor, H. A., & Terhaar, M. (2013). Development of an institutional review board preapproval process for doctor of nursing practice students: process and outcome. *Journal of Nursing Education, 52*(1), 51–55. doi:10.3928/01484834-20121212-01

REFERENCES

American Nurses Association. (2015). *Code of ethics with interpretative statements.* Silver Spring, MD: Author. Retrieved from https://www.nursingworld.org/practice-policy/nursing-excellence/ethics/code-of-ethics-for-nurses/coe-view-only

Beecher, H. K. (1966). Ethics and clinical research. *New England Journal of Medicine, 274*(24),1354–1360. doi:10.1056/nejm196606162742405

Beskow, L. M. (2016). Lessons from HeLa cells: The ethics and policy of bio-specimens. *Annual Review of Genomics Human Genetics, 17*(1), 395–417. doi:10.1146/annurev-genom-083115-022536

Brenan, M. (2018, Dec. 20). Nurses again outpace other professions for honesty and ethics. Gallup. Politics. Retrieved from https://news.gallup.com/poll/245597/nurses-again-outpace-professions-honesty-ethics.aspx

Caplan, A. L. (2014). Foreword. In S. Rubenfeld & S. Benedict (Eds.), *Human subjects research after the Holocaust.* Basel, Switzerland: Springer International Publishing.

Centers for Disease Control and Prevention. (2013). *U.S. Public Health Service Syphilis Study at Tuskegee.* Atlanta, GA: Author. Last modified December 11.

Collaborative Institutional Training Initiative. (2019). CITI Program. https://about.citiprogram.org/en/homepage

Czarnowski, G. (2014). Involuntary abortion and coercive research on pregnant forced laborers in national socialism. In S. Rubenfeld & S. Benedict (Eds.), *Human subjects research ater the Holocaust.* Basel, Switzerland: Springer International Publishing.

Fansiwala, K. (2016). The duality of medicine: The Willowbrook state school experiments. Retrieved from http://www.thereviewatnyu.com/all/2016/2/20/the-duality-of-medicine-the-willowbrook-state-school-experiments

Federal Policy for the Protection of Human Subjects: Six Month Delay of the General Compliance Date of Revisions While Allowing the Use of Three Burden-Reducing Provisions During the Delay Period, 83 Fed. Reg. 118 (June 19, 2018) Rules and Regulations 28497–28520.

Ferrari, M. (2014). No exceptions, no excuses: A testimonial. In S. Rubenfeld & S. Benedict (Eds.), *Human subjects research after the Holocaust.* Basel, Switzerland: Springer International Publishing.

Goldby, S., Krugman, S., Pappworth, M. H., & Edsall, G. (1971). The Willowbrook letters: Crticism and defense. *Lancet.* Retrieved from http://science.jburroughs.org/mbahe/BioEthics/Articles/WillowbookLetters.pdf

Grady, C. (2015). Institutional review boards: Purpose and challenges. *Chest,* 148 (5), 1148–1155. doi:10.1378/chest.15-0706

Kor, E. M. (2014). Twin experiments at Auschwitz: A first-person account. In S. Rubenfeld & S. Benedict (Eds.), *Human subjects research after the Holocaust.* Basel, Switzerland: Springer International Publishing.

The National Commission for the Protection of Human Subjects of Biomedical and Behavioral Research. (1979). *The Belmont report: Ethical principles and guidelines for the protection of human subjects of research.* Rockville, MD: Office of Human Research Protections.

Protection of Human Subjects, 45 C.F.R. part 46 (2009).

Ratzan, R.M. (1981). The experiment that wasn't: A case report in clinical geriatric research. *The Gerontologist, 21*(3), 297–302. doi:10.1093/geront/21.3.297

Roelcke, V. (2014). Sulfonamide experiments on prisoners in Nazi concentration camps: Coherent scientific rationality combined with complete disregard of humanity. In S. Rubenfeld & S. Benedict (Eds.), *Human subjects research after the holocaust.* Basel, Switzerland: Springer International Publishing.

Rubenfeld, S. (2014). Introduction: How did it go so wrong? In S. Rubenfeld & S. Benedict (Eds.), *After the holocaust.* Basel, Switzerland: Springer International Publishing.

Szanton, S. L., Taylor, H. A., & Terhaar, M. (2013). Development of an institutional review board preapproval process for doctor of nursing practice students: process and outcome. *Journal of Nursing Education, 52*(1), 51–55. doi:10.3928/01484834-20121212-01

U. S. Department of Health and Human Services. (2017). *Final rule enhances protections for research participants, modernizes oversight system.* Rockville, MD: Office of Human Protections.

U. S. Department of Health and Human Services. (2019). *Common Rule 2019: Federal policy for the protection of human subjects.* Office of Human Research Protections. Rockville, MD.

U. S. Department of Health and Human Services, Office for Human Research Protections. (1998). *OHRP expedited review categories.* Retrieved from https://www.hhs.gov/ohrp/regulations-and-policy/guidance/categories-of-research-expedited-review-procedure-1998/index.html

U. S. Government Printing Office. (1949a). *Trials of war criminals before the Nuremberg military tribunals under control council law No. 10 ("Green Series")* (Vol. 1). Washington, DC: Author.

U. S. Government Printing Office. (1949b). *Trials of war criminals before the Nuremberg military tribunals under control council law No. 10 ("Green Series")* (Vol. 2). Washington, DC: Author.

Westfall, J. M., Mold, J., & Fagnan, L. (2007). Practice based research-"Blue Highways" on NIH roadmap. *Journal of the American Medical Association*. 297(4), 403–406.

CHAPTER ELEVEN

Data Management and Evaluation of Translation

Martha Sylvia

What gets measured gets improved.
—Peter Drucker

A DNP Translates evidence into practice on a systems, large-scale level, with the result being an improvement in quality of health-related outcomes (American Association of Colleges of Nursing, 2015; Mundinger, Starck, Hathaway, Shaver, & Woods, 2009). *Improvement* implies *defining, measuring, analyzing,* and *demonstrating* a positive change in outcomes that is carried out through monitoring and evaluating the translation project.

■ EVALUATION APPROACH

Understanding the impact of translation requires a flexible, grounded, iterative, contextualized, and participatory approach and can be referred to as *learning evaluation* (Balasubramanian et al., 2015). Although the project is in the implementation phase, *monitoring* of program outcomes is taking place. During the monitoring phase, data are gathered, analyzed, and interpreted to inform project implementation and to improve processes. *Evaluation* of the project takes place when data collection and project implementation are completed and these adhere to a protocol established during the project-planning phase. Use of a rigorous monitoring protocol leads to an evaluation that is streamlined and efficiently executed with preconceived expectations of results. Predetermined outcome measures are used for both the monitoring and evaluation phases.

Principles of a learning evaluation include:

- Gathering data to describe the changes made and how the changes are implemented
- Collecting relevant process and outcome data

- Assessing multilevel factors affecting implementation, process, outcome, and transportability
- Assisting organizations in using data for continuous quality improvement
- Operationalizing common measurement strategies to generate transportable results (Balasubramanian et al., 2015)

■ EVALUATION RIGOR

Evaluation of translation projects must be rigorous, scholarly, and, most important, provide convincing evidence that changes in outcomes are a result of the intervention project, which translates evidence into practice (Terhaar, Taylor, & Sylvia, 2016). Flexible, scientifically rigorous study designs are necessary to evaluate translation projects (Balasubramanian et al., 2015). Although it is often not feasible for quality- improvement/translation projects to use randomized control trials mainly due to time, financial, and equitability constraints, evaluation of translation can use the tools of research to attain a high level of rigor (Terhaar, 2018).

Internal Validity and Generalizability

In research, *internal validity* refers to the extent to which a study avoids confounding, or the possibility that a factor other than the intervention itself contributed to a change in outcomes. Strong internal validity allows a higher level of confidence that a desired change in outcomes is due to the intervention. Generalizability, or *external validity*, is the degree to which the results of a study can be generalized to similar settings and circumstances (Polit & Beck, 2018). In applying the same concepts to translation projects, internal validity is of utmost importance. Generalizability is not expected; however, *transportability*, the ability to implement the translation intervention in a different setting, is important. Evaluation of translation projects includes an assessment of internal validity and transportability (Balasubramanian et al., 2015).

■ PREPARING FOR EVALUATION

Evaluation Plan

Planning for evaluation takes place during the project planning phase. The original problem statement informs project aims and subsequent objectives and measures. For instance, if the original problem statement purported a high readmission rate for a population of patients with congestive heart failure, then the aims, objectives, and measures would focus on reducing readmission rates as a result of the translation project.

There may be nuances in the definitions of aims and objectives for a translation project. For instance, in some cases aims may be written in broader terms that describe aspirations for the translation project overall, such as "improving the health of patients with congestive heart failure (CHF)." Aims may also be written more specifically using the SMART framework: Are they specific, measurable, achievable, realistic, and time-phased (Centers for Disease Control and Prevention, 2017)? If the aims are in more general, overarching terms, it is usually the objectives that follow each aim that describe the specifics about translation achievements. Regardless of terminology, either the aims or the objectives should describe measurable results. For example, "within 3 months of implementation, patients with CHF who received the intervention will have a 10% lower readmission rate than patients with CHF who did not receive the intervention."

Evaluation takes place in seven phases: (a) planning; (b) data collection; (c) data cleansing; (d) data manipulation; (e) exploratory analysis; (f) outcomes analysis; and (g) dissemination, reporting, and presentation (Sylvia & Terhaar, 2014).

■ OUTCOMES

Measuring Successful Implementation

Multilevel factors affect successful implementation of evidence-based health innovations and can be measured in constructs that are important for evaluation, derived from the field of dissemination and implementation science (Chaudoir, Dugan, & Barr, 2013). These factors, their description, and measurement examples are described in Table 11.1. Multiple instruments exist for specific measures in each of the factors (Chaudoir et al., 2013; Lewis et al., 2015).

TABLE 11.1 Multilevel Evaluation Factors

Factor	Description	Measurement Example
Structural/outer setting	Constructs representing the external structure of the broader sociocultural context or community within which a specific organization is situated	Description of the political climate, social climate, policy, economic climate, or infrastructure (workforce, transportation)
Organizational/inner setting	Constructs that represent aspects of the organization in which an innovation is being implemented	Leadership effectiveness, culture, innovation climate (extent to which organization values and rewards evidence-based practice or innovation)
Innovation	Constructs that represent aspects of the innovation that will be implemented	Adaptability, complexity, cost, advantage of the choice of one innovation above another/relative advantage, quality of evidence supporting the innovation's efficacy/evidence strength and quality, process for the innovation/design quality and packaging

(continued)

TABLE 11.1 Multilevel Evaluation Factors (*continued*)

Factor	Description	Measurement Example
Provider level	Constructs that represent aspects of the individual provider/clinician who implements the innovation with a patient or client	Attitudes toward evidence-based practice, perceived behavioral control for implementing the innovation
Patient level	Constructs representing patient characteristics or characteristics of the recipient of the intervention	Health-relevant beliefs, motivation, personality traits, health literacy, trust of medical practices
Transferability	Constructs that determine the ability of an intervention to be transferred to another setting and can be used in two situations: (1) prior to deciding on transferring an intervention to a new setting, (2) when evaluating the replica intervention to help explain the effects of the intervention that has been replicated	The ASTAIRE tool, which has four categories of analyzing the transferability with 23 structured criteria • Population • Environment • Implementation • Support for transfer
Patient/client outcomes	These are outcomes that the intervention is meant to directly or indirectly impact	Functional status, quality of life, perceived health status

ASTAIRE, *AnalySe de la Transférabilité et accompagnement à l'Adaptation des Interventions en pRomotion de la santE.*

Sources: From Cambon, L., Minary, L., Ridde, V., & Alla, F. (2013). A tool to analyze the transferability of health promotion interventions. *BMC Public Health, 13*, 1184. doi:10.1186/1471-2458-13-1184; Chaudoir, S. R., Dugan, A. G., & Barr, C. H. (2013). Measuring factors affecting implementation of health innovations: A systematic review of structural, organizational, provider, patient, and innovation level measures. *Implementation Science, 8*, 22. doi:10.1186/1748-5908-8-22; Lewis, C. C., Stanick, C. F., Martinez, R. G., Weiner, R. G., Kim, M., Barwick, M., & Comtois, K. A. (2015). The Society for Implementation Research Collaboration instrument review project: A methodology to promote rigorous evaluation. *Implementation Science, 10*(1), 2. doi:10.1186/s13012-014-0193-x

Value

The concept of *value* in healthcare varies depending on the perspective of the stakeholder. Patients may describe value in terms of the quality of their relationship with their provider, meeting personal goals, or living normal lives. Providers may suggest that *value improvement* means developing diagnostic and treatment tools that offer them more confidence in the effectiveness of the services they offer. Employers discuss value improvements in terms of keeping workers and their families healthier and more productive at lower costs, whereas health insurers perceive *value* as the delivery of interventions that have a substantial evidence base for effectiveness and efficiency. Finally, health product innovators value improved products for patients that are more profitable, differentiated, and innovative (Institute of Medicine, 2009).

The Triple Aim goals, as outlined by Berwick and colleagues through the Institute of Health Improvement (IHI), offer an established and accepted framework for determining value in health innovation with three goals:

1. Improving the individual experience of care
2. Improving the health of populations
3. Reducing the per capita costs of care for populations (Berwick, Nolan, & Whittington, 2008)

A suggested set of outcome measures designed to address the three domains are as follows:

- Mortality
  - Years of potential life lost, life expectancy, standardized mortality ratio
- Health and functional status
  - Health- related quality of life (HRQOL-4) or multidomain assessment such as the Patient Reported Outcomes Measurement Information System (PROMIS)
- Health life expectancy
- Disease burden
  - Incidence and/or prevalence of major chronic conditions
  - Morbidity burden
- Behavioral and psychological factors
  - Behaviors such as smoking, alcohol consumption, physical activity, and diet
  - Physiological factors such as blood pressure, body mass index, cholesterol and blood glucose levels
- Experience of care
  - Consumer Assessment of Healthcare Providers and Systems (CAHPS)
  - Likelihood to recommend
  - Measures based on the Institute of Medicine's six aims for improvement—Safe, effective, timely, efficient, equitable, and patient-centered
- Cost
  - Total cost
  - Utilization of services, that is, hospital and emergency department (Stiefel & Nolan, 2012)

■ DESIGNS FOR MEASURING TRANSLATION INTERVENTION OUTCOMES

Certain analysis designs are commonly used for measuring the impact of evidence translation projects. Each of these designs are described with the appropriate statistics.

Qualitative Analysis

Qualitative analysis can be used to describe the conditions in which the translation project takes place, the types of changes that are taking place, how the changes are made, facilitators and barriers to the process, and key stakeholders' experiences with the translation (Balasubramanian et al., 2015). To achieve transportability of practice innovations it is imperative to document and understand the complexity of implementation, including the experience of patients and staff.

Methods that allow for the observation of events, relationships, and context over time are well suited for qualitatively evaluating translation projects. Guided reflection through the application of periodic reflection is one way to determine structure and process complexity. The purpose of periodic reflection is to ensure documentation of important activities occur over the course of the project. These reflections can be completed though 30- to 60-minute guided discussions with team members to determine role-specific activities and relationships with those in separate roles participating in unique one-on-one discussions with the interviewer. Patients are also interviewed in a similar structure (Finley et. al., 2018)

Descriptive Design

Descriptive evaluation designs are used most often when the cohort receiving the intervention is small and/or when there is no comparison group. This is most often used in feasibility and pilot translation projects. Descriptive designs are the sole way to present the results of a project that does not use any type of comparisons, but the same type of descriptive information is used as the initial way to present the results of a project that does use a comparison group.

A descriptive design provides information about a group receiving the translation intervention and about the outcome metrics. Information about a group might include demographic characteristics such as age, gender, and ethnicity; geographical characteristics such as Zip Code, city, county, and state; psychosocial characteristics such as marital status or social support; or financial characteristics such as income level. The outcome metric would be presented without any comparisons within the project itself but may be compared to similar outcomes in the literature. When a translation intervention is meant to impact an event, for example, when trying to decrease the wait time for an ED visit, the descriptive information is about that certain event as opposed to describing the characteristics of a group. Descriptive information for an event might include the date and time; staff involved in the event; and the patient involved in the event.

Univariate statistics are used in descriptive evaluation designs; mean, median, mode, and proportions are used to present aggregated information about the group or set of events exposed to the intervention. In addition, distributions of the values for an outcome may be presented using histograms and box plots. Because there is no comparison group, there is no independent or dependent variable.

Pre–Postmeasurement in One Cohort

Paired-grouping evaluation designs measure the same outcome in one cohort over two or more points in time. The comparison is within the same cohort with one measurement representing a time period when the cohort was not exposed to the intervention and the comparison measurement representing a time period when the cohort was exposed to the intervention. The independent variable is the exposure to the intervention and is represented by the time period (pre or post). The dependent variable is the outcome.

If the dependent outcome variable is continuous (e.g., weight, diastolic blood pressure), the mean, standard deviation, and distributions are used to describe the outcome. A paired *t*-test is used to determine whether the differences in means are statistically significant. When a dichotomous outcome variable is used (e.g., weight loss achieved: yes/no, diastolic blood pressure less than 80: yes/no), then proportions are used to describe the outcome and McNemar's test of proportions is the appropriate test used to determine statistically significant differences. In the case of an ordinal outcome variable (e.g., Likert scales), proportions are still used to describe the outcome and the Wilcoxon signed-rank test is used to determine statistically significant differences.

Comparison of Two Different Cohorts

Different cohorts can be compared either during the time of intervention delivery or at different time periods. When comparing cohorts in the same time period, a cohort is selected, using inclusion and exclusion criteria, to receive the intervention and is referred to as the *intervention cohort*. A second cohort is selected using the same inclusion and exclusion criteria but does not receive the intervention and is referred to as the *comparison cohort*.

Or a comparison cohort may be selected prior to the delivery of the intervention, sometimes referred to as *causal comparative design* (Brewer & Kubin, 2010). When selecting a cohort from a previous time period, the same consideration must be given to inclusion and exclusion criteria as when selecting a comparison cohort from the same time period. In addition, special consideration should be given to the impact of time on the outcomes. For instance, when measuring costs as an outcome, changes in policy or inflation rates could account for changes in cost aside from the intervention itself, and could have a negative or positive impact on the outcome.

Because translation projects do not commonly use randomization to assign individuals to intervention and comparison cohorts, careful attention is given to determining whether the groups differ on known characteristics other than receipt of the intervention. An evaluation of the differences in known characteristics, such as age, gender, ethnicity, and so on between groups, is necessary to determine whether there are reasons other than the intervention that may account for the realized changes in outcomes. This is accomplished by testing for statistical significance between groups on these characteristics. For instance, if the mean difference in age between the intervention group and the comparison group is statistically significant, then consideration of age as a confounder is necessary when statistically testing the differences in the outcome between groups (Sylvia & Murphy, 2018).

When describing the characteristics of each cohort and the outcomes, univariate statistics are used. Proportions and means are used for categorical and continuous variables, respectively, as previously described in the Descriptive Design section. In addition, bivariate statistics are used to determine whether the differences in cohort characteristics and in the outcomes are statistically significantly between groups. The independent *t*-test for continuous variables and the chi-square test for dichotomous and categorical variables are most commonly used. If confounding variables are discovered in the evaluation of the differences in characteristics between groups, then multivariate analysis, most often using logistic or linear regression, is used to determine statistically significant differences in outcomes between groups due to the translation intervention.

Ongoing Monitoring Using Run Charts and Statistical Process Control

Run charts and/or statistical process control (SPC) are designs used to understand the outcomes of implementation in close to real time in order to continuously inform decisions and improve processes (Sherry & Sylvia, 2018). These designs allow for the distinction between *natural cause variation*, which occurs naturally due to individual differences, temporal factors (e.g., seasonality), or other factors, and *special cause variation*, which occurs because of the intervention (Carey, 2003).

The run chart is used to plot data points of a process over time and displays each point chronologically, with a median line delineated on the graph. A *run* is defined as one or more consecutive points that are on the same side of the median line. SPC is a more sensitive and powerful way of displaying data over time that involves taking various methods for monitoring processes and combining them to determine whether changes seen in the data over time are statistically significantly different from normal variation (indicative of special cause variation). The charts are useful for monitoring processes, identifying early signs of correlation between processes and outcomes, identifying differences across groups, or aiding in self-management interventions (Marsteller, Huizinga, & Cooper, 2013).

Once control charts are plotted, there is typically a set of tests used to determine significance. The following tests are usually used to test for significance on SPC charts (Benneyan, Lloyd, & Plsek, 2003):

- One point outside the upper or lower control limits
- Two of three successive points more than 2 sigma from the mean on the same side of the center line
- Four out of five successive points more than 1 sigma from the mean on the same side of the center line
- Eight successive points on the same side of the center line
- Six successive points increasing or decreasing (a trend)
- Obvious cyclical behavior

See Exemplar 21.3, Rapid Access to Tertiary Care: Mitigating Barriers Impacting Clinical, Financial, and Operational Outcomes, by Scott Newton in which a run chart to report the outcomes of a translation project is used.

Other Designs

Other design elements with more sophistication can be incorporated to adjust for biases that may be inherent due to the comparison and intervention cohort selection process, the correlation of multiple time-dependent measurements of the same outcome in the same cohort, and non-normal distributions of outcome data. A statistician should be consulted in these instances.

Power Analysis for Determining Adequate Numbers

Power analysis can be a great tool used during the translation project planning phase to determine the number of individuals (or events) needed in each of the comparison groups to find statistically significant differences in outcomes, if they do exist. Using power analysis for sample-size determination adds to the internal validity of the overall translation project. Information needed to use power analysis includes (a) the statistical significance level, or the percentage chance that the intervention is determined to be successful when it actually is not (usually 0.05 or 5%); (b) the level of statistical power, or the chance that the intervention is determined not to be successful when it actually is (usually 0.80% or 80%); (c) the degree of difference in the outcome between the intervention and comparison groupings (i.e., mean or proportion expected in the outcome metric for each group); and (d) the appropriate statistical test (Sylvia, 2018). Many sample-size calculators are available online.

■ CONCLUSIONS

The evaluation of translation is an integral part of translating evidence into practice. A sound, rigorous evaluation plan developed during the project-planning phase will pave the way to solid outcomes that describe success of the intervention on multiple levels for multiple stakeholders, of which the patient is the utmost important one.

■ REFERENCES

American Association of Colleges of Nursing. (2015). *The doctor of nursing practice: Current issues and clarifying recommendation*. Washington, DC: Author.

Balasubramanian, B. A., Cohen, D. J., Davis, M. M., Gunn, R., Dickinson, L. M., Miller, W. L., . . . Stange, K. C. (2015). Learning evaluation: Blending quality improvement and implementation research methods to study healthcare innovations. *Implementation Science, 10*(1), 31. doi:10.1186/s13012-015-0219-z

Benneyan, J., Lloyd, R., & Plsek, P. (2003). Statistical process control as a tool for research and healthcare improvement. *Quality and Safety in Health Care, 12(6)*, 458–464. doi:10.1136/qhc.12.6.458

Berwick, D. M., Nolan, T. W., & Whittington, J. (2008). The Triple Aim: Care, health, and cost. *Health Affairs, 27*(3), 759–769. doi:10.1377/hlthaff.27.3.759

Brewer, E. W., & Kubin, J. (2010). Causal comparative design. In N. J. Salkind (Ed.), *Encyclopedia of research design* (pp. 124–131). Thousand Oaks, CA: Sage.

Cambon, L., Minary, L., Ridde, V., & Alla, F. (2013). A tool to analyze the transferability of health promotion interventions. *BMC Public Health, 13*, 1184. doi:10.1186/1471-2458-13-1184

Carey, R. G. (2003). *Improving healthcare with control charts: Basic and advanced SPC methods and case studies*. Milwaukee, WI: ASQ.

Centers for Disease Control and Prevention. (2017, April). *Writing SMART objectives* Retrieved from https://www.cdc.gov/dhdsp/evaluation_resources/guides/writing-smart-objectives.htm

Chaudoir, S. R., Dugan, A. G., & Barr, C. H. (2013). Measuring factors affecting implementation of health innovations: A systematic review of structural, organizational, provider, patient, and innovation level measures. *Implementation Science, 8*, 22. doi:10.1186/1748-5908-8-22

Finley, E. P., Huynh, A. K., Farmer, M. M., Bean-Mayberry, B., Moin, T., Oishi, S. M., . . . Hamilton, A. B. (2018). Periodic reflections: A method of guided discussions for documenting implementation phenomena. *BMC Medical Research Methodology, 18*(1), 153. doi:10.1186/s12874-018-0610-y

Institute of Medicine. (2009). *Value in health care: Accounting for cost, quality, safety, outcomes, and innovation.* Washington, DC: National Academy of Sciences.

Lewis, C. C., Stanick, C. F., Martinez, R. G., Weiner, R. G., Kim, M., Barwick, M., & Comtois, K. A. (2015). The society for implementation research collaboration instrument review project: A methodology to promote rigorous evaluation. *Implementation Science, 10*(1), 2. doi:10.1186/s13012-014-0193-x

Marsteller, J., Huizinga, M., & Cooper, L. (2013). *Statistical process control: Possible uses to monitor and evaluate patient-centered medical home models.* Rockville, MD: Agency for Healthcare Research and Quality.

Mundinger, M., Starck, P., Hathaway, D., Shaver, J., & Woods, N. (2009). The ABCs of the doctor of nursing practice: Assessing resources, building a culture of clinical scholarship, curricular models. *Journal of Professional Nursing, 25*(2), 69–74. doi:10.1016/j.profnurs.2008.01.009

Polit, D. F., & Beck, C. T. (2018). *Essentials of nursing research: Appraising evidence for nursing practice generating and assessing evidence for nursing practice* (9th ed.). Philadelphia, PA: Wolters Kluwer.

Sherry, M., & Sylvia, M. (2018). Ongoing monitoring. In M. Sylvia & M. Terhaar (Eds.), *Clinical analytics and data management for the DNP* (pp. 281–308). New York, NY: Springer Publishing Company.

Stiefel, M. S., & Nolan, K. (2012). *A guide to measuring the triple aim: Population health, experience of care, and per capita cost.* Cambridge, MA: Institute for Health Improvement.

Sylvia, M. (2018). Basic statistical concepts and power analysis. In M. Sylvia & M. Terhaar (Eds.), *Clinical analytics and data management for the DNP* (pp. 11–25). New York, NY: Springer Publishing Company.

Sylvia, M., & Terhaar, M. (2014). An approach to clinical data management for the doctor of nursing practice curriculum. *Journal of Professional Nursing, 30*(1), 56–62. doi:10.1016/j.profnurs.2013.04.002

Sylvia, M. L., & Murphy, S. (2018). Outcomes data analysis. In M. Sylvia & M. Terhaar (Eds.), *Clinical analytics and data management for the DNP* (pp. 229–254). New York, NY: Springer Publishing Company.

Terhaar, M. (2018). Introduction to clinical data management. In M. Sylvia & M. Terhaar (Eds.), *Clinical analytics and data management for the DNP* (pp. 1–9). New York, NY: Springer Publishing Company.

Terhaar, M., Taylor, L., & Sylvia, M. (2016). The doctor of nursing practice: Shifting from start-up to impact. *Nursing Education Perspectives 37(1), 3–9.*

CHAPTER TWELVE

Dissemination of Evidence

Sharon Dudley-Brown

The overall purpose of dissemination is the utilization of knowledge.
—Cronenwett (1995), Ordonez and Serrat (2009)

Dissemination Is an Important Component of Translation of evidence because if the translation is not disseminated, then no change in care will occur and innovations will not be adopted. *Dissemination* is the communication of clinical, research, and theoretical findings for the purpose of transitioning new knowledge to the point of care (Brown & Schmidt, 2009). This chapter describes the methods and issues in dissemination of evidence.

■ RESEARCH DISSEMINATION

Funk, Tornquist, and Champagne (1989) framed a model of research dissemination that outlined three factors that are important and necessary for research to be disseminated:

1. Qualities of the research: These include the topic, relevance, applicability, availability of research, scientific merit, significance, level of control the practitioners have over their own practice, and the gap between research and practice.
2. Characteristics of the communication: These include the use of nontechnical language, clarification on limits of generalizability, strategies for implementation, demonstration of new techniques, broad dissemination, and discussion between researchers and clinicians.
3. Facilitation of utilization: This factor includes the reinforcement of new knowledge, ongoing dialog between researchers and clinicians, updates on research in the area, sharing of experiences, and giving support during implementation experiences. Attention to these categories can increase dissemination in any area. These can be easily transitioned to factors that

influence how evidence-based practice (EBP) is disseminated. For example, the quality of the translation is probably the most important. Is it a topic of significance to many healthcare providers or many institutions? Did the translation solve a meaningful clinical problem? Does this contradict other evidence or research?

Levels of Dissemination

Dissemination occurs at multiple levels. Once the translation project is complete, the first area for dissemination is internal, at the site of the adoption or innovation. This is usually institutionally based and can include clinical staff as well as administrative staff. The translation can also be disseminated to upper management. Presentation at clinical or grand rounds can be accomplished through small or largegroup presentations. The focus of each of these may be different in order to meet the needs of the audience. After the translation is disseminated at the site, it should be disseminated at the institutional level. This can be accomplished by hospital or organizational professional committee meetings or journal clubs. It can also be reported through a variety of media such as print flyers, news updates, or via a closed-circuit TV system. Many institutions now have an EBP day to showcase EBP projects using posters and podium presentations. One must also consider how and in what venue to disseminate the translation externally—beyond the institution or both nationally and internationally (see the three Ps in the section, The Three Ps of Dissemination). In addition, external dissemination to influence policy may occur through the use of media or through government advocacy. Dissemination is most successful if multiple methods are used over time (Brown & Schmidt, 2009).

Highlighting the challenges in the dissemination of evidence internally, Oermann, Roop, Nordstrom, Galvin, and Floyd (2007) described an intervention for disseminating Cochrane reviews to nurses. The authors sought to determine whether short summaries of a systematic review that presented the findings without requiring a background in research and statistics were effective in increasing nurses' awareness of research results and understanding of the evidence. Subjects included staff and advanced practice nurses (APNs) in seven hospitals, and subjects either received the intervention or served as a control. Although the number of nurses who completed the posttest was small, results support the feasibility of disseminating the findings of systematic reviews to bedside nurses and APNs. Nurses reported increased awareness of the research evidence, which was most apparent in the staff nurses.

Indeed, because dissemination and diffusion of evidence within an organization is influenced by the organization's contextual factors, external dissemination is influenced by larger organizational and social systems and values.

Strategies for Improving Dissemination

In a recent brief by the Commonwealth Fund on the dissemination of EBPs in healthcare, Yuan et al. (2010) cited key strategies to improve the dissemination of best practices in quality improvement (QI). These include (a) highlighting the evidence base and the relative simplicity of recommended practices; (b) aligning the campaigns with strategic goals of adopting organizations; (c) increasing the recruitment by integrating opinion leaders into the enrollment process; (d) forming a coalition of credible campaign sponsors; (e) generating a threshold of participating organizations, which maximizes network exchanges; (f) developing practical implementation tools and guides for key stakeholder groups; (g) creating networks to foster learning opportunities; and (h) incorporating monitoring and evaluation of milestones and goals (Yuan et al., 2010).

Kreuter and Bernhardt (2009) describe the challenge in dissemination of evidence as a marketing and distribution problem. They describe a lack of infrastructure necessary to move public health programs from research to practice and propose recommendations for building that needed infrastructure within the public health system.

Dissemination, in fact, is an expectation of all DNP students, as it is described in the American Association of Colleges of Nursing's (AACN) Essential III. How this occurs and how often are just beginning to be explored. In a study aimed at examining the publication record across eight cohorts of post-master's DNP students at one university, the authors found variability across the cohorts, but that more than half (51%) of the graduates contributed a peer-reviewed publication to the literature (Becker, Johnson, Rucker & Finnell, 2017). Their conclusion was that "expecting, rather than encouraging a publishable-ready manuscript as a course deliverable would further the student's motivation to disseminate their scholarship" (p. e1395).

Other strategies for improving dissemination include the use of various translation frameworks, such as the RE-AIM (reach, effectiveness, adoption, implementataion, maintenance) framework and the knowledge-to-action (KTA) cycle (see Chapter 2, The Science of Translation and Major Frameworks; Chambers, 2018). Both of these, according to Chambers (2018), focus on impact and activities that are necessary to influence practice and to see the importance of moving scientific knowledge into practice. Moreover, the KTA model now has an online counterpart, CAN-IMPLEMENT.PRO (Lockwood, Stephenson, Lizarondo, van Den Hoek, & Harrison, 2016). In fact, there has been a lot of focus on dissemination as defined slightly differently than in the dissemination of translation (the focus of this chapter). In fact, Dobson (2018) reports on dissemination science, which promotes EBP and uses scientific principles in the dissemination of evidenced-based treatments. These include diffusion and then implementation of the translated practice, which is really the uptake of evidence into practice. This is slightly different from the dissemination of translation or EBP, which is to get the results of the translation out to providers and end users (patients), with the goal to improve patient outcomes.

The Three Ps of Dissemination

There are three main methods of (external) dissemination, also known as the *three Ps*: posters, presentations, and papers (manuscripts). All three may require an abstract for acceptance. A good abstract targets the audience and aim (whether it be a poster or presentation at a conference, or a manuscript) and provides key information in a clear manner. Formatting is important and depends on the use of the abstract, but using the recommended fonts and word limit are crucial to acceptability. An abstract should be written in the past tense, and the American Psychological Association (APA) publication manual has clear and useful guidelines for both a research and a nonresearch abstract (APA, 2009). The APA suggests that an abstract be accurate, self-contained, concise and specific, nonevaluative, and coherent and readable. It suggests an abstract be less than 120 words, but the conference organizing committee or journal more likely dictates this length.

Poster

A poster is a versatile medium, and is used to disseminate research or nonresearch at a conference or other venue, such as in the community. The primary purpose of a poster presentation is to facilitate scholarly dialog among colleagues (Betz, Smith, Melnyk, & Rickey, 2005). One advantage is that work presented on a poster can (usually) still be in progress. Posters also need to be prepared to guidelines provided by the organizer. The message needs to be scholarly, straightforward, and clear. Incomplete sentences can be used, and bulleting of items is recommended. Posters should be more detailed than a speech, less detailed than a presentation, but more interactive than either (Schaffner, 2008). The use of charts and graphs provides visual stimulation as well as complements the data presented in verbal form. The reader's eye (in the United States) moves from top to bottom and from left to right, and, therefore, the individual sections of the poster need to be structured in this way. It has been suggested that the font of the title be more than 96 points and the font of the text be more than 24 to 36 points. A suggested guide is to make the text large enough to read from 3 to 6 feet away, or be able to read the material easily while standing, when the poster is laid on the ground. A prominent title can also help lure people to the poster. There are numerous resources with suggested guidelines and methods for poster designs and construction available via the Internet (Box 12.1). Using a search engine to search "poster presentation guidelines" will undoubtedly provide numerous options. The website www.posterpresentations.com provides (free) templates for varying sizes of posters, and (for a fee) will print and ship the poster to you, your hotel, or to your meeting site.

Content will vary depending on whether the authors are presenting a research project, an EBP project, or a clinical case or review. For a research poster, categories might include *background, research aims/hypothesis, review of the literature, design/methods, sample and setting, data analysis, results, limitations, discussion,* and *conclusion/implications*. For a poster on an EBP project, topics might include *background/significance, clinical question, search methods, appraisal of the evidence, method of grading the evidence, synthesis of findings, translation of evidence/intervention, findings, evaluation,* and *discussion* (Table 12.1).

Once the poster is made, the author has to fulfill the obligations of a presenter because poster viewing and presentation involve communication and networking among colleagues. The author should be prepared to learn from the viewers and should consider a poster as a way to market his or her work. For example, the authors need to be available near their poster at stated times. The author or representative should bring handouts, an abstract, and business cards. Smith and Mateo (2009) suggest the author(s) evaluate the poster after the poster session. In addition, the

BOX 12.1 Helpful Websites for Posters and Oral Presentations

www.ncsu.edu/project/posters • This site provides tips on how to create effective poster presentations, has a quick reference guide, and has start-to-finish instructions.

www.csun.edu/plunk/documents/poster_presentation.pdf • This site offers a pdf on tips for scientific poster presentations, including an ethics section.

www.youtube.com/watch?v=Ilr22p0jWjQ • This is a YouTube video from the University of California at Berkeley, with tips for poster presentations.

gradschool.unc.edu/academics/resources/postertips.html • This site from the University of North Carolina, contains tips and links for developing and delivering both poster and oral presentations.

pages.cs.wisc.edu/~markhill/conference-talk.html • This site, although dated, provides advice on giving an effective oral presentation.

www.nwlink.com/~donclark/leader/leadpres.html • This leadership site contains useful information on presentations.

go.owu.edu/~dapeople/ggpresnt.html • This site, from the library at Ohio Wesleyan University, offers tips on oral presentations, including presentation handouts, delivery, how to handle fear, and the role of the audience.

enterprisersproject.com/article/2018/9/7-ted-talks-how-improve-your-presentations • This site offers seven notable TED (technology/entertainment/design) talks on how to improve presentations; particularly notable for healthcare professionals is the one on data visualization or how to get people to better appreciate your data.

TABLE 12.1 Poster Content

Research Poster	Evidence-Based Practice Project Poster
Background	Background/significance
Research aims/hypotheses	Clinical question
Review of the literature	Search methods
Methods/design	Appraisal of evidence
Sample and setting	Method of grading evidence
Data analysis	Synthesis of findings
Results	Translation of evidence/intervention
Limitations	Findings
Discussion	Evaluation
Conclusions/implications	Discussion

author(s) should jot down the feedback received from viewers, whether related to that project or to ideas for future projects.

Presentation

Oral presentations can be invited or juried. If juried, an abstract is necessary and is crucial for acceptance. Conference sponsors usually solicit presenters by announcing a call for abstracts. Typically, an invited speaker does not need to prepare an abstract. An oral presentation is better than a poster for dissemination of philosophical and theoretical topics. Oral presentations must be of completed work, and thus, the abstract is completed in the past tense.

Once an abstract is accepted for an oral presentation, the author(s) need to ascertain the target audience, the room setting (size and seating arrangement), and the time allotted (both for the presentation as well as questions), and whether the presentation (frequently in PowerPoint) needs to be submitted in advance, taking note of the date of submission.

In preparation, the content of the presentation needs to be dictated by what was submitted in the abstract. Developing an outline from the abstract is one method used to begin preparation. Because the purpose of the slides is to enhance the presentation of the content (Smith & Mateo, 2009), the author(s) must decide the number and type of slides (words, pictures/graphs, or both), depending on the content and audience. The recommendation is a maximum of one slide per minute of talk. This also requires that the presenter understand the exact time he or she has to present, as well as ant time needed to entertain questions or discussion. Considerations for developing slides include the following: (a) use contrasting colors (such as navy blue background and yellow lettering); (b) keep a consistent template and font throughout; (c) choose a simple font (Arial, sans serif, or Times New Roman); (d) keep the number of words per slide to a minimum; (e) left-justify the text; and (f) when using graphs, orient the audience (Betz et al., 2005; Smith & Mateo, 2009). As with posters, there are numerous resources on the Internet to assist not only in preparing the slides, but also with tips on presenting them (see Box 12.1).

Once the presentation is completed, follow the conference guidelines for submission, if requested. Because most presentations are done on computer software (as opposed to actual slides), make and bring another copy of the presentation to the conference (e.g., on a flash drive), as well as a printed copy of the slides, for use in the event of a technological malfunction.

Public speaking is a skill, and thus requires learning and practice (Englehart, 2004). Rehearsing the presentation is a must, especially for those new to oral presentations. Presenting to colleagues at work is an excellent way to not only rehearse, but also to obtain any suggestions and feedback on the content and to enhance clarity. A common pitfall in oral presentations is not being able to keep within the allotted time. The sole responsibility of staying on time lies with the presenter.

Another type of oral presentation is a panel presentation. The style and purpose of panel presentations vary widely (Melnyk & Fineout-Overholt, 2011). Typically, the panel includes a moderator, who may serve as a coordinator, and who provides commentary after individual panelists. In addition, typical panels take questions from the audience. Sometimes panelists will be expected to have slides, but more frequently, panelists are not required to have slides. Again, as a panelist, pay attention to time allotted.

Publication

Papers or manuscripts for publication can be written about research, EBP projects, or case studies or clinical reviews. Manuscripts are usually required to be written about completed work. All posters and presentations should also be considered for a manuscript submission at a later date. Whereas posters and presentations are only for the people in attendance, a manuscript is considered a permanent contribution and method of dissemination to the profession. Publication options include books, professional journals, electronic journals, the Internet (including list serves, Twitter, and blogs), newsletters, and newspapers.

In developing a manuscript for a professional journal, the journal intended for publication needs to be considered early on. Peer-reviewed journals publish more rigorously reviewed manuscripts than non-peer-reviewed journals. Both the target audience and the target journal need to be defined. Authorship should also be decided and agreed upon in advance. The author(s) need to review the author guidelines from the specific journal and comply with suggested length, reference style, and other specific manuscript details. Most of this information is now available online. Many journals will accept and respond to queries from authors, usually submitted electronically through the journal/editor website, or via email. In a query to the editor, the author(s) must succinctly explain their plans for the structure and content of the manuscript. This can save authors considerable time and effort.

Just as there are guidelines for the publication of randomized controlled trials (RCTs; consolidated standards of reporting trials [CONSORT]) and preferred reporting items for systematic reviews and meta-analyses (PRISMA), there are also guidelines for the publication of QI projects in healthcare (Altman et al., 2001; Liberati et al., 2009). Standards for Quality Improvement Reporting Excellence (SQUIRE) guidelines have been developed for authors describing the development and testing of interventions to improve the quality and safety of healthcare (Davidoff et al., 2008). Journals, such as the *Journal of Nursing Care Quality* and *The Joint Commission Journal on Quality and Patient Safety*, have adopted these guidelines for reporting QI projects to ensure that the project is sufficiently reported, so that readers can understand the problem, intervention, setting, and outcomes (Oermann, 2009). The SQUIRE guidelines assist in the reporting of QI projects, including details of the intervention and circumstances leading to the need for the change, and the setting and local conditions that could influence the outcomes. In addition, as Oermann (2009) points out, these guidelines can be used to educate nurses and other healthcare professionals on the QI process and as a framework for the project plan (p. 94). Categories include the following sections (and subsections): (a) title and abstract (title, abstract), (b) introduction (background knowledge, local problem, intended improvement, study question), (c) methods (ethical issues, setting, planning the intervention, planning the study of the intervention, methods of evaluation, and analysis), (d) results (outcomes), (e) discussion (summary, relation to other evidence, limitations, interpretation, and conclusions), and (f) other information (funding; Davidoff et al., 2008; Table 12.2).

TABLE 12.2 SQUIRE Guidelines for Reporting QI Studies

Section of Paper	Description
Title and abstract	Did you provide clear and accurate information for finding, indexing, and scanning your article?
1. Title	a. Indicate that the article is on improvement of quality.
	b. State aim or intervention.
	c. Indicate the study method.
2. Abstract	Summarize key information using journal's abstract format.
Introduction	Why did you start?
3. Background knowledge	Provide a brief summary of the current knowledge of the problem being addressed in the project; include characteristics of setting.
4. Local problem	Describe the specific local problem addressed in the project.
5. Intended improvement	a. Describe changes/improvements in processes and outcomes of the proposed intervention.
	b. Specify who and what led to the decision to make changes, include why the project is done now (timing).
6. Study question	State primary and other questions that QI study was intended to answer.
Methods	What did you do?
7. Ethical issues	Indicate the ethical concerns of implementing the improvement and study and how they are addressed.
8. Setting	Specify the elements and characteristics of the setting most likely to influence change/improvement.
9. Planning the intervention	a. Describe the intervention in enough detail for others to reproduce it.
	b. Indicate the factors that contributed to the decision about specific intervention to implement.
	c. Describe the plans for how the intervention was to be implemented: What was done, how tests of change would be used to modify the intervention, and by whom?
10. Planning the study of the intervention	a. Outline plans for assessing how well the intervention was implemented.
	b. Describe mechanisms by which the intervention components were expected to cause changes, and plans for testing if they were effective.
	c. Identify the study design for measuring the effects of intervention.
	d. Discuss plans for implementing essential aspects of the study design.
	e. Describe the aspects of study design that addressed internal validity (integrity of data) and external validity (generalizability).

(continued)

TABLE 12.2 SQUIRE Guidelines for Reporting QI Studies (*continued*)

Section of Paper	Description
11. Methods of evaluation	a. Describe the instruments and procedures used to assess effectiveness of implementation, contributions of intervention components and context factors to effectiveness of intervention, and outcomes.
	b. Report validity and reliability of assessment instruments.
	c. Explain methods to ensure data quality and adequacy.
12. Analysis	a. Provide details of qualitative and quantitative (statistical) methods.
	b. Align unit of analysis with the level at which the intervention was implemented, if applicable.
	c. Specify the degree of variability expected in implementation, change expected in primary outcome (effect size), and ability of the study design (including size) to detect those effects.
	d. Describe the analytic methods to demonstrate the effects of time as a variable.
Results	What did you find?
13. Outcomes	a. Nature of setting and improvement intervention:
	i. Indicate the relevant elements of setting and structures and patterns of care that provided context for the intervention.
	ii. Explain the actual course of intervention.
	iii. Document success in implementing intervention components.
	iv. Describe how and why the initial plan evolved and the lessons learned.
	b. Changes in processes of care and patient outcomes associated with intervention:
	i. Present data on changes observed in the care delivery process.
	ii. Present data on changes observed in patient outcomes.
	iii. Consider benefits, harms, unexpected results, problems, and failures.
	iv. Present evidence on the strength of association between observed changes/improvements and intervention components/context factors.
	v. Include summary of missing data for intervention and outcomes.
Discussion	What do the findings mean?
14. Summary	a. Summarize the most important successes and difficulties in implementing intervention and the main changes observed.
	b. Highlight the strengths of the study.

(*continued*)

TABLE 12.2 SQUIRE Guidelines for Reporting QI Studies (*continued*)

Section of Paper	Description
15. Relation to other evidence	Compare and contrast study results with relevant findings of others.
16. Limitations	a. Consider the possible sources of confounding, bias, or imprecision in design, measurement, and analysis that might affect study outcomes.
	b. Explore the factors that could affect generalizability.
	c. Address likelihood that observed gains may weaken over time, and describe plans for sustainability.
	d. Review efforts to minimize study limitations.
	e. Assess the effect of limitations on interpretation and application of results.
17. Interpretation	a. Explore the possible reasons for differences between observed and expected outcomes.
	b. Draw inferences consistent with strength of data about causal mechanisms and size of observed change.
	c. Suggest steps that might be modified to improve future performance.
	d. Review issues of cost of intervention (opportunity and financial).
18. Conclusions	a. Consider practical usefulness of the intervention
	b. Suggest implications for healthcare and other QI studies.
Other information	Were there other factors relevant to the conduct and interpretation of the study?
19. Funding	List funding sources, if any, and the role of funding organization in design, implementation, interpretation, and publication.

QI, quality improvement; SQUIRE, Standards for Quality Improvement Reporting Excellence.

Source: Adapted from Davidoff, F., Batalden, P., Stevens, D., Ogrinc, G., Mooney, S., & SQUIRE Development Group. (2008). Publication guidelines for improvement studies in health care: Evolution of the SQUIRE project. *Annals of Internal Medicine, 149*(9), 670–676. doi:10.7326/0003-4819-149-9-200811040-00009; Oermann, M. H. (2009). SQUIRE guidelines for reporting improvement studies in healthcare: Implications for nursing publications. *Journal of Nursing Care Quality, 24*(2), 91–95. doi:10.1097/01.ncq.0000347445.04138.74

Developing the manuscript content, proofreading it, and responding to suggestions all take time, perseverance, and a positive attitude (Betz et al., 2005). To increase the chances that a manuscript will be accepted, the following guidelines are recommended: Select the appropriate audience, select the appropriate journal, query the editor about the topic, include implications for practice and significance of your project, conform to submission requirements, adhere to copyright laws, use recent references, maintain organization, use tables and graphs, determine authorship in advance, acknowledge assistance appropriately, and conform to ethical practice (Smith & Matteo, 2009).

■ ETHICAL CONCERNS

Ethical issues in publication have recently come to the forefront. Siedlecki, Montague, and Schultz (2008) describe common ethical pitfalls that authors may encounter during the preparation and submission of a manuscript and how to avoid them. These include plagiarism, failure to cite sources correctly, dual publications, and authorship decisions. Plagiarism can be intentional or unintentional, but involves stealing (knowingly or unknowingly) another person's work or ideas and using them as your own. This also includes self-plagiarism, which occurs when an author borrows extensively from one of his or her prior works and does not properly acknowledge the original source through a citation. Although citation errors are common in the healthcare literature, they connote sloppiness by the author and may greatly hinder the reader's ability to locate a source. The use of online citation management software programs, such as EndNote or Refworks, can help eliminate this problem and can easily convert from APA format to other reference styles. Dual publication, or salami publishing, is the publication of multiple manuscripts for one project or study (Baggs, 2008; Siedlecki et al., 2008). Authorship problems can arise when several individuals submit an article as a group. Everyone who made a "substantial contribution" to the project should be listed as an author, and conversely, all individuals listed as authors should be involved in writing and reviewing the manuscript (Baggs, 2008; Broome, 2008; Graf et al., 2007; Siedlecki et al., 2008). Clear guidelines on authorship can be found on the website of the International Committee of Medical Journal Editors at www.icmje.org (Table 12.3).

Another component of ethical issues in dissemination concerns the ethical issues surrounding the dissemination of sensitive data and information from an organization. For example, if the translation of evidence identifies an improvement in outcomes, safety, or cost, some may view the preimplementation data as a poor outcome. A good rule to follow is to be sure administrators at the site of the translation are aware of outcome preimplementation and postimplementation of a translation project prior to any dissemination. Another suggestion is to disseminate the information at the institutional level first prior to any dissemination outside of the institution.

Dissemination may be conducted with the purpose of influencing health policy. There is a need for healthcare professionals to write policy briefs based on the translation of evidence, in a way that legislators can understand. The key to writing a policy brief is to be succinct and direct in the communication (Melnyk & Fineout-Overholt, 2011).

TABLE 12.3 **Guidelines on Authorship in Healthcare Literature**

www.icmje.org/icmje-recommendations.pdf	ICMJE offers recommendations for the conduct, reporting, editing, and publication of scholarly work in medical journals.
www.icmje.org/recommendations/browse/roles-and-responsibilities/defining-the-role-of-authors-and-contributors.html	Here, ICMJE defines the role of authors and contributors.

ICMJE, International Committee of Medical Journal Editors.

The media offer other avenues for dissemination of translation, which may include both written (e.g., a magazine or newsletter) and face-to-face interviews. Interviews can be a powerful method to use to get the findings disseminated to the public. However, for the inexperienced, it is recommended to contact a public relations specialist, if available through the organization, to assist with this type of dissemination (Melnyk & Fineout-Overholt, 2011).

■ CONCLUSIONS

In sum, dissemination is the final phase of translation and is imperative for moving evidence into practice. Preparation for dissemination for any venue and by any method will enhance the success of any dissemination and translation initiative (Betz et al., 2005).

■ REFERENCES

Altman, D. G., Shulz, K. F., Moher, D., Egger, M., Davidoff, F., Elbourne, D., . . . CONSORT Group. (2001). The revised CONSORT statement for reporting randomized trials: Explanation and elaboration. *Annals of Internal Medicine, 134(8),* 663–694.

American Psychological Association. (2009). *Publication manual of the American Psychological Association* (6th ed.). Washington, DC: Author.

Baggs, J. G. (2008). Issues and rules for authors concerning authorship versus acknowledgements, dual publication, self plagiarism, and salami publishing. *Research in Nursing and Health, 31*(4), 295–297. doi:10.1002/nur.20280

Becker, K. D., Johnson, S., Rucker, D. & Finnell, D. S. (2017). Dissemination of scholarship across eight cohorts of doctor of nursing practice graduates. *Journal of Clinical Nursing, 27*(7–8), e1395–e1401. doi:10.1111/jocn.14237

Betz, C. L., Smith, K., Melnyk, B. M., & Rickey, T. (2005). Disseminating evidence. In B. M. Melnyk & E. Fineout-Overholt (Eds.), *Evidence-based practice in nursing and healthcare: A guide to best practice* (pp. 361–403). Philadelphia, PA: Lippincott, Williams & Wilkins.

Broome, M. E. (2008). The "truth, the whole truth and nothing but the truth." *Nursing Outlook, 56*(6), 281–282. doi:10.1016/j.outlook.2008.10.001

Brown, J. M., & Schmidt, N. A. (2009). Sharing the insights with others. In N. A. Schmidt & J. M. Brown (Eds.), *Evidence-based practice for nurses: Appraisal and application of research* (pp. 399–417). Sudbury, MA: Jones & Bartlett.

Chambers, C. T. (2018). From evidence to influence: Dissemination and implementation of scientific knowledge for improved pain research and management. *Pain, 159,* S56–S64. doi:10.1097/j.pain.0000000000001327

Cronenwett, L. R. (1995). Effective methods for disseminating research findings to nurses in practice. *Nursing Clinics of North America, 30*(3), 429–438.

Davidoff, F., Batalden, P., Stevens, D., Ogrinc, G., Mooney, S., & SQUIRE Development Group. (2008). Publication guidelines for improvement studies in health care: Evolution of the SQUIRE project. *Annals of Internal Medicine, 149*(9), 670–676. doi:10.7326/0003-4819-149-9-200811040-00009

Dobbson, K. S (2018). Dissemination: Science and sensibilities. *Canadian Psychology, 59*(2), 120–125. doi:10.1037/cap0000143

Englehart, N. (2004). Giving effective presentations. *Canadian Operating Room Nursing Journal, 22*(1), 22–24.

Funk, S. G., Tornquist, E. M., & Champagne, M. T. (1989). A model for improving the dissemination of nursing research. *Western Journal of Nursing Research, 11*(3), 361–367. doi:10.1177/019394598901100311

Graf, C., Wagner, E., Bowman, A., Flack, S., Scott-Lichter, D., & Robinson, A. (2007). Best practice guidelines on publication ethics: A publisher's perspective. *International Journal of Clinical Practice, 61*(Suppl. 152), 1–26. doi:10.1111/j.1742-1241.2006.01230.x

Kreuter, M. W., & Bernhardt, J. M. (2009). Reframing the dissemination challenge: A marketing and distribution perspective. *American Journal of Public Health, 99*(12), 2123–2127. doi:10.2105/ajph.2008.155218

Liberati, A., Altman, D. G., Tetzlaf, J., Mulrow, C., Gotzsche, P. C., Ioannidis, J. P. A., . . . Moher, D. (2009). The PRISMA statement for reporting systematic reviews and meta-analysis of studies that evaluate health care interventions: Explanation and elaboration. *Journal of Clinical Epidemiology, 62(10)*, e1–e34. doi:10.1016/j.jclinepi.2009.06.006

Lockwood, C., Stephenson, M., Lizarondo, L., van Den Hoek, J., & Harrison, M. (2016). Evidence implementation: Development of an online methodology from the knowledge-to-action model of knowledge translation. *International Journal of Nursing Practice, 22*(4), 322–329. doi:10.1111/ijn.12469

Melnyk, B. M., & Fineout-Overholt, E. (2011). *Evidenced-based practice in nursing & healthcare: A guide to best practice* (2nd ed.). Philadelphia, PA: Lippincott Williams & Wilkins.

Oermann, M. H. (2009). SQUIRE guidelines for reporting improvement studies in healthcare: Implications for nursing publications. *Journal of Nursing Care Quality*, *24*(2), 91–95. doi:10.1097/01.ncq.0000347445.04138.74

Oermann, M. H., Roop, J. C., Nordstrom, C. K., Galvin, E. A., & Floyd, J. A. (2007). Effectiveness of an intervention for disseminating Cochrane reviews to nurses. *Medsurg Nursing*, *16*(6), 373–377.

Ordonez, M., & Serrat, O. (2009). Disseminating knowledge products. *Asian Development Bank: Knowledge Solutions, 43*, 1–6.

Schaffner, M. (2008, May). *Preparing a research poster*. Paper presented at the 35th annual course of the Society of Gastroenterology Nurses and Associates, Salt Lake, UT.

Siedlecki, S. L., Montague, M., & Schultz, J. (2008). Writing for publication: Avoiding common ethical pitfalls. *Journal of Wound, Ostomy, and Continence Nursing*, *35*(2), 147–150. doi:10.1097/01.won.0000313636.83881.22

Smith, S. P., & Matteo, M. A. (2009). Reporting results through publication. In M. A. Mateo & K. T. Kirchhoff (Eds.), *Research for advanced practice nurses: From evidence to practice* (pp. 441–455). New York, NY: Springer Publishing Company.

Yuan, C. T., Nembhard, I. M., Stern, A. F., Brush, J. E., Krumholz, H. M., & Bradley, E. H. (2010). Blueprint for the dissemination of evidence-based practices in health care . *Commonwealth Fund Issue Brief*, *1399*(86), 1–14.

PART FOUR

Enablers of Translation

CHAPTER THIRTEEN

Education: An Enabler of Translation

Mary F. Terhaar and Marisa L. Wilson

Tell me and I forget.
Teach me and I learn.
Involve me and I remember.
—Benjamin Franklin

Translation Can Be Understood as Moving Science from awareness through acceptance and into adoption, in order to address a need or gap. In the end, it is all about changing the behavior of clinicians, individuals, and communities as a means of improving health and related outcomes. Changing behavior of any kind requires both motivation and the acquisition of new knowledge and these are the goals of education (Bandura, 1997). As a result, effective translation is predicated on understanding and competence that is developed through education.

Just as every translation effort, every practice change, every new program will rely on education at its foundation, so, too, the impact of education relies on translation of new evidence into its practice. There is great potential to increase the impact, contain expense, broaden reach, and decrease delay between discovery of new instructional methods and technologies and their application so long as those who teach adopt strong evidence in their design and instruction. To do so can be expected to benefit individual learners and the society.

Such transformation depends on the ability of those providing instruction to anticipate the needs of the learner and the market, understand the technologies that can briskly advance dissemination and learning, and transform educational practices.

As healthcare systems increase in size and complexity, learners within those organizations become increasingly diverse. Such diversity is a feature of the society and an important characteristic of learners across higher education as well. In these contexts, there is evidence to guide educators seeking to offer effective and impactful instruction.

Many of the translation frameworks presented in Chapter 2, The Science of Translation and Major Frameworks, highlight the critical role of education in the translation process. To be effective, the design and execution of that education requires thoughtful application of evidence and best practice from the field of education and knowledge acquisition. This chapter skims the surface of that best evidence and practice.

It is useful to begin with the end in mind and then plan backward from there (Wiggins & McTighe, 2004). The characteristics of the learner, the context of learning, and the nature of the change to be accomplished all factor in decisions about design, deployment, and evaluation of learning. The purpose of this chapter is to address each of these aspects of education and provide a guide to help clinicians whose translation efforts depend on changing knowledge, attitudes, and beliefs.

Upon completion of this chapter, the reader will have an understanding of:

1. The evolving diversity in learners that is relevant for those who would teach effectively
2. The most impactful and broadly adopted educational theories that can be applied to support translation
3. A set of evidence-based practices adopted by effective educators engaged in translation
4. A set of metrics that can be used to evaluate educational interventions and innovations

■ DIVERSITY AMONG LEARNERS

Nurses routinely educate three groups of learners: patients, their families, and the healthcare team members charged with the provision of care. Although the focus of the instruction may differ for each group, the diversity of characteristics of the learners cuts across all three.

With respect to patients and their families, accountable care charges clinicians and systems with keeping patients and their goals in the center of all planning and caregiving. From this perspective, patients are partners in care, which is a long-standing and familiar approach in nursing. Likewise, with regard to education, it is useful to keep the student at the center of all planning and teaching (Cox & Naylor, 2013).

With respect to healthcare team members, the pace of change in science and technology demands everyone engaged in the provision of healthcare remain current. This includes unlicensed personnel, technicians, paraprofessionals, and professionals from a broad range of disciplines and specialties.

The age, life experience, and learning style of the learner must be taken into consideration when developing an educational experience. If the educator does not factor these into the development of the material, the platform, and/or the learning activities, then there is a risk that all or a portion of the targeted learners will be disengaged, resulting in less-than-effective learning. This section begins with a description of the influence of age and experience on learning and ends with a review of learning styles. Remember, individual differences influence learning: A young learner may be more attuned to certain educational experiences (online learning and apps), whereas an adult learner may prefer others (reading and writing papers). Effective education will be designed and deployed if these individual differences and learning characteristics are kept in mind.

Education for the Young Learner

Pedagogy refers to the act of teaching together with the knowledge, skill, and judgment to practice it. According to Merriam-Webster, pedagogy is *the art, science, and profession of teaching* (merriam-webster.com). As a noun, it has been described as *any conscious activity by one person designed to enhance the learning of another* (Watkins & Mortimer, 1999). A broader definition explains that *pedagogy is the act of teaching together with its attendant discourse. It is what one needs to know, and the skills one needs to command in order to make and justify the many different kinds of decisions of which teaching is constituted* (Alexander, 2003). When one teaches, one develops and practices a pedagogy and there are many different models to consider.

Traditional pedagogy framed the educator as the repository of information to be conveyed. In this model, the educator is the adult and the learner is the child. The educator is *the sage on the stage* and the learner is the recipient of the teaching (King, 1993). Learners are framed as relatively passive, the classroom is controlled, and the teacher has authority. Lectures, readings, and films are common strategies used to convey information, and tests are commonly used to evaluate learning. This is the one-way pedagogy many educators recall from their youth as experienced during K–12 education.

Young learners rely on an authority to decide what they need to learn. These learners expect that what they are learning to be useful some time in the future. They bring minimal life experience to the learning and typically do not question instruction or authority.

Education for the Adult Learner

Andragogy differentiates the adult learner from the child (Knowles, 1980). This adult learner is understood to bring life experience to the educational activity, coming to the educational session with clear goals and wanting to put what is learned into use immediately. This changes everything. The adult learner can be expected to be engaged, to have goals for the learning experience, and to require that the learning be applicable and relevant. Passivity is not the expected norm. This learner expects the educator to acknowledge and respect the knowledge and accomplishments the learner brings to the classroom (whatever its form) and expects to contribute to the learning experience (Branson et al., 1975). Self-directed learning, group activities, and project-based learning are commonly used to convey content. More diverse means to evaluate learning are also used, including discussions, papers, projects, and reports (King, 1993).

Because translation may require instructional programs for children and adults, the educator facilitating that translation will need to be able to employ both andragogic and pedagogic approaches. It will be useful to frame education as a supported learning experience, regardless of the age of the participant, and to provide experiences in which the educator facilitates learning.

Adult learners decide for themselves what they consider important to learn. They rely on their own beliefs and experiences to validate what they are learning. They expect to immediately use what they learn and want to serve as a resource for the educator. It is important to reflect on the aspects of pedagogy and andragogy when creating educational events for young and adult learners (Mazzolini & Maddison, 2003; Wick, Pollock, Jefferson, & Flanagan, 2006).

Diversity of Learning Styles

When preparing educational programming and resources to support translation, it is helpful to consider that learners may vary with respect to their levels of motivation, attitudes, experiences, and goals. Evidence demonstrates three categories of potential diversity that have important implications for achieving a desired outcome. Learners will differ in style (the way one takes in and processes information), approach (surface, deep, or strategic), and intellectual development (the attitude the learner has about the nature of knowledge). All inform the development of the educational event.

Learning styles have historically been categorized as cognitive, affective, and psychological in nature and are stable indicators of how learners perceive, interact with, respond to, and engage with the learning experience (Keefe, 1979). For example, some learners may be interested only in theory and abstraction; others may want just the facts; some may want observables with which they can interact; and still others may want to have visual presentations of information (Felder & Brent, 2005). One style is neither better nor worse than the other: They are simply different. Considering approaches to learning that appeal to the different sensibilities is fundamental to developing an effective educational event.

Learners may be more receptive to predominantly visual, auditory, or kinesthetic sensory experiences. Visual learners prefer seeing what they are learning. So pictures and images will help them understand the information better than just verbal explanation (Russell, 2006). Written material, notes, diagrams, and pictures are most effective for visual learners. Auditory learners prefer to hear the message or instruction that is being given. These learners prefer to be talked through the process. They learn through listening. Lecture, discussion, and podcasts work well for auditory learners. Kinesthetic learners want to "do something." These learners use touch, movement, and space. These kinesthetic learners require the hands-on approach and learn by imitation and practice. When preparing the educational event, the developer has to consider multiple modalities, so that the strengths and weaknesses of each type of learning style are addressed.

Learners use different approaches to learning. Some rely only on memorization, taking in only what they need to know. These are the surface learners. Others dive into the material, questioning and exploring everything that is offered. These are the deep learners. Others pick and choose the approach, depending on their perceived need for the material and the situation in which they find themselves. These are the strategic learners. The effective educator provides opportunities for those learners who want that "deep dive" to question and probe, while at the same time providing other learners who prefer a more strategic or more surface-learning experience with facts that can quickly be assimilated (Felder & Brent, 2005).

Learners also differ in their intellectual development. For some, at a basic stage of learning, knowledge is considered to be certain and authorities are viewed as omniscient. For others, at a higher stage, knowledge is considered to be uncertain and a sense of personal responsibility to determine the truth is valued (Felder & Brent, 2005). Learners at a still higher level of intellectual development can be expected to question the educator, to challenge logic, and to offer alternative positions and solutions.

Historically, in healthcare, the many disciplines have been educated in parallel streams, even silos, where specialized knowledge, language, culture, and reasoning grow discretely with little opportunity for shared meaning, shared goals, and shared problem-solving (World Health Organization, 2010). This tremendous legacy of missed opportunity has been shown to contribute to error, compromise quality of care, and diminish patient satisfaction. Translation brings many disciplines together to improve outcomes. Education that facilitates translation will be most effective if it includes learners from many disciplines joined together for a common purpose in a collaborative learning environment and experience (Interprofessional Education Collaborative Expert Panel, 2011).

Greater and more transformative learning occurs when teaching styles and learning styles are matched as fully as is practical (Hayes & Allinson, 1996). Although it can be difficult to identify all of the styles, stages, and preferences of the learners, the best practice would ensure a diversity of approaches be used to respond to a diversity of learners. The educator can and should include order, structure, creativity, group work, and practical exercises to appeal to most learning styles. Table 13.1 presents some basic considerations for developing the educational event.

Distance Between Learner and Instructor

Depending on the indication for the instruction and the size of the system, the distance between the teacher and the learner may vary. In some cases, learners may meet with instructors face-to-face either one-on-one or in groups. Depending on the way the teacher and learner connect, the instructional materials and platforms may vary, but the outcome cannot.

Depending on the indication for the instruction and the size of the system, the teacher and learner may engage across different time zones or have different availability for interaction. They may participate remotely in a live session in which everyone is engaged at the same time (synchronously) or may participate remotely even spanning different times (asynchronously). Each format requires development of instructional materials and technologies to reliably, consistently, and effectively deliver information

TABLE 13.1 Considerations for Developing Educational Content

Prelearning preparation	Know what prior knowledge is assumed and communicate this to the learners.
Development of learning objectives	Develop objectives, so that all participants are working toward the same goal.
Organization of the content	Ensure that content is organized in such a way as to allow building of knowledge.
Inclusion of emotion	When learning includes not only the intellect but also appeals to the emotion, it becomes more influential and lasting.
Opportunities for participation	Participation allows the learner to internalize material. This requires development of activities.
Reinforcement	Learners have to receive indications of success in order to ensure motivation.
Feedback	Learners have to be periodically informed of their progress.
Application	The learner has to be able to demonstrate application or the transfer of learning to the new problem or situation.

Source: Adapted from the University College Dublin Adult Education Centre. (2019). *Our work. UDA access and lifelong learning*. Dublin, Ireland: University College Dublin. Retrieved from http://www.ucd.ie/all/ourwork

and achieve the intended understanding. Again, the instruction must accomplish the same outcomes regardless of the platform for its presentation and use. Many educators and administrators in post-secondary education in the United States have come to understand that learner outcomes from online programs can and must match, if not exceed, those of more traditional face-to-face offerings (Allen & Seaman, 2015).

Although the debate about distance learning in higher education is passionate, its application for industry and healthcare is less so. Any platform that instructs and informs patients and has the potential to increase self-care and improve outcomes is an approach worth implementing.

■ DESIGN OF INSTRUCTION

Instructional design refers to the process the educator applies to determine and develop the outcomes, methods, materials, content, and approaches that will constitute the learning experience (Lowyck & Poysa, 2001). It is the process and prescription that will facilitate learning. When the instruction to be offered is a component of translation, the process begins with the evidence and closes with action based upon it.

ADDIE Model For Instructional Design

Several models can be used to guide the instructional-design process and prominent among them is the ADDIE model, which was developed at Florida State University in 1975. ADDIE stipulates five phases in the design process: **a**nalysis, **d**esign,

development, **i**mplementation, and **e**valuation. These phases are used to organize the content in this chapter.

Analysis

The first phase in the ADDIE model is assessment. Just as high-impact writing targets a particular audience, the same is true of high-impact instruction. Both begin with an understanding of the learner(s), which can be developed in many ways. The goal here is to evaluate baseline knowledge, skill, and learning goals, as well as preferred learning style, all of which inform the instruction.

Assessment can be formal or informal, qualitative or quantitative, individual or aggregate. The approach to assessment is based on the nature of the information required to support effective instruction and impactful translation. For example, if a translation project focuses on changing practice and ensuring that caregivers are aware of evidence, then the assessment would measure caregiver's knowledge of that evidence.

Interviews or focus groups could also be used as an assessment. This approach leads to an understanding of the needs of a group and has the potential to yield rich qualitative data. It also allows the evaluator to adapt the assessment based on feedback from the group. Exemplar 20.5 provides a summary of a translation project that involved focus groups, which helped to identify learning needs of individuals in the target population.

Assessment might also take the form of a test that could be presented online or on paper. This approach would provide quantitative data to measure individual knowledge as well as the collective knowledge of a group. It can be used to identify gaps in knowledge, which focuses the content and instructional design. Useful to assess patients and caregivers alike, this approach provides data that can be linked before and after instruction to evaluate its effectiveness. Exemplar 20.6 provides an example of a translation project that began with a knowledge assessment in the form of a test.

If testing is to be conducted, the construction of that test is important. Test items are most effective and most fair when they relate directly to the learning objectives and evidence. This allows assessment of the knowledge, beliefs, and attitudes relevant to the evidence and goals of the translation project. Assessment of important knowledge should be the focus of the test. Generally, it is useful to ensure that each item evaluates a different concept from the evidence to be translated. Presenting a set of questions with multiple options (multiple-choice questions) enables the evaluation of each learner's ability to discriminate knowledge of the evidence-based practice from those practices no longer supported by evidence. Exhibit 13.1 presents a checklist of the best practices for test construction.

The learner is also to be considered in the development of the test. Specifically, the reading level and experience of the learner are relevant. A common practice is to prepare test questions and educational materials at a sixth-grade reading level, which can be accomplished using one of many online text-readability resources.

It is during the assessment phase that pedagogy is determined, based on the needs and preferences of the learner. Context must be considered during the initial

EXHIBIT 13.1 **Test Construction Checklist for Multiple-Choice Items**

The Stem	Notes
Use clear simple language.	
Test important information.	
Be grammatically correct.	
Make a positive assertion.	
Present a single coherent idea.	
Answer Options	
Avoid hints in grammar.	
Be sure there is a correct or best option.	
Make distractors plausible.	
Avoid "all of the above."	
Avoid "none of the above."	
Length of options should be consistent.	
Randomly place correct option among distracters.	
Make items independent.	

Source: Adapted from Brame, C. J. (2013). *Writing good multiple choice test questions*. Nashville, TN: Vanderbilt University. Retrieved from https://cft.vanderbilt.edu/guides-sub-pages/writing-good-multiple-choice-test-questions

assessment as well. The designer needs to understand the available resources (people, material, technology), competing priorities or confounding concerns (e.g., concurrent introduction of electronic health record or physical relocation), timeline, and fiscal pressures. All inform decisions about design, development, and implementation.

Design

The second phase in the ADDIE model involves design of the instruction. Here, learning objectives are set. The learning experience (which includes content based on the evidence; methods, materials, and media to be used for instruction and evaluation of learning; and the instruction plan) is developed during this phase. All design is conducted with the learner and the desired end in mind.

Learning Objectives

Clear objectives are set based on the identified gaps between the actual and the target knowledge base. These lead to planning the learning experience and then follow to execution and evaluation. Well-written learning objectives clearly state what the learner will accomplish as a result of the education. They undergird all instructions and help to convey the nature of the change to be accomplished. Bloom identified three kinds of related learning and referred to these as *learning domains*: cognitive, affective, and psychomotor (Bloom, 1994; Bloom, Engelhart, Furst, Hill, & Krathwohl, 1956; Krathwohl, Bloom, & Masia, 1964). According to Bloom and colleagues, some learning is cognitive in nature, which means its purpose is to change knowledge, understanding, application, analysis, synthesis, or evaluation. Other learning is affective, which means its intent is to change the way one receives, responds to, values, organizes, or characterizes information. Still other learning is psychomotor in nature, which means its intent is to change perception and guide physical response. Psychomotor learning targets change in behavior or action. Commonly based on Bloom's taxonomy, learning objectives establish the domain of the learning to be targeted. Having specified whether the intended learning is cognitive, affective, or behavioral in nature, the instruction can be designed to accomplish the intended learning and to elicit evidence of the targeted change as an evaluation of learning as well as an evaluation of instruction. A recent version of Bloom's taxonomy is presented in Figure 13.1.

Design of Instruction and the Learning Experience

The learning objectives direct design of the instruction and promote an effective experience for the intended learner. Gagné, Briggs, and Wagner (1988) and Gagné (1985) described a nine-step process to structure the learning experience and support

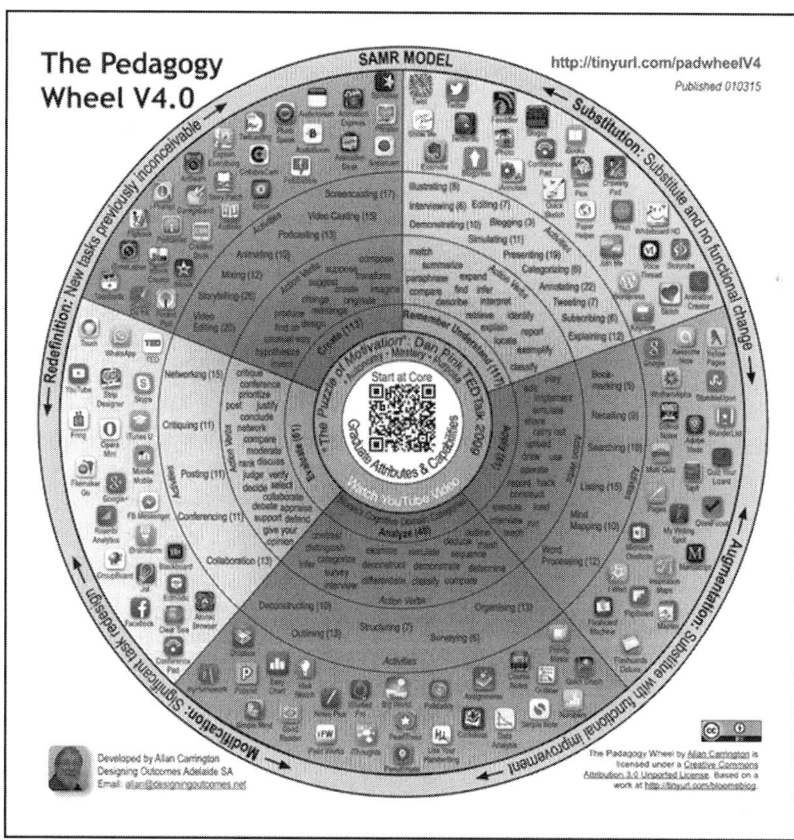

FIGURE 13.1 Bloom's taxonomy as updated.SAMR, substitution, augmentation, modification, redefinition; TED, technology/education/design.

Source: From Carrington, A. (n.d.). The pedagogy wheel, v4.0. Retrieved from https://designingoutcomes.com/the-padagogy-wheel-its-a-bloomin-better-way-to-teach

design. This approach remains popular today because it has been so effective over time. The nine steps lead to both development and deployment of instruction. They guide the educator through a logical approach based on cognitive theory.

Gain the Learner's Attention

The first step is to gain the attention of the learner. Common approaches include telling a story, presenting a case, showing a video, introducing a problem, describing a challenge, taking a survey online, or posing a question. All these examples are activities that bring the focus of the learner to the intended learning. These activities are commonly called *icebreakers* and are used to gain attention and energize the learner. Like all aspects of the instructional design, these opening activities will be most effective when directly related to the learning objectives. Any opening activity or icebreaker should be carefully selected, well planned, and well executed to ensure that the time devoted to the activity adds value to the learning.

Present the Learning Objective

The second step is to present the learning objective. This involves making explicit what is to be learned or mastered during the instruction. This step provides the opportunity to set expectations about the information to be covered and can be accomplished using discussion, survey, planned activity, or some other approach. Presenting the objective helps move learning from the abstract to the specific and allows refinement of the objective if necessary.

Recall Prior Learning

The third step is to recall prior learning. This involves activating memory with which to link new information and experience. In this step, what is known by the learner is reviewed and recognized by the instructor. This can be accomplished using images, documents, discussions, cases, simulations, or other strategies. The act of recalling prior learning helps the learner to ground new knowledge in memory and experience; it facilitates making connections between the familiar and the unfamiliar. In the case of translation, it helps identify assumptions and biases based on experience, so that the review of the evidence can directly replace outdated science or knowledge.

Present Learning Stimulus

The fourth step is to present the stimulus, which involves a more precise and detailed presentation of new information or experience. This step could involve introduction of a definition, a tool, an instrument, or some other practical, tangible item that represents the new information. In the case of translation, the stimulus is the new evidence. New tools, resources, documents, or other methods for translation could be presented at this point. It is critical that the learner have the opportunity to hear the new evidence to be translated.

Guide Learning

The fifth step is to guide learning. This is the experience planned to amplify, clarify, and expand understanding. Therefore, the learner is able to interact more deeply with the stimuli presented in step 4. This might involve group discussion, simulation, practice, lecture, or another instructional method. In the case of translation, especially with professionals, it is constructive to facilitate some conversation about the practices that the evidence refutes or displaces. Adult learners may be challenged to replace traditional practices they have used over time. They need to engage in a variety of learning experiences suited to their learning styles and goals because the intent will be to change knowledge and behavior, and this requires deep learning.

Assess Performance

The sixth step is to assess performance. In this step, the instructor provides a challenge that requires the learner to demonstrate learning or mastery. This might be a test, a discussion, or a simulation. Its focus will be to determine the learner's understanding or mastery of the important content or skills. This assessment then can lead the instructor to clarify, amplify, correct, or reinforce the content to be learned.

The final step is to enhance retention and transfer of knowledge. Commonly forgotten, this step provides an opportunity to reinforce learning with a focus on sustained change. This might involve review of content, simulation, group activity, or a debriefing.

All steps in the process are linked to the learning objectives. Beginning with gaining attention and ending with enhancing retention, the entire instructional design is developed and deployed with a clear focus that is learner specific and essential to changing practice and outcomes.

Development

The third phase in the ADDIE model is development. This phase involves creation of the content and materials to be used during instruction. When the instruction is intended to support translation, these materials and tools must ensure that strong evidence is accurately transmitted. These materials may be used by a number of teachers across a variety of settings and must ensure fidelity to the translation plan. It is useful to describe each learning objective, map the related content derived from the evidence, assign the time to be allocated to presenting that content, describe in detail the method for conveyance, make explicit any tools or technology associated with each learning objective, and describe all associated learner engagement or activities. A planning guide is presented in Exhibit 13.2.

Implementation

The fourth phase in the ADDIE model is implementation. This phase involves presentation of the content in keeping with the instructional design plan. Individuals who will present the education must be introduced to the instructional design through some form of training event. They will require opportunities to experience the plan

EXHIBIT 13.2 Tool for Planning Instruction

Learning Objective	Time	Evidence-Based Content	Method of Instruction	Learning Activities	References
1					
2					
3					
4					

and interact with the materials in advance of presenting it. The goal is to ensure consistency in instruction, fidelity to the design and the evidence, and delivery of high-quality instruction.

Face-to-face, online, and blended instructions are widely used to deliver content and support learning. All have widely penetrated higher education and professional development. In healthcare, self-paced learning, print materials, and multimedia approaches are commonly used as well. Regardless of the mode of delivery, the goal is to support substantial learner engagement with the content and always maintain the expectation of providing safe, contemporary, quality care (Phillips, 2005). In professional development, it is common that all the participants have access to a common information system, which makes online instruction practical, accessible, and user-friendly. Online instruction can be made available across shifts and disciplines, and the metrics available through the technology platforms are useful to support compliance with regulatory requirements. These are all important considerations when planning and deploying instruction (Niebuhr, Niebuhr, Trumble, & Urbani, 2014).

The goal is always to provide a learner-centered experience that facilitates active engagement with the instruction (Phillips, 2005). This active and engaged learning is based on seven principles described by Chickering and Gamson (1987), who encourage all educators to do the following:

1. Be ambitious and set high expectations.
2. Promote reciprocity and cooperation with and between learners to deepen learning.
3. Ensure engagement, which accelerates learning.
4. Stay on task and help learners do the same because time engaged with new content is key to success.
5. Give feedback, do it regularly, make it interactive, and focus on growth.
6. Interact with the learner, do so often, keep it on point, and connect to learners' goals.
7. Respect diversity and actively demonstrate respect for differences in race, ethnicity, age, learning style, experience, and much more.

Keeping these foundational principles in mind, the instructional methods and designs should be informed and improved by ongoing feedback from learners.

Evaluation

The final phase in the ADDIE model is evaluation. This involves providing some challenge that asks the learner to demonstrate attainment of the learning objectives. Evaluation helps to determine both the effectiveness of the instruction and the readiness of the learner for the change in practice that is the goal of translation. Qualitative methods (focus groups or interviews) or quantitative methods (testing) may be used during evaluation, just as they were used during preliminary assessment. When the challenge presented following instruction matches the challenge presented during analysis in phase 1, then comparison of scores allows robust evaluation commonly conducted using some comparison of means.

With online learning, a variety of metrics are available, including the number of posts, the length of the posts, and the extent to which these posts meet the intent of the discussion board. These measures, easily gathered using technology, may not be the best indicator of learning, but may be valuable in determining the number of people who participated in an educational program (Mazzolini & Maddison, 2007).

■ INSTRUCTIONAL TECHNOLOGY

Dramatic and expansive changes in healthcare, the swift pace at which science proceeds, and the explosion of technology at our fingertips define the context of healthcare today. It has become easy to access facts, but tricky to find trustworthy, actionable information in the perpetual stream of data. Public forums outside healthcare, like TED (technology/education/design) Talks, have transformed education and the expectations of learners forever. These programs have simultaneously stepped up the game for educators and appealed to the skills and affinities of millennials and nexters, who have grown up in a world of technology and information that is available with just a few key strikes. Today, learners want education to be accessible, scholarly, current, and interactive. They expect high production value in the materials and rock stars for educators. They expect learning opportunities to be available on demand, precisely when and where they are needed; to be offered in ways that appeal to different learning styles; and to allow selection of content that connects directly to an immediate need or interest. Learners expect education to be useful, culturally respectful, and engaging. That it should be scholarly, reliable, and accurate is assumed.

Learning can happen one-on-one during interactions between caregivers and learners or it can happen in groups of varying sizes. It can happen at bedsides, in classrooms, or online. Instruction can be provided face-to-face when time with and proximity to the learner are possible. Otherwise, it can happen over great distance, allowing healthcare professionals to teach or reinforce teaching to remote patients and caregivers. Regardless, the context and purpose of the instruction inform its design, implementation, and evaluation.

Technology can be used to teach, remind, influence, practice, shape, and monitor both knowledge and health behavior. Though less familiar and often less comfortable, technology can also serve the same function for those not so young. Then, when it is viewed as useful, it will become less peculiar and even more useful.

■ ONLINE LEARNING

The young have grown up with technologies that were designed for them, improved by their feedback, and suited precisely to their needs and habits. They are natives of digital culture, language, and ways of thinking. Many academics are more likely to be immigrants to the tech culture and have been slow to embrace online learning in higher education. Inexperience with learning technologies and bias toward familiar systems have contributed to this discrepancy in proficiency and comfort with technology-enabled and distance learning modalities.

Online learning can be framed as simply the latest step in the evolution of distance education, which originated in the form of correspondence programs (via postal service in 1728 and 1840), morphed into radio programming (1894 and 1936) and subsequently television programming when President Hoover (1927) proclaimed that "*Human genius has now destroyed the impediment of distance in a new respect, and in a manner hitherto unknown,*" and most recent, online or Internet programming holds promise to transform ("Hoover Seen and Heard," 1927, p. 10; Kentnor, 2015). Regardless of the target population, the goal is to provide information that is accessible, convenient, and controlled for quality. The idea suits the needs of disabled and homebound (patients), the overextended (parents, working students, family members of the sick, and healthcare providers alike), and the geographically challenged (those in military service or members of other diaspora).

CONCLUSIONS

Instruction of patients, families, communities, and clinicians is routinely essential to effective translation work. This chapter presents a set of practices, supported by evidence and expert opinion, that are useful in efforts to change the knowledge, attitudes, and practices of clinicians and those in our care. These include working backward from clear learning objectives suited precisely to the learner, using a methodical approach to planning and design, developing instruction that achieves optimal engagement with the content and the experience of learning, making the most of technologies and media, and creating a safe and respectful environment in which to learn.

The evidence applies to instruction in all its forms: face-to-face, online, and blended. In each situation, the means by which the evidence is applied may vary. For example, on-line instruction is making advances in organization, design, and engagement that can benefit face-to-face instruction. On the other hand, face-to-face instruction can set the bar for expectations of engagement with faculty and classmates. Each can inform and improve the other. Each form can advance the purposes and aims of the teams engaged in translation.

Nonetheless, it is important to keep in mind that providing instruction about what is to be learned from the evidence is often essential to successful translation and to ensuring fidelity with the recommendations of strong evidence. However, education alone cannot be expected to change practice or to improve clinical outcomes. For this reason, education on its own does not suffice as a translation project.

REFERENCES

Alexander, P. A. (2003). Development of expertise: The journey from acclimation to proficiency. *Educational Researcher*, *32*(8), 10–14. doi:10.3102/0013189x032008010

Allen, E., & Seaman, J. (2015). *Grade level: Tracking online education in the United States*. Babson Park, MA: Babson Survey Research Group & Quahog Research Group.

Bandura, A. (1997). *Social learning theory*. Englewood Cliffs, NJ: Prentice Hall.

Bloom, B. S. (1994). Reflections on the development and use of the taxonomy. In K. J. Rehage, L. W. Anderson, & L. A. Sosniak (Eds.), *Bloom's taxonomy: A forty-year retrospective* (*Yearbook of the National Society for the Study of Education*). Chicago, IL: National Society for the Study of Education.

Bloom, B. S., Engelhart, M. D., Furst, E. J., Hill, W. H., & Krathwohl, D. R. (1956). *Taxonomy of educational objectives: The classification of educational goals. Handbook I: Cognitive domain*. New York, NY: David McKay Company.

Brame, C. J. (2013). *Writing good multiple choice test questions*. Nashville, TN: Vanderbilt University. Retrieved from https://cft.vanderbilt.edu/guides-sub-pages/writing-good-multiple-choice-test-questions

Branson, R. K., Rayner, G. T., Cox, J. L., Furman, J. P., King, F. J., & Hannum, W. H. (1975). *Interservice procedures for instructional systems development*. (5 vols.) (TRADOC Pam 350-30 NAVEDTRA 106A). Ft. Monroe, VA: U.S. Army Training and Doctrine Command, August 1975. (NTIS No. ADA 019 486 through ADA 019 490).

Carrington, A. (n.d.). The pedagogy wheel, v4.0. Retrieved from https://designingoutcomes.com/the-padagogy-wheel-its-a-bloomin-better-way-to-teach

Chickering, A. W., & Gamson, Z. F. (1987). Seven principles for good practice in undergraduate education. *American Association for Health Education Bulletin*, *39*(7), 3–6.

Cox, M., & Naylor, M. (2013). *Transforming patient care: Aligning interprofessional education with clinical practice redesign*. New York, NY: Josiah Macy Jr. Foundation.

Felder, R. M., & Brent, R. (2005). Understanding student differences. *Journal of Engineering Education, 94*(1), 57–72. doi:10.1002/j.2168-9830.2005.tb00829.x

Gagné, R. (1985). *The conditions of learning and the theory of instruction* (4th ed.). New York, NY: Holt, Rinehart, & Winston.

Gagné, R. M., Briggs, L. J., & Wagner, W. W. (1988). *Principles of instructional design*. New York, NY: Holt, Rinehart, & Winston.

Hayes, J., & Allinson, C. W. (1996). The implications of learning styles for training and development: A discussion of the matching hypothesis. *British Journal of Management, 7(1)*, 63–73. doi:10.1111/j.1467-8551.1996.tb00106.x

Hoover seen and heard 200 miles: Test of television may mean general use of seeming miracle. (1927, April 8). *Cleveland Plain Dealer*, p. 10.

Interprofessional Education Collaborative Expert Panel. (2011). *Core competencies for interprofessional collaborative practice: Report of an expert panel*. Washington, DC: Interprofessional Education Collaborative.

Keefe, J. W. (1979). Learning style: An overview. In J. W. Keefe (Ed.), *Student learning style: Diagnosing and prescribing programs*. Reston, VA: National Association of Secondary School Principals.

Kentnor, H. (2015). Distance education and the evolution of online learning in the United States. *Curriculum & Teaching Dialogue*. 17(1 & 2), 21–000.

King, A. (1993). From sage on the stage to guide on the side. *College Teaching, 41*(1), 30–35. doi:10.1080/87567555.1993.9926781

Knowles, M. S. (1980). *The modern practice of adult education: From pedagogy to andragogy*. Chicago, IL: Follett.

Krathwohl, D. R., Bloom, B. S., & Masia, B. B. (1964). Taxonomy of educational objectives: The classification of educational goals. In *Handbook II: The affective domain*. New York, NY: David McKay Company.

Lowyck, J., & Poysa, J. (2001). Design collaborative learning environments. *Computers in Human Behavior, 17(5–6)*, 507–516. doi:10.1016/s0747-5632(01)00017-6

Mazzolini, M., & Maddison, S. (2003). Sage, guide, or ghost? The effect of instructor intervention on student participation in online discussion forums. *Computers & Education, 40*(3), 237–253. doi:10.1016/s0360-1315(02)00129-x

Mazzolini, M., & Maddison, S. (2007). When to jump in: The role of the instructor in online discussion forums. *Computers & Education, 49*(2), 193–213. doi:10.1016/j.compedu.2005.06.011

Niebuhr, V., Niebuhr, B., Trumble, J., & Urbani, M. J. (2014). Online faculty development for creating e-learning materials. *Education for Health, 27*(3), 255–261. doi:10.4103/1357-6283.152186

Phillips, J. M. (2005). Strategies for active learning in online continuing education. *Journal of Continuing Education in Nursing, 36*(2), 77–83. doi:10.3928/0022-0124-20050301-08

Russell, S. S. (2006). An overview of adult-learning processes. *Urologic Nursing, 26*(5), 349–370.

University College of Dublin Adult Education Centre. (2019). *Our work. UDA access and lifelong learning*. Dublin, Ireland: University College of Dublin. Retrieved from http://www.ucd.ie/all/ourwork

Watkins, C., & Mortimer, P. (1999). Pedagogy: What do we know? In P. Mortimer (Ed.), *Understanding pedagogy and its impact on teaching* (pp. 1–19). London, UK: Chapman.

Wick, C., Pollock, R., Jefferson, A., & Flanagan, R. (2006). *Six disciplines of breakthrough learning: How to turn training and development into business results*. San Francisco, CA: Pfeiffer.

Wiggins, G., & McTighe, J. (2004). What is backward design? In *Understanding design: Professional development workbook*. Alexandria, VA: Association for Supervision and Curriculum Development .

World Health Organization. (2010). *Framework for action on interprofessional education and collaborative practice*. Geneva, Switzerland: Author.

CHAPTER FOURTEEN

Information Technology: A Foundation for Translation

Marisa L. Wilson

By focusing on "meaningful use," we recognize that better health care does not come solely from the adoption of technology itself, but through the exchange and use of health information to best inform clinical decisions at the point of care.
—David Blumenthal, MD

The Use of Health Information Technology (HIT) and informatics processes is fundamental to the collection of data, creation of information, and development and dissemination of knowledge, all of which are critical to safe and effective patient care. It is essential that the DNP leader understand that the use of information technology will be fundamental to her or his work in justifying the existence of an issue or gap, determining the best evidence to support a solution, measuring and monitoring impact, and supporting the dissemination of best practices. As this text focuses on translation, this chapter specifically describes the ability of HIT and informatics processes to support translation of evidence into practice.

Information technology comprises the tools to create and store evidence. The information technology infrastructure of hardware, software, networks, and databases allows clinicians to collect, store, and transmit data from the point of care to other providers who are essential in the support of the patient or consumer. Information technology assists the DNP to find evidence through focused searches. The large databases housing publications, systematic reviews, electronic textbooks, and decision-support systems are used by the DNP leader to generate translatable evidence. Informatics processes that denote the representation, processing, and communication of data are tools for the DNP to convert data collected at the point of care into information and knowledge that drive better, higher quality, safer care.

Current legislation and federal mandates, including *Meaningful Use (MU),* required by the Health Information Technology for Economic and Clinical Health (HITECH) Act under the American Recovery and Reinvestment Act of 2009, supported efforts to design and implement interoperable HIT systems across all phases of the patient–consumer trajectory. These HIT systems constitute the backbone of healthcare reform and promote patient engagement. They are vital to the success of the Triple Aim: improved quality, better efficiency, and cost reduction.

MU is the name of the three-stage process for healthcare reform based on technology and innovation. The first stage promoted the capture and sharing of patient data through the adoption of certified electronic health records (EHRs); the second applied the data to improve processes through clinical decision support (CDS), care coordination, and patient engagement; and the third delivered outcomes through increased use of CDS and health information exchange (HealthIT.gov, 2019b). MU had significant impact on the proliferation of EHRs in acute care and office-based settings, which provides a foundation for the ability to collect data and dissemination of DNP evidence. According to the Office of the National Coordinator (2019), in 2017, nearly nine out of 10 providers had adopted an EHR and over 96% of all nonfederal acute care facilities had adopted an EHR (HealthIT.gov, 2019a). Therefore, as a result of the phases of MU, the tools that are available in most clinical spaces have been further strengthened with the introduction of the Medicare Access and CHIP Reauthorization Act (MACRA). MACRA transitioned MU into one of the four components of the Merit-Based Incentive Payment System (MIPS), which promotes quality, cost, interoperability, and improvement activities (HealthIT.gov, 2019b).

As part of Stages 1 and 2 of MU, these certified EHRs must be able to incorporate CDS tools. CDS interventions in the second stage of MU were required to address four or more clinical quality measures that help quantify healthcare processes and outcomes. These include patient perceptions, organizational structures, and/or systems associated with the provision of high-quality healthcare, and relate to one or more quality goals for healthcare (Centers for Medicare & Medicaid Services [CMS], 2014). The mandate of MU, together with the open definition of *quality measures* proffered by the CMS, justifies the use of CDS beyond generation of basic alerts. Well designed and deployed, the CDS tools offer providers a viable means to insert evidence where it is needed, which is in the provision of direct patient care.

This chapter explains CDS in the context of the healthcare process and also explains how CDS can facilitate technologically mediated translation for the uptake of evidence at the point of care. Familiar to many clinicians as drug alerts that "pop up" during the order entry process, CDS has far greater potential to deliver evidence to guide care because the variety of tools is far more nuanced and complex. CDS tools that go beyond these familiar alerts are introduced. The technological and organizational considerations required to create CDS tools for translation are briefly described. Finally, the role CDS can play in improving care is highlighted using examples.

■ WORKING DEFINITION OF *CDS*

CDS has been defined as software that directly facilitates clinical decisions. The logic is simple. Characteristics of an individual patient are matched to a clinical knowledge base. Then, recommendations are presented to the clinician and/or patient, who retain responsibility for a decision and plan of action (Sim et al., 2001). CDS systems provide users with alternatives as well as information on which to base an informed decision.

CDS encompasses a broad set of HIT functions that build on the repository of information in the EHR to provide persons involved in the care process with evidence-based, clinically appropriate, person-specific knowledge based on patient information that has been intelligently filtered and presented at the appropriate time in the workflow to enhance care (Department of Health and Human Services [HHS], 2010; Osheroff, Pifer, Teich, Sittig, & Jenders, 2005).

CDS should not be viewed simply as a technology or as a substitute for critical thinking, but as a complex intervention that requires careful consideration of the goals, the delivery, the recipient, and the point in time when it appears, for maximum impact (Berner, 2009). This definition indicates that CDS tools can be developed not only for doctors, nurse practitioners, and nurses, but also for the support staff, patients, caregivers, and populations. Consider the use of alerts sent electronically to patients reminding them of tests that need to be conducted based on their demographics or messages sent to provide instruction on home medication regimens.

The Health and Medicine Division (of the National Academies of Sciences, Engineering, and Medicine) has long recognized problems with healthcare quality in the United States and has, for over a decade, advocated the use of HIT applications with CDS to improve care (Institute of Medicine [IOM], 2001). When applied effectively, CDS can increase the quality of care, improve health outcomes, reduce the chance of errors and adverse events, improve efficiency, reduce cost, and increase patient satisfaction (CMS, 2014; Osheroff et al., 2007).

CDS tools can support care across a variety of settings, including acute, post-acute, ambulatory, and long term. They can be used in population and public health settings. Innovative CDS tools that meet the criteria for MU include those that support care in all settings.

CDS TOOLS

CDS is not just an alert, notification, or care plan, but encompasses a variety of tools that need to be selected based on the individual clinical situation (CMS, 2014). As technology develops and becomes more pervasive in practice, CDS tools and interventions will mature and change. At this time, with the current state of product development, CDS tools include the following (Osheroff et al., 2012):

1. Immediate alerts for patients and providers offering warnings or critiques
2. Event-driven alerts and reminders for patients and providers
3. Parameter guidance for providers
4. Condition- or diagnosis-specific order sets, care plans, and protocols
5. Smart documentation forms and templates
6. Condition-specific guidelines

7. Single patient-relevant data summaries
8. Multipatient real-time monitors and dashboards
9. Predictive and retrospective data-analytics reports
10. Contextually relevant and filtered reference information and knowledge resources
11. Expert workup advisories

In addition to the variety of tools available, there are varying information technology architectures for CDS that influence design, build, implementation, and adoption. Decisions related to architecture have to be made in consultation with the chief information officer and other stakeholders in the information technology department who oversee the EHR and available resources. CDS architectures are described by Velickovski et al. (2014) as follows:

1. Stand-alone and not integrated at all with the EHR or HIT, thus requiring the user to input all patient-specific data
2. Integrated completely within the EHR or HIT, thus requiring fewer data-input demands on the user and promoting a more proactive approach
3. Standards based, which separates the CDS from the EHR but requires interoperability through the standardization of computer-interpretable guidelines
4. Service oriented, which separates the CDS from the EHR but integrates the functions by interfacing the CDS and the EHR through data transfer, often through a web-service protocol handling the data exchange

Architecture affects each user, the technology, and cognitive processes differently. Regardless of tool or architecture, CDS is intended to remind users of things that need to be done, provide information for those who are unsure, correct errors, and/or make recommendations in real time and within an appropriate workflow supporting decision-making (Berner, 2009).

■ THE FIVE Rs OF CDS

As one thinks about the CDS options that may be appropriate for a specific patient or population or clinician, consideration of a CDS best practice framework is helpful. Just as there are a set of rights that guide medication administration, so, too, there are rights to guide CDS. The five Rs of CDS should guide selection of the specific tool to be used as a translation method and include the following (Osheroff et al., 2012):

1. The *right information* in the form of correct guidance or response to a clinical need must be provided in a usable format.
2. The *right person* or *people* must receive the information and this may include providers, support staff, teams, the patient or consumer, and other caregivers.
3. The *right channel* or platform must be developed (consider the EHR, mobile device, monitor, report, portal).

4. The *right intervention* must be selected and this may include order sets, templates, flow sheets, dashboards, lists, alerts, and reminders.
5. Information must be provided at the *right point* in the workflow when making decisions or planning an action.

CDS has to be relevant for those affected by the decision and those who can act on the information. As the CDS is planned and developed, one must consider what the type of evidence to be translated is, who will act on that information, how they will act on it, and in what way the evidence will be used to complete or trigger an action.

When deciding on a CDS tool, one must consider the timing of information provided. CDS can be interruptive, informative, or targeted. The CDS tool can interrupt the decision maker in the process, it can just inform the decision maker about population parameters in either a push-or-pull format, or it can be targeted to a specific patient about whom the clinician is making a decision. In addition, the CDS tool design can differ with respect to how much control the user will have to see the information or not and to use the information or override it. CDS can be set up to display information on demand, allowing the user full control over the choice to access it, the circumstances under which to view the information, and the choice to accept it (Berner, 2009).

CDS tools can be either active or passive. An active CDS presents or "pushes" information to the clinician. This information compares available patient information with programmed rules, protocols, and guidelines by utilizing a knowledge base, available patient information, or inference engine (McCartney, 2007). A passive CDS presents resources for the clinician to access through a link if further information is desired. This passive CDS is initiated by the clinician, on demand, or "pulled" by clicking on links or guidelines (Horsky et al., 2012; McCartney, 2007).

■ OPERATIONALIZING CDS

In preparing to create a CDS as a method to translate evidence into care, some preliminary steps have to be taken. First, a scope of the clinical question has to be developed. Knowledge around clinical concern has to be identified, synthesized, and rated (Lang, 2008). Data have to be gathered, analyzed, and presented in a way that suggests how the problem is framed and allows the problem to be identified when it presents (Roberts & Tsevat, 2011). The developer of the CDS tool has to be very clear about the parameters around which the system will "know" the presenting problem for which a decision is needed. This will require the developer/practitioner to clearly stipulate the data cues that perhaps will include things like specific diagnoses, laboratory results, radiology results, assessments, and other pertinent findings. Knowledge then has to be synthesized into something that can quickly be presented, based on the application of that data. Then, from the synthesis, a determination of action has to be developed and translated into discreet, meaningful, and actionable data elements that represent the response options for clinicians (Lang, 2008). This may be interventions, medications to be prescribed, or education to be delivered. The developer/practitioner will then need to decide whether the decision support offered can be overridden and how this override is to be documented.

This means clinicians who want to use CDS as a method for translation need access to reliable, accurate patient data to trigger the CDS when needed. Patient demographics, diagnosis codes, test results, or medication lists may be the data triggers. All need to be accurately, completely, and efficiently captured in a standardized format that can be read by the computer. This process requires the clinician to investigate the appropriate standardized terms and data elements that will be used to capture the problem and response. If data are not being captured in a discreet way within the EHR, then this must be changed because CDS relies on discreet, standardized, trustworthy data elements.

Next, the clinical problem has to be structured into a decision model that represents the core components of the problem and the actions from which to choose when confronted with the problem. In a clinical situation, this may include not one, but several alternative solutions (Roberts & Tsevat, 2011). This process of developing the decision model will create a decision tree with sufficient detail to allow construction, validation, and presentation of the CDS model to support meaningful user interactions (Roberts & Tsevat, 2011). Probabilities need to be assigned to the pathways on the tree, so that the most advantageous responses can be clearly presented and, conversely, gaps can be identified and addressed. Creation of an EHR-based CDS requires substantial modeling activity. Modeling includes deciding what clinical data and patient data are relevant. These data are used to identify concepts and relationships among the concepts relevant to decision-making and then to ascertain the problem strategy that can use clinical knowledge to reach an appropriate conclusion (Musen, Shahar, & Shortliffe, 2006). This synthesized knowledge is transformed into practice recommendations, interventions, and outcomes. Synthesized knowledge becomes actionable in this modeling process (Lang, 2008).

■ ORGANIZATIONAL PROCESS FOR CDS IMPLEMENTATION

In order for CDS to be optimally used to deliver evidence at the point of care, it has to fit into the workflow. CDS prompts have to be presented at a point in time when decisions are being made (Castillo & Kelemen, 2013). *Workflow* refers to the structure or work system features and processes that support care (Carayon et al., 2006). CDS cannot be placed into an existing workflow without proper attention to what is actually happening during the care process, how decisions are being made, who is making the decisions, and how all of the participants, including the patient, can be involved. This requires a thorough study of current and potential actions that are occurring with the understanding that this will most likely result in an iterative-process redesign. Redesign efforts mandate concerted analysis of existing flows and development of new flows that will exist after the CDS has been implemented with the participation of clinicians involved to ensure uptake (Al-Badareen, Selamat, Samat, Nazira, & Akkanat, 2014). Often, during preliminary study, it is determined that the workflow has to be adapted, particularly if the baseline is inefficient or ineffective. This is essential when the CDS introduces new patterns of communication or decision-making into the process. Moreover, CDS has to be minimally disruptive to cognitive processes in order to support critical thinking and must neither disrupt nor overwhelm. The unintended consequences of overwhelming cognitive processes have been well documented in the phenomenon of alert fatigue, which often results in a CDS being turned off or ignored. The prevalence of disruptions that are minimally important interferes with the thinking and the action of the clinician (Cvach, 2012; Cvach, Currie, Sapirstein, Doyle, & Pronovost, 2013).

Developing, engineering, and maintaining currency of knowledge, guidelines, and best practices that must evolve over time become critical organizational challenges (Wright, Sittig, Ash, Bates, et al., 2011). Maintenance of knowledge that is embedded within the CDS has to be managed over time. Because knowledge and evidence are always expanding, because new drugs and treatments are being developed, and because guidelines change over time (Berner, 2009), knowledge management processes have to be planned in order to keep the CDS and what is driving it updated and relevant (Ash et al., 2010).

■ EVALUATION OF CDS

A plan for continuous evaluation has also to be organized. Results from CDS alerts or interventions must be tracked and refined over time. In determining what to evaluate and measure, one must be sure to think inclusively. Evaluation measures must align with the original aims of the translation and correspond to other organizational goals, objectives, and activities in order to determine direct and indirect impact of the CDS. For each CDS intervention, a plan for identifying, tracking, and addressing the availability, use by the target, and usability is essential (Osheroff et al., 2012). Looking for unintended consequences, unintended behavior, workarounds, and indirect outcomes is integral to good evaluation. Evaluation is an ongoing process that has to be considered from the initial planning stages of the translation and intervention.

■ EXAMPLES OF CDS

There are currently excellent examples of CDS used to translate the work of the DNP as a method of best practice dissemination. Alford, Alexander, and Barr (2018), optimized CDS tools to improve the care of older adults with diabetes mellitus type 2. Kirby, Kruger, Jaine, O'Hair, and Granger (2018) utilized the power of CDS tools to improve referral rates for patients with symptomatic aortic stenosis. Both of these projects embedded a synthesis of evidence into an information technology with consideration to the workflow, message, audience, and the evaluation strategy. The CDS tool selected was a method of translation that has a target phase of care that may be prevention, diagnosis, treatment, intervention, or follow-up. Each target requires different knowledge and workflow considerations. Table 14.1 outlines some examples of CDS tools with their targets.

TABLE 14.1 Clinical Decision-Support Targets and Actions

CDS Target of Care	CDS Example
Prevention	Immunization, screenings, disease management, guidelines for care, cessation reminders, order reminders
Diagnosis	Comparison of patient data to system knowledge base in order to present potential diagnoses from which to choose
Treatment	Treatment guidelines for specific diagnoses, daily or lifetime drug dose recommendations, alerts, choosing among alternatives
Follow-up	Appointment reminders, adverse event reporting, ancillary orders triggered by primary order (lab tests following medication administration)
Provider efficiency	Care plans, order sets, documentation templates, smart templates
Cost reduction	Duplicate test alerts, drug formulary guidelines

CDS, clinical decision support.

Source: Adapted from Berner, E. S. (2009, June). *Clinical decision support systems: State of the art* (Publication number 09-0069-EF). Rockville, MD: Agency for Healthcare Research and Quality.

The target CDS tool selected will also be categorized into decision-support type. Medication ordering, order-process facilitators, alerts, information displays, workflow support, and expert decision-making are some of the categories. Table 14.2 lists these categories and some corresponding CDS tools.

The state, context, and technology of CDS are not static and continue to develop as advances are made. Some specific resources will provide guidance over time despite change and should be considered as decision support for CDS development. Table 14.3 provides a list of CDS resources.

TABLE 14.2 Clinical Decision-Support Categories and Tools

CDS Category	CDS Tool Example
Medication dosing support	Dose recommendations and adjustments
	Formulary checking against an order
	Single-dose range checking
	Maximum daily dose checking
	Maximum lifetime dose checking
	Default doses for specific drugs based on diagnosis or reason
	Indication-based dosing

(continued)

TABLE 14.2 Clinical Decision-Support Categories and Tools (*continued*)

CDS Category	CDS Tool Example
Ordering facilitators	Medication order sentences
	Corollary orders that must go with a primary order
	Indication-based ordering based on assessment or diagnosis
	Service-specific order sets based on specialty
	Condition-specific order sets based on diagnosis
	Procedure-specific order sets based on CPT code
	Condition-specific treatment protocols
	Transfer order sets such as when a patient is moved from ICU to lower level of care or at discharge
	Nonmedication order sets
Point-of-care alerts	Drug–condition interaction reminders
	Drug–drug interaction
	Drug–allergy interactions
	Plan-of-care alerts such as the need for glucose monitoring
	Critical lab values alerts
	Duplicate order checking
	Care reminders
	Tickler lists for tasks needing to be done
	Radiology ordering support
	High-risk-state monitoring
Relevant information display	Context-sensitive information retrieval
	Patient-specific relevant data displays
	Medication/test cost displays
	Context-sensitive user interface
Expert systems	Antibiotic-ordering support
	Ventilator support
	Diagnostic support
	Risk assessment tools
	Transfusion support
	Nutrition-ordering support
	Lab test interpretation
	Syndromic surveillance
	Image recognition and interpretation

(*continued*)

TABLE 14.2 Clinical Decision-Support Categories and Tools (*continued*)

CDS Category	CDS Tool Example
Workflow support	Order routing
	Registry functions
	Medication reconciliation
	Automatic orders termination
	Order approval processing
	Documentation templates

CDS, clinical decision support; CPT, Current Procedural Terminology.

Source: Adapted from Wright, A., Sittig, D. F., Ash, J. S., Feblowitz, J., Meltzer, S., McMullen, C., . . . Middleton, B. (2011). Development and evaluation of a comprehensive clinical decision support taxonomy: Comparison of front-end tools in commercial and internally developed electronic heath record systems. *Journal of the American Medical Informatics Association, 18*, 232–242.

■ CONCLUSIONS

CDS is a tool that can address gaps in care and improve quality, safety, and outcomes. CDS allows one to create a synthesis of evidence into actionable knowledge for clinicians to use at the point of care in which decisions are made. However, all aspects of the CDS need to be carefully considered as type, placement, and cognitive load can have significant impact on the efficacy of the CDS message.

TABLE 14.3 Clinical Decision-Support Resources

Resource	URL
AHRQ	healthit.ahrq.gov/ahrq-funded-projects/clinical-decision-support-initiative/glides
AMIA—clinical decision-support working group	www.amia.org/programs/working-groups/clinical-decision-support
CMS—CDS rules	www.cms.gov/Regulations-and-Guidance/Legislation/EHRIncentivePrograms/downloads/11_Clinical_Decision_Support_Rule.pdf
HIMSS	www.himss.org/library/clinical-decision-support
Office of the National Coordinator for Health IT—CDS policy	www.healthit.gov/policy-researchers-implementers/clinical-decision-support-cds
Plan for Successful CDS Development, Design, and Deployment	https://www.healthit.gov/sites/default/files/3-4-3-successful-cds.pdf

AHRQ, Agency for Healthcare Research and Quality; AMIA, American Medical Informatics Association; CDS, clinical decision support; CMS, Centers for Medicaid & Medicare Services; HIMSS, Health Information Management Systems Society; IT, information technology.

■ REFERENCES

Al-Badareen, Selamat, M. H., Samat, M., Nazira, Y., & Akkanat, O. (2014). A review on clinical decision support systems in healthcare. *Journal of Convergence Information Technology*, *9*(2), 125–135.

Alford, D., Alexander, S. & Barr, R. (2018). Optimization of clinical decision support tools for the care of older adults with diabetes mellitus type 2. *CIN: Computers, Informatics, Nursing, 36*(6), 259–264. doi:10.1097/CIN.0000000000000452

Ash, J. A., Sitting, D. F., Dykstra, R., Wright, A., McMullen C., Richardson, J., & Middleton, B. (2010). Identifying best practices for clinical decision support and knowledge management in the field. In C. Saffran, S. Reti, & H. F. Marin (Eds.), *Medinfo 2010* (Studies in Health Technology and Informatics, Vol. 160, Pt. 2, pp. 806–810). Amsterdam, The Netherlands: IOS Press. doi:10.3233/978-I-60750-588-4-806

Berner, E. S. (2009, June). *Clinical decision support systems: State of the art* (Publication number 09-0069-EF). Rockville, MD: Agency for Healthcare Research and Quality.

Carayon, P., Schoofs Hundt, A., Karsch, B. T., Gurses, A. P., Alvarado, C. J., Smith, M., & Flatley Brennan, P. (2006). Work system design for patient safety: The SEIPS model. *Quality and Safety in Health Care*, *15*(1), i50–i58. doi:10.1136/qshc.2005.015842

Castillo, R. A., & Kelemen, A. (2013). Considerations for a successful clinical decision support system. *CIN: Computers, Informatics, Nursing*, *31*(7), 319–326. doi:10.1097/nxn.0b013e3182997a9c

Centers for Medicare & Medicaid Services. (2014). *Clinical decision support: More than just alerts tipsheet*. Retrieved from http://www.cms.gov/Regulations-and-Guidance/Legislation/EHRIncentivePrograms/Downloads/ClinicalDecisionSupport_Tipsheet-.pdf

Cvach, M. (2012). Monitor alarm fatigue: An integrative review. *Biomed Instrument & Technology, 46*(4), 268–277. doi:10.2345/0899-8205-46.4.268

Cvach, M. M., Currie, A., Sapirstein, A., Doyle, P. A., & Pronovost, P. (2013). Managing clinical alarms: Using data to drive change. *Nursing Management, 44*(11), 8–12. doi:10.1097/01.numa.0000437594.58933.ce

Department of Health and Human Services. Centers for Medicare & Medicaid Services. (2010). Medicare and Medicaid programs: Electronic health record incentive program; final rule. *Federal Register*, *75*(144), 44350. Retrieved from http://www.gpo.gov/fdsys/pkg/FR-2010-07-28/html/2010-17207.htm

HealthIT.gov. (2019a). HealthIT Dashboard. Retrieved from https://dashboard.healthit.gov/quickstats/quickstats.php

HealthIT.gov. (2019b). Meaningful use and MACRA. Retrieved from https://www.healthit.gov/topic/meaningful-use-and-macra/macra

Horsky, J., Schiff, G. D., Johnston, D., Mercincavage, L., Bell, D., & Middleton, B. (2012). Interface design principles for usable decision support: A targeted review of best practices for clinical prescribing intervention. *Journal of Biomedical Informatics*, *45*(6), 1202–1216. doi:10.1016/j.jbi.2012.09.002

Institute of Medicine. (2001). *Crossing the quality chasm: A new health system for the 21st century*. Washington, DC: National Academies Press.

Kirby, A. M., Kruger, B., Jain, R., O'Hair, D. P., & Granger, B. B. (2018). Using clinical decision support to improve referral rates in severe symptomatic aortic stenosis: a quality improvement initiative. *CIN: Computers, Informatics, Nursing, 36*(11), 525–539. doi:10.1097/CIN.0000000000000471

Lang, N. M. (2008). The promise of simultaneous transformation of practice and research with the use of clinical information systems. *Nursing Outlook*, *56*(5), 232–236. doi:10.1016/j.outlook.2008.06.011

McCartney, P. R. (2007). The new networking: Clinical decision support systems. *American Journal of Maternal–Child Nursing*, *32*(1), 58. doi:10.1097/00005721-200701000-00014

Musen, M. A., Shahar, Y., & Shortliffe, E. H. (2006). Clinical decision-support systems. In E. H. Shortliffe & J. J. Cimino (Eds.), *Biomedical informatics* (pp. 698–736). New York, NY: Springer Publishing Company.

Osheroff, J. A., Pifer, E. A., Teich, J. M., Sittig, D. F., & Jenders, R. A. (2005). *Improving outcomes with clinical decision support: An implementer's guide*. Chicago, IL: Healthcare Information and Management Systems Society.

Osheroff, J. A., Teich, J. M., Levick, D., Saldana, L., Velasco, F. T., Sittig, D. F., . . . Jenders, R. A. (2012). *Improving outcomes with clinical decision support: An implementer's guide* (2nd ed.). Chicago, IL: Healthcare Information and Management Systems Society.

Osheroff, J. A., Teich, J. M., Middleton, B., Steen, E. B., Wright, A. B., & Detmer, D. E. (2007). A roadmap for national action on clinical decision support. *Journal of the American Medical Informatics Association, 14*(2), 141–145. doi:10.1197/jamia.m2334

Roberts, M. S., & Tsevat, J. (2011). Decision analysis. In M. D. Aronson (Ed.), *UpToDate*. Retrieved from https://www.uptodate.com/contents/decision-analysis

Sim, I., Gorman, P., Greenes, R. A., Haynes, R. B., Kaplan, B., Lehmann, H., & Tang, P. C. (2001). Clinical decision support systems for practice of evidence-based medicine. *Journal of the American Medical Informatics Association*, *8*(6), 527–534. doi:10.1136/jamia.2001.0080527

Velickovski, F., Ceccaroni, L., Roca, J., Burgos, F., Galdiz, J. B., Marina, N., & Lluch-Arlet, M. (2014). Clinical decision support systems (CDSS) for preventive management of COPD patients. *Journal of Translational Medicine*, *12*(Suppl. 2), S9. doi:10.1186/1479-5876-12-s2-s9

Wright, A., Sittig, D. F., Ash, J. S., Bates, D. W., Feblowitz, J., Fraser, G., . . . Middleton, B. (2011). Governance for clinical decision support: Case studies and recommended practices from leading institutions. *Journal of the American Medical Informatics Association*, *18*(2), 187–194. doi:10.1136/jamia.2009.002030

Wright, A., Sittig, D. F., Ash, J. S., Feblowitz, J., Meltzer, S., McMullen, C., . . . Middleton, B. (2011). Development and evaluation of a comprehensive clinical decision support taxonomy: Comparison of front-end tools in commercial and internally developed electronic heath record systems. *Journal of the American Medical Informatics Association*, *18*(3), 232–242. doi:10.1136/amiajnl-2011-000113

CHAPTER FIFTEEN

Interprofessional Collaboration and Teamwork for Translation

Kathleen M. White

We can assure our patients that their care is always provided by a team of experts, but we cannot assure our patients that their care is always provided by expert teams.
—A. S. Frankel, M. W. Leonard, and C. R. Denham (2006)

Interprofessional Collaboration (IPC) Among Healthcare Professionals is a critical challenge in today's healthcare environments. A growing body of literature recommends strategies to improve collaboration, communication, and respect among healthcare professionals. The gap in time between the creation of evidence and the translation of that evidence into healthcare practice is well documented to be 17 years. To lessen this time frame requires the involvement and commitment of an interprofessional team in order to identify problems in healthcare that need correction, identify possible solutions using evidence, and cooperate to implement that evidence to improve practice.

■ WHY IPC?

IPC is a process during which different professional groups work together to positively impact healthcare processes and delivery; each values the expertise and contributions that others bring to the team (Zwarenstein, Goldman, & Reeves, 2009). Petri (2010) identified the terms *interdisciplinary collaboration, interdisciplinary team, multidisciplinary collaboration, interdisciplinary teamwork, interdisciplinary practice*, and *teamwork* as surrogate concepts for IPC that are often used interchangeably by authors. Petri also found related terms: *team, integrated team, cooperative work, cooperation, joint practice, working group, teamwork, cooperation, competition, compromise, avoidance, accommodation*, and *conflict resolution*. The need to define the terms became important. The World Health Organization (WHO; 2010) defined *interprofessional collaborative practice* as multiple health workers from different professional backgrounds working together with patients, families, caregivers, and communities to deliver the highest quality of care. The WHO further distinguished interprofessional teamwork as levels of cooperation, coordination, and collaboration characterizing the relationships among professionals in delivering patient-centered care.

Research in the area of IPC is complicated by the use of varied terms, such as *collaboration, communication, coordination*, and *teamwork*, as well as the overlap of the field with other fields of study that also examine how healthcare is organized and delivered. For example, *shared care* has been defined as the joint participation of primary care physicians and specialty care physicians in the planned delivery of care, informed by an enhanced information exchange over and above routine discharge and referral notices (Smith, Allwright, & O'Dowd, 2007). IPC also involves issues that arise due to different professionals working together, such as problematic power dynamics, poor communication patterns, lack of understanding of one's own and others' roles and responsibilities, and conflicts caused by varied approaches to patient care (Suter et al., 2009). In a recent scoping review of interprofessional healthcare practices, three types of interprofessional practice were identified: interprofessional education (IPE), interprofessional practice collaboration, and interprofessional organizational interventions (Goldman, Zwarenstein, Bhattacharyya, & Reeves, 2009).

The WHO (2010) has called for the development of a collaborative practice-ready health workforce to be the main determinant of successful IPC. A collaborative practice-ready health worker is a practitioner who has learned how to work in an interprofessional team and who is competent to do so (WHO, 2010). The report points out that reading about working in teams is not the answer. Many health workers believe themselves to be practicing collaboratively, simply because they work together with other health workers. In reality, they may simply be working within a group in which each individual has agreed to use his or her own skills to achieve a common goal (WHO, 2010). The goal of every healthcare system is to provide evidence-based practice, and healthcare teams, working collaboratively, are at the heart of an evidence-based practice.

■ BACKGROUND—TEAMWORK AND EVIDENCE-BASED PRACTICE

The Health and Medicine Division (of the National Academies of Sciences, Engineering, and Medicine) has been an advocate of interprofessional team approaches to healthcare for almost 40 years. The Health and Medicine Division report *Crossing the Quality Chasm: A New Health System for the 21st Century* (Institute of Medicine [IOM], 2001), identified that cooperation among health professionals must be a priority and that collaboration and communication to ensure exchange of information and coordination of care is paramount. In 2003, the Health and Medicine Division further defined five core competencies for health profession education for the future: provide patient-centered care, apply quality improvement, employ evidence-based practice, utilize informatics, and work in interdisciplinary

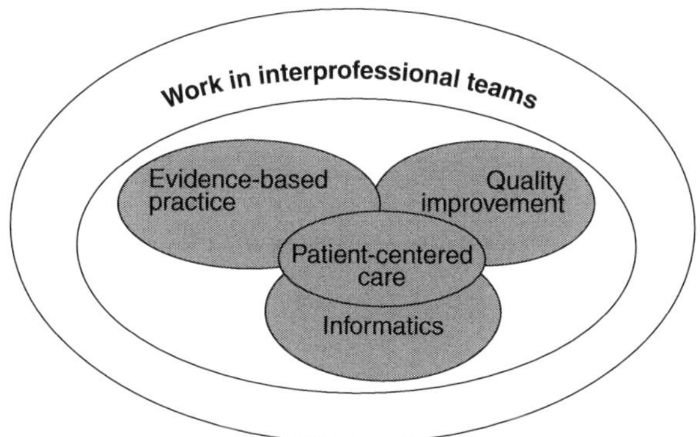

FIGURE 15.1 Health professional competencies—working in interprofessional teams.

Source: From the Institute of Medicine. (2003). *Health professions education: A bridge to quality*. Washington, DC: National Academies Press.

teams (IOM, 2003). These competencies are depicted in Figure 15.1. The report suggested that health profession education should prepare health profession students to work together, fostering interprofessional collaborative practice, in order to build a safer and improved healthcare system.

However, 15 years later, IPC remains a challenge for most healthcare teams. The research to date shows that interprofessional teams demonstrate higher quality efficient healthcare delivery and better outcomes when compared to care provided by individuals in silos (IOM, 2013).

Zwarenstein and Bryant (2000), in a systematic review of the literature assessing the effects of interventions designed to improve doctor–nurse collaboration, found only two studies that met the inclusion criteria, but concluded that increasing collaboration improved outcomes of importance to patients and healthcare managers. However, these improvements were seen in process outcomes rather than clinical outcomes. In a later review, Zwarenstein, Goldstein, and Reeves (2009) again performed a systematic review of the literature to assess the impact of practice-based interprofessional collaborative interventions on professional practice and healthcare outcomes. The review of only five studies suggested that IPC can improve healthcare processes and outcomes; but with a limited number of studies, small sample sizes, and different settings, it was difficult to generalize the effectiveness of any of the interventions.

In a 2012 meta-analysis, Abu-Rish et al. (2012) found 83 studies that reviewed IPE strategies and found that translating IPE into interprofessional practice and team-based care is not well defined. They attempted to identify emerging trends in successful IPE strategies that would provide an understanding of different health profession roles and scopes of responsibilities, and improved communication among the professions. Because deficiencies in communication and collaboration have been shown to have a negative impact on healthcare and patient outcomes, Martin, Ummenhofer, Manser, and Spirig (2010) attempted to identify interventions that facilitate IPC. They reviewed 14 studies that tested new models of practice, including care coordination, individualized treatment plans, health-status monitoring, and coaching and promotion of community-based services, which all used IPC team approaches to care management. All but one study identified at least one positive and statistically significant effect of IPC. Barnsteiner, Disch, Hall, Mayer, and Moore (2007), in discussing the challenges to IPC, reported that interprofessional learning takes place within a context in which differences in culture, beliefs, and prior healthcare experiences among learners of various professions often exist. Exploring the differences and similarities among professional groups as a part of the interprofessional learning process helps learners to build a solid foundation of understanding upon which future healthcare partnerships can be built. Although this research to date is positive, consistent among the studies is the recommendation for additional rigorous research among different patient populations and across settings and providers in order to identify interventions that improve patient clinical outcomes.

The challenge to IPC in healthcare is an international concern. In 2008, the WHO conducted a survey among its members to assess the penetration of IPE into practice globally; identify best practices; and illuminate examples of successes, barriers, and enabling factors in IPE (WHO, 2010). Forty-two countries from each of the six WHO regions of the world representing 396 respondents answered the survey to provide information about their IPE. The results of the survey indicated that IPE is occurring among students from medicine, nursing, midwifery, social work, and allied health. In many countries, IPE is compulsory and they have experienced educational and health policy benefits from implementing IPE. For example, respondents reported that students have real-world experience and insight and that students learn about the work of other practitioners. In terms of health policy benefits, the respondents reported improved workplace practices and productivity, improved patient outcomes, increased staff morale, improved patient safety, and better access to healthcare. However, many reported that significant effort is still required to ensure that interprofessional initiatives are developed, delivered, and evaluated in keeping with internationally recognized best practice (WHO, 2010). The report summarized the current evidence that interprofessional collaborative practice maximizes the strengths and skills of each member of the healthcare team, but recommended that more research is needed (WHO, 2010). The report also found that collaborative practice can improve: access to and coordination of health services, appropriate use of specialist clinical resources, health outcomes for people with chronic diseases, and patient care and safety. It also reported from the evidence that collaborative practice can decrease: total patient complications, length of hospital stay, tension and conflict among caregivers, staff turnover, hospital admission, clinical error rates, and mortality rates (WHO, 2010). As a result of this work, the WHO proposed the Framework for Action on IPE and Collaborative Practice that highlighted the current state of IPC in healthcare education and practice and identified successful strategies for collaborative teamwork (WHO, 2010; Figure 15.2).

In 2011, the Health Resources and Services Administration (HRSA) convened a meeting of the Interprofessional Education Collaborative (IPEC), the Josiah Macy Foundation, and the Robert Wood Johnson Foundation to advance IPE as a priority and to develop core competencies for interprofessional collaborative practice (IPEC Expert Panel, 2011). In 2012, the HRSA, in collaboration with the Josiah Macy

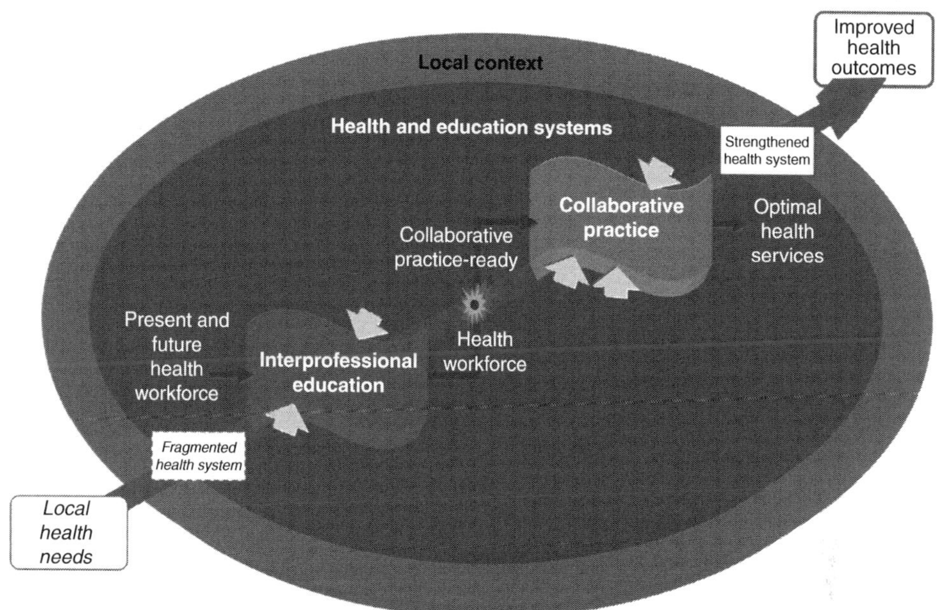

FIGURE 15.2 The WHO Framework for Action on Interprofessional Education and Collaborative Practice.

WHO, World Health Organization.

Source: From World Health Organization. (2010). *The Framework for Action on Interprofessional Education and Collaborative Practice*. Geneva, Switzerland: WHO Health Professions Networks Nursing & Midwifery Human Resources for Health.

Foundation, the Robert Wood Johnson Foundation, the John Hartford Foundation, and the Gordon and Betty Moore Foundation, established the National Coordinating Center for Interprofessional Education and Collaborative Practice at the University of Minnesota. IPEC published the Core Competencies for Interprofessional Collaborative Practice (2011), which describe four competency domains each containing a set of specific and related competency statements (the Core Competencies for Interprofessional Collaborative Practice [2011] are available at aamc-meded.global.ssl.fastly.net/production/media/filer_public/70/9f/709fedd7-3c53-492c-b9f0-b13715d11cb6/core_competencies_for_collaborative_practice.pdf). The American Association of Colleges of Nursing (AACN) has incorporated IPC competencies in the Essentials of Baccalaureate Education for Professional Nursing Practice (AACN, 2008), Essentials of Master's Education in Nursing (AACN, 2011), Essentials of Master's Education for Advanced Practice Nursing (AACN, 1996), and the Essentials of Doctoral for Advanced Nursing Practice (AACN, 2006). In addition, quality and safety competencies for pre-licensure and graduate-level nurses that integrate teamwork and team-based care were developed by the Quality and Safety Education for Nursing (Cronenwett et al., 2007, 2009). The Accreditation Council for Graduate Medical Education has identified interpersonal and communication skills as one of its six core competencies for graduate medical education (2015; www.acgme.org/acgmeweb). The Joint Commission has continued to emphasize the need for effective communication among health professionals in its National Patient Safety Goals program. Both 2015 and 2016 have the goal to improve staff communication (The Joint Commission, 2015), central to IPC.

Similarly, the UK's Centre for the Advancement of Interprofessional Education (CAIPE) and the Canadian Interprofessional Health Collaborative (CIHC) have also convened professionals to deliberate on the need for IPE and collaborative practice. The CAIPE developed a report titled, *Creating an Interprofessional Workforce: An Education and Training Framework for Health and Social Care in England* (Department of Health, 2007). This report makes 12 recommendations to stakeholders, such as policy makers at different levels, educators, providers, employers, professional bodies, patients, users, and caregivers. An outcome of the report was the development and validation of a comprehensive framework, The Continuum of Interprofessional Collaborative Practice in Health and Social Care (Figure 15.3), to illustrate five types of collaborative practices that vary depending on four situations (Careau et al., 2015). The four components of IPC are the situation of the client and family, the intention underlying the collaboration, the interaction among practitioners, and the combination of disciplinary knowledge. The five types of collaborative practice are independent practice, parallel practice, consultation/reference practice, concerted practice, and shared healthcare practice. These practice types increase in complexity and intensity as practitioners advance toward the right on the continuum.

In the fall of 2008, the CIHC convened a workgroup to encourage shared thinking around the foundations for interprofessional competency and to develop a Canadian competency framework for IPC. The workgroup defined *IPC* as the process of developing and maintaining effective interprofessional working relationships with learners, practitioners, patients/clients/families, and communities to enable optimal health outcomes and identified six competency domains: (a) interprofessional communication, (b) patient/client/family/community-centered care, (c) role clarification, (d) team functioning, (e) collaborative leadership, and (f) interprofessional conflict resolution. It further defined elements of collaboration to include respect, trust, shared decision-making, and partnerships. See Figure 15.4 for the CIHC National Interprofessional Competency Framework.

One final development in promoting the critical importance of interprofessional collaborative approaches among healthcare providers was the creation of the *Journal of Interprofessional Care* in 1992. The journal had previously been called the *Holistic Medicine Journal*, but with the increasing focus on interprofessional approaches to healthcare delivery, a scholarly vehicle was needed to disseminate research and new developments measuring the impact and benefits of these interprofessional educational and practice collaborations.

■ STRATEGIES TO FACILITATE IPC FOR TRANSLATION OF EVIDENCE TO PRACTICE

The WHO's call for a "collaborative practice-ready health workforce" is one possible solution to mitigate the challenges faced by our healthcare systems today. As Frankel,

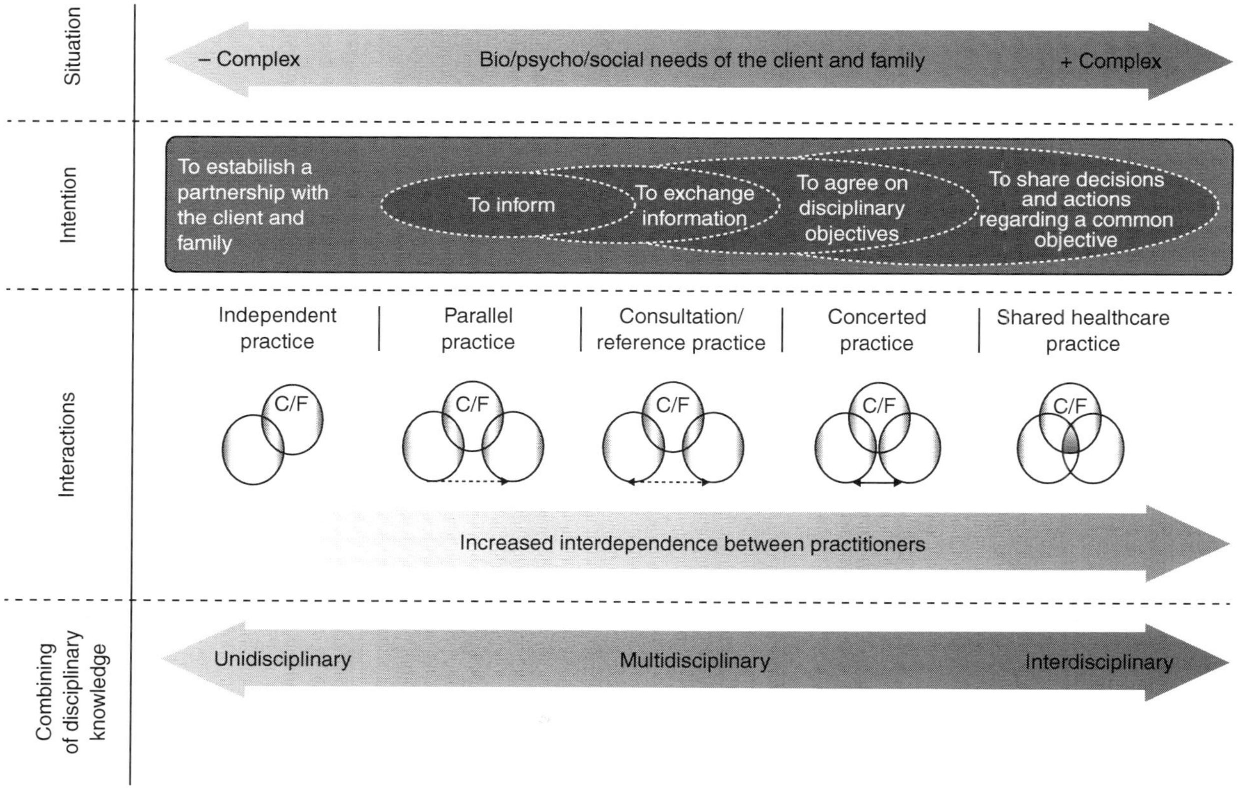

FIGURE 15.3 The Continuum of Interprofessional Collaborative Practice in Health and Social Care.

C/F, client and family.

Source: From Careau, E., Brière, N., Houle, N., Dumont, S., Vincent, C., & Swaine, R. B. (2014). Interprofessional collaboration: Development of a tool to enhance knowledge translation. *Disability and Rehabilitation*, *14*, 1–7.

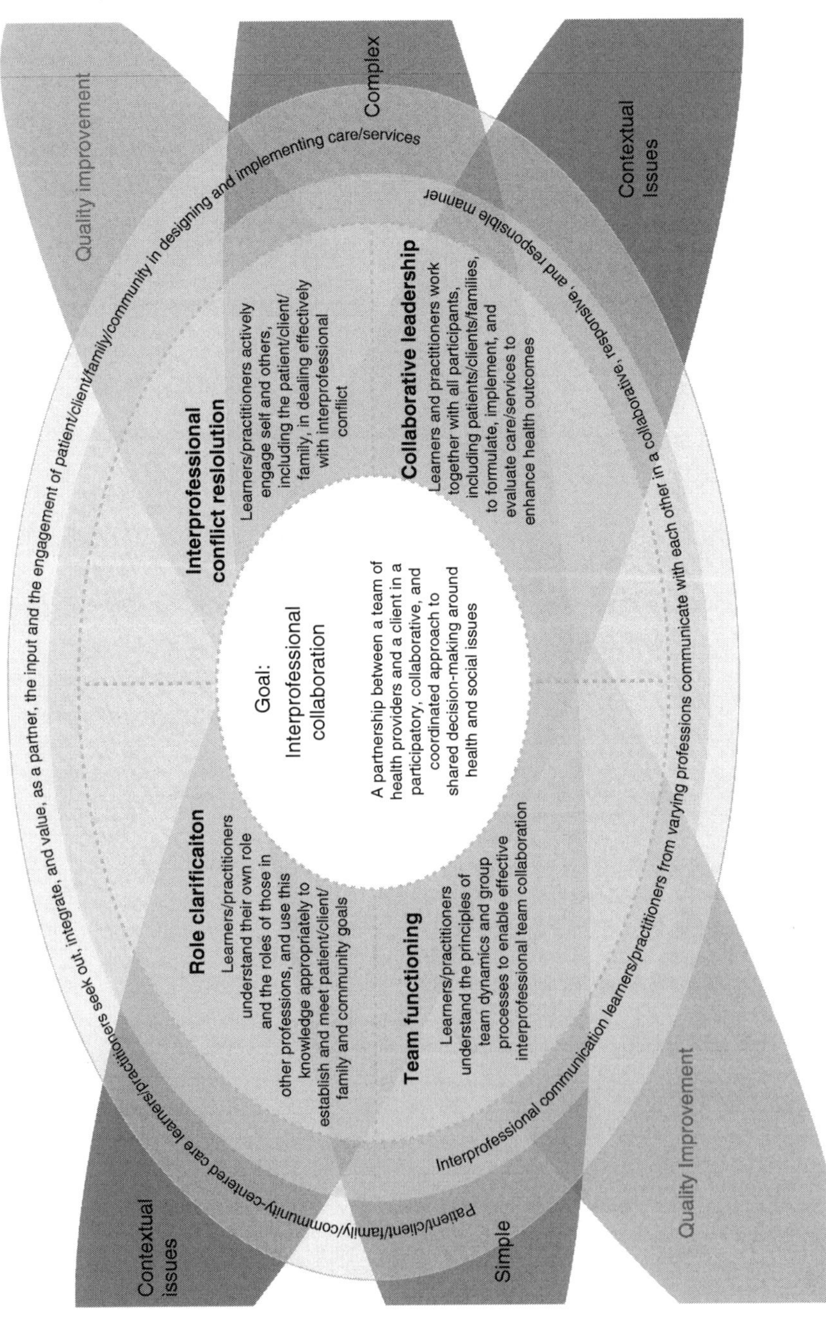

FIGURE 15.4 The CIHC National Interprofessional Competency Framework.

CIHC, Canadian Interprofessional Health Collaborative.

Source: From Canadian Interprofessional Health Collaborative. (2010). *A National Interprofessional Competency Framework*. Retrieved from www.cihc.ca/files/CIHC_IPCompetencies_Feb1210.pdf

Leonard, and Denham (2006, p. 1700) said, "we can assure our patients that their care is always provided by a team of experts, but we cannot assure our patients that their care is always provided by expert teams."

The WHO Framework for Action on IPE and Collaborative Practice proposed a series of action steps (WHO, 2010) that were not meant to be prescriptive, but rather used to develop and facilitate the transition to full commitment to interprofessional collaborative practice:

1. Agree on a common vision and purpose for IPE with key stakeholders across all faculties and organizations.
2. Develop IPE curriculum according to principles of good educational practice.
3. Provide organizational support and adequate financial and time allocation for the development and delivery of IPE and staff training in IPE.
4. Introduce IPE into health worker training programs.
5. Ensure the staff responsible for developing, delivering, and evaluating IPE are competent in this task, have expertise consistent with the nature of the planned IPE, and have the support of an IPE champion.
6. Ensure the commitment to IPE by leaders in educational institutions and all associated practice and work settings.

Bainbridge, Nasmith, Orchard, and Wood (2010) suggest a systems approach to IPC that includes:

1. Role clarification—Health professionals understand their own role and the roles of those in other professions, and use this knowledge appropriately to establish and meet patient/client/family and community goals.
2. Patient/client/family/community-centered care—Health professionals seek out, integrate, and value, as a partner, the input and the engagement of patient/client/family/community in designing and implementing care/services.
3. Team functioning—Health professionals understand the principles of team dynamics and group processes to enable effective interprofessional team collaboration.
4. Collaborative leadership—Health professionals understand and can apply leadership principles that support a collaborative practice model.
5. Interprofessional communication—Health professionals from varying professions communicate with each other in a collaborative, responsive, and responsible manner.
6. Dealing with interprofessional conflict—Health professionals actively engage self and others, including the client/patient/family, in positively and constructively addressing interprofessional conflict as it arises.

The frameworks and action step models just described are helpful in developing systems of IPC that are critical to the implementation of new discoveries and best practices to create evidence-based systems of care. The active participation of all health professionals is needed to identify and resolve healthcare problems through a problem-solving approach to clinical decision-making that recognizes the contributions, roles, and responsibilities of all healthcare providers involved in that clinical care. Active participation requires that health professionals be involved in and committed to team building, improved communication processes, consideration of organizational context, active leadership, and careful management and planning of the translation.

Team Building

Interprofessional team building and teamwork are critical for implementing practice changes and knowledge translation. Teams play a critical role in the delivery of healthcare, but effective teams and true IPC involve commitment, respect, and nurturing in order to be successful. IPC team building is a dynamic process, and it is perfectly normal for teams to go through the stages of team development: forming, storming, norming, and performing (Tuckman, 1965). The four stages create a helpful framework for recognizing a team's behavioral patterns; they are most useful as a basis for team discussion.

Building a team among a diverse group of professionals is a challenge that requires the development of trust and finding a balance among differing perspectives. First and foremost, the team must include and appreciate the diversity of its members. *Workforce diversity* refers to the personal and/or functional heterogeneity of the workgroup as a whole (Jehn, Northcraft, & Neale, 1999). Viewed as both a liability and an asset, diversity influences work and outcomes, and can be harnessed to improve outcomes, which translate to competitive advantage. *Personal diversity* refers to attributes of individuals that are associated with culture, ethnicity, gender, age, generation, cognitive processing, learning style, emotional intelligence, spirituality, belief, and motivations. Functional heterogeneity refers to the training, role, skill, experience, and goals of those same workforce members.

The topics of personal diversity and functional heterogeneity both emanate from the current management literature on mental models, a critical concept in team building in organizations. What are mental models? Mental models are beliefs and assumptions that influence our actions; they are deeply held internal images of how the world works (Senge, 1990). They form out of our experiences in life and, as we process data and deal with observations, we make assumptions and draw conclusions based on those experiences. They are often unconscious and act as a filter for our minds. Mental models can limit data and facts and ultimately skew factual information. Recognizing your mental model is difficult because it is often seen as reality instead of perception. Overcoming mental models and focusing on your strengths allow for productive conversations about complex and controversial issues.

Mental models that skew our view of the role and contributions of other health professionals in the team are a major topic for discussion in the positive psychology of organizations today and a significant contributor to team building for translation of evidence to practice. The current literature on positive psychology for team building suggests that team members consider and discuss how they can create collaborative relationships in the work setting (Muha, 2015). Asking questions, such as "What ideas do you have for creating great teamwork?" and "Who could you count on to help build a high-functioning team?" can start the dialog.

Satisfying the challenge of using effective teamwork to translate evidence into practice takes both time and effort. It requires a process of reflection and skill building over time and also needs effective leadership and buy-in of the stakeholders and team members.

Now, consider that each functional group is educated separately in its own school, which has historically been another discrete functional unit. Consider that each has traditions of learning and socialization, each has a specialized language, and each learns to target a particular aspect of care. Just as differences in culture, background, and other personal attributes influence what each individual brings to collaboration, so does education, experience, and competence. The approach to providing the best care, promoting safety, and developing innovations that improve outcomes must engage all members of the healthcare workforce and exploit the talent, knowledge, and experience each brings.

The challenge of getting a group of professionals to collaborate along the accountable care continuum is a wonderful example. Consider the number of specialists and subspecialists involved in a patient's care across this continuum. There are outpatient services and resources, inpatient departments in a hospital, supportive services/units, and outpatient follow-up services such as urgent, emergency, tertiary, rehabilitative, palliative, ongoing care, and public health. Some collaborations might be common, but others are less so. Bringing these individuals, services, and resources together as team members to participate together to solve a clinical problem by defining the issue, searching and appraising current evidence, and making recommendations to translate evidence into practice or generate new knowledge to solve the problem are daunting tasks.

Communication

Skilled communication becomes the key to this team building. The development of interprofessional relationships characterized by collaboration and partnership leads to improved patient experience of care (including quality and safety), improving the health of populations and decreasing the cost of healthcare (e.g., Centers for Medicare & Medicaid Services's [CMS] Triple Aim). However, two additional measures of improvement, increased satisfaction and implementation/translation of evidence-based care, are also essential.

Why is skilled communication among health professionals so difficult to achieve? Years of silo education and practice are at the root of this challenge for healthcare improvement. The "physician as captain of the ship" mentality that permeated healthcare delivery for years is slowly eroding. The Joint Commission has found that more than 60% of medication errors are a result of miscommunication among health professionals. Research, such as that revealed in *Silence Kills* (Maxfield, Grenny, McMillan, Patterson, & Switzler, 2005), indicates that healthcare professionals are often afraid to speak up and challenge practices of other healthcare professionals for fear of retaliation.

Investigators explored specific concerns of physicians and nurses when communicating that may contribute to avoidable errors and other chronic problems in healthcare. They indicated that when emotionally and politically risky topics are addressed in the healthcare setting, it has key results like patient safety and improved quality of care. The study found seven categories of conversations that are especially difficult and, at the same time, appear to be especially essential for people in healthcare to master: broken rules, mistakes, lack of support, incompetence, poor teamwork, disrespect, and micromanagement. The authors concluded that it is critical for hospitals to create cultures of safety where healthcare professionals are able to speak up about their concerns.

The Agency for Healthcare Research and Quality (AHRQ) and the Department of Defense (DoD) developed an evidence-based program, Team Strategies and Tools to Enhance Performance and Patient Safety (TeamSTEPPS); it was intended to improve communication, collaboration, and teamwork skills among healthcare professionals. Teamwork and IPC have been found to be successful in transforming the culture within healthcare. TeamSTEPPS identifies five key principles based on team structure and four skills necessary for a team to function effectively: communication, team leadership, situation monitoring, and mutual support (see Figure 15.5).

TeamSTEPPS has been implemented widely and offers great promise as a practical approach for use in IPE and facilitation of collaborative practice. However, communication remains the number one issue facing teams in healthcare.

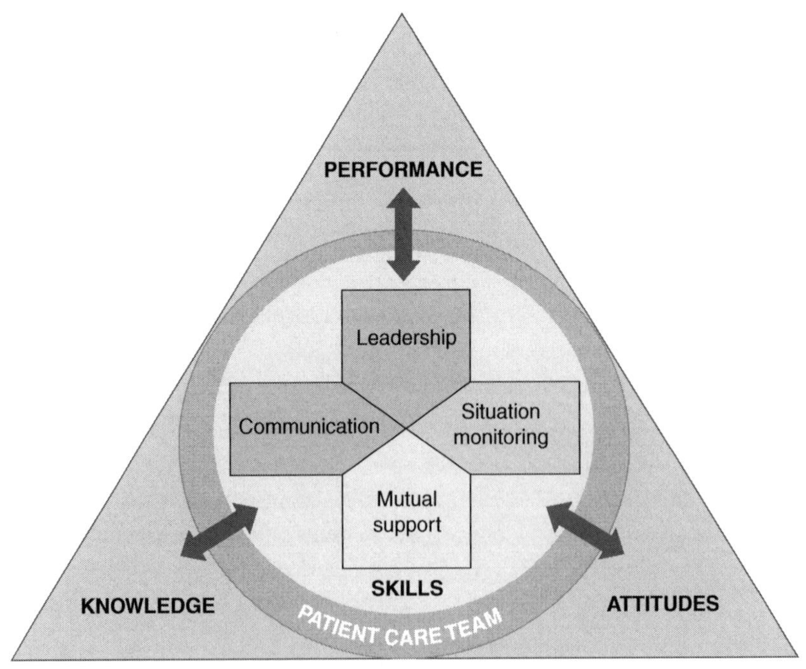

FIGURE 15.5 TeamSTEPPS—team structure.

TeamSTEPPS, Team Strategies and Tools to Enhance Performance and Patient Safety.

Source: From the Agency for Healthcare Research and Quality. (n.d.). TeamSTEPPS fundamentals course: Team structure. Retrieved from www.ahrq.gov/teamstepps/index.html

Fostering positive and constructive communication among interprofessional healthcare team members is just one part of effective communication. It is also necessary to develop an interprofessional communication plan that identifies each participating profession/discipline that will be involved, the goals for the communication, and what type of information will be communicated. Final consideration should be given to the mode and vehicle to be used for the communication. Different interprofessional groups may have preferred modes of communication and the leadership of those groups may have a preferred method of communicating. Sensitivity to those differences and preferences is fundamental to a successful communication plan.

Challenge of Context

Why is context so difficult in translation? Context is addressed in several chapters in this book. Context is also important when considering IPC and translation. Major efforts using educational strategies to foster interprofessional collaborative practice are a great start. However, translation efforts in the organization, whether a small or large facility, must involve the interprofessional team. Essential to the translation is the development of ongoing and sustained relationships and partnerships, true IPC, to capitalize on the knowledge and skills that each member brings to the team. This requires effective communication among partners with an understanding of the contextual environment of the organization, including healthcare professionals' commitment to core values, and the mission and vision of the organization. Adaptation of the evidence, new knowledge, or best practice to the local context is the responsibility of the IPC team and requires that the team provide input and expertise about the fit and feasibility of the translation within the organization's context.

Interprofessional Leadership

Facilitating team building, communication, and understanding the context also requires supportive and visible leadership that facilitates a culture of shared learning and practice. This leadership, modeling IPC at all levels of the organization, requires articulating a clear, valued, and shared vision of collaboration among health professionals with a common and understandable purpose of that collaboration for translation and practice improvement. How is this actually accomplished? Fundamental to success is visible leadership that supports evidence-based practice initiatives by setting priorities, identifying and optimizing resources, diagnosing barriers and facilitators, and "walking the talk." The executive leader who asks what evidence and best practices exist to solve an identified problem, and then supports the management team to solve problems, evaluate evidence, and make recommendations for change, is walking the talk. However, these efforts must involve not only the immediate management team, but also collaboration with multiple internal and external stakeholders, the interprofessional team.

What about the leadership of the interprofessional team? There is a current emphasis in many healthcare organizations/systems on leadership assessment. For the interprofessional team to be collaborative, consideration should be given to the leader's fit for the team, the work to be done, and the organization's culture. An outside hiring approach would match the talents of the individual, looking for the leader's fit with the organization's culture and the position. However, the work of translation, more often than not, will involve individuals who are already in place/positions in the organization. It is essential that each leader understand his or her leadership style, strengths and weaknesses, in relation to the IPC team. Balancing leadership strengths for different IPC teams is necessary for success.

Plan, Plan, Plan

Involving the team in planning a successful translation of evidence into practice is the keystone of IPC. Experience suggests that the amount of time and effort needed for most translation projects is often underestimated. Central to any project plan is flexibility, especially in terms of timelines and responsibilities.

In putting the plan together, the first step is identifying and creating the translation team, ensuring representation from all key professional and stakeholder groups. The IPC team should begin with agreement on the definition of the practice problem, goals of the project, and translation methods. These decisions must be communicated to the interprofessional team for their buy-in and participation. Involving the whole team in the early project plan, as discussed in Chapter 9, Project Management for Translation, should eliminate the predictable bumps and barriers to translation success.

Evaluation of the translation's project plan includes monitoring the status of the project, reviewing the team's participation and performance, and identifying any unintended consequences to the project or to the IPC team. For example, has the team lost any members from key professional groups who need to be replaced for the translation to be successful? Have responsibilities changed for any professional group/discipline critical to the translation? Have there been any key leadership changes in the organization that could affect the translation? Are resources stable in the environment? These and other questions/concerns, depending on the translation project, should be continuously monitored during the translation in relation to and for their effect on the IPC team. Most professionals involved with this type of work consider evaluation methods carefully from the beginning of the translation project. However, with the emphasis on IPC teams for translation, monitoring, and evaluation of the project, the team, the context, and organizational leadership add critical dimensions to oversight for the translation. An "ear to the ground" approach is required throughout.

■ CONCLUSIONS

IPC is necessary because of the current complexity of the healthcare environment. There is general agreement that the silo approach to healthcare education and practice no longer works. Problems in the healthcare environment must be examined and approached from a team, organizational, or systems perspective. As concluded by the WHO (2010), there is a great need for healthcare to embrace IPE and collaborative practice to implement strategies that promote IPC to improve outcomes and move from fragmented healthcare to strong healthcare systems throughout the world (Reeves et al., 2009; Reeves & Hean, 2013). Henry Ford is credited with saying, "coming together is a beginning; keeping together is progress; working together is success"—this is true for interprofessional collaborative teams facilitating quality, safety, and evidence-based healthcare practice. We have made progress, but there is much more to do for effective IPC in healthcare.

■ REFERENCES

Abu-Rish, E., Kim, S., Choe, L., Varpio, L., Malik, E., White, A., . . . Zierle, B. (2012). Current trends in interprofessional education of health sciences students: A literature review. *Journal of Interprofessional Care, 26*(6), 444–451. doi:10.3109/13561820.2012.715604

Accreditation Council for Graduate Medical Education. (2015). *Core competencies for graduate medical education*. Retrieved from https://www.acgme.org/acgmeweb

Agency for Healthcare Research and Quality. (n.d.). TeamSTEPPS fundamentals course: Team structure. Retrieved from www.ahrq.gov/teamstepps/index.html

American Association of Colleges of Nursing. (1996). *Essentials of master's education for advanced practice nursing*. Washington, DC: Author.

American Association of Colleges of Nursing. (2006). *Essentials of doctoral for advanced nursing practice*. Washington, DC: Author.

American Association of Colleges of Nursing. (2008). *Essentials of baccalaureate education for professional nursing practice*. Washington, DC: Author.

American Association of Colleges of Nursing. (2011). *Essentials of master's education in nursing*. Washington, DC: Author.

Bainbridge, L., Nasmith, L., Orchard, C., & Wood, V. (2010). Competencies for interprofessional collaboration. *Journal of Physical Therapy Education, 24*(1), 6–11. doi:10.1097/00001416-201010000-00003

Barnsteiner, J. H., Disch, J. M., Hall, L., Mayer, D., & Moore, S. M. (2007). Promoting interprofessional education. *Nursing Outlook, 55*(3), 144–150. doi:10.1016/j.outlook.2007.03.003

Canadian Interprofessional Health Collaborative. (2010). *A National Interprofessional Competency Framework*. Retrieved from www.cihc.ca/files/CIHC_IPCompetencies_Feb1210.pdf

Careau, E., Briere, N., Houle, N., Dumont, S., Vincent, C., & Swaine, B. (2015). Interprofessional collaboration: Development of a tool to enhance knowledge translation. *Disability and Rehabilitation, 37*(4), 372–378. doi:10.3109/09638288.2014.918193

Cronenwett, L., Sherwood, G., Barnsteiner, J., Disch, J., Johnson, J., Mitchell, P., . . . Warren, J. (2007). Quality and Safety Education for Nurses. *Nursing Outlook, 55*(3), 122–131. doi:10.1016/j.outlook.2007.02.006

Cronenwett, L., Sherwood, G., Pohl, J., Barnsteiner, J., Moore, S., Sullivan, D., . . . Warren, J., (2009). Quality and safety education for advanced nursing practice. *Nursing Outlook, 57*(6), 338–348. doi:10.1016/j.outlook.2009.07.009

Department of Health. (2007). Creating an interprofessional workforce—An education and training framework for health and social care in England (CIPW). Retrieved from file:///C:/Users/kwhite2/Downloads/Department-of-Health-2007-Creating-an-Interproferssional-Workforce-An-Education-and-Training-Framework-for-Health-and-Social-Care-in-England-CIPW..pdf

Frankel, A. S., Leonard M. W., & Denham, C. R. (2006). Fair and just culture, team behavior, leadership engagement: The tools to achieve high reliability. *Health Services Research, 41*(4p2), 1690–1709. doi:10.1111/j.1475-6773.2006.00572.x

Goldman, J., Zwarenstein, M., Bhattacharyya, O., & Reeves, S. (2009). Improving the clarity of the interprofessional field: Implications for research and continuing interprofessional education. *Journal of Continuing Education in the Health Professions, 29*(3), 151–156. doi:10.1002/chp.20028

Institute of Medicine. (2001). *Crossing the quality chasm: A new health system for the 21st century*. Washington, DC: National Academies Press.

Institute of Medicine. (2003). *Health professions education: A bridge to quality.* Washington, DC: National Academies Press.

Institute of Medicine. (2013). *Interprofessional education for collaboration: Learning how to improve health from interprofessional models across the continuum of education to practice: Workshop summary*. Washington, DC: National Academies Press.

Interprofessional Education Collaborative Expert Panel. (2011). *Core competencies for interprofessional collaborative practice: Report of an expert panel.* Washington, DC: Interprofessional Education Collaborative.

Jehn, K. A., Northcraft, G. B., & Neale, M. A. (1999). Why differences make a difference: A field of study of diversity, conflict, and performance in workgroups. *Administrative Science Quarterly, 44*(4), 741–763. doi:10.2307/2667054

Martin, J. S, Ummenhofer, W., Manser, T., & Spirig, R. (2010). Interprofessional collaboration among nurses and physicians: Making a difference in patient outcomes. *Swiss Medical Weekly,* 140, w13062.

Maxfield, D., Grenny, J., McMillan, R., Patterson, K., & Switzler, A. (2005). *Silence kills: The seven crucial conversations for healthcare.* Provo, UT: VitalSmarts.

Muha, T. (2015). *Creating a positive culture with the PROPEL principles.* Retrieved from http://www.thepropelprinciples.com/2015/10/04/create-a-positive-culture-with-the-propel-principles

Petri, L. (2010). Concept analysis of interdisciplinary collaboration. *Nursing Forum, 45*(2), 73–82. doi:10.1111/j.1744-6198.2010.00167.x

Reeves, S., & Hean, S. (2013). Why we need theory to help us better understand the nature of interprofessional education, practice and care. *Journal of Interprofessional Care,* 27(1), 1–3. doi:10.3109/13561820.2013.751293

Reeves, S., Zwarenstien, M., Goldman, J., Barr, H., Freeth, D., Hammick, M., & Koppel, I. (2009). Interprofessional education: Effects on professional practice and health care outcomes [Review]. *Cochrane Library,* (4). Chichester, UK: Wiley.

Senge, P. (1990). *The fifth discipline: The art and practice of the learning organization.* New York, NY: Doubleday/Currency.

Smith, S. M., Allwright, S., & O'Dowd, T. (2007). Effectiveness of shared care across the interface between primary and specialty care in chronic disease management. *Cochrane Database of Systematic Reviews, 18*(3), CD00491.

Suter, E., Arndt, J., Arthur, N., Parboosingh, J., Taylor, E., & Deutschlander, S. (2009). Role understanding and effective communication as core competencies for collaborative practice. *Journal of Interprofessional Care,* 23(1), 41–51. doi:10.1080/13561820802338579

The Joint Commission. (2015). *2016 National Patient Safety Goals.* Retrieved from http://www.jointcommission.org/standards_information/npsgs.aspx

Tuckman, B. W. (1965). Developmental sequence in small groups. *Psychological Bulletin, 63*(6), 384–399. doi:10.1037/h0022100

World Health Organization. (2010). *Framework for action on interprofessional education & collaborative practice.* Geneva: WHO Health Professions Networks Nursing & Midwifery Human Resources for Health.

Zwarenstein, M., & Bryant, W. (2000). Interventions to promote collaboration between nurses and doctors, *Cochrane Database Systematic Review, 2000*(2), CD000072.

Zwarenstein, M., Goldman, J., & Reeves, S. (2009). Interprofessional collaboration: Effects of practice-based interventions on professional practice and healthcare outcomes. *Cochrane Database of Systematic Reviews, 2009*(3), CD000072.

CHAPTER SIXTEEN

Creating a Culture That Promotes Translation

Joyce P. Williams and Sharon Dudley-Brown

Culture does not change because we desire to change it. Culture changes when the organization is transformed; the culture reflects the realities of people working together every day.
— Frances Hesselbein, Former CEO of Girl Scouts of the USA

Culture plays a large part in the success of translation of evidence into practice. Whether it is the culture of the individual, the culture of the unit, the culture of the leadership, or the culture of the organization, attention to culture when planning the translation will help ensure its success.

We know that evidence-based practice (EBP) is adopted at low rates and this has been found to be in direct correlation to organizational culture (Kaplan, Zeller, Damitio, Culbert, & Bayley, 2014). *Organizational culture* is recognized as the basic pattern of attitudes, beliefs, and values that serve to stabilize and provide structure and meaning to an organization (Schein, 2010, p. 3). Each organization has its own cultural DNA; core values shape the invisible architecture of the environment and provide a powerful cornerstone of culture for developing capacities, attitudes, and behaviors (Osborne & Plastrik, 1997). Educational initiatives enable practitioners to translate knowledge into practice adding interprofessional education and collaboration, which is now emphasized and encouraged as part of organizational culture (Mann, Sargeant, & Hill, 2009)

The cultures within health organizations may constrain implementation of new ideas. Redirecting the climate of the organization and embracing its beliefs and core values is one method used to strengthen the organization. Core values should be authentic and should inspire; they should be powerful to quash invalid assumptions that may have become embedded in the institutional culture.

■ CULTURE

Broadly, *culture* can be defined as a blueprint for our way of living, thinking, behaving, and feeling. It circumscribes and guides the ways in which societies and ethnic groups solve their problems and derive meaning from their lives. Culture contains and regulates our daily behavior, attitudes, and values in many latent and manifest ways. Kavanagh and Kennedy (1992) defined *culture* as an identifiable group whose members operate on the assumptions that they share beliefs, experiences, and patterns of meanings. Culture is learned and is made up of shared beliefs and behaviors by members of a group.

Cultural relativism, which can be defined as cultures being equal, neither inferior nor superior to each other, is an important concept in translation. In cultural relativism, other ways of being are different, but equally valid. Customs, beliefs, and practices must be understood relative to the context, in order to understand the behavior. The opposite of cultural relativism is *ethnocentrism*, which is the belief that your culture is superior to all others, and all others are inferior. The consequence of ethnocentrism is cultural imposition: imposing one's beliefs onto others.

In working with other cultures, Kleinman (1988) proposed eight questions to help one understand another person's culture, when it comes to health. These include the following:

- What is the problem?
- What do you think caused the problem?
- Why do you think it started when it did?
- What do you think the sickness does/how does it work?
- How severe is the sickness?
- What kind of treatment should be given? What results do you want to achieve?
- What problems has the sickness caused?
- What do you fear the most about the sickness?

In dealing with two (or more) different organizational cultures, one can extrapolate these questions to help people from two different settings understand each other and work together, improving cultural relativism and decreasing ethnocentrism. For example, in beginning an EBP project, one may ask others their perspective of the problem. If coming in at the point of translation, asking, "What results do you want to achieve?" may be relevant in agreeing on common outcomes for the project. Substituting *problem* for *sickness* in Kleinman's eight questions may provide the common ground to begin translation.

Culture, in an organization or subsystem (such as an individual unit), is really the shared knowledge and behavior of the people who interact in that system. In nursing, many times it is defined as "the way things are done around here." This culture is manifested through values, beliefs, and assumptions imbedded in institutions and organizations.

Therefore, *organizational culture* can be defined as a pattern of shared basic assumptions invented, discovered, or developed by a given group as it learns to cope with its problem of external adaptation and internal integration. This has to have worked well enough to be considered valid, and therefore, to be taught to new members as the correct way to perceive, think, and feel, in relation to those problems (Schein, 1985).

Organizations, by their very nature, possess essential goals that are intrinsic, built into the system, and witnessed in protocols and procedures that contribute to the undertakings of the system. The success of any organization occurs because of its culture; it is one of an organization's most important and predictable aspects, but the hardest to change. The collective attitudes and behaviors of the people who work in the organization are responsible for shaping its culture.

Culture is the vehicle by which the organization shares modes of behavior. Value is a major link between culture and action. Causal effects of any organization are demonstrated in strategic plans in which the beliefs and assumptions influence the cohesion and unity among staff and match its core values, becoming a part of the cultural plan.

Structure and culture collectively guide the internal workings of organizational systems and are conduits for individuals to achieve successful outcomes. Explicit knowledge created by researchers is highly valued. Essential to learning, according to Peter Senge, are clarifying the vision and objectives, creating an organizational model, indicating what it stands for, building shared visions from leaders to the whole organization, learning in teams, and linking each element into a cohesive existence (Gray, 2001). The whole organization must focus on learning. Senge also submits that leaders help develop new understandings, part of collective learning and subsequent implementation (Lannon, 2018).

Adopting EBP depends on context—the environment where practice occurs (Wente & Kleiber, 2013). Indicators of effective context are clearly defined boundaries, transparent decision-making processes, adequate resources, reflective evaluation, and willingness to change (Wente & Kleiber, 2013). Lack of engagement indicates poor morale and fosters an unhealthy environment. Any organization with hierarchical management and little flexibility will be challenged to adapt satisfactorily to innovations. Staff members who appreciate progress identify barriers and develop ways to remain positive when coworkers are resistant to change. Among the potential barriers to EBP engagement are a lack of EBP knowledge and skills, unsupportive organizational cultures, a paucity of administrative support, lack of EBP mentors, and absence of tools and resources to assist implementation of EBP (Melnyk, Fineout-Overholt, Giggleman, & Cruz, 2010). Other barriers to dissemination and implementation can be described as primary, secondary, and tertiary defenses. *Primary obstacles* refer to staff behavior and practice unfamiliarity, lack of education and training, inexperience, and lack of competency (Kojo Asamoah, 2014). *Secondary obstacles* are systemic-level influences, and *tertiary obstacles* refer to environmental impediments (Kojo Asamoah, 2014). In contrast, organizations with positive perceptions report culture, leadership, evaluation of social capital, informal interactions, formal interactions, structural and electronic resources, and organizational slack as movement to adopt EBP and research utilization; context is important to the unit culture and is a predictor of EBP adoption (Wente & Kleiber, 2013).

Research informs us that EBP beliefs and implementation are inextricably linked to perceived organizational culture (Kaplan et al., 2014). In an integrative review of organizational context, authors found that organizational features, specifically staffing and culture, facility structure, and quality-improvement experiences, together make up the organizational context (Li, Jeffs, Barwick, & Stevens, 2018).

■ PARADIGMS

Change can be viewed in terms of paradigms. This involves knowing the identity of an organization. Paradigms are found in the unwritten rules and behaviors that manifest between peers and supervisors, employees and consumers. They advise us in actions and in thought. Shifting a paradigm is necessary to change a culture and, thus, requires shifting the the assumptions and perceptions that embody the establishment. This requires knowing the obstacles in the current methodology. One must identify the gap between those who "know" and those who "implement," to eliminate the "know–do" gap. This enables practitioners to reach beyond current care models and provide comprehensive evidence-based approaches to healthcare that will influence the socioeconomic determinants of health and well-being (Bergstrom, Peterson, Namusoko, Waiswa, & Wallin, 2012; Havemann, 2008).

Improvements to EBP are founded in scientific research and may require shifting paradigms by articulating an action plan and providing concrete benchmarks and buffers to aid in the process. Shifting paradigms involves following a strategy in which needs are identified to improve current therapies and to reach outcomes that will be positive for the consumers and that underscore the importance of sustained advancements in care. Sometimes it may be easier to work within existing paradigms and remodel them to move current standards forward. One of the many challenges noted in translation is the "knowledge-to-action gap," whereby incomplete transfer occurs because of passivity among clinicians; this is resolved through transactional worldviews, whereby the focus is on participation, a paradigm shift that encourages learning (Rogoff, 2016). Establishing rapport between researchers and clinicians is a means of promoting a model of active engagement to avert translational barriers (Morris & Taub, 2014).

On occasion, a paradigm becomes trendy or fashionable. If such a paradigm is present in an organization, it requires a robust examination of whether the desired outcome will be achieved. Notable leaders often create new paradigms to add a fresh outlook to an organization and to revitalize stagnant groups with the hope of improvement in verifiable results.

Going through this transitional period is not always easy; but over time, individuals become accustomed to the new blueprint and let go of the old model. Changing the habits of employees is more efficient when you meet them halfway. This is accomplished by using a design in which all are encouraged to learn and participate, followed by offering opportunities in which the redesign is shared and short group exercises follow. Good knowledge management offers time for listening and enables free flow of ideas, thus forming a connection between leaders and staff. This develops the capacity to create, find, appraise, use, and store evidence basic to informative decision-making.

ORGANIZATIONAL CULTURE

Culture is distinguished as something that an "organization is as well as something that the organization *has*" and solidifies its values and beliefs (Bergstrom et al., 2012). The comparison can be made that the purpose, incentive, accountability, and power of organization culture are the DNA designers seek to change (Osborne & Plastrik, 1997, p. 2).

When we examine organizational culture, we identify the existing processes to understand the major elements comprising the environment. The factors that shape a culture are the aggregate of attitudes and behaviors of those working within the organization. The introduction of new ideas to promote growth within the practice comes from the people (Tye, n.d.). There is interdependency in the system beginning with the core operations, leading to outcomes for the users that are based on strategic plans. Important to shaping the culture are objectives for which accountability is strong, whether hierarchical, cultural, or personal, to achieve positive results.

It is important to understand the organization's readiness for EBP implementation: The culture will either impede or facilitate the adoption (Thiel & Ghosh, 2008). One tool used to ascertain the organization's cultural readiness for EBP is the Organizational Culture and Readiness for System-wide Integration of Evidence-based Practice (OCRSIEP) scale. Calculating which cultural factors influence implementation is central to optimal evidence-based translation (Melnyk et al., 2010).

Culture is collective in nature and evolves over time through interaction, development, and sharing of common beliefs and values (Bowditch, Buono, & Stewart, 2007). Within each organization are individual and self-governing characteristics that shape the ways staff perform and work together and strategize toward common goals. Culture may be amenable to innovations; positive support is integral to influence adoption of EBP (Halm, 2010). The promotion of evidence-based decision-making responsibilities encompasses behavior and language and is shared by leaders and staff alike. Culture represents value, regard for individuals, consistency, teamwork, power, recognition, and challenges and commitment to transform research for effective impact in healthcare (Bergstrom et al., 2012). The interaction within these groups is an evolutionary process followed by nterrelated professionals to convey EBP and translation into practice.

■ ORGANIZATIONAL CULTURE VERSUS CLIMATE

Organizational climate is frequently viewed as an environment of information sharing and interrelated experiences (Hann, Bower, Campbell, Marshall, & Reeves, 2007; Schneider, Ehrhart, & Macey, 2013). Organizational climate more closely reflects the employees' perception of the organization's culture (Gershon, Stone, Bakken, & Larson, 2004). Organizational climate is easy to measure by viewing policies and procedures. On the other hand, organizational culture is difficult to assess, as values and beliefs are intangible. Both organizational culture and climate are associated with morale, stress, and adverse events in an organization (Gershon et al., 2004).

Core problems within organizations are a lack of integration, collaboration, and adaption. Power distribution and breakdown confront the very culture of contemporary organizations. Tension among staff plus ambiguous control and coordination are predictors of unstable environments and lead to uncertainty and necessitate rapid changes in values and goals within the process culture (Shafritz & Hyde, 1997). Empirical relationships are implicit among EBP beliefs, EBP implementation, group cohesion, organizational culture, and provider job satisfaction, guiding the context of practice in healthcare. Further analysis of the dynamics among clinicians, researchers, and managers identifies organizational shortcomings and offers recommendations to achieve organizational readiness and support for EBP (Melnyk et al., 2010).

Negative aspects of organizational culture (little or no value for individual responsibility) and climate (rigid leadership styles and poor communication channels) are associated with lower rates of worker morale, higher levels of work stress, higher accident rates, and higher rates of adverse events. Organizations receptive to a progressive environment strive to reduce barriers and promote optimal cultures and climate. Interdependency, along with work values, increase motivation in adaptive structures. Estrada (2009) explored the perceptions to engagement and the ability to implement EBP and found that organizational infrastructure either supports or facilitates research utilization through its leadership. Rycroft-Malone et al. (2004, p. 922) support this environment by proposing the subelements of "receptive context, culture, leadership, and evaluation" as cornerstones of translation. Without synergy, the context is lost and, subsequently, EBP failure ensues. One of the seminal organizational leaders, stated, "Every organization is a product of how its members think and interact" (Rycroft-Malone et al., 2004). An infrastructure in which nursing quality and EBP have a natural synergy is needed to support a learning culture, whereas absence of a learning culture can act as a major hindrance to successful implementation (Li et al., 2018).

Capacity development provides skills and a learning environment that will engage stakeholders to produce and share knowledge, thus promoting accountability, inclusion, participation, and cohesion (Havemann, 2008). Moving from passive involvement in education and training toward active participation of translation enriches the training environments (Estabrooks et al., 2009; Kislov, Waterman, Harvey, & Boaden, 2014). Training and learning improve employee motivation with a part of training providing evaluation and feedback, which reflects a more conducive environment for change (Bergstrom et al., 2012). The extent to which learning occurs is based on opportunities, inquiry, collaboration, sharing, empowerment, environmental support, and leadership with expansive vision (Estrada, 2009). Leaders must be role models for transformation at the individual, team, and organizational levels. An effort to moderate a culture throughout the process increases acceptance and collaboration and fosters a willingness to participate in change.

Teamwork fosters vision, interaction, commitment, and cooperation to develop new ideas. Perceived team effectiveness affects competing values, participation, achievement, openness to innovation, and adherence to rules. Quality of care depends on the balance between flexibility and control and how opportunities are measured and improved, using protocols and teamwork (Bosch, Dijkstra, Wensing, van der Weijden, & Grol, 2008). Beliefs are formed, maintained, and transformed by the organization; knowing them is primary before they can be communicated openly. Leadership may have additional or differing ideas from staff; however, it is the fusion of both levels that articulates the common ground and values demonstrated in the organization. Recognition of the culture and practicing its norms exemplifies value and acceptance by those that again are reflected in the core values.

The workplace atmosphere is evident among the various layers of the organization. Social interaction and communication reflect positively or negatively. Leadership, staff, and support personnel promote an undeniable camaraderie, which is apparent in the morale of groups and individuals. A perspective employee may find a false feeling during the initial interview and on further interactions will be able to identify the bonds and connection between staff. Understanding individual behaviors is helpful to ascertain the right fit for a new employee. Promoting value toward members and emphasizing rich modes of communication enhance the landscape for new employees and show a best-fit strategy.

■ NORMS, VALUES, AND BASIC ASSUMPTIONS OF AN ORGANIZATION

An organization's underlying system of beliefs and values must transform EBP for it to be sustainable (Denhardt, 1999; Schein, 1997; Senge, 1990). Values and beliefs are the essence of the organization's philosophy for achieving success. They reflect "the way things should be" (Bowditch et al., 2007, p. 327), and direct acceptable behaviors in clinical care. Karl Popper's (1958) principle for making scientific progress through explicit attempts to refute, refine, and thus improve fundamental principles and theories remains significant in EBP and translation. Promoting an evidence-based management matrix includes the three main topics: inform, change, and monitor (Gray, 2001), with the patient as the center of implementation of care.

An organization's context includes internal as well as external factors. Examples of internal contextual features are receptiveness by leaders and clinicians, clear strategic vision, good managerial relations, and a climate conducive to implementation of EBP and research. Contextual factors are embedded in the governance of the organization; context matters when setting priorities for research.

Value statements are part of the checks-and-balances system that holds leadership responsible and provides a framework about the organization. Values reflect commitment to professionalism, integrity, service, and quality. Sharing values from the top down is one means of disseminating and collaborating for best practice and provides the link between ideas and actions. When value is not recognized or supported, formative processes are stunted.

Cultures develop as organizations learn to manage the problems of external adaptation and internal integration (Hann et al., 2007). Personal attitudes and beliefs are integral to clinicians and directly affect patient care. This can be seen in outcome-based and result-driven care. Therapeutic relationships between patient and clinician support trusting relationships. Furthermore, partnerships among practitioners correlate with the underpinnings of capacity building and foster opportunities for evaluation and research within the organization. Standards in the workplace set the quality and are predicated on the conceptualization of knowledge transfer, the process that influences EBP interventions.

The social system or context of care within the organization is reflected in the attitude of the employees. How the employee views the organization's purpose may differ between leaders and coworkers. Equating the goals of administration with the individuals in the organization requires communication to articulate shared thinking. Theoretical constructs and scientific analysis in healthcare have led to EBP initiatives. Decoding the phenomena of an employee's perception within the culture contributes to the environment of culture and climate.

Collaboration and communication help identify systems within healthcare organizations and trace the energy exchange in provision of care. Von Bertalanffly describes the model of general system theory: a system consists of interacting elements that are open to and affected by their environments. Using this premise, relationships depend on the external environment (Shafritz & Hyde, 1997). We can deduce that knowledge and experience sharing reflect positively on the organization and lead to homeostasis and equilibrium in the structure.

Organizational processes are viewed as organic with flexibility and spontaneity dominant, as opposed to following mechanistic processes, in which control or stability prevail. Activities that ensure smooth functioning are another important aspect in an organization, in which internal components relate to the outside world. This is in contrast to organizations with an external view, where competition is notable.

Bosch et al. (2008) describe independent factors that measure an organization's culture. Organizations understand that more than one culture exists within it; the mix of cultures is organized into internal and external, or stable versus flexible components. Further delineation produces at least four types of cultures. One group value consists of teamwork, cohesiveness, and sharing. Environments that are considered culturally developmental encourage leaders to examine the positive aspects of practice and take sound risks to stimulate growth and promote innovative creativeness. A rational culture strives for achievement; it uses champions to achieve goals, whereas hierarchical cultures exhibit rules, regulations, stability, and coordination (Bosch et al., 2008). Processes involve collecting and recording outcome measurements. Within an environment, the following characteristics can predict and validate quality of care: participation, which demonstrates safety of decision-making; support for innovation; discussion and review of procedures; quality monitoring; clarity of objectives; and teamwork (Hann et al., 2007).

Both culture and climate are important determinants of healthcare performance (Hann et al., 2007). Three determinants of performance are appropriate in assessing organization effectiveness. These are goals that are clear, measurable, and consensual (Bowditch et al., 2007). The mission and the operational practices on a day-to-day basis reflect appropriate goal setting. Organizational goals are viewed as being consistent for appraising organizational performance. Goals and values serve as the foci for assurances of success in moving knowledge to practice and can be observed in successful outcomes, the morale of employees, and their passion as work is performed.

■ ASSUMPTIONS OF ORGANIZATIONAL CULTURE

First, healthcare organizations possess discernible cultures that affect quality and performance. Second, although cultures are resistant to change, they are, to some extent, malleable and manageable. The strength of an organization is promulgated in shared beliefs and existing values. Cohesiveness among staff can be viewed as solid and strong when collective values dominate. Likewise, bendable relationships yield weakness and offer little to affect the overall philosophy of institutions. Bosch et al. (2008) described teamwork as elementary to improving patient care as sharing common goals, distributing work, training, and communicating benefit patients. Historically, positive associations working in teams demonstrate improved outcomes in clinical performance and turnover rates. Support for teamwork and quality of care is effective and results in achieving high levels of success, and is associated with organization culture and performance.

Organizations may have group cultures that tend to be "inward looking" (Bowditch et al., 2007), which lack flexibility, sharing, and collaboration. To reach desired outcomes, acquiring the appropriate balance between control-oriented and flexible cultures requires continuous measurement, improvement, and teamwork. Lack of a strong culture limits effectiveness, whereas openness to innovation is associated with team worth.

Third, it is possible to identify particular cultural attributes that facilitate or inhibit good performance. The culture of an organization is directly related to job satisfaction in nursing (Melnyk et al., 2010), reminding leaders to establish cultures that facilitate EBP implementation.

Fourth, any benefits accruing from a cultural change will outweigh any dysfunctional consequences. Thus, cultural changes are usually for the best.

Positive changes are instituted to align with the accepted goals to benefit the organization. Disruption occurs when changes are not in accord with the desired outcome and reflect less-than-optimal morale. To combat any negativity, decentralized decision-making is recommended, wherein leaders serve as conduits to demonstrate the significance of the outcome and why this opportunity will be advantageous for the group. Use of a dedicated change agent is a practical way to facilitate acceptance and management support to sustain change (Atchan, Davis, & Foureur, 2014).

Major Dimensions in the Assessment of Organizational Culture or Climate

First, organizational success or failure is predicated on the quality of the leaders (Boone & Bowen, 1987). Leader behavior and effectiveness are directly correlated with staff performance. Leadership is a method through which influence is directed toward individuals and groups to attain specific goals (Bowditch et al., 2007). Organizational heroes or role models are identified as those who clarify the values and beliefs essential for success.

Leaders can exert power and use it for prestige, reward, or to control groups. Referent power attracts individuals who identify with their leader's characteristics, which dominate in the organization. A combination of different types of leaders is known as *emergent leadership*, which is ideal for optimal culture and climate in most organizations. The effectiveness of leaders is demonstrated in their motivation and the ways in which they use power. Their ability to inspire speaks to the culture and climate because without this talent, groups will not engage and provide the permission to lead (Bowditch et al., 2007). This power is measured slowly through proposals, assessments, relationships, vision, building networks, open communication, and sensitivity.

Second, operational groups demonstrate high group loyalty; defend efficiency, communication, and respect for each other; and welcome support that contributes to performance goals. Within these organizations, interlocking groups communicate allegiance, favorable attitudes, and trust.

Third, communications are an important aspect of organizational culture. Communications should be sensitive, efficient, and effective (Boone & Bowen, 1987). The characteristics integral to effective translation are principles that support problem-solving activities with optimal standards. Consistent with relationships are those individuals who possess great knowledge and insight, providing opportunity to influence the advancement of practice common among leaders. Conveying essential information permits strong bonds to be built within group relationships.

Effective weapons for organizational communication consist of maintaining perspective, involving employees in the model, selecting pioneers to promote the idea, and committing to this for the duration. Maintaining these communication skills helps employees to see the value in the recognized need, understand execution of the need, and facilitate implementation of the need. Culture change is continuous, challenging, and powerful.

Fourth, the quality of work life (QWL) is another dimension of organizational culture. The notion of QWL was introduced in the late 1960s as a means to facilitate a holistic wellness approach to the employee in the long term. It encompasses the physical and mental health of the person, including the social and behavioral aspects of a person's being. Prospective knowledge expansion, worker safety, and protection of rights, and differentiating accountability are all aspects included in QWL. Breaking this down further, one looks at how effective employees are within the organization, whether open communications between management and subordinates improve or resolve issues, and the use of collaborative incentive programs for improvement in outcomes.

The fifth dimension of organization culture involves the effect of the culture on the healthcare workers; employees should feel a sense of belonging and that they are needed by the organization. Anticipated healthcare worker outcomes are belief in the system and synergistic relationships to support the culture and climate in the organization. Important to the philosophy are wellness and whole-person QWL, integration and communication, and optimizing substantive goals within the environment. Secondary objectives are openness to practice ideals, opportunities for research, and organizational resources with appropriate compensation for services. Linkages and partnerships afford opportunities for skill and knowledge development, minimize staff turnover, and create balance, enhancing worker outcomes.

COMPETING-VALUES FRAMEWORK

Competing values speak to the philosophy of the organization and are the essence for success. Some organizations have divergent cultures and subcultures that muddy opportunities for maintaining strong values. Organizational development is the application of knowledge to improve processes leading to organizational effectiveness (Erhardt, 2018). It also supports human potential, development, and performance.

Within each organization, cultures emerge and are viewed in connection to imagery, symbols, events, values, and beliefs. A friendly and social environment promotes a clannish culture. The contrast to this would be a market culture where product is outcome oriented. Additional components of culture include the hierarchical characteristics, which mean the flexibility or not of the organization, its structure, and whether it is process driven. This particular aspect of culture restricts autonomy and empowerment. The creation or evolution of cultures is known as *developmental culture*, where learning is conducive and begins with setting short- and long-term goals.

The competing-values framework (CVF) of organizational culture is a four-quadrant model of value systems set within two axes, reflecting different value orientations (Quinn & Rohrbaugh, 1981; Scott-Cawiezell, Jones, Moore, & Vojir, 2005). The first axis depicts flexibility versus control, where determinants influence organizational structure. The second axis represents concern for internal and external foci. Choices must be made that include concentration and integration or separation and distribution. Most organizations function on multiple cultures that have merged over time, with certain characteristics dominating the others.

Six content dimensions are used to frame the questions for the assessment. These dimensions consider the dominant organizational characteristic, administration, management style, organizational "glue," strategic emphasis, and criteria for success (Scott-Cawiezell et al., 2005). The valuation makes obvious both positive or negative cultures and the components linked to their values and beliefs. Although the CVF was originally developed as a way to assess organizational effectiveness, more recently, it has been used to understand the impact of organizational culture and QWL (Goodman, Zammuto, & Gifford, 2001).

Translation and the Role of Culture

Translation of evidence and culture remain important concepts, and are directly and positively related to EBP implementation. Research gaps exist despite the data supporting change; to achieve this in an organization is contingent on the culture and environment of the organization. Several factors account for this from technical issues to governance (unsupportive culture), funding, and operationalization. Translation interventions that target known barriers to change can be effective if they are based on identified barriers (Bennett et al., 2016). Translation can be limited by singular approaches and individual behaviors of decision makers, rather than the context to support the organization as a whole, strengthening systems and optimizing effectiveness (Armstrong et al., 2013).

Another way to optimize translation is through the evidence: through a combination of getting the evidence straight and getting the evidence used (Gaddis, Greenwald, & Huckson, 2007). Getting the evidence straight is the first approach of a two-part plan toward translation. Ample evidence exists in clinical practice. It is how this knowledge is implemented that strategically influences change in practice. The fact is that research studies have been identified, conducted, and published resulting in support for EBP; however, the degree of incorporation into practice is inconsistent. The evidence must be centered around a specific clinical question, and one must also determine and interpret the quality of evidence.

The second part of the strategy is to integrate the evidence, or get it used, in order to improve outcomes. Before implementation of a practice change, an assessment of the environment and culture must take place in the organization. Examining the mission, vision, and core values will inform those committed to the transformation. Beyond this action is knowledge of the leadership and management tier, plus those responsible for the education and training.

Do they display the commitment necessary to push this movement forward? In addition, are they capable and diverse enough to work with staff to support the team on all levels? Last, do the educators comprehend EBP knowledge and skills, do they have additional resources and access to technological methodologies (computers, Internet, and databases), information science professionals, and integrated health organization information systems as well as library access to augment the training and workshops needed to customize and share the path toward change?

The change process can begin once the assumptions have been carefully examined for the organization. These include the value and belief system of the organization and the connectedness of the professionals about to make the transition. Intrinsic to the process is proactive leadership that steps forward and leads by example, demonstrating the positive components of EBP, and facilitates the exchange of information needed each step of the way. Introducing the change in phases limits the hurdles because large drastic changes are harder to tolerate, whereas incremental modifications are less contested. Using this philosophy reinforces affirmative trust and creates further interest in the concept. When executing a change among great numbers in an organization, it is often prudent to divide the efforts and transition from one area to another if possible. This can be done by starting with one unit and following a systematic path, moving from one location to another until all areas have been approached.

Elements for Successful Change

Change is an integral part of any organization's culture. The process follows an incremental progression and redirection of pathways to care. All establishments should have well-delineated visions and goals, describing the tenets that support the mission. The most effective way to create and transfer knowledge is through development of a comprehensive plan to educate, followed by evaluation tools and methods, collaboration, and experience to reach desired outcomes.

Management must demonstrate confidence in the plan and have a well-thought-out protocol to change the landscape (i.e., maintain consistency of terms and data definitions). This shift has to be persistent, include the potential barriers that might hinder the progression of the movement, and dispel fears of misperceptions germane to EBP. There is overwhelming support for shifting the current paradigm to one that contributes effective patient-centered care. Defining the concept within the organization and communicating this vision contained in the strategic plan will compel professionals to come on board with energy, exercising teamwork and synergy to reach optimal outcomes. Case studies are also an innovative way to report on progress toward a specific objective or cluster objectives on a particular topic.

Clear goals articulate what needs are shared, the training needed, and act as advanced communication portals to conduct and contribute to improvement to the vision of the organization. In addition, structural changes lead to quality improvement that contributes to high-quality care. An organization is not complete without its resources or logistical and administrative support. These individuals are those people who make the work of groups manageable. They also help organize workflow, receive reports, and provide the behind-the-scenes continuity possible. There will always be resistance somewhere in the process, but this can usually be managed by individual or small-group assistance. Optimism is highly recommended to achieve buy-in from everyone.

Creating a Culture for Translation

The process of culture change involves a shift in philosophy and practice toward patient-directed, consumer-driven health promotion and quality of life (White-Chu, Graves, Godfrey, Bonner, & Sloane, 2009). Creating a culture for translation includes building the infrastructure (including human resources: champions, mentors, and leaders), technical resources, and medical information resources. In addition, stakeholder involvement is important, as is the importance of context.

During translation, it is advantageous to identify the resources that will contribute to efficiency throughout the process. Potential resources are leaders and mentors who develop opportunities and educational programs for staff and create communication networks and forums where good discussion can take place and where people become engaged in issues that shed light on their skills, sharing personal expertise and skills. Other tangible resources are timelines, libraries with a bank of information pertinent to translational knowledge and change, case examples, access to technological equipment, and experienced professionals. Building the infrastructure requires evaluation at regular intervals to measure and track targeted achievements. A successful EBP culture will demonstrate evidence of resources to enable nurses to engage in EBP; this is also articulated in the mission statement (Thiel & Ghosh, 2008).

Champions

Organizational heroes are role models within the subset of an organization's infrastructure who personify the cultural value system and define the organization's concept in noticeable ways. These individuals may be leaders or practitioners, and they represent and reinforce the values of culture by underscoring models of improvement in outcomes of patient care, thus providing a standard of performance while motivating organizational members (Greiner & Knebel, 2003). This is in direct contrast to those who circulate myths, thus undermining the cultural values abandoning the organization's needs and creating dysfunction. Stopping this behavior requires cultivation of a positive environment by featuring champions, and establishes a joint effort toward positive change. Research has shown that identifying committed champions strengthens the adoption of EBP. Effective knowledge transfer (KT) involves having one executive-level champion to be an advocate for the project, who is supported by an executive assistant responsible for logistics and scheduling, who generally keeps the task alive (Tye, n.d.). Encouragement by peers, positive work relationships, and academic detailing foster a work environment that is ready to implement EBP (Kaplan et al., 2014). A sustaining culture imposes engagement to sustain quality and outcomes inclusive of EBP (Roberts, 2013).

Mentors

Capacity-building measures also include mentorships that incorporate protocol design, analysis of results, journal clubs that introduce relevant literature-noting gaps, and, finally, creating linkages within the clinical arena (Verhoef, Mulkins, Kania, Findlay-Reece, & Mior, 2010). EBP mentors are commonly cited as important aspects to sustaining a culture of inquiry for EBP (Breckenridge-Sproat et al., 2015; Fitzsimons & Cooper, 2012; Patterson, Mason, & Duncan, 2017). Mentors provide mentoring to clinical teams, as well as to individual staff, and although frequently these are advanced practice providers, they can be staff nurses who have experience on an EBP team. Supportive environments identify mentors who will embrace the implementation of EBP, which is also indicative of readiness for change within an organizational culture; they will encourage the search for evidence, foster journal clubs, and actively participate in approaches based on research (Thiel & Ghosh, 2008). Improvements in patient care are indicative of the positive outcomes accomplished by EBP mentors utilized in healthcare systems.

Another form of advisement is the use of knowledge brokers (KBs), who work closely with leaders and staff to facilitate systems change and establish connections between researchers and users (Dobbins et al., 2009). KBs facilitate a decision-making culture and stress the value of EBP to energize knowledge translation strategies. They hold the role of "knowledge manager," performing functions to transfer and exchange information across health-related contributors, venues, and sectors.

Leaders

Changes in healthcare require strong leadership to help staff move good evidence into practice and optimize patients' outcomes (Gawlinski & Rutledge, 2008). Facilitating a supportive culture with leaders is instrumental to reaching the Health and Medicine Division (of the National Academies of Sciences, Engineering, and Medicine)'s 2020 goal that 90% of clinical decisions should be evidence based (Melnyk, Fineout-Overholt, Gallagher-Ford, & Kaplan, 2012). Through the use of participative leadership styles (Fisher & Sheeron, 2014) and transformational leadership (Gallagher-Ford, 2014), the nurse manager can have significant influence on overcoming barriers to implementation and use of EBP. There is a tremendous need for nurse leaders to expand the scope so that EBP strategies are embedded in the culture of organizations and results reflect the best patient outcomes. Leader acceptance must demonstrate that the organizational structure is ready by facilitating organizational acumen. Their input to the value of EBP is reflected in providing team goals, resource materials, ongoing communication forums, EBP-focused grand rounds, outcome measures to evaluate evidence-based initiatives (Melnyk et al., 2012), and future meetings. Strong leaders model behaviors and attitudes throughout processes and understand that good ideas come from everywhere, and they provide encouragement and support to everyone to reach the objective. Leaders who are innovative, empowering, and focused on learning are receptive to changing practice, building effective teams, and implementing EBP. Sustaining EBP requires leaders to embed a culture of inspiration for EBP.

Technical and Medical Information Resources

A strong component of any organization is data mining and information technology. The informatics system must be able to yield appropriate surveillance and collection of trends internally and externally, with the ability to locate reports on disease treatment protocols to determine what works and what does not. In addition, access to outside web-based resources via the Internet will connect medical information resources locally, regionally, nationally, and internationally. This opportunity provides the necessary means to remain connected to other professionals and translates well to future publications and media news bytes.

Stakeholder Involvement

Stakeholder awareness and involvement are critical components of translation. In creating a culture for translation, one must consider all stakeholders. These include anyone who will be affected by the translation, as well as anyone who can influence it, but who is not directly involved with the work of the translation. Stakeholder roles include that of consultant (provides input, but has no decision-making authority responsible for carrying out tasks or making recommendations); approval (signs off on recommendations, but may veto); and informed (needs to be notified on progress, but no input into decisions). Thus, a stakeholder analysis needs to be conducted as part of the planning process (see Chapter 9, Project Management for Translation).

Care must be continuous, customized, and personalized to meet the needs of the patient. Translation makes users aware of knowledge and facilitates its use. It closes the gap between what we know and what we do, and moves knowledge into action (Graham & Tetroe, 2009). Health professionals support patient care through knowledge acquisition and use of EBP guidelines. Safe care is a priority and prevents errors that interfere with identified patient outcomes. While acknowledging the needs of the patient, transparency in the decisions made in patient care promotes the central worth of the patient. None of this can be accomplished without collaboration, communication, delegation of responsibilities, and exchange of information in coordination of care (Institute of Medicine, 2003). These principles relate to the importance of stakeholder involvement in the care of the patient.

Fostering Professionalism and Autonomy

Professionalism is cultivated through excellent informal and formal communication. Providing a culture and environment conducive to innovative practice stimulates practitioners to offer patient-centered care. EBP and KT focus on transdisciplinary, holistic, global partnerships in research, knowledge generation, translation, and action (Shahab & Ghaffar, 2008). Engagement of the team of caregivers and using established good EBP methodology endorse robust networks that are valuable to all. Evaluative criteria are demonstrated by documenting "progress" in assessments and changes from baseline measures toward the targeted outcomes, and often result in cost-effectiveness.

Importance of Context and Utilization of a Model

Both Kitson, Harvey, and McCormack (1998) and the Promoting Action on Research Implementation in Health Services Model; PARiHS; Kitson et al., 2008; Rycroft-Malone et al., 2004a, 2004b) focus on context, noting that *context* is defined as the environment or setting in which the translation of evidence is to be implemented. Context comprises three components: organizational culture, leadership, and evaluation. Thus, the context and the culture of the organization as the setting of translation are important. Melnyk, Fineout-Overholt, Giggleman, and Choy (2017) showed that by implementing the Advancing Research and Clinical Practice Through Close Collaboartion (ARCC) Model, healthcare systems can enhance clinicians' beliefs and implementation of evidenced-based care, improve patient outcomes, and move organizational culture toward EBP.

In a literature review on promoting the implementation of EBP, the authors found that three factors were vital to implementing EBP: characteristics of the leader, characteristics of the organization, and characteristics of the culture (Sandstrom, Borglin, Nilsson, & Williams, 2011).

■ CONCLUSIONS

Culture is an important part of translation of evidence into practice. Engineering change in healthcare systems and groups (Straus, Tetroe, & Graham, 2009a, 2009b) is interrelated in the culture cycle in organizations. Integrating knowledge from research and linking the exchange between researchers and practitioners is the objective of translation in organizations. An accepting organizational culture is pivotal to translation, and has a direct impact on the success of the organization, as well as on the success of the translation.

■ REFERENCES

Armstrong, R., Waters, E., Dobbins, M., Anderson, L., Moore, L., Petticrew, M., . . . Swinburn, B. (2013). Knowledge translation strategies to improve the use of evidence in public health decision making in local government: Intervention design and implementation plan. *Implementation Science, 8,* 121. doi:10.1186/1748-5908-8-121

Atchan, M., Davis, D., & Foureur, M. (2104). Applying a knowledge translation model to uptake of the Baby Friendly Health Initiative in the Australian health care system. *Women and Birth, 27*(2), 79–85. doi:10.1016/j.wombi.2014.03.001

Bennett, S., Whitehead, M., Eames, S., Fleming, J., Low, S., & Caldwell, E. (2016). Building capacity for knowledge translation in occupational therapy: Learning though participatory research. *BMC Medical Education, 16*(1), 257–268. doi:10.1186/s12909-016-0771-5

Bergstrom, A., Peterson, S., Namusoko, S., Waiswa, P., & Walin, L. (2012). Knowledge translation in Uganda: A qualitative study of Ugandan midwives' and managers' perceived relevance for the sub-elements of the context cornerstone in the PARIS framework. *Implantation Science, 7*(1), 117–130. doi:10.1186/1748-5908-7-117

Boone, L. E., & Bowen, D. D. (1987). *The great writings in management and organizational behavior* (2nd ed.). Boston, MA: McGraw-Hill.

Bosch, M., Dijkstra, R., Wensing, M., van der Weijden, T., & Grol, R. (2008). Organizational culture, team climate, and diabetes care in small office-based practices. *BMC Health Services Research, 8,* 180–188. doi:10.1186/1472-6963-8-180

Bowditch, J. L., Buono, A. F., & Stewart, M. (2007). *A primer on organizational behavior* (7th ed.). New York, NY: John Wiley & Sons.

Breckenridge-Sproat, S., Throop, M. D., Raju, D., Murphy, D. A., Loan, L. A., & Patrician, P. A. (2015). Building a unit-level mentored program to sustain a culture of inquiry for evidenced-based practice. *Clinical Nurse Specialist, 29*(6), 329–337. doi:10.1097/nur.0000000000000161

Denhardt, R. B. (1999). *Public administration: An action orientation* (3rd ed.). Fort Worth, TX: Harcourt Brace College.

Dobbins, M., Hanna, S. E., Ciliska, D., Manske, S., Cameron, R., Mercer, S., . . . Robeson, P. (2009). A randomized controlled trial evaluating the impact of knowledge translation and exchange strategies. *Implementation Science, 4,* 61. doi:10.1186/1748-5908-4-61

Erhardt, R. (2018). *Cultural analysis of organizational development units: A comprehensive approach based on the competing values framework* (Doctoral dissertation). Georgia State University, Atlanta, GA. Retrieved from https://scholarworks.gsu.edu/bus_admin_diss/107

Estabrooks, C. A., Hutchinson, A. M., Squires, J. E., Birdsell, J., Cummings, G. G., Degner, L., . . . Norton, P. G. (2009). Translating research in elder care: An introduction to a study protocol series. *Implementation Science, 4,* 51. doi:10.1186/1748-5908-4-51

Estrada, N. (2009). Exploring perceptions of a learning organization by RNs and relationship to EBP beliefs and implementation in the acute care setting. *Worldviews on Evidence-Based Nursing, 4*(6), 200–209. doi:10.1111/j.1741-6787.2009.00161.x

Fisher, C. A., & Sheeron, J. (2014). Creating a culture of EBP: What's a manager to do? *Nursing Management, 45*(10), 21–23. doi:10.1097/01.numa.0000453943.62534.03

Fitzsimons, E., & Cooper, J. (2012). Embedding a culture of evidenced-based practice. *Nursing Management, 19*(7), 14–19. doi:10.7748/nm2012.11.19.7.14.c9370

Gaddis, G., Greenwald, P., & Huckson, S. (2007). Toward improved implementation of evidence-based clinical algorithms: Clinical practice guidelines, clinical decision rules, and clinical pathways. *Academic Emergency Medicine, 14*(11), 1015–1022. doi:10.1197/j.aem.2007.07.010

Gallagher-Ford, L. (2014). Implementing and sustaining EBP in real world healthcare settings: Transformational evidenced-based leadership: Redesigning traditional roles to promote and sustain a culture of EBP. *Worldviews on Evidenced-Based Nursing, 11*(2), 140–142. doi:10.1111/wvn.12033

Gawlinski, A., & Rutledge, D. (2008). Selecting a model for evidence-based practice changes: A practical approach. *AACN Advanced Critical Care, 19*(3), 219–300. doi:10.1097/01.aacn.0000330380.41766.63

Gershon, R. R., Stone, P. W., Bakken, S., & Larson, E. (2004). Measurement of organizational culture and climate in healthcare. *Journal of Nursing Administration, 34*(2), 33–40. doi:10.1097/00005110-200401000-00008

Goodman, E. A., Zammuto, R. F., & Gifford, B. D. (2001). The competing values framework: Understanding the impact of organizational culture on the quality of work life. *Organization Development Journal, 19*(3), 58–67.

Graham, I. D., & Tetroe, J. M. (2009). Getting evidence into policy and practice: Perspective of a health research funder. *Journal of the Canadian Academy of Child and Adolescent Psychiatry, 18*(1), 46–50.

Gray, J. A. M. (2001). *Evidence-based health care: How to make a health policy and management decisions* (2nd ed.). London, UK: Churchill Livingstone.

Greiner, A., & Knebel, E. (Eds). (2003). *Health professions education: A bridge to quality*. Washington, DC: The National Academies Press.

Halm, M. (2010). "Inside looking in" or "Inside looking out"? How leaders shape cultures equipped for evidence-based practice. *American Journal of Critical Care, 19*(4), 375–378. doi:10.4037/ajcc2010627

Hann, M., Bower, P., Campbell, S., Marshall, M., & Reeves, D. (2007). The association between culture, climate, and quality care in primary health care teams. *Family Practice, 24*(4), 323–329. doi:10.1093/fampra/cmm020

Havemann, K. (2008). The changing landscape of research for health. *Global Forum Update for Health, 5*, 59–63.

Institute of Medicine. (2003). *The learning healthcare system: Workshop summary (IOM Roundtable on Evidence-Based Medicine)*. Retrieved from http://books.nap.edu/catalog.php?record_id=11903

Kaplan, L., Zeller, E., Damitio, D., Culbert, S., & Bayley, K. (2014). Improving the culture of evidence-based practice at a Magnet hospital. *Journal for Nurses in Professional Development, 30*(6), 274–280. doi:10.1097/nnd.0000000000000089

Kavanagh, K., & Kennedy, P. H. (1992). *Promoting cultural diversity: Strategies for health care professionals*. Newbury Park, CA: Sage.

Kislov, R., Waterman, H., Harvey, G., & Boaden, R. (2014). Rethinking capacity building for knowledge mobilization: Developing multilevel capabilities in healthcare organizations. *Implementation Science, 9*, 166. doi:10.1186/s13012-014-0166-0

Kitson, A., Harvey, G., & McCormack, B. (1998). Enabling the implementation of evidence-based practice: A conceptual framework. *Quality in Health Care, 7*(3), 149–158. doi:10.1136/qshc.7.3.149

Kitson, A. L., Rycroft-Malone, J., Harvey, G., McCormack, B., Seers, K., & Titchen, A. (2008). Evaluating the successful implementation of evidence into practice using the PARIHS framework: Theoretical and practical challenges. *Implementation Science, 3*, 1. doi:10.1186/1748-5908-3-1. Retrieved from http://www.implementationscience.com/content/pdf/1748-5908-3-1.pdf

Kleinman, A. (1988). *The illness narratives: Suffering, healing, and the human condition*. New York, NY: Basic Books.

Kojo Asamoah, S. (2014, Feb/March). Dissemination and translation of evidenced-based guidelines to practices for nurses: A systematic review of literature. *Virginia Nurses Today*, p. 11. Retrieved from www.VirginiaNurses.com

Lannon, C. P. (Ed). (2018). Rethinking leadership in the learning organization. Retrieved from https://thesystemsthinker.com/rethinking-leadership-in-the-learning-organization

Li, A., Jeffs, L., Barwick, M., & Stevens, B. (2018). Organizational contextual features that influence the implementation of evidence-based practices across healthcare settings: A systematic integrative review. *Systematic Reviews, 7*, 72–91. doi:10.1186/s13643-018-0734-5

Mann, K., Sargeant, J., & Hill, T. (2009). Knowledge translation in interprofessional education: What difference does interprofessional education make to practice? *Learning in Health and Social Care, 8*(3), 154–164. doi:10.1111/j.1473-6861.2008.00207.x

Melnyk, B., Fineout-Overholt, E., Gallagher-Ford, L., & Kaplan, L. (2012). The state of evidence-based practice in US nurses. *Journal of Nursing Administrators, 42*(9), 410–417. doi:10.1097/nna.0b013e3182664e0a

Melnyk, B., Fineout-Overholt, E., Giggleman, M., & Cruz, R. (2010). Correlates among cognitive beliefs, EBP implementation, organizational culture, cohesion and job satisfaction in evidence-based practice mentors from a community hospital system. *Nursing Outlook, 58*, 301–308. doi:10.1016/j.outlook.2010.06.002

Melnyk, B. M., Fineout-Overholt, E., Giggleman, M., & Choy, K. (2017). A test of the ARCC model improves implementation of evidenced-based practice, healthcare culture and patient outcomes. *Worldviews on Evidenced-Based Nursing, 14*(1), 5–9. doi:10.1111/wvn.12188

Morris, D., & Taub, E. (2014). Training model for promoting translation from research to clinical settings: University of Alabama at Birmingham training for constraint-induced movement therapy. *Journal of Rehabilitation Research and Development, 51*(2), xi–xviii. doi:10.1682/jrrd.2014.01.0008

Osborne, D., & Plastrik, P. (1997). *Banishing bureaucracy: The five strategies for reinventing government*. Reading, MA: Addison-Wesley.

Patterson, A. E., Mason, T. M., & Duncan, P. (2017). Enhancing a culture of inquiry. *Journal of Nursing Administration, 47*(3), 154–158. doi:10.1097/nna.0000000000000458

Popper, K. (1958). *The logic of scientific discovery*. London, UK: Hutchinson.

Quinn, R. E., & Rohrbaugh, J. (1981). A competing values approach to organizational effectiveness. *Public Productivity Review, 5*(2), 122–140. doi:10.2307/3380029

Roberts, D. (2013). What's the problem with EBP? *Medical Surgical Nursing, 22*(5), 279.

Rogoff, B. (2016). Culture and participation: A paradigm shift. *Current Opinion in Psychology, 8*, 182–189. doi:10.1016/j.copsyc.2015.12.002

Rycroft-Malone, J., Harvey, G., Seers, K., Kitson, A., McCormack, B., & Titchen, A. (2004a). An exploration of the factors that influence the implementation of evidence into practice. *Journal of Clinical Nursing, 13*(8), 913–924. doi:10.1111/j.1365-2702.2004.01007.x

Rycroft-Malone, J., Seers, K., Titchen, A., Harvey, G., Kitson, A., & McCormack, B. (2004b). What counts as evidence in evidence-based practice? *Journal of Advanced Nursing, 47*(1), 81–90. doi:10.1111/j.1365-2648.2004.03068.x

Sandstrom, B., Borglin, G., Nilsson, R., & Williams, A. (2011). Promoting the implementation of evidenced-based practice: A literature review focusing on the role of nursing leadership. *Worldviews on Evidenced-Based Nursing, 8*(4), 212–223. doi:10.1111/j.1741-6787.2011.00216.x

Schein, E. (1985). *Organizational culture and leadership*. San Francisco, CA: Jossey-Bass.

Schein, E. (2010). *Organizational culture and leadership* (p. 3). New York, NY: John Wiley & Sons.

Schneider, B., Ehrhart, M. G., & Macey, W. H. (2013). Organizational climate and culture. *Annual Review of Psychology, 64*, 361–388. doi:10.1146/annurev-psych-113011-143809

Scott-Cawiezell, J., Jones, K., Moore, L., & Vojir, C. (2005). Nursing home culture: A critical component in sustained improvement. *Journal of Nursing Care Quality, 20*(4), 341–348. doi:10.1097/00001786-200510000-00010

Senge, P. (1990). *The fifth discipline: The art and practice of the learning organization*. Retrieved from http://www.infed.org/thinkers/senge.htm

Shafritz, J. M., & Hyde, A. C. (1997). *Classics of public administration* (4th ed.). Fort Worth, TX: Harcourt Brace College.

Shahab, S., & Ghaffar, A. (2008). Strengthening the base: Innovation and convergence in climate change and public health. *Global Forum Update on Research for Health, 5*, 36–40.

Straus, S. E., Tetroe, J., & Graham, I. (2009a). Knowledge translation is the use of knowledge in health care decision-making. *Journal of Clinical Epidemiology, 61*(1), 6–10. doi:10.1016/j.jclinepi.2009.08.016

Straus, S. E., Tetroe, J., & Graham, I. D. (Eds). (2009b). *Knowledge translation in health care: Moving from evidence to practice*. Hoboken, NJ: Blackwell Publishing.

Thiel, L., & Ghosh, Y. (2008). Determining registered nurses' readiness for evidence-based practice. *Worldviews on Evidence-Based Nursing, 5*, 182–192. doi:10.1111/j.1741-6787.2008.00137.x

Tye, J. (n.d). Transforming people through the power of values. Retrieved from http://www.valuescoachinc.com/wp-content/uploads/2012/05/The-Business-Case-for-Values-Training-A-Special-Report-from-Values-Coach1.pdf

Verhoef, M. J., Mulkins, A., Kania, A., Findlay-Reece, B., & Mior, S. (2010). Identifying the barriers to conducting outcomes research in integrative health care clinic settings—a qualitative study. *BMC Health Services Research, 10*, 14. doi:10.1186/1472-6963-10-14. Retrieved from http://www.biomedcentral.com/1472-6963/10/14

Wente, S., & Kleiber, C. (2013). An exploration of context and the use of evidence-based nonpharmacological practices in emergency departments. *Worldviews on Evidence-Based Nursing, 10*(4), 187–197. doi:10.1111/wvn.12010

White-Chu, E. F., Graves, W. J., Godfrey, S. M., Bonner, A., & Sloane, P. (2009). Beyond the medical model: The culture change revolution in long-term care. *Journal of the American Medical Directors Association, 10*(6), 370–378. doi:10.1016/j.jamda.2009.04.004

PART FIVE

Issues in Translation

CHAPTER SEVENTEEN

Best Practices in Translation: Challenges and Barriers in Translation

Sharon Dudley-Brown

When written in Chinese, the word "crisis" is composed of two characters: one represents danger, and the other represents opportunity.

—JOHN F. KENNEDY

WE KNOW THAT THERE ARE MANY CHALLENGES and barriers in the translation of evidence, as seen in the lag time in adoption and the general lack of translation of evidence in healthcare. According to McGlynn et al. (2003), only one half of evidence reaches widespread use. This has been documented across healthcare fields, countries, and settings (Harding, Porter, Horne-Thompson, Donley, & Taylor, 2014; Williams, Perillo, & Brown, 2015), including nursing (Omer, 2012; Yadav & Fealy, 2011), occupational therapy (Lyons, Brown, Tseng, Casey, & McDonald, 2011), and medicine (Sadeghi-Bazargani, Sadegh, & Azami-Aghdash, 2014).

To translate evidence into practice, a cascade framework can be used—which is an adaptation of a knowledge translation cascade created by the World Health Organization (WHO; Tugwell, Robinson, Grimshaw, & Santesso, 2006). The first step is the identification of barriers and facilitators, the second is the prioritization of the barriers, the third is choosing a model for translation to address key barriers, the fourth is using that model and developing appropriate interventions to address the barriers, the fifth is the evaluation of the translation, and the sixth is the dissemination of the translation. This chapter addresses steps one through four because the final two steps are covered in later chapters.

IDENTIFICATION OF BARRIERS RELATED TO EVIDENCE TRANSLATION

The identification of barriers and facilitators is suggested to be completed a priori in any translation project. Both challenges and barriers can be broken down via the process described by Funk, Champagne, Wiese, and Tornquist (1991a) and Funk, Tornquist, and Champagne (1995) as barriers to research utilization. However, one can argue that these are the same categories of barriers seen when exploring those related to evidence translation. These categories include the characteristics of the adopter, organization or institution, innovation, and communication.

These categories were initially developed from a factor analysis of the BARRIERS Scale, developed by Funk et al. (1991a, 1995). The characteristics of the adopter are essentially the characteristics of the individual who will adopt the evidence, for example, the nurse. This category takes into consideration the nurse's knowledge, skills, values, and awareness of the evidence, as well as the nurse's willingness to change or try new ideas. The second category includes the characteristics of the organization, which address the organization's role in the translation process as well as the setting. This includes authority to make changes, administrative support for implementation, facilities, and time for implementation. The third category, characteristics of the innovation, involves the qualities of the evidence and prior research. This also includes the "innovation" to borrow from Rogers's (1983) work on diffusion of innovations, which is defined as the idea, practice, or object that is new to the potential adopter. The last category focuses on the characteristics of the communication (another category borrowed from Rogers's work). This includes the accessibility of the evidence and channels of communication.

Use of the BARRIERS Scale

A systematic review of the BARRIERS Scale (Funk, Champagne, Wiese, & Tornquist, 1991b; Funk et al., 1995) explored the state of knowledge from use of the scale and recommendations made about the future use of the scale. The authors included 63 studies, most of which were cross-sectional in design but of weak to moderate quality. The scale was found to be reliable, as assessed by internal consistency. However, the validity of the scale to accurately capture barriers was lacking. One possible contributory factor is the fact that the scale was developed in the late 1980s to early 1990s, and the healthcare environment and the nursing profession have changed over the past 30 years. For example, patient participation in decision-making has increased, and patients' preferences and opinions may present a barrier to research utilization. The initial scale did not contain any questions related to patients' opinions; however, Greene (1997) added this to the patients' scale and measured barriers toward pain management in oncology. In that study, the item "patients will not take medication or follow the recommendations" was ranked as the third highest barrier by nurses.

The main barriers reported from this systematic review (Funk et al., 1995) were related to the setting and the presentation of research findings. Overall, despite varying geographic locations, sample size, response rate, study setting, and assessment of study quality, identified barriers were consistent. Of the top 10 barriers, the items "there is insufficient time on the job to implement new ideas," "the nurse does not have time to read research," "the nurse does not have enough authority to change patient care procedures," "the statistical analyses are not understandable," together with "the relevant literature is not compiled in any place" were the most frequently reported. Six of the top 10 barriers belonged to the Setting subscale. Few studies reported associations between reported research use and perceptions of barriers to research utilization.

Carlson and Plonczynski (2008) conducted an integrative review on whether the BARRIERS Scale has changed practice. To be specific, they looked at whether the identification of perceived barriers to research utilization influences nurses' use of research: Whether the extent of nurses' perceived barriers to research utilization and most frequently cited barriers have changed over time and whether nurses' most frequently cited barriers differ across countries. Findings included that there was no evidence that identification of barriers to nurses' use of research influenced nursing practice; that the most frequently cited barriers have not changed over time; and that there were some differences in most frequently cited barriers by country, for all three categories (characteristics of the organization, communication, and adopter; Carlson & Plonczynski, 2008).

More recent use of the BARRIERS Scale has provided similar results. Lyons et al. (2011) explored perceived research knowledge, attitudes and practices, and barriers among Australian pediatric occupational therapists. From the use of the BARRIERS Scale, they found the most barriers on the communication subscale and then the organization subscale. Omer (2012) used the BARRIERS Scale to explore barriers and facilitators of research utilization among nurses in Saudi Arabia and found that the highest perceived barriers were on the Organization subscale, followed by the Communication subscale. Athanasakis (2013) reviewed some of the literature on use of the BARRIERS Scale alone or combined with another instrument and found that the barriers came mainly from the clinical characteristics of the clinical setting. More recent, the BARRIERS Scale was administered to critical care nurses in Jordan (Hweidi, Tawalbeh, Al-Hassan, Alayadeh, & Al-Smadi, 2017). Results included the findings that nurses did not feel they had time to even read research at work, that organizational barriers were the greatest, and that factors hindering research use are multidimensional.

In addition, a study was conducted to determine whether the BARRIERS Scale discriminated between research users and nonresearch users on perceptions of barriers (Bostrom, Kajermo, Nordstrom, & Wallin, 2008). They found that the BARRIERS Scale revealed differences in the perception of barriers between research users and nonresearch users among nurses and concluded that the scale appears to be useful to identify some barriers of research utilization but not organizational barriers.

Other Scales of Use

Although Funk and colleagues' BARRIERS Scale has been used to explore reasons why nurses do not use research (Funk et al., 1991a, 1995), there have been more recent studies looking at barriers and facilitators to use of evidence-based practice (EBP). Leasure, Stirlen, and Thompson (2008) specifically wanted to identify the presence or absence of provider and organizational variables associated with the use of EBP among nurses. Using a researcher-developed instrument on perceived internal and external organizational processes related to implementation of EBP changes. Questionnaires were mailed to nurse executives, who then gave the questionnaires to staff nurses. Results from 119 nurses revealed the following facilitators: reading journals that publish original research, journal club, nursing research committee, a facility research committee, and facility access to the Internet. Barriers found included lack of staff involvement in projects, no communication about projects that were completed, no knowledge of outcomes, and the fact that most job descriptions did not include a research component. Although there is a methodological flaw (bias) of sending the questionnaires first to nurse managers who distributed them to their staff, the findings are similar to those of Funk et al. (1991a, 1995).

The Promoting Action on Research Implementation in Health Services (PARiHS) framework was developed to represent essential determinants of successful implementation of research into clinical practice (Kitson, Harvey, & McCormack, 1998) and can be dually used to explore challenges and barriers in translation. The PARiHS framework posits three core elements that determine the success of research implementation:

1. Evidence—The strength and nature of the evidence as perceived by multiple stakeholders
2. Context—The quality of the context or environment in which the research is implemented
3. Facilitation—Processes by which implementation is facilitated

Each of these three core elements, in turn, comprise multiple, distinct components (for frameworks on translation, see Chapter 2, The Science of Translation and Major Frameworks and Chapter 3, Change Theory and Models: Framework for Translation). Because of its focus on these three areas critical in translation, PARiHS can be used to determine, a priori, potential barriers to translation.

Meijers's Work on Contextual Factors

Exploring contextual factors and research utilization, Meijers et al. (2006) conducted a systematic review exploring the relationship between contextual factors and research utilization and mapped results to the PARiHS model. In 10 papers, six contextual factors were identified as having a statistically significant relationship with research use, namely, the role of the nurse, multifaceted access to resources, organizational climate, multifaceted support, time for research activities, and provision of education. The contextual factors could successfully be mapped to the dimensions of context in the PARiHS framework (context, culture, leadership), with the exception of evaluation. However, the authors found that few studies of sufficient quality were found because of methodological limitations, and the results in reviewed studies were mixed. They concluded that the strength of the relationship among the six contextual factors and research utilization by nurses is still largely unknown; however, findings do provide support that the PARiHS framework allows for better understanding of the impact of context on research use.

Facilitators to Translation of Evidence

Although challenges and barriers are both individual and institutional, facilitators to translation of evidence largely depend on the organization or institution. Cummings, Estabrooks, Midodzi, Wallin, and Hayduk (2007) developed and tested a theoretical model of organizational influences on research use, based on the PARiHS framework, and assessed the influence of less positive to contexts that are more positive on research use. Findings of hospital characteristics that positively influenced research use by nurses were staff development, opportunity for nurse-to-nurse collaboration, and staffing and support services. Increased emotional exhaustion led to a reduction in reported research use and higher rates of nurse- and patient-reported events. Nurses working in contexts that had a more positive culture, leadership, and evaluation reported significantly more research use, staff development, and lower rates of patient and staff adverse events. The authors conclude that the findings highlight the combined importance of culture, leadership, and evaluation to increase research use and improve patient safety. Findings also strengthen the PARiHS framework and its use to guide research into practice and translation (Cummings et al., 2007)

Foxcroft and Cole (2004) conducted a Cochrane review to determine to what extent organizational infrastructures are effective in promoting the implementation of research evidence on the promotion of evidence-based nursing (EBN) practice. The authors found no studies rigorous enough to be included, and obtained seven case studies. They concluded that conceptual models on organizational processes used to promote EBP need to be better evaluated and suggested time-series designs to further explore this topic. Clearly, although organizational infrastructure is important, there are no clear guidelines on its implementation in terms of the promotion of EBP.

Newhouse, Dearholt, Pugh, and White (2007) explored ways in which institutions could build infrastructure to support EBP. These include leadership, establishing a structure for building and sustaining EBP such as shared governance committees, developing an EBP skill set with the availability of EBP experts and mentors, developing material resources, setting expectations (revising job descriptions), collaborating with a school of nursing, and continuing to revise and update tools.

Mohide and Coker (2005) also described their organizational interventions to increase the rate of research dissemination and uptake. They used an EBN committee as an organizational strategy to shift the culture toward scholarship. Specific strategies and activities used included organizational commitment to EBP, strategic positioning of the EBN committee within nursing's administrative structure, articulation of a mission, conceptualization of a model for EBN practice, learning on the job, selection and adoption of an evidence-based model for implementing change, and marketing for a change in culture toward clinical scholarship.

Measuring knowledge, attitude, and perceived barriers to EBP in faculty, researchers used the BARRIERS Scale and an EBP questionnaire (Stichler, Fields, Kim, & Brown, 2011). Results indicated that master's- prepared faculty had significantly higher mean scores in the practice of EBP as compared with doctorally prepared faculty, and that attitude was more positive than their knowledge/skills and practice of EBP. The influence of faculty's knowledge, attitudes, and perceived barriers needs to be explored more with the issue of translation, their experience in the translation of evidence, and in conducting EBP projects.

■ PRIORITIZATION OF BARRIERS

After identifying the barriers and facilitators of EBP, one must prioritize the barriers. One way to do so has been proposed by Tugwell et al. (2006), by prioritizing across the six Ps: public/community, patient, press, practitioner, policy maker, and private sector (as discussed in Chapter 12, Dissemination of Evidence). Barriers "must be prioritized as to whether they are modifiable, which are 'mission critical,' and how to address them" (Tugwell et al., 2006, p. 646). Tugwell et al. (2006) go on to describe how to identify key barriers based on three criteria: modifiability, available interventions, and "bottleneck issues," but state that barriers need to be prioritized based on local settings and relevant stakeholders. At an institutional level, this is where stakeholders can be asked to assist in prioritization, realizing that each stakeholder may identify a different barrier.

■ CHOOSING A MODEL TO ADDRESS KEY BARRIERS

Models used for translation, such as the PARiHS framework, can be used not only to explore and assess challenges and barriers to translation, but also to address the challenges and barriers found. This is the next step in the cascade framework for translation previously mentioned. For example, the category of context, which includes culture, leadership, and evaluation, is important in translation. Although culture can be assessed and described (see Chapter 16), evaluation (see Chapter 11) and assessment of leadership (see Chapter 6) are also important. Leadership can be used to address any barriers or challenges found in assessment. In addition to leadership, an organization's readiness to change is a key factor in addressing barriers to translation.

An Organizational Readiness to Change Assessment (ORCA) instrument, organized according to the core elements and subelements of the PARiHS framework, was developed (Helfrich, Li, Sharp, & Sales, 2009). The instrument comprises three major scales corresponding to the core elements of the PARiHS framework: (a) strength and extent of evidence for the clinical practice changes represented by the quality-improvement (QI) program, assessed with four subscales; (b) quality of the organizational context for the QI program, assessed with six subscales; and (c) capacity for internal facilitation of the QI program, assessed with nine subscales. Each subscale comprised between three and six items, assessing a common dimension of the given scale. Although the authors found general support for the reliability and factor structure of the ORCA, there was poor reliability among measures of evidence, factor analysis results for measures of general resources; and the clinical champion role did not conform to the PARiHS framework. Additional validation is needed, including criterion validation.

■ USING THE MODEL TO DEVELOP INTERVENTIONS TO ADDRESS BARRIERS

The aforementioned strategies for assessing and acting on challenges and barriers to translation of evidence have primarily focused on organizations. From the perspective of an individual provider, one can use Pathman's pipeline (Diner et al., 2007; Glasziou & Haynes, 2005; Pathman, Konrad, Freed, Freeman, & Koch, 1996) to move evidence into action and to assess and address potential challenges and barriers. This pipeline, linear in fashion, focuses on translation of knowledge and includes the following: clinician awareness, acceptance, applicability, ability, action, agreement, and then adherence to the evidence. Specifically, these are provider-oriented and patient-focused strategies to assist in translation of evidence into practice. Although the initial proposed pipeline was to address physician adherence to guidelines, Pathman et al. (1996) described four stages from evidence to action: the clinician needs to be aware, agree, adopt, and then adhere. Diner et al. (2007) later proposed a revised Pathman's pipeline, and an adaptation by Glasziou and Haynes (2005), to address the path to optimal patient outcomes, moving from evidence to practice. Diner and colleagues' adaptation includes the "leaks" along the pipeline. The leaks, the droplets of water, provide illustrative examples of information loss, misuse, or inapplicability at each level. The first five leaks deal with the physician and healthcare team, whereas the last two leaks are specific to the patient's environment. This model addresses how to "slow the leaks" and thus improve the flow of information from high-quality, clinically relevant evidence to the achievement of optimal patient outcomes. Unlike previous models, this model is more individually than institutionally based.

Diner et al. (2007) also addressed barriers to change of practice for the individual practitioner. These include self-motivation and incentives that reinforce old behavior, the environment (budget, liability, and peer group influence), recommendations that contradict previously accepted standards of care, and competing nonprovider influences such as pharmaceutical marketing, hospital administration, concern over costs, and The Joint Commission mandates. Removing barriers to translation for an individual practitioner may indeed prove more difficult than addressing those barriers from an institutional perspective. Individual concerns, values, and motivation may be more difficult to change, and strategies for change are scarce in the literature.

Kulier, Gee, and Khan (2008) described five steps to guide implementation of new research findings into practice, using the pipeline metaphor, adapted from Glasziou and Haynes (2005).

1. *Knowledge and awareness*—This step helps the clinician to be aware of new clinically useful and applicable evidence. It suggests institutional interventions such as journal club meetings and ward rounds.
2. *Acceptance and persuasion*—This step focuses on persuading the clinician about the potential benefit for the patient. One proposed intervention strategy is the use of key opinion leaders and providing information from multiple sources.

3. *Decision-making*—This step involves choice in implementing research findings. The authors again suggest more institutional strategies, such as the use of clinical directors or persons in a position of power, to bring about change within the organization. This decision-making phase truly depends on the individual, and here is where values and motivation are able to bring about any change.
4. *Implementation*—This step focuses on all the variables needed to actually implement a change. Here, the authors suggest such interventions as the use of clinical protocols and clinical practice guidelines.
5. *Continuation*—This step focuses on maintaining the change. This can occur through regular monitoring, audits, and ongoing feedback.

Although assessment of challenges and barriers in translation is acknowledged by many, it is the unforeseen challenges and barriers that occur during translation that may pose more of a problem and may be difficult to overcome. It is knowledge, through frameworks, that can assist the translation by identifying and addressing as many barriers in advance.

Another challenge in translation of evidence rests with the consumer. Carman et al. (2010, p. 2) explored how making healthcare decisions based on evidence of effectiveness could be translated into a language that consumers would understand and embrace, as part of the development of a "communication toolkit" to help consumers communicate more effectively about evidence-based healthcare. Using focus groups, interviews, and an online survey with healthcare consumers, the researchers found many beliefs, values, and knowledge to be at odds with what policy makers prescribe as evidence-based healthcare. Few consumers understood terms such as *medical evidence* or *quality guidelines*, and many believed that more healthcare and state-of-the-art care meant higher quality, better care. Thus, translation of evidence-based healthcare into understandable concepts and activities that support and motivate consumers must occur at the provider level, the institutional level, as well as with employers, health plans, and policy makers.

■ CONCLUSIONS

In summary, the translation of evidence is fraught with challenges and barriers, although the imperative to succeed is strong. The translation of knowledge has been promoted by the Institute of Medicine, now called the *National Academy of Medicine*, and has been linked to healthcare quality. The translation of knowledge has been linked to the concept of a paradigm shift by Thomas Kuhn, in that science does not progress linearly, but periodically undergoes paradigm shifts. Now is the time for a paradigm shift. However, barriers still exist to the application of knowledge, specifically in the area of risk versus benefit, comfort with current practice versus outcomes, cost, rewards, lack of experience, values, contexts, and others. As individual practitioners we need to acknowledge and address these challenges and barriers, and institutions must also promote translation and address both individual and institutional barriers to both translation of evidence and to the practice of EBP.

REFERENCES

Athanasakis, E. (2013). Nurses' research behavior and barriers to research utilization into clinical nursing practice: A closer look. *International Journal of Caring Sciences, 6*(1), 16–28.

Bostrom, A., Kajermo, K. N., Nordstrom, G., & Wallin, L. (2008). Barriers to research utilization and research use among registered nurses working in the care of older people: Does the BARRIERS scale discriminate between research users and non-research uses on perception of barriers? *Implementation Science, 3*, 24. doi:10.1186/1748-5908-3-24

Carlson, C. L., & Plonczynski, D. J. (2008). Has the BARRIERS scale changed nursing practice? An integrative review. *Journal of Advanced Nursing, 63*(4), 322–333. doi:10.1111/j.1365-2648.2008.04705.x

Carman, K. L., Maurer, M., Yegian, J. M., Dardess, P., McGee, P., Evers, M., & Marlo, K. O. (2010). Evidence that consumers are skeptical about evidence-based health care. *Health Affairs, 29*(7), 1400–1406. doi:10.1377/hlthaff.2009.0296

Cummings, G. G., Estabrooks, C. A., Midodzi, W. K., Wallin, L., & Hayduk, L. (2007). Influence of organizational characteristics and context on research utilization. *Nursing Research, 56*(Suppl 4), S24–S39. doi:10.1097/01.nnr.0000280629.63654.95

Diner, B. M., Carpenter, C. R., O'Connell, T., Pang, P., Brown, M. D., Seupaul, R. A., . . . KT-CC Theme IIIa Members. (2007). Graduate medical education and knowledge translation: Role models, information pipelines, and practice change thresholds. *Academic Emergency Medicine, 14*(11), 1008–1014. doi:10.1197/j.aem.2007.07.003

Foxcroft, D., & Cole, N. (2004). Organizational infrastructures to promote evidence-based nursing practice. *Cochrane Database of Systematic Reviews, 2004*(4), CD002212. doi:10.1002/14651858.cd002212

Funk, S. G., Champagne, M. T., Wiese, R. A., & Tornquist, E. M. (1991a). Barriers to using research findings in practice: The clinician's perspective. *Applied Nursing Research, 4*(2), 90–95. doi:10.1016/s0897-1897(05)80062-x

Funk, S. G., Champagne, M. T., Wiese, R. A., & Tornquist, E. M. (1991b). Barriers: The barriers to research utilization scale. *Applied Nursing Research, 4*(1), 39–45. doi:10.1016/s0897-1897(05)80052-7

Funk, S. G., Tornquist, E. M., & Champagne, M. T. (1995). Barriers and facilitators of research utilization. An integrative review. *Nursing Clinics of North America, 30*(3), 395–407.

Glasziou, P., & Haynes, B. (2005). The paths from research to improved health outcomes. *Evidence-Based Nursing, 8*(2), 36–38. doi:10.1136/ebn.8.2.36

Greene, P. E. (1997). *Diffusion of innovations in cancer pain management and barriers to changing practice: A study of office practice oncology nurses* (Unpublished doctoral dissertation). Georgia State University, School of Nursing, Georgia.

Harding, K. E., Porter, J., Horne-Thompson, A., Donley, E., & Taylor, N. F. (2014). Not enough time or low priority? Barriers to evidence-based practice for allied health clinicians. *Journal of Continuing Education in the Health Professions, 34*(4), 224–231. doi:10.1002/chp.21255

Helfrich, C. D., Li, Y. F., Sharp, N. D., & Sales, A. E. (2009). Organizational Readiness to Change Assessment (ORCA): Development of an instrument based on the Promoting Action on Research in Health Services (PARIHS) framework. *Implementation Science, 4*, 38. doi:10.1186/1748-5908-4-38

Hweidi, I. M., Tawalbeh, L. I., Al-Hassan, M. A., Alayadeh, R. M., & Al-Smadi, A. M. (2017). Research use of nurses working in the critical care units: Barriers and facilitators. *Dimensions of Critical Care Nursing, 36*(4), 226–233. doi:10.1097/dcc.0000000000000255

Kitson, A., Harvey, G., & McCormack, B. (1998). Enabling the implementation of evidence-based practice: A conceptual framework. *Quality in Health Care, 7*(3), 149–158. doi:10.1136/qshc.7.3.149

Kulier, R., Gee, H., & Khan, K. S. (2008). Five steps from evidence to effect: Exercising clinical freedom to implement research findings. *British Journal of Obstetrics & Gynecology, 115*(10), 1197–1202. doi:10.1111/j.1471-0528.2008.01821.x

Leasure, A. R., Stirlen, J., & Thompson, C. (2008). Barriers and facilitators to the use of evidence-based best practices. *Dimensions of Critical Care Nursing, 27*(2), 74–82. doi:10.1097/01.dcc.0000311600.25216.c5

Lyons, C., Brown, T., Tseng, M. H., Casey, J., & McDonald, R. (2011). Evidence-based practice and research utilization: Perceived research knowledge, attitudes, practices and barriers among paediatric occupational therapists. *Australian Occupational Therapy Journal, 58*, 178–186. doi:10.1111/j.1440-1630.2010.00900.x

McGlynn, E. A., Asch, S. M., Adams, J., Keesey, J., Hicks, J., DeCristofaro, A., & Kerr, E. A. (2003). The quality of health care delivered to adults in the United States. *New England Journal of Medicine, 348*(26), 2635–2645. doi:10.1056/nejmsa022615

Meijers, J. M., Janssen, M. A., Cummings, G. G., Wallin, L., Estabrooks, C. A., & Halfens, R. Y. G. (2006). Assessing the relationships between contextual factors and research utilization in nursing: Systematic literature review. *Journal of Advanced Nursing, 55*(5), 622–635. doi:10.1111/j.1365-2648.2006.03954.x

Mohide, E. A., & Coker, E. (2005). Toward clinical scholarship: Promoting evidence-based practice in the clinical setting. *Journal of Professional Nursing, 21*(6), 372–379. doi:10.1016/j.profnurs.2005.10.003

Newhouse, R. P., Dearholt, S., Pugh, L. C., & White, K. M. (2007). Organizational change strategies for evidence-based practice. *Journal of Nursing Administration, 37*(12), 552–557. doi:10.1097/01.nna.0000302384.91366.8f

Omer, T. (2012). Research utilization in a multicultural nursing setting in Saudi Arabia: Barriers and facilitators. *Journal of Nursing Research, 20*(1), 66–73. doi:10.1097/jnr.0b013e31824777d8

Pathman, D. E., Konrad, T. R., Freed, G. L., Freeman, V. A., & Koch, G. G. (1996). The awareness-to-adherence model of the steps to clinical guideline compliance. The case of pediatric vaccine recommendations. *Medical Care, 34*(9), 873–889. doi:10.1097/00005650-199609000-00002

Rogers, E. M. (1983). *Diffusion of innovations.* New York, NY: Free Press.

Sadeghi-Bazargani, H., Sadegh, J., & Azami-Aghdash, S. (2014). Barriers to evidenced-based medicine: A systematic review. *Journal of Evaluation in Clinical Practice, 20*, 793–802. doi:10.1111/jep.12222

Stichler, J. F., Fields, W., Kim, S. C., & Brown, C. E. (2011). Faculty knowledge, attitudes, and perceived barriers to teaching evidenced-based nursing. *Journal of Professional Nursing, 27*(2), 92–100. doi:10.1016/j.profnurs.2010.09.012

Tugwell, P., Robinson, V., Grimshaw, J., & Santesso, N. (2006). Systematic reviews and knowledge translation. *Bulletin of the World Health Organization, 84*(8), 643–651. doi:10.2471/blt.05.026658

Williams, B., Perillo, S., & Brown, T. (2015). What are the factors of organizational culture in health care settings that act as barriers to the implementation of evidence-based practice? A scoping review. *Health Education Today, 35*, e34–e41. doi:10.1016/j.nedt.2014.11.012

Yadav, B. L., & Fealy, G. M. (2011). Irish psychiatric self-reported barriers, facilitators and skills for developing evidence-based practice. *Journal of Psychiatric and Mental Health Nursing, 19*, 116–122. doi:10.1111/j.1365-2850.2011.01763.x

CHAPTER EIGHTEEN

Legal Issues in Translation

Sharon Dudley-Brown

The very first requirement in a hospital is that it should do the sick no harm.
—Florence Nightingale, *Notes on Nursing: What It Is, and What It Is Not*

Whether Evidence Is Translated Into Clinical Practice is contingent on the overarching social, legal, ethical, and political climate (Larkin et al., 2007). Researchers and clinicians alike must address questions of legal risk in translation of evidence. Just as providers are seeking to provide evidence-based care, so, too, have the courts begun to demand more and better evidence (Morreim, 2001). Moreover, it is evidence that is essential to any lawsuit, from presenting actions and circumstances to providing context for judging whether the standard of care was met (Gibson, 2004). However, although the same word may be used (*evidence*), clinicians and lawyers understand and apply it very differently, and it is the patient who is caught in the middle (Eisenberg, 2001).

■ LEGAL ISSUES IN TRANSLATION

Legal considerations in the translation of evidence include Food and Drug Administration (FDA) regulations, patent laws, the tort system, standard of care, and the current malpractice environment. The FDA has specific regulations for investigation of new drugs and devices that widen the evidence-to-practice gap by potentially delaying the use of newer drugs and devices that may improve outcomes. Along the same line is the potential delay for a patented treatment that may produce better outcomes than what is standard. The tort system, which varies from state to state in the United States, may delay translation as well. The standard of care can be used to show actual practice patterns, or how a standard was violated.

In a typical lawsuit for malpractice, the patient must establish that the provider owed a duty of care to the patient, that there was a breach of that duty, that injury resulted, and that the breach led to or caused the injury. This breach of duty has been interpreted to question whether there was a failure to meet the standard of care (Gibson, 2004).

Clinical Practice Guidelines as the Standard of Care

The issue of standard of care and development and use of clinical practice guidelines (CPGs) are and have been at the center of malpractice issues in translation. An adversarial legal milieu promotes clinical inertia and delays translation because early adoption of evidence often seems as a deviation from the prevailing standard of care. However, ignorance of evidence may promote inertia, but many people do not practice according to guidelines because of worries of deviating from them, even if based on patient- and situation-specific issues that should be taken into consideration. Because the prevailing standard of care is based on what care is customary at a given place and time, providers are lulled into complacency, which may result in a delay in translation of evidence into practice (Larkin et al., 2007). Practicing clinicians typically respond to threats to malpractice over adherence to CPGs.

CPGs have been developed, disseminated, and used to advance evidence-based practice. However, even the definition and development of a CPG has been debated. *CPGs* have been defined as "systematically developed statements to assist practitioner and patient decisions about appropriate healthcare for specific clinical circumstances" (Field & Lohr, 1990, p. 38). Moreover, a more recent definition suggests they are statements that include recommendations intended to optimize patient care that is informed by a systematic review of evidence and an assessment of the benefits and harms of alternative care options (Institute of Medicine [IOM], 2011). In addition, CPGs may be developed using evidence-based methodology, or they may document customary or common practice, the opinions of an individual or group of experts (Taylor, 2014). Terminology found in the publications may vary, from CPG to standards, guidelines, and options. In addition to the issue of CPGs, the use of a checklist, again commonly based on evidence, has been debated for use in improving quality and minimizing legal liability (Howie & McMullen, 2010). Although in nursing, the care pathway has been noted to be both a legal sword and a shield (Griffith, 2008).

However, CPGs appear to be a double-edged sword. Whereas they can guide clinicians in the diagnosis and management of a particular problem, they can be, and are used by third-party payers, regulatory bodies, and courts in the determination of whether care was appropriate and adequate (Rosoff, 2001). Some argue that a "standard of care," which presumes that the same care is used for all patients, goes against the principles of evidence-based practice, whereby patient preferences and values are taken into consideration. Moreover, in some cases, "the standard of care lags behind best practices" (Oberman, 2017, p. 25). Oberman (2017) goes on to argue that the law demands only that the treatment provided is no less than what could be expected from a reasonable professional, meaning a minimally competent professional, when dealing with malpractice or liability. Therefore, the conflict between standard of care and litigation may be similar to that between a standard of care and the practice of evidence-based care. However, it seems that most can argue that the evidence-based care can be practiced using the best available evidence without referring to CPGs (Taylor, 2014). Taylor (2014) concludes "CPGs considered alone and in isolation of the facts of the case do not represent the standard of care" (p. 290).

Expert Witness Testimony: CPGs Versus Customary Practice

Expert testimony is frequently used to deal with quality-of-care issues that arise in the courts. The main issues calling for expert testimony are (a) an applicable standard of care; (b) causation; and (c) the assessment of damages, which often involves (d) medical prognosis (Rosoff, 2001). Whereas the type of issue dictates the nature and scope of the expert witness's testimony, the last three issues (causation, assessment of damages, and prognosis) usually require the expert witness to apply his or her expertise directly to the question at hand; however, in the first issue, the standard of care is different. In this situation, the expert witness does not testify to what he or she thinks is the proper way to treat the case but, rather, to what others in the profession would commonly do in such a situation. Thus, the expert witness's contribution is his or her knowledge of how professional peers commonly handle similar situations. The issue of whether CPGs are evidence based and whether they are synonymous with customary practice still remains to be seen.

However, newly developed CPGs may differ substantially from prevailing practice, and thus, if *customary practice* is the legal standard, CPGs would not be used extensively in the legal system. However, according to Rosoff (2001), whereas CPGs have been used as evidence of customary practice, they have also been used as evidence of a respectable majority, evidence of reasonable prudence, evidence of acceptable practice, and as a legal standard of care. Usually, the existence of a duty to care is straightforward. Most actions of medical negligence hinge on questions of standard of care or in determination of causation. CPGs, therefore, may affect both of these elements of negligence. However, standards of care can vary greatly geographically, and a CPG can be either a minimum or maximum standard of care. Both negligence and causation are issues in U.S., Canadian, and U.K. laws (Hurwitz, 1994; McDonagh & Hurwitz, 2003; Rosoff, 2001).

The Debate: CPGs as a Sword or a Shield for the Practitioner

CPG can be used as a sword or a shield (Gibson, 2004; Rosoff, 2001; Ruhl & Siegal, 2017). As a sword, CPG can be used by a patient plaintiff to place blame by establishing that there was a guideline that the defendant should have used or followed but did not. In contrast, a defendant (the provider) can use it as a shield by showing that he or she acted in conformity with an established guideline, and thus met the requisite standard of care (Gibson, 2004; Rosoff, 2001). Rosoff (2001) goes on to state that CPGs are more commonly used by plaintiffs. Certain states (Minnesota, Maine) have adopted laws that provide only for defensive use of a CPG, and the American Medical Association (AMA) has declared that there is insufficient evidence to show that CPGs can be developed specifically enough to be used as a defense in medical liability litigation (AMA, 1993). Thus, the AMA opposes direct adoption of CPGs as a legal standard and urges that they should be used as evidence of *standards of practice* and that their degree of authority depends on their degree of acceptance among peers.

Whether CPGs are accepted as evidence of standards of practice among peers is debatable. According to Tanenbaum (1994), who has conducted research on how physicians reason about their clinical care, learn from their experiences, and pass information along to colleagues, physicians have two different ways of processing information: deterministic reasoning, which searches out mechanisms of illness based on the sciences, and probabilistic reasoning, which is drawn from past experiences. Tanenbaum concludes that a clinician's decisions are not likely to be influenced by outcomes research and, thus, the physician is skeptical about the information that forms the basis of evidence-based medicine. "The probabilists play the odds, while the determinists imagine the process" (Tanenbaum, 1994, pp. 30–31). Taylor (2014) provides some examples of when guidelines are either considered or allowed into evidence, when they have been excluded, as well as when a guideline was entered into evidence by the plaintiff but then was subsequently used by the defense to support its position.

The Debate: CPGs and the Provider's Autonomy

Another pressing issue in the use of CPGs is their potential to be in conflict with provider judgment and autonomy, either of the individual or the collective autonomy of a professional group. In addition to erosion of autonomy, there is a greater risk of liability and how relevant CPGs are to an individual's practice.

The law has two functions: litigation, the settlement of disputes, which is retrospective in orientation, and regulation, which is prospective and more forward looking. The law's regulatory function is more compatible with the notion of evidence-based practice, which is more probabilistic. Regulation, which deals with what might happen (a probabilistic notion) rather than trying to determine what actually did happen in a spat or incident, is the focus of litigation (Rosoff, 2001).

In terms of legal issues, most center on the individual provider, and much of that has focused on CPGs. However, on an institutional and organizational basis, legal issues in translation center on policies and procedures: the evidence used to develop policies and procedures, when the policies and procedures are updated, and who should follow them are all pertinent.

Protecting Yourself

One way to protect oneself, as a nurse, from a lawsuit is through documentation. Although proper documentation is requisite to a number of issues, namely, continuity and provision of care and care coordination, it also helps to protect the nurse (and healthcare providers) from litigation. Some of this documentation allows for acknowledgment of following the standard of care, but can provide facts and protect against negligence (Ferrell, 2007). Essentially, "if there is no documentation, there's no evidence" (Ferrell, 2007, p. 62).

Another way to protect oneself is through documentation of reason(s) for not adhering to CPGs, especially if a particular CPG has been adopted for use at a facility. Many guidelines may not be appropriate for every patient in every situation, and thus it falls to the providers to provide judgment on them. In addition, patient's values and beliefs may not be in agreement with that of any CPG, so here documentation is again important. Providers then clearly need to evaluate all CPGs that they are asked to use, prior to their use or implementation into policies and procedures. For example, using evaluation criteria by the AGREE (Appraisal of Guidelines for Research and Evaluation) Collaboration (Brouwers et al., 2010), a clinician, or preferably a group of clinicians, can follow the criteria to determine whether that particular guideline meets quality standards and is worthy of its use in a particular organization or with a particular population of patients.

CONCLUSIONS

In conclusion, because of the legal issues inherent in translation, it is incumbent upon all nurses to be knowledgeable of the intersection between healthcare and the law, and to understand the potential ramifications of the use of all CPGs and their place in evidence-based practice.

REFERENCES

American Medical Association. (1993). Statement to Committee on Health, Committee on Ways and Means, 103d Cong., 1st sess., Ser. No. 103–123.

Brouwers, M., Kho, M. E., Browman, G. P., Cluzeau, F., Feder, G., Fervers, B., . . . AGREE Next Steps Consortium. (2010). AGREE II: Advancing guideline development, reporting and evaluation in healthcare. *Canadian Medical Association Journal, 182*, E839–E842. doi:10.1503/cmaj.090449

Eisenberg, J. M. (2001). What does evidence mean? Can the law and medicine be reconciled? *Journal of Health Politics, Policy and Law, 26*(2), 369–381. doi:10.1215/03616878-26-2-369

Ferrell, K. G. (2007). Documentation, Part 2: The best evidence of care. *American Journal of Nursing, 107*(7), 61–64. doi:10.1097/01.naj.0000279271.41357.fa

Field, M. J., & Lohr, K. N. (Eds.). (1990). *Clinical practice guidelines: Directions for a new program*. Washington, DC: National Academies Press.

Gibson, E. (2004). Clinical practice guidelines: Their influence on the standard of care in malpractice. *Journal of Evidenced Based Dental Practice, 4*, 96–99. doi:10.1016/j.jebdp.2004.02.011

Griffith, R. (2008). Care pathways: Legal sword or legal shield? *British Journal of Healthcare Management, 14*(4), 156–160. doi:10.12968/bjhc.2008.14.4.29117

Howie, W. O., & McMullen, P. C. (2010). Can checklists minimize legal liability and improve the quality of patient care? *Journal for Nurse Practitioners, 6*(9), 694–697. doi:10.1016/j.nurpra.2010.07.006

Hurwitz, B. (1994). Clinical guidelines: Proliferation and medicolegal significance. *Quality and Safety in Health Care, 3*(1), 37–44. doi:10.1136/qshc.3.1.37

Institute of Medicine. (2011). *The future of nursing: Leading change, advancing health*. Washington, DC: National Academies Press. Retrieved from https://doi.org/10.17226/12956

Larkin, G. L., Hamann, C. J., Monico, E. P., Degutis, L., Schuur, J., Kantor, W., & Graffeo, C. S. (2007). Knowledge translation at the macro level: Legal and ethical considerations. *Academic Emergency Medicine, 14*(11), 1042–1046. doi:10.1197/j.aem.2007.07.006

McDonagh, R. J., & Hurwitz, B. (2003). Lying in the bed we've made: Reflection on some unintended consequences of clinical practice guidelines in the courts. *Journal of Obstetrics Gynaecology Canada, 25*(2), 139–143. doi:10.1016/s1701-2163(16)30210-9

Morreim, E. H. (2001). From the clinics to the courts: The role evidence should play in litigating health care. *Journal of Health Politics, Policy and Law, 26*(2), 410–427. doi:10.1215/03616878-26-2-409

Oberman, M. (2017). The sticky standard of care. *Hastings Center Report, 47*(6), 25–26. doi:10.1002/hast.782

Rosoff, A. J. (2001). Evidence-based medicine and the law: The courts confront clinical practice guidelines. *Journal of Health Politics, Policy, and Law, 26*(2), 327–368. doi:10.1215/03616878-26-2-327

Ruhl, D. S., & Siegal, G. (2017). Medical malpractice implications of clinical practice guidelines. *Otolaryngology—Head and Neck Surgery, 157*(2), 175–177. doi:10.1177/0194599817707943

Tanenbaum, S. (1994). Knowing and acting in medical practice: The epistemological politics of outcomes research. *Journal of Health Politics, Policy and Law, 19*, 27–44. doi:10.1215/03616878-19-1-27

Taylor, C. (2014). The use of clinical practice guidelines in determining standard of care. *Journal of Legal Medicine, 35*, 273–290. doi:10.1080/01947648.2014.913460

PART SIX

Translation Exemplars

CHAPTER NINETEEN

Population Health Exemplars

Mary F. Terhaar

The Well-Being of Individuals in the Community has long been a concern of science and the health professions. Initially, scientists worked to develop an understanding of the conditions that contributed favorably or detrimentally to the health of individuals in society. The goal was to identify, understand, and influence the social determinants of health (Braveman, Egert, & Williams, 2010). More recent, the concept of population health *has evolved to include health outcomes, social determinants, interventions, and policies that relate to the health of individuals and groups of individuals in society (Armitage, Suter, Oelke, & Adair, 2009).*

Successful advancement of the health of individuals in society depends on the ability of health professions to set meaningful targets for improvement and to reliably and consistently evaluate performance. Meaningful improvement spans communities, practices, facilities, payers, and providers. It cannot be effective if restricted to tertiary care. Success is intensely data dependent. As a result, population health relies heavily on data, informatics, and analytics.

In this chapter, five examples of translation projects that focus on improving the health of individuals in society are presented. Each exemplar summarizes scholarship conducted by a DNP in partial fulfillment of requirements for graduation. These students are the authors of the work presented here, and the primary sources are provided within the text. Each exemplar addresses a different clinical challenge, engages different members of the healthcare team, employs different methods, and uses different approaches to evaluation. Each exemplar provides the following:

- *The* ***title*** *of the project*
- *The* ***team*** *that participated in the work*
- *A* ***statement of the problem*** *in a particular site or setting*
- ***Background*** *describing a brief overview of the problem, including baseline data*
- ***Aims****, which are measurable, directional statements of what will be better once the project is complete*
- ***Translation framework****, which provides an overview of the framework(s) used to conceptualize the work and process*
- ***Translation method(s)****, which explains the strategy or approach used to accomplish change while ensuring fidelity with the evidence and adaptation to the setting*
- ***Results****, which describe whether the aims were achieved*
- ***Impact****, which explains the significance, implications, and sustainability of the work*

- ***Dissemination**, which credits the primary publication of the work and conferences at which it has been presented*
- ***Additional references**, which cite translated evidence*

References

Armitage, G. D., Suter, E., Oelke N. D., & Adair, C.E. (2009). Health systems integration: State of the evidence. *International Journal of Integrated Care, 9*(e82), 316–372.

Braveman, P., Egerter, S., & Williams, D. R. (2010). The social determinants of health: Coming of age. *Annual Review of Public Health, 2011*(32), 381–398.

■ EXEMPLAR 19.1: ADHERENCE TO GUIDELINES FOR NON-HIGH-DENSITY LIPOPROTEIN SCREENING

Deborah S. Croy

Team

Nurse practitioner

Nurses

Administrative staff

Medical director

Nursing faculty

Bland County Medical Clinic

Johns Hopkins University School of Nursing

Problem

Inconsistent implementation of clinical practice guidelines (CPGs) for screening of non-high-density lipoproteins.

Background

Emerging evidence suggests the use of non-high-density lipoprotein cholesterol (non-HDL-C) as a predictor of cardiovascular disease (CVD) is a more robust indicator of atherogenic risk than low-density lipoprotein cholesterol (LDL-C), particularly in patients with CVD, hypertension, hyperlipidemia, and diabetes. Adherence to non-HDL-C CPGs remains low, with primary care providers continuing to focus on LDL-C only. Implementation of new guidelines is especially challenging in low-resourced environments.

Aims

1. To increase adherence to CPGs
2. To increase provider adherence to the testing and treatment of elevated non-HDL-C in patients with diabetes, hypertension, hyperlipidemia, and CVD in a rural Appalachian federally qualified community health center (FQHC)

Translation Framework

The Agency for Healthcare Research and Quality's (AHRQ) Knowledge Transfer Framework Model recommends multifaceted interventions when different partnerships, end users, and types of professionals such as healthcare providers, administrators, and support staff are involved in the change process (Exhibit 19.1.1). The premise is that motives, needs, and constraints of each group of participants are different, so interventions need to be designed to meet the individual needs of the members of the group. The project to improve provider adherence to the CPGs in the testing and treatment of non-HDL-C was multifaceted for the same reasons identified by the AHRQ.

EXHIBIT 19.1.1 **Adaptation of AHRQ Framework**

	Knowledge Creation and Distillation	Diffusion and Dissemination	Adoption, Implementation, and Institutionalization
Processes	Systematic review	Partnerships	Clinical practice guideline
	Guideline review	Primary care medical home teams	Implementation model
		Professional organizations	
Sources	AHA	SPSS reports	BCMC management
	ACC	Feedback reports	Federally qualified health centers
	American Association of Clinical Endocrinologists		State organizations
	European cardiology associations		National organizations
	Canadian cardiology associations		
	NLA		
Actors	Providers	CMS	CMS
	Patients	Patient-centered medical home	Private payers
	CMS	Affordable Care Act	Regulatory boards
	Virginia Health Care Foundation	Meaningful use	Stakeholders

(*continued*)

EXHIBIT 19.1.1 Adaptation of AHRQ Framework (*continued*)

	Knowledge Creation and Distillation	Diffusion and Dissemination	Adoption, Implementation, and Institutionalization
Target audience		BCMC stakeholders	Federally Qualified Health Centers
		Media	• State
		Federally Qualified Health Centers	• National
		Professional organizations: ACC, AHA, NLA, PCNA, AANP	Primary care facilities
Activities	Chart audits	Adherence strategies	Analysis
		• Academic detailing	• Effectiveness
		• Algorithms	• Cost benefit
		Feedback reports	Policies for future guidelines

AANP, American Association of Nurse Practitioners; ACC, American College of Cardiology; AHA, American Heart Association; AHRQ, Agency for Healthcare Research and Quality; BCMC, Bland County Medical Clinic; CMS, Centers for Medicare & Medicaid Services; NLA, National Lipid Association; PCNA, Primary Care Nursing Association; SPSS, Statistical Package for Social Sciences.

The AHRQ's model has three steps; the first step is knowledge creation and distillation. New knowledge from research must be evaluated for rigor and appropriateness for use in a setting. The distillation process involved reviewing the findings and developing the message into one that is relevant to the intended targets. A systematic review showed that unrecognized and untreated elevated non-HDL-C levels was a patient safety issue. A retrospective chart audit provided new knowledge on the status of adherence at Bland County Medical Clinic (BCMC). The second step is diffusion and dissemination using teams, mass diffusion, and targeted dissemination. The multidisciplinary team in place at BCMC targeted all staff, patients, and other identified stakeholders. The final step in the knowledge transfer framework is to design interventions, adopt evidence-based practices, and implement the model. The interventions implemented in the project were the ones identified from the literature search. Throughout the framework and the translational project, continual assessment and modification were necessary to ensure success of the program. The project as well as the AHRQ model can be replicated by other organizations.

Translation Methods

Academic detailing, a simple algorithm, and written feedback reports were used to increase compliance. First, a chart audit was conducted on 134 patient charts of seven providers to evaluate the frequency of lipid testing and patient education regarding diet, exercise, and smoking cessation. Then, the project lead reviewed audit findings with each of the seven providers. Discussion focused on areas of compliance and the challenges each experienced in adhering to the guidelines. All providers identified strategies they could use to increase compliance based on the evidence as described by the project lead.

A decision support and reminder tool was provided to each provider in the form of an algorithm (Figure 19.1.1). The algorithm was used to help providers remember the important findings from the evidence and key points from the practice guidelines. Finally, an audit was repeated and the success of the aims was evaluated.

Results

Provider adherence to the testing and treatment of elevated non-HDL-C in patients with diabetes, hypertension, hyperlipidemia, and CVD increased. Providers were more likely to provide dietary education (47.8%, p = .000), medication prescriptions (38.7%, p = .004), and exercise instruction (76.8%, p = .000) following academic detailing and audit and feedback. Smoking-cessation education improved minimally (05.50%, p = 1.00).

The chart audit for each group was conducted for 3 months (one fiscal quarter) to drive quality improvement, but the sample size is not sufficient for the findings to be powered at this time.

Impact

Evidence suggests that when guidelines are followed, non-HDL-C is reduced, along with risk of CVD, complications, and death. Previous investigations have explored provider adherence to guidelines in primary care, but few address strategies to achieve adherence in a rural Appalachian FQHC.

This project used a combination of academic detailing and audit and feedback to increase compliance. Outcomes encourage the use of a systematic approach for the implementation of CPGs where providers treat the underserved vulnerable high-risk patients.

Dissemination

Croy, D. S. (2015, Feb. 15). Member spotlight: Deborah Croy, DNP, RN, ANP-BC, AGPCNP-BC, CLS, AAC. (2015, February 15). NLA community. *LipidSpin*. Retrieved from https://www.lipid.org/node/1411

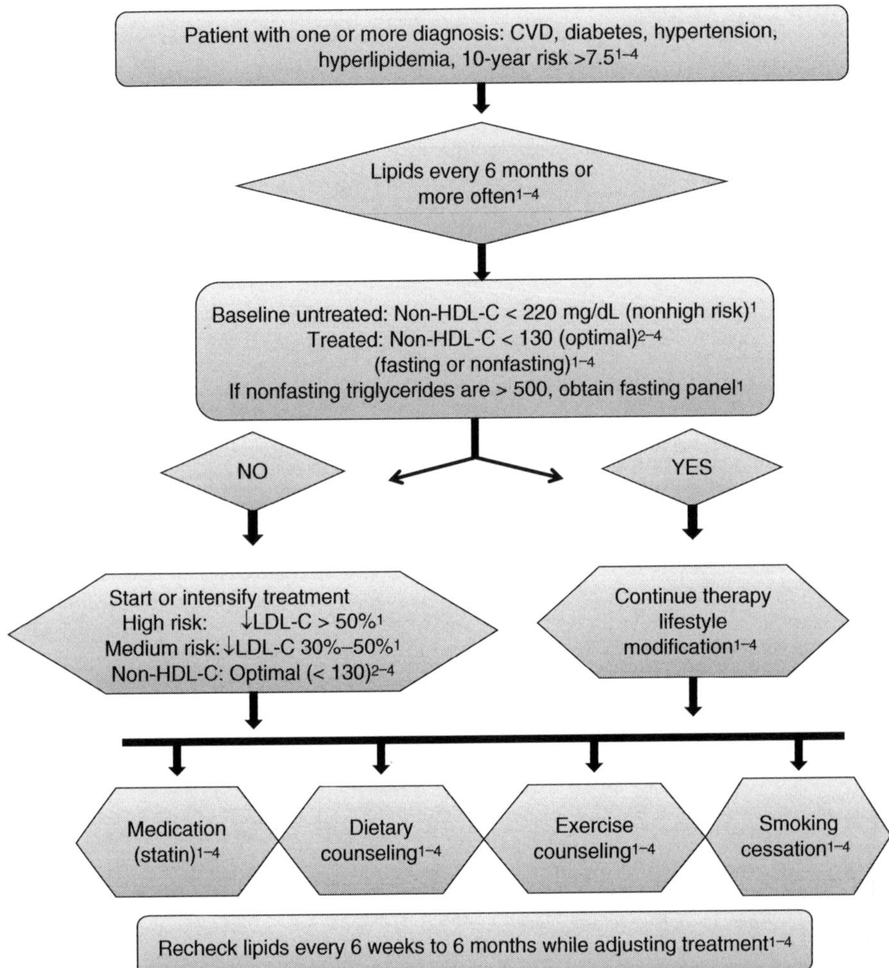

FIGURE 19.1.1 Non-HDL algorithm.

CVD, cardiovascular disease; HDL, high-density lipoprotein; LDL-C, low-density lipoprotein cholesterol; non-HDL-C, non-high-density lipoprotein cholesterol.

[1] Stone, N. J., Robinson, J., Lichtenstein, A. H., Merz, N. B., Blum, C. B., & Eckel, R. H. (2014). 2013 ACC/AHA guideline on the treatment of blood cholesterol to reduce atherosclerotic cardiovascular risk in adults: A report of the American College of Cardiology/American Heart Association task force on practice guidelines. *Journal of the American College of Cardiology, 65*(25), 2889–2934. doi:10.1016/j.jacc.2013.11.002

[2] Grundy, S. M., Cleeman, J. I., Merz, C. N., Brewer, H. B., Clark, L. T., Hunninghake, D. B., . . . Stone, N. J. (2004). Implications of recent clinical trials for the national cholesterol education program adult treatment panel III guidelines. *Journal of the American College of Cardiology, 44*(3), 720–732. doi:10.1016/j.jacc.2004.07.001

[3] Grundy, S. M. (2013). An international atherosclerosis society position paper: Global recommendations for the management of dyslipidemia. *Journal of Clinical Lipidology, 7*(6), 561–565. doi:10.1016/j.jacl.2013.10.001

[4] Jellinger, P. S., Smith, D. A., Mehta, A. E., Gando, O., Handlesman, Y., Rodbard, H. W., . . . Seibel, J. A. (2012). American association of clinical endocrinologists' guidelines for management of dyslipidemia and prevention of atherosclerosis. *Endocrine Practice, 18*, 1–78. doi:10.4158/ep.18.s1.1

Additional References

Agency for Healthcare Research and Quality. (2011). *Slide 42. Project overview: AHRQ's patient-centered outcomes research dissemination and implementation activities.* Retrieved from http://www.ahrq.gov/news/events/nac/2011-11-nac/slutsky/slutskysl42.html

Assmann, G., Benecke, H., Neiss, A., Cullen, P., Schulte, H., & Bestehorn, K. (2006). Gap between guidelines and practice: Attainment of treatment targets in patients with primary hypercholesterolemia starting statin therapy. Results of the 4E-registry (efficacy calculation and measurement of cardiovascular and cerebrovascular events including physicians' experience and evaluation). *European Journal of Cardiovascular Prevention & Rehabilitation, 13*(5), 776–783. doi:10.1097/01.hjr.0000189805.76482.6e

Bertoni, A. G., Bonds, D. E., Chen, H., Hogan, P., Crago, L., Rosenberger, E., . . . Goff, D. C. (2009). Impact of a multifaceted intervention on cholesterol management in primary care practices: Guideline adherence for heart health randomized trial. *Archives of Internal Medicine, 169*(7), 678–686. doi:10.1001/archinternmed.2009.44

Bloom, B. S. (2005). Effects of continuing medical education on improving physician clinical care and patient health: A review of systematic reviews. *International Journal of Technology Assessment in Health Care, 21*(3), 380–385. doi:10.1017/s026646230505049x

Boaz, A., Baeza, J., & Fraser, A. (2011). Effective implementation of research into practice: An overview of systematic reviews of the health literature. *British Medical College Research Notes, 4*(1), 212. doi:10.1186/1756-0500-4-212

Brusamento, S., Legido-Quigley, H., Panteli, D., Truk, E., Knai, C., Saliba, V., . . . Busse, R. (2012). Assessing the effectiveness of strategies to implement clinical guidelines for the management of chronic diseases at primary care level in EU member states: A systematic review. *Health Policy, 107*, 168–183. doi:10.1016/j.healthpol.2012.08.005

Davidson, M. H., Maki, K. C., Pearson, T. A., Pasternak, R. C., Deedwania, P. C., McKenney, J. M., . . . Ballantyne, C. M. (2005). Results of the national cholesterol education (NCEP) program evaluation project utilizing novel e-technology (NEPTUNE) II survey and implications for treatment under the recent NCEP writing group recommendations. *American Journal of Cardiology, 96*(4), 556–563. doi:10.1016/j.amjcard.2005.04.019

DeGuzman, P. B., Akosah, K. O., Simpson, A. G., Barbieri, K. E., Megginson, G. C., Goldberg, R. I., & Beller, G. A. (2012). Sub-optimal achievement of guideline-derived lipid goals in management of diabetes patients with atherosclerotic cardiovascular disease, despite high use of evidence-based therapies. *Diabetes and Vascular Disease Research, 9*(2), 138–145. doi:10.1177/1479164111431471

Eaton, C. B., Parker, D. R., Borkan, J., McMurray, J., Roberts, M. B., Goldman, R., & Ahern, D. K. (2011). Translating cholesterol guidelines into primary care practice: A multimodal cluster randomized trial. *Annals of Family Medicine, 9*(6), 528–537. doi:10.1370/afm.1297

Elshazly, M. B., Martin, S. S., Blaha, M. J., Joshi, P. H., Toth, P. P., McEvoy, J. W., . . . Jones, S. R. (2013). Non–high-density lipoprotein cholesterol, guideline targets, and population percentiles for secondary prevention in 1.3 million adults: The VLDL-2 study (very large database of lipids). *Journal of the American College of Cardiology, 62*(21), 1960–1965. doi:10.1016/j.jacc.2013.07.045

Feifer, C., Ornstein, S. M., Jenkins, R. G., Wessell, A., Corley, S. T., Nementh, L. S., . . . Liszka, H. (2006). The logic behind a multi-method intervention to improve adherence to clinical practice guidelines in a nationwide network of primary care practices. *Evaluation Health Professions, 29*(1), 65–88. doi:10.1177/0163278705284443

Francke, A. L., Smit, M. C., de Veer, A. J., & Mistiaen, P. (2008). Factors influencing the implementation of clinical guidelines for health care professionals: A systematic meta-review. *British Medical College: Medical Informatics and Decision Making, 8*(1), 38. doi:10.1186/1472-6947-8-38

Gandara, E., Moniz, T. T., Dolan, M. L., Mellia, C., Dudley, J., Smith, A., & Kachalia, A. (2009). Improving adherence to treatment guidelines: A blueprint. *Critical Pathways in Cardiology, 8*(4), 139–145. doi:10.1097/hpc.0b013e3181bc8074

Grundy, S. M. (2013). An international atherosclerosis society position paper: Global recommendations for the management of dyslipidemia. *Journal of Clinical Lipidology, 7*(6), 561–565. doi:10.1016/j.jacl.2013.10.001

Grundy, S. M., Cleeman, J. I., Merz, C. N., Brewer, H. B., Clark, L. T., Hunninghake, D. B., . . . Stone, N. J. (2004). Implications of recent clinical trials for the national cholesterol education program adult treatment panel III guidelines. *Journal of the American College of Cardiology, 44*(3), 720–732. doi:10.1016/j.jacc.2004.07.001

Hysong; S. J. (2009). Meta-analysis: Audit and feedback features impact effectiveness on care quality. *Medical Care, 47*(3), 356–363. doi:10.1097/mlr.0b013e3181893f6b

Jamtvedt, G., Young, J., Kristoffersen, D., O'Brien, M., & Oxman, A. (2006). Audit and feedback: Effects on professional practice and health care outcomes. *Cochrane Database of Systematic Reviews, 2*(2). doi:10.1002/14651858.cd000259.pub2

Jaspers, M. W., Smeulers, M., Vermeulen, H., & Peute, L. W. (2011). Effects of clinical decision-support systems on practitioner performance and patient outcomes: A synthesis of high-quality systematic review findings. *Journal of the American Medical Informatics Association, 18*(3), 327–334. doi:10.1136/amiajnl-2011-000094

Jellinger, P. S., Smith, D. A., Mehta, A. E., Gando, O., Handlesman, Y., Rodbard, H. W., . . . Seibel, J. A. (2012). American association of clinical endocrinologists' guidelines for management of dyslipidemia and prevention of atherosclerosis. *Endocrine Practice, 18*, 1–78. doi:10.4158/ep.18.s1.1

Kumar, A., Fonarow, G. C., Eagle, K. A., Hirsch, A. T., Califf, R. M., Albertz, M. J., . . . Cannon, C. P. (2009). Regional and practice variation in adherence to guideline recommendations for secondary and primary prevention among outpatients with atherothrombosis or risk factors in the United States: A report from the REACH registry. *Critical Pathways in Cardiology, 8*(3), 104–111. doi:10.1097/hpc.0b013e3181b8395d

Mansouri, M., & Lockyer, J. (2007). A meta-analysis of continuing medical education effectiveness. *Journal of Continuing Education for Health Professions, 27*(1), 6–15. doi:10.1002/chp.88

Naughton, C., Feely, J., & Bennett, K. (2007). A clustered randomized trial of the effects of feedback using academic detailing compared to postal bulletin on prescribing of preventative cardiovascular therapy. *Family Practice, 24*(5), 475–480. doi:10.1093/fampra/cmm044

Nieva, V. F., Murphy, R., Ridley, N., Donaldson, N., Combes, J., Mitchell, P., . . . Carpenter, D. (2005). From science to service: A framework for the transfer of patient safety research into practice. In K. Henriksen, J. B. Battles, E. Marks, & D. Lewin (Eds.), *Advances in patient safety: From research to implementation* (Vol. 2). Rockville, MD: Agency for Healthcare Research and Quality.

Ornstein, S., Nietert, P. J., Jenkins, R. G., Wessell, A. M., Nemeth, L. S., & Rose, H. L. (2008). Improving the translation of research into primary care practice: Results of a national quality improvement demonstration project. *The Joint Commission Journal on Quality and Patient Safety, 34*(7), 379–390. doi:10.1016/s1553-7250(08)34048-3

Ostini, R., Hegney, D., Jackson, C., Williamson, M., Mackson, J. M., Gurman, K., . . . Tett, S. E. (2009). Systematic review of interventions to improve prescribing. *Annals of Pharmacotherapy, 43*(3), 502–513. doi:10.1345/aph.1l488

Prior, M., Guerin, M., & Grimmer Somers, K. (2008). The effectiveness of clinical guideline implementation strategies: A synthesis of systematic review findings. *Journal of Evaluation of Clinical Practice, 14*(5), 888–897. doi:10.1111/j.1365-2753.2008.01014.x

Soumerai, S. B., & Avorn, J. (1990). Principles of educational outreach ("academic detailing") to improve clinical decision making. *Journal of the American Medical Association, 263*(4), 549–556. doi:10.1001/jama.263.4.549

Stafford, R. S., Bartholomew, L. K., Cushman, W. C., Cutler, J. A., Davis, B. R., Dawson, G., . . . Whelton, P. K. (2010). Impact of the ALLHAT/JNC7 dissemination project on thiazide-type diuretic use. *Archives of Internal Medicine, 170*(10), 851–858. doi:10.1001/archinternmed.2010.130

Stone, N. J., Robinson, J., Lichtenstein, A. H., Merz, N. B., Blum, C. B., & Eckel, R. H. (2014). 2013 ACC/AHA guideline on the treatment of blood cholesterol to reduce atherosclerotic cardiovascular risk in adults: A report of the American College of Cardiology/American Heart Association task force on practice guidelines. *Journal of the American College of Cardiology, 65*(25), 2889–2934. doi:10.1016/j.jacc.2013.11.002

Virani, S. S., Steinberg, L., Murray, T., Negi, S., Nambi, V., Woodard, L. D., & Ballentyne, C. M. (2011). Barriers to non-HDL cholesterol goal attainment by providers. *American Journal of Medicine, 124*(9), 876–880. e2. doi:10.1016/j.amjmed.2011.02.012

Virani, S. S., Woodard, L. D., Landrum, C. R., Pietz, K., Wang, D., Ballantyne, C. M., & Petersen, L. A. (2011). Institutional, provider, and patient correlates of low-density lipoprotein and non-high-density lipoprotein cholesterol goal attainment according to the adult treatment panel III guidelines. *American Heart Journal, 161*(6), 1140–1146. doi:10.1016/j.ahj.2011.03.023

■ EXEMPLAR 19.2: SCREENING OF GERIATRIC BEHAVIORAL HEALTH ISSUES IN THE EMERGENCY ROOM

Lisa M. Sgarlata

Team

Chief administrative officer

Physicians

Chief nursing officer

Chief foundation officer

Vice president for oncology services

Lee Memorial Health System

Johns Hopkins University School of Nursing

Problem

Inadequate screening of behavioral health issues within the geriatric population who present to the ED in southwest Florida.

Background

Rates of ED visits for people with psychiatric diagnoses have increased more than overall ED visits, providing evidence that EDs are primary portals for the system (Cunningham, McKenzie, & Taylor, 2006).

In an update to their 2012 report, *Assessing the Needs of Elder Floridians*, the Florida Department of Elder Affairs reported that 11% of geriatric individuals had to go without treatment for emotional and mental health problems in the state compared to 19% within the Lee County service area (Bureau of Planning and Evaluation, 2013).

Local southwest Florida hospitals have seen an increase in the number of geriatric patients presenting to local EDs with exacerbation of both their physical and psychiatric issues. In 2013, local EDs saw an increase of 17.3% in admission rates and a 24.8% increase in total cost for these patients since 2010 (Lee Memorial Health System, 2013).

Evidence strongly recommends the need for implementation of a cadre of interventions to improve outcomes for geriatric behavioral health patients, which includes a collaborative care model and utilization of specialty personnel to provide a geriatric behavioral health screening (National Council for Behavioral Health, 2014).

Aims

The purpose of this project was to identify co-occurring behavioral health issues within the geriatric population that presents to the EDs within southwest Florida. There were two aims:

1. To increase screening for co-occurring behavioral health issues (delirium, depression, and substance use) for all geriatric patients who present in the ED of the pilot campus.

2. To increase behavioral health referrals (psychiatric or substance use) for geriatric patients seen in the ED at the pilot campus.

Translation Framework

The project utilized the RE-AIM framework for translation into nursing practice (Figure 19.2.1). *RE-AIM* stands for reach, effectiveness, adoption, implementation, and maintenance. Supported by the Substance Abuse and Mental Health Services Administration (SAMHSA), this framework recognizes essential elements of behavioral health practices that support sustainability of services (Substance Abuse and Mental Health Services Administration, 2013).

Translation Methods

This project is a retrospective cohort study of ED visits from a public, not-for-profit Level-II trauma and acute care facility that occurred between August 1 and November 30, 2014. Approved by the Nursing Research Council and Investigational Review Committee of the health system, the project was overseen by the Geriatric Behavioral

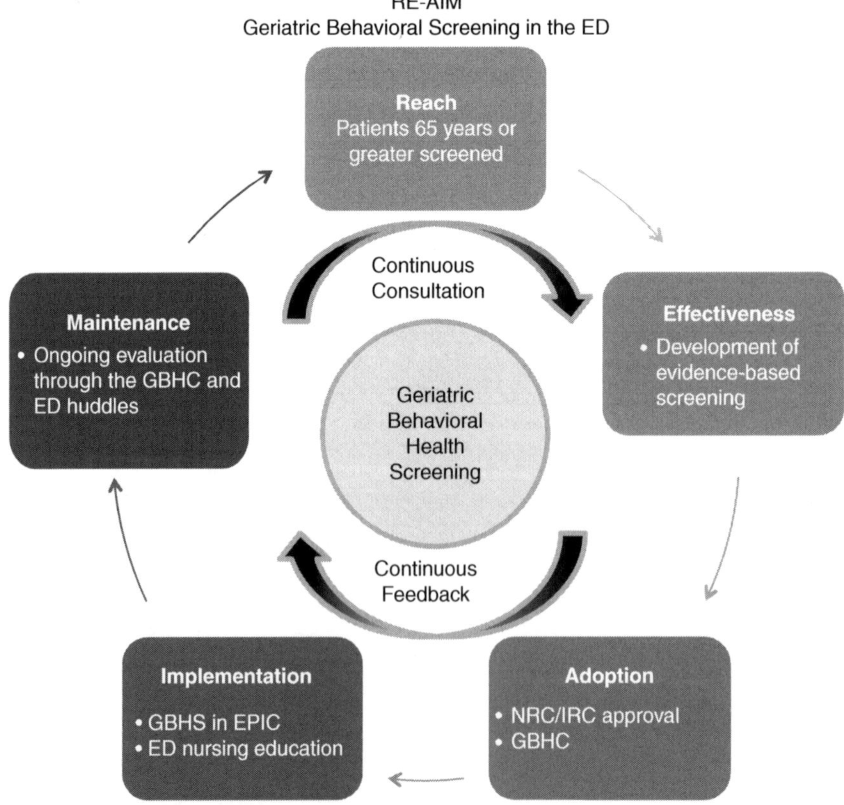

FIGURE 19.2.1 Adapted RE-AIM framework.

EPIC, education, prevention, intervention, counseling; GBHC, Geriatric Behavioral Health Council; GBHS, geriatric behavior health screening; IRC, Investigational Review Committee; NRC, Nursing Research Council; RE-AIM, reach, effectiveness, adoption, implementation, and maintenance.

Health Council (GBHC), an interdisciplinary team of physicians and nurses, as well as ancillary psychiatric and community personnel. The GBHC provided oversight on all aspects of the project from implementation up to and including ongoing maintenance consistent with the aims of increased screening, identification, and referrals for geriatric patients with co-occurring behavioral health disorders.

Results

Aim 1: On the pilot campus, 57% of the patients received screening for behavioral health comorbidities as compared to none at the comparison campus (p = .0001).

Aim 2: Early referral for behavioral health comorbidities increased to 14% on the pilot campus as compared to 1% at the comparison campus (p = .0001); 85.3% of the population screened positive using the Delirium Triage Screening (DTS), providing early detection of delirium, depression, and substance use in the screened population (Figure 19.2.2).

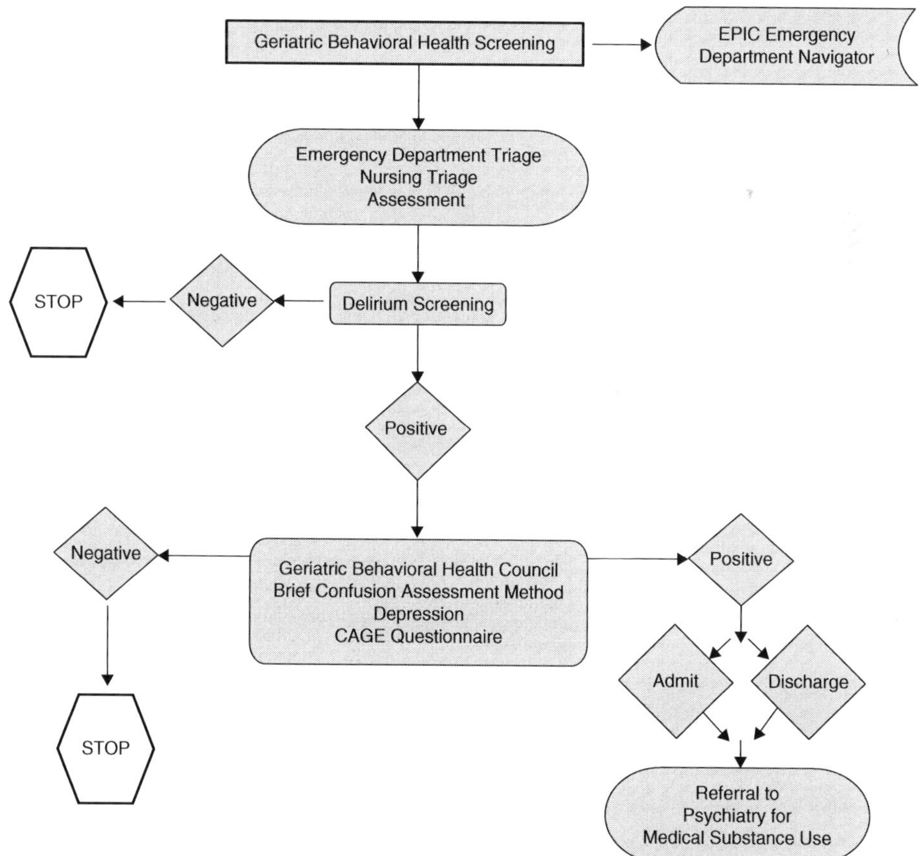

FIGURE 19.2.2 Implementation: Geriatric behavioral health screening algorithm and specialty ED nursing assessment.

CAGE, cut down, annoyed, guilty, eye-opener; EPIC, education, prevention, intervention, counseling.

Additional References

Bureau of Planning and Evaluation. (2013). *Assessing the needs of elder Floridians*. State of Florida: Department of Elder Affairs. Retrieved from http://elderaffairs.state.fl.us/doea/needs_assessment.php

Cunningham, P., McKenzie, K., & Taylor, E. F. (2006). The struggle to provide community-based care to low-income people with serious mental illness. *Health Affairs*, *25*, 694–705. doi:10.1377/hlthaff.25.3.694

Lee Memorial Health System. (2013). *FY 2012 consolidated Lee Memorial Health System community benefit report*. Retrieved from www.leememorial.org

National Council for Behavioral Health. (2014). *Medicare to rescind Part D mental health drug restrictions*. Retrieved from www.thenationalcouncil.org

Substance Abuse and Mental Health Services Administration. (2013). *Using the RE-AIM implementation framework to improve behavioral health*. Retrieved from www.samhsa.org

■ EXEMPLAR 19.3: A SYSTEMATIC APPROACH INCORPORATING FAMILY HISTORY IMPROVES IDENTIFICATION OF CARDIOVASCULAR DISEASE RISK

Mariam Kashani

Team

Nurse practitioners

Medical staff

Sonographer

Integrative Cardiac Health Project, Walter Reed National Military Medical Center

Johns Hopkins University School of Nursing

Problem

Heart disease is the leading cause of death in the United States. Current assessment strategies underestimate risk of cardiovascular disease (CVD), and as a result, patients are prescribed suboptimal therapies incongruent with their true risk.

Background

Primary care providers routinely evaluate risk for heart disease using the Framingham Risk Score (FRS). The FRS is the most broadly used cardiovascular risk assessment instrument available. Yet, FRS has been found to underestimate risk by as much as 50% (Lee et al., 2010).

Family history (FH) of premature CVD is a robust predictor of heart disease and is commonly collected in routine visits (Chow et al., 2011). Accuracy of risk assessment may be improved by as much as 40% by incorporating FH (Qureshi et al., 2012). Awareness of FH alone does not lead to risk-reducing behaviors (Elis, Pereg, Shochat, Tekes-Manova, & Lisher, 2008). Risk reductions that emphasize self-care efficacy have proven to be successful (Adams, 2010). However, as FH is not included in the FRS, there is potential to underestimate risk and offer less than optimal care and instruction to patients.

Carotid intima–media thickness (CIMT) testing is a useful and objective method to evaluate CVD by measuring the thickness of the inner lining of carotid artery walls. The thicker the lining of the intima, the greater the risk of stroke or heart disease.

The purpose of this project is to improve CVD risk assessment by using a clinical decision support tool to increase risk identification and awareness in patients with positive FH in a military healthcare system.

Aims

This project had two aims:

1. To increase identification of high-risk patients, using CIMT as a measure of subclinical atherosclerosis to validate the reclassification (retrospective analysis)
2. To increase self-efficacy for CVD prevention in patients with positive FH of premature CVD (prospective rapid cycle improvement)

Translation Framework

The Knowledge-to-Action Framework was adapted to organize this project (Figure 19.3.1). It describes the cycle of work that moves evidence into practice and outcomes.

Translation Methods

Two methods were used in this project: decision support and rapid cycle performance improvement.

Decision Support (Retrospective Arm)

A novel evidence-based clinical decision support tool was developed to combine FH with the FRS to generate a new risk assessment as an adjunct to current strategies.

First, a retrospective chart audit was performed and the FRS was identified for each of 413 consecutive patients who had been prospectively enrolled in the Integrative Cardiac Health Project Registry before initiation of the second project. Charts of 239 patients who had been classified as "low" or "intermediate" risk using the FRS were reviewed to identify positive FH. For the purpose of this project, positive FH was defined as "a first-degree relative having a CVD event before the age of 55 years in men and 65 years in women." Next, risk scores for this subgroup were reclassified as high risk to account for the combined risk.

CIMT testing data were available for all clinic patients. These CIMT data were used to generate independent risk scores by a separate reviewer who had been blinded to the calculated risk assessments.

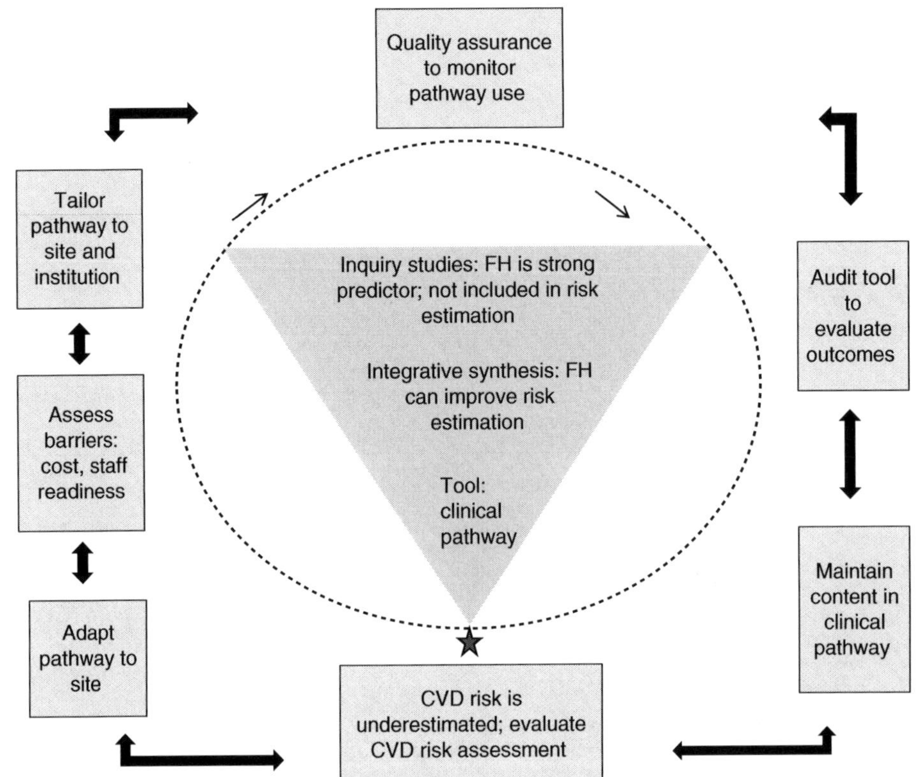

FIGURE 19.3.1 Adapted Knowledge-to-Action Framework.

CVD, cardiovascular disease; FH, family history.

Source: Adapted from Graham, I., Logan, J., Harrison, M., Straus, S. E., Tetroe, J., Caswell, W., & Robinson, N. (2006). Lost in knowledge translation: Time for a map? *Journal of Continuing Education for Health Professions, 26*, 13–24.

In this way, validity of the modified risk assessment could be evaluated. The decision-support tool presented in the following text is the result of this process.

Rapid Cycle Performance Improvement (Prospective Arm)

This decision-support tool, which incorporated positive FH with the FRS, was then used systematically by providers in the CVD prevention clinic visits (Figure 19.3.2). Clinicians engaged in empowering conversations with patients and families directed at informing their self-care decisions based on the refined risk assessment.

A self-efficacy questionnaire (SEQ) for CVD prevention was used before and after measurement.

Results

Modified Risk Assessment

Of 239 patients who had been classified as low risk using FRS, 115 (48%) were found to have positive FH of premature CVD. Patients with negative FH were younger (44.9 compared to 54.3 years, p = .02) and FRS scores were lower, though

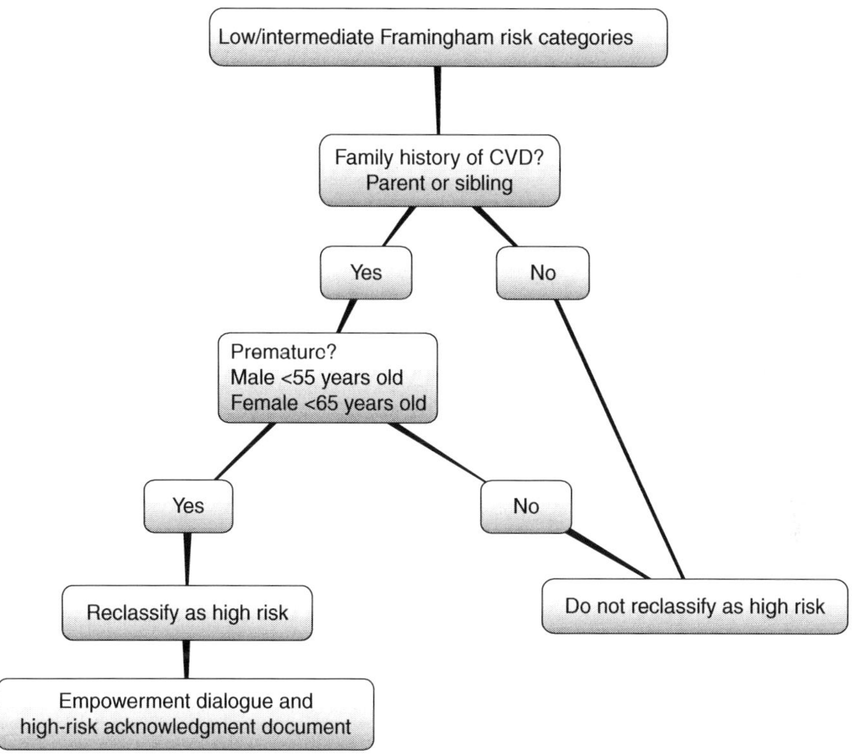

FIGURE 19.3.2 CVD risk decision-support tool.

CVD, cardiovascular disease.

insignificantly so, as both groups were classified as low risk (3.01 vs. 4.5, p <.001). Fewer patients with negative FH were found to have abnormal CIMT (55% vs. 75%, p < .001) (Figure 19.3.3). Patients with positive FH were more likely to have abnormal CIMT and CVD.

Self-Efficacy

Patients classified as high risk using the revised risk assessment (decision-support tool) demonstrated greater change in self-efficacy scores than those who were not classified as high risk (7.5 vs. 3.9, p <.001; Figure 19.3.4).

Impact

Translation of evidence into practice is dynamic, and mechanisms to help clinicians accomplish translation continue to evolve. Recent evidence indicates that positive FH has predictive validity (Chow et al., 2011). This project demonstrates that a reproducible systematic approach for adding FH to current practice enhances prediction and identifies more high-risk patients who, at present, are not captured. Moreover, patients who received scores more accurately capturing true risk demonstrated increased self-efficacy, which declares the value and potential impact of accurate risk assessment.

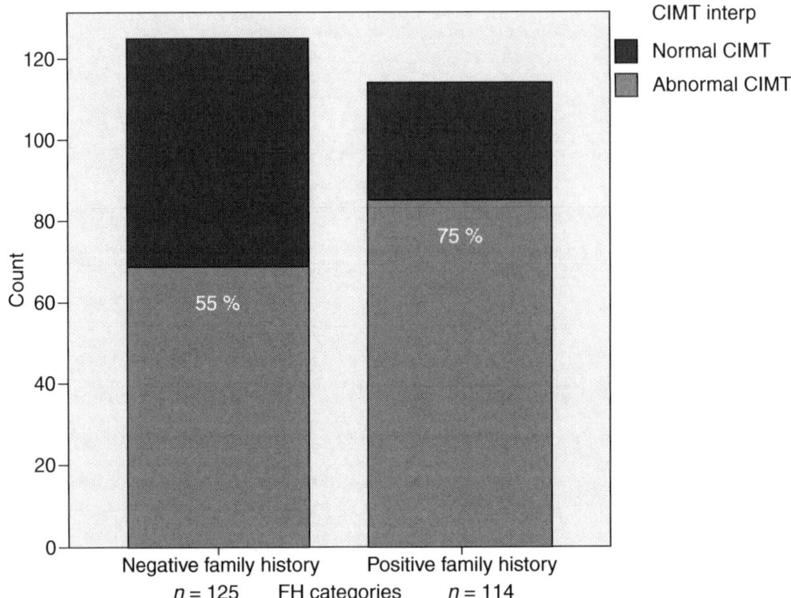

FIGURE 19.3.3 Aim 1: Proportion of abnormal CIMT within family history categories.

CIMT, carotid intima–media thickness; FH, family history; interp, interpretation.

Analysis in Low-Risk Patients

n = 39	Pre-SEQ mean (±*SD*)	Post-SEQ mean (±*SD*)	*Change in SEQ (mean)
Positive family history *n* = 22	34.8 (5.74)	42.3 (3.31)	7.5
Negative family history *n* = 17	37.5 (5.01)	41.4 (3.00)	3.9

FIGURE 19.3.4 Aim 2: Change in self-efficacy.

SD, standard deviation; SEQ, self-efficacy questionnaire.

*$p < .001$. Independent *t*-test.

This report describes a mechanism to address a gap in clinical practice. The findings are sufficiently promising to warrant further emphasis on evidence translation and validation of these instruments used in other settings.

Dissemination

Kashani, M., Eliasson, A., Bailey, K., Vernalis, M., & Terhaar, M. (2015). A systematic approach incorporating family history improves identification of cardiovascular disease risk. *Journal of Cardiovascular Nursing, 30*(4), 292–297. doi:10.1097/JCN.0000000000000163

Kashani, M., Eliasson, A., Vernalis, M., Costa, L., & Terhaar, M. (2013). Improving assessment of cardiovascular disease risk by using family history: An integrative literature review. *Journal of Cardiovascular Nursing, 28*(6), E18–E27. doi:10.1097/JCN.0b013e318294b206

Abstracts

Kashani, M., Eliasson, A., Bailey, K., Vernalis, M., & Terhaar, M. (2013). Systematic inquiry of family history improves cardiovascular risk assessment. *Circulation Cardiovascular Quality and Outcomes, 6*, A314.

Kashani, M., Eliasson, A., Walizer, E., Fuller, C., Engler, E., Villines, T., & Vernalis, M. (2015). Early empowerment strategies boost self-efficacy to improve health outcomes. *Circulation Cardiovascular Quality and Outcomes, 8*(2), A331.

Additional References

Adams, R. J. (2010). Improving health outcomes with better patient understanding and education. *Risk Management Healthcare Policy, 2010*(3), 61–72.

Chow, C. K., Islam, S., Bautista, L., Rumboldt, Z., Yusufali, A., Xie, C., . . . Yusuf, S. (2011). Parental history and myocardial infarction risk across the world: The INTERHEART study. *Journal of the American College of Cardiology, 57*(5), 619–627. doi:10.1016/j.jacc.2010.07.054

Elis, A., Pereg, A., Shochat, T., Tekes-Manova, D., & Lisher, M. (2008). Family history of cardiovascular disease does not predict risk-reducing behavior. *European Journal of Cardiovascular Prevention and Rehabilitation, 15*, 325–328. doi:10.1097/hjr.0b013e3282f50ed8

Lee, G. K., Lee, L. C., Liu, C. W., Lim, S. L., Shi, L. M., Ong, H. Y., . . . Yeo, T. C. (2010). Framingham risk score inadequately predicts cardiac risk in young patients presenting with a first myocardial infarction. *Annals of the Academy of Medicine of Singapore, 39*(3), 163–167.

Qureshi, N., Armstrong, S., Dhiman, P., Saukko, P., Middlemass, J., Evans, P. H., Kai, J., & ADDFAM (Added Value of Family History in CVD Risk Assessment) Study Group. (2012). Effect of adding systematic family history enquiry to cardiovascular disease risk assessment in primary care: A matched-pair, cluster randomized trial. *Annals of Internal Medicine, 156*(4), 253–262. doi:10.7326/0003-4819-156-4-201202210-00002

Sol, B., Graaf, Y., Bijl, J., Goessens, N. B., & Visseren, F. L. (2005). Self-efficacy in patients with clinical manifestations of vascular diseases. *Patient Education and Counseling, 61*, 443–448. doi:10.1016/j.pec.2005.05.011

■ EXEMPLAR 19.4: DEVELOPING A SYSTEM OF CARE FOR THE TRANSIENT ISCHEMIC ATTACK PATIENT

Mary Marshman

Team

Emergency services

Hospitalist

Neurology

Radiology

Nursing

Centra Lynchburg General Hospital

Problem

Up to 40% of patients who experience a first-time stroke have had a prior transient ischemic attack (TIA). The care these patients receive is inconsistent, which increases the risk of stroke, disability, and mortality. The burden of illness is high as is the cost of care (Easton et al., 2009; Ovbiagele et al., 2012).

Background

The Johns Hopkins Nursing Evidence-Based Practice Model was used to prosecute the evidence. Several strong recommendations flowed from this review (Figure 19.4.1).

Aims

This project had two aims:

1. To reduce the recurrence of TIA
2. To reduce recurrence of stroke

Translation Framework

The Quality Enhancement Research Initiative (QUERI) framework guided this effort (Figure 19.4.2).

Translation Methods

An algorithm was developed to facilitate evidence-based clinical management of TIA. The work was done by an interdisciplinary team. It was implemented within the ED and shared with the Virginia Stroke Systems Taskforce to assist in addressing gaps in stroke prevention at a state level.

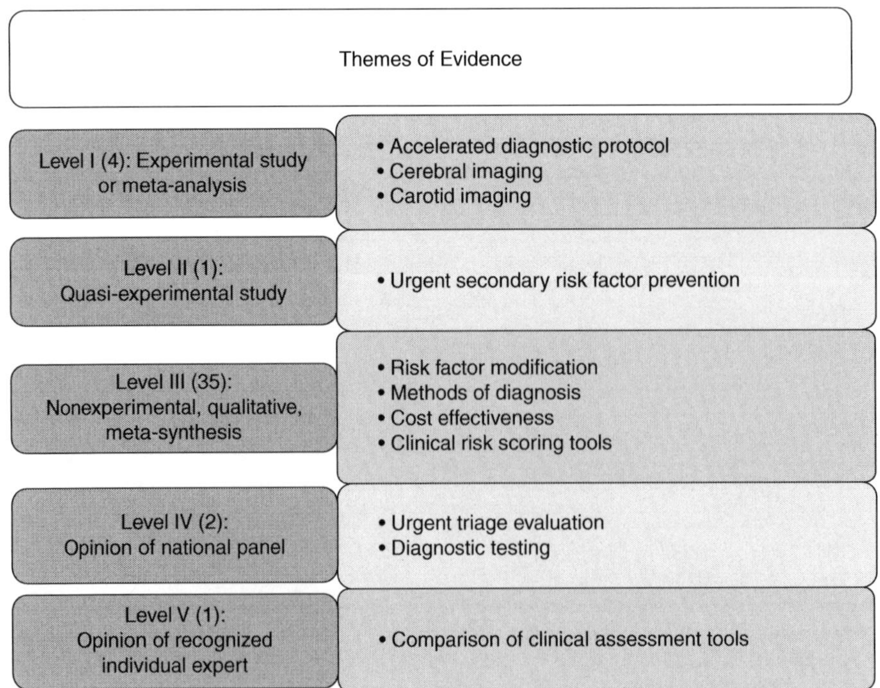

FIGURE 19.4.1 Themes of evidence.

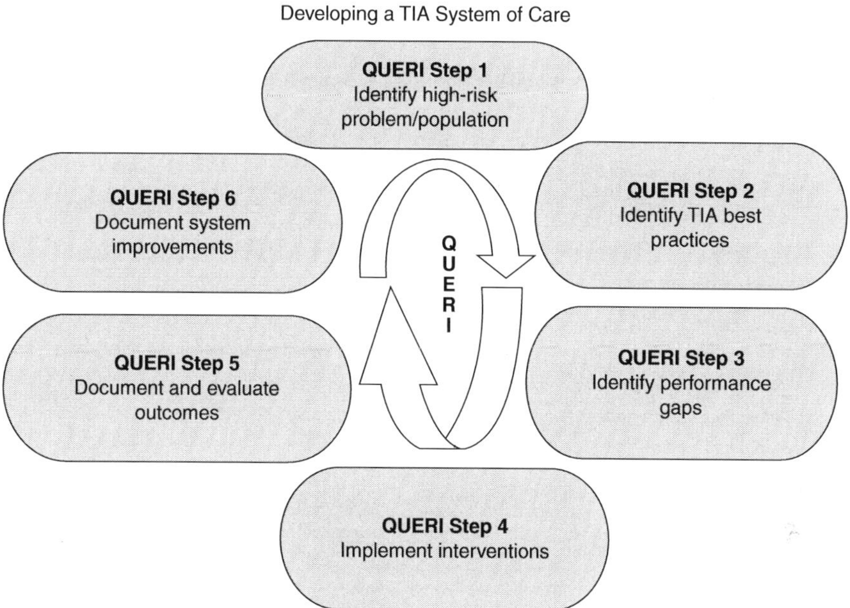

FIGURE 19.4.2 Adapted QUERI framework.
QUERI, Quality Enhancement Research Initiative; TIA, transient ischemic attack.

Results

Aims 1 and 2 were achieved.

Recurrent TIA was reduced from 2.5% in the baseline group to no occurrence in the intervention group, and recurrent stroke was reduced from 10.1% to 2.9% (Exhibit 19.4.1).

EXHIBIT 19.4.1 TIA Project Outcomes

Algorithm Patient Outcomes	Mean (*SD*) or Percentage	
	Comparison Group (*n* = 80)	Intervention Group (*n* = 67)
Postindex ischemic events		
Recurrent TIA	2.5%	0%
Recurrent stroke	10.1%	2.9%

Statistical significance $p < .05$.

Chi-square analysis was used for categorical variables.

A description of algorithm-based patient outcomes is found in the comparison and intervention study. Although trends were noted in reduction of ischemic events postintervention, findings were not statistically significant between groups ($p = .093$).

SD, standard deviation; TIA, transient ischemic attack.

EXHIBIT 19.4.2 TIA Project Financial Outcomes

	Mean (*SD*)				(95% CI)
	Comparison Group (*n* = 80)	Intervention Group (*n* = 67)	*p* Value*	Mean Difference	Confidence Interval
Total length of stay (hours measured)	40.5 (19.67)	33.7 (14.31)	.018*	6.8	(1.19, 12.31)
Total cost of cerebral imaging	$5,331 ($2904)	$2,889 ($1800)	.001*	$2,442	($1,667, $3,218)
Total cost of carotid imaging	$3,511 ($1986)	$1,682 ($758)	.001*	$1,829	($322, $2,337)
Total direct cost overall	$11,094 ($4728)	$6,710 ($2420)	.001*	$4,384	($3,185, $5,583)

*Statistically significant $p < .05$.

Independent samples *t*-test for continuous variables. Total direct cost overall includes cost for cerebral imaging, carotid imaging, and disposition mean cost per patient based on length of stay.

Relevant cost findings of the study outcomes demonstrating effectiveness of the TIA algorithm.

SD, standard deviation; TIA, transient ischemic attack.

Impact

Favorable clinical outcomes translated to favorable financial performance (Exhibit 19.4.2).

Dissemination

This work was presented at the 2015 International Stroke Conference in Nashville, Tennessee, on February 10, 2015.

Additional References

Easton, J. D., Saver, J. L., Albers, G. W., Alberts, M. J., Chaturvedi, S., Feldmann, E., . . . Sacco, R. L. (2009). Definition and evaluation of transient ischemic attack: A scientific statement for health care professionals from the American Heart Association/American Stroke Association Stroke Council, Council on Cardiovascular Surgery and Anesthesia, Council on Cardiovascular Radiology and Intervention, Council on Cardiovascular Nursing, and the Interdisciplinary Council on Peripheral Vascular Disease. *Stroke, 40*, 2276–2293. doi:10.1161/strokeaha.108.192218

Marshman, M. (2015, February). Algorithm development to improve transient ischemic attack outcomes: Application of evidence based practice and quality. *Stroke, 46*, ANS24. The International Stroke Conference in Nashville, TN.

Ovbiagele, B., Goldstein, L. B., Higashida, R. T., Howard, V. J., Claiborne Johnston, S., Khavjou, O. A., . . . Trogdon, J. G. on behalf of the American Heart Association Advocacy Coordinating Committee and Stroke Council (2013). Forecasting the future of stroke in the United States: A policy statement from the American Heart Association and American Stroke Association. *American Heart Association Journal, 2013*(44), 2361–2375. doi:0.1161/STR.0b013e31829734f2

EXEMPLAR 19.5: A NUTRITIONAL INTERVENTION TO ADDRESS METABOLIC SYNDROME IN THE NAVAJO

Lorenzo T. Nava

Team

Clinical staff

Nutrition support

Nursing staff

Public health staff

Community leaders

Crownpoint Healthcare

Johns Hopkins University School of Nursing

Problem

Metabolic syndrome affects nearly half of the Navajo adults on a reservation, greatly increasing their risk for negative cardiovascular events. The modern Navajo diet, heavy in fat and refined carbohydrates, has been identified as an important contributing factor to the high rates of metabolic syndrome in this area.

Background

Metabolic syndrome is defined by the presence of at least three out of five cardiovascular risk factors: impaired fasting blood glucose level, elevated triglycerides, low-serum high-density lipoprotein, elevated blood pressure, and central obesity. Individuals with metabolic syndrome have a cardiovascular disease risk as high as 2.35 times that of the general population (Go et al., 2013).

Metabolic syndrome affects Navajo adults at rates disproportionately higher than the rest of the U.S. population. Between 2004 and 2006, metabolic syndrome was estimated to affect 43.2% of Navajo men and 47.3% of Navajo women (Schumacher et al., 2008). During the same period, 35.1% of U.S. men and 32.6% of U.S. women met the criteria for metabolic syndrome (Go et al., 2013). Nutrition plays an important role in the pathogenesis of metabolic syndrome, and an estimated 30% to 41% of calories in the modern Navajo diet are from foods high in fat and refined carbohydrates (Schumacher et al., 2008; Sharma et al., 2009).

The cultural and socioeconomic conditions present in the Navajo reservation are unique. The reservation is largely undeveloped, with limited access to electricity, running water, telephone service, and paved roads (University of Arizona, 2008; U.S. Census, 2010, U.S. Department of Agriculture, 2014). Despite these challenges, the area has remained culturally wealthy through the preservation of the Navajo language, beliefs, and rituals (Plawecki, Sanchez, & Plawecki, 1994). Previous researchers have identified a need for culturally relevant educational strategies to address components of metabolic syndrome in the Navajo (Cunningham-Sabo et al., 2008).

Aims

The purpose of this translation project was to design a nutrition curriculum to be implemented in the Navajo Nation. The aims were that the program be:

1. Evidence based
2. Culturally appropriate
3. Age appropriate

Translation Framework

Multiple theoretical frameworks were used to develop a curriculum to address the problem of metabolic syndrome in the Navajo. Each of these complementary frameworks was used for a distinct part of the evidence translation process. A culturally adapted version of the Knowledge-to-Action (KTA) Framework was used as a guide in the definition of the problem and the selection of an intervention appropriate for the community. After the selection of an intervention, the logic model was used for adapting the curriculum to meet the needs of the community. During the adaptation phase, Bloom's taxonomy was used as a guide to establish appropriate learning objectives for educational modules and the program as a whole. Finally, the concepts of adult learning theory were used as a guide for designing educational activities within the curriculum.

Translation Methods

Two methods were applied in this translation project: process redesign and instructional design.

Process Redesign

Ongoing meetings with community leaders led to the development of a curriculum to be used across the community. Community leaders emphasized the importance of using visual examples to help learners understand abstract concepts such as serving sizes. Thus, the curriculum strongly incorporates the use of visuals in place of written materials whenever possible. Community leaders also emphasized the importance of simplifying concepts discussed as well as dietary recommendations. Scientific terminology and complex dietary recommendations are avoided wherever possible, and analogies to everyday situations are used to explain complex concepts like glycemic load. Community leaders also emphasized the cultural and local appropriateness of any dietary recommendations made within the curriculum. Careful thought and effort went into identifying and including ingredients that participants are familiar with and able to obtain within the community. Furthermore, recipes sampled and recommendations made within the curriculum are done so with the consideration of affordability and cultural acceptability.

Instructional Design

Three interventions supported by the evidence were identified as suitable to address metabolic syndrome in the target community: the Ke `Ano Ola (KAO) program, the

Family Education Diabetes Series (FEDS), and the Wai`anae Diet (WDP) program (Gellert, Aubert, & Mikami, 2010; Mendenhall et al., 2010).

The KAO program was a 12-week healthy lifestyle program emphasizing nutrition, exercise, and community involvement (Gellert et al., 2010). The FEDS program was a 6-month intervention emphasizing community gatherings; healthy, affordable, and available traditional foods; and cultural activities (Mendenhall et al., 2010). The WDP was a 3-week culturally appropriate, community-based intervention based on the traditional Hawaiian diet (Shintani et al., 1994).

Based on the KTA model, the WDP was determined to be the most appropriate and feasible intervention for the target population due to its implementation in a similar population, a similar location, the documented efficacy, and the duration of the intervention. The WDP curriculum was selected as a template to be adapted with integration of elements of the KAO and FEDS programs.

After selecting a curriculum template, a logic model was developed to guide the adaptation phase. Available resources were identified as inputs, activities using those inputs were identified as outputs, and the overall program goals were identified as outcomes. After consultation with community leaders and content experts in nutrition and the Navajo culture, the WDP curriculum was adapted to be able to convert the available inputs into the outputs necessary to produce the intended outcomes.

After the initial adaptation of the WDP curriculum, the curriculum was further refined through the use of a modified, consensus-building approach. The curriculum was distributed to Navajo community leaders as well as content experts in nutrition with a four-item questionnaire using open-ended questions such as: What did you like about this module? What could be improved? What do you think are the most important points to focus on? What do you think are the least important points? Qualitative feedback received was compiled and used to develop a second questionnaire, in which community leaders and experts were asked to rank intervention concepts, themes, and methods in order of importance. Cumulative scores for each item were then reviewed, and adaptations to the curriculum were made based on the feedback received through the questionnaires.

Results

The final result of the program development and instructional design process is the Diné Ch`iyáán curriculum, a 3-week curriculum that includes nutrition and wellness modules, cooking demonstrations, grocery-shopping tours, and cultural activities. Concepts of adult-learning theory are integrated into the curriculum with an emphasis on practicality, relevancy, experiential learning, interactivity, and mutual respect (Keating, 2011). The curriculum is designed to promote the consumption of traditional Navajo foods, particularly those consumed prior to European contact, with an emphasis on availability, affordability, and palatability. Wherever possible, the Navajo language is used to list food ingredients and recipes discussed in the curriculum. Cooking demonstrations feature traditional Navajo recipes from community members as well as those collected from the National Center for Native

American Aging at the Center for Rural Health at the University of North Dakota (Goodwin & Hall, 2004).

Meetings take place in the evening to allow for the participation of working individuals. After checking in, community members participate in a 30-minute interactive learning module on nutrition followed by 15 minutes of discussion. Following the nutrition module, participants share a meal prepared following traditional Navajo recipes that are distributed in the form of a cookbook. During the meal, participants learn how to prepare the foods they are eating through a cooking demonstration given by the facilitators. After the meal, community members participate in a second 30-minute learning module on the Navajo Wellness model, followed by 15 minutes of discussion. Class meetings take place on weeknights, following the two-lesson format on Monday to Thursday, with Fridays reserved for open discussion and cultural activities.

Impact

The Diné Ch`iyáán curriculum is distinct in the manner in which it was developed. Extensive collaboration of community leaders and content experts ensured that elements deemed important by all parties were present in the final product, thus producing an evidence-based curriculum that is culturally and socially appropriate. The curriculum is congruent with the Navajo concept of wellness and designed to reinforce the concept of life in balance with nature.

Dissemination

Nava, L. T. (2014). *Nutrition-based interventions to address metabolic syndrome in the Navajo: A systematic review.* Charleston, SC: Transcultural Nursing Society Annual Conference.

Nava, L. T., Zambrano, J. M., Arviso, K. P., Brochetti, D., & Becker, K. L. (2014a). Nutrition-based interventions to address metabolic syndrome in the Navajo: A systematic review. *Journal of Clinical Nursing, 24*(21–22), 3024–3045. doi:10.1111/jocn.12921

Nava, L. T., Zambrano, J. M., Arviso, K. P., Brochetti, D., & Becker, K. L. (2014b). *Nutrition-based interventions to address metabolic syndrome in the Navajo: A systematic review.* Washington, DC: Minority and Health Disparities Conference.

Additional References

Cunningham-Sabo, L., Bauer, M., Pareo, S., Phillips-Benaly, S., Roanhorse, J., & Garcia, L. (2008). Qualitative investigation of factors contributing to effective nutrition education for Navajo families. *Maternal Child Health Journal, 12*, S68–S75. doi:10.1007/s10995-008-0333-5

Gellert, K. S., Aubert, R. E., & Mikami, J. S. (2010). Ke 'Ano Ola: Moloka'i's community-based healthy lifestyle modification program. *American Journal of Public Health, 100*(5), 779–783. doi:10.2105/AJPH.2009.176222

Go, A. S., Mozaffarian, D., Roger, V. L., Benjamin, E. J., Berry, J. D., Borden, W. D., . . . Turner, M. B. (2013). Heart disease and stroke statistics—2013 update: A report from the America Heart Association. *Circulation, 127*(1), e6–e245.

Goodwin, J., & Hall, J. (2004). *Healthy traditions: Recipes of our ancestors.* Grand Forks, ND: National Center for Native American Aging at the Center for Rural Health, University of North Dakota School of Medicine and Health Sciences. Retrieved from http://ruralhealth.und.edu/publications/resources/archive

Keating, S. (2011). *Curriculum development and evaluation in nursing* (2nd ed.). New York, NY: Springer Publishing Company.

Mendenhall, T. J., Berge, J. M., Harper, P., GreenCrow, B., LittleWalker, N., WhiteEagle, S., & BrownOwl, S. (2010). The Family Education Diabetes Series (FEDS): Community-based participatory research with a midwestern American Indian community. *Nursing Inquiry, 17*(4), 359–372. doi:10.1111/j.1440-1800.2010.00508.x

Plawecki, H., Sanchez, T., & Plawecki, J. (1994). Cultural aspects of caring for Navajo Indian clients. *Journal of Holistic Nursing, 12*(3), 291–306. doi:10.1177/089801019401200307

Schumacher, C., Ferucci, E., Lanier, A., Slattery, M., Schraer, C., Raymer, T., . . . Tom-Orme, L. (2008). Metabolic syndrome: Prevalence among American Indian and Alaska Native people living in the southwestern United States and in Alaska. *Metabolic Syndrome and Related Disorders, 6*(4), 267–273. doi:10.1089/met.2008.0021

Sharma, S., Yacavone, M., Cao, X., Pardilla, M., Qi, M., & Gittelsohn, J. (2009). Dietary intake and development of a quantitative FFQ for a nutritional intervention to reduce the risk of chronic disease in the Navajo Nation. *Public Health Nutrition, 13*(3), 350–359. doi:10.1017/s1368980009005266

Shintani, T., Beckham, S., Tang, J., O'Connor, H., Hughes, C., & Sato, A. (1994). The Waianae Diet Program: A culturally sensitive, community-based obesity and clinical intervention program for the Native Hawaiian population. *Hawaii Medical Journal, 53*(5), 136–147.

University of Arizona. (2008). *The Navajo Nation quick facts.* Retrieved from https://indiancountryextension.org/sites/indiancountryextension.org/files/publications/files/u6/Navajo%20Nation%20Quick%20Facts%20Oct08.pdf

U.S. Census. (2010). *American fact finder.* Retrieved from http://factfinder.census.gov/faces/tableservices/jsf/pages/productview.xhtml?pid=ACS_10_SF4_DP02&prodType=table

U.S. Department of Agriculture. (2014). *Food access research atlas.* Retrieved from http://www.ers.usda.gov/data-products/food-access-research-atlas/go-to-the-atlas.aspx#.VFbto_nF-55

CHAPTER TWENTY

Specialty Practice Exemplars

Mary F. Terhaar

SPECIALIZATION IS A DEFINING CHARACTERISTIC OF HEALTHcare in this century. It has driven the advancement of science; focused careers, knowledge, skill, and judgment; increased efficiency; and led to impressive innovation. This progress is the result of expertise developed within one domain such as cardiac surgery, radiation oncology, or forensic psychiatry.

Limitations and challenges have accompanied impressive progress in specialization. The base of evidence available to inform practice is burgeoning. As a result, clinicians who seek to base their practice in evidence find it difficult to sift through the large number of papers and publications to find out which is relevant and useful.

In this chapter, you will find eight examples of translation projects that focus on translation of evidence in specialty practice. Each exemplar summarizes scholarship conducted by a DNP in partial fulfillment of requirements for graduation. These students are the authors of the work presented here and the primary sources are provided within the text. Each exemplar addresses a different clinical challenge, engages different members of the healthcare team, employs different methods, and uses different approaches to evaluation. Each exemplar provides the following:

- *The* ***title*** *of the project*
- *The* ***team*** *that participated in the work*
- *A* ***statement of the problem*** *in a particular site or setting*
- ***Background*** *describing a brief overview of the problem, including baseline data*
- ***Aims****, which are measurable, directional statements of what will be better once the project is complete*
- ***Translation framework****, which provides an overview of the framework(s) used to conceptualize the work and process*
- ***Translation method(s)****, which explains the strategy or approach used to accomplish change while ensuring fidelity with the evidence and adaptation to the setting*
- ***Results****, which describe whether the aims were achieved*
- ***Impact****, which explains the significance, implications, and sustainability of the work*

- ***Dissemination****, which credits the primary publication of the work and conferences at which it has been presented*
- ***Additional references****, which cite translated evidence*

■ EXEMPLAR 20.1: THE TOXIGEN INITIATIVE

Charlene M. Deuber

Team

Staff nurses

Neonatal nurse practitioners

Quality-improvement officers

Neonatologists

Residents

Respiratory therapists

Children's Hospital of Philadelphia

Johns Hopkins University School of Nursing

Problem

Supplemental oxygen (SpO2) plays a critical role in the management of infants born at the limits of viability, but carries the risk of morbidity associated with high blood oxygen concentrations and/or prolonged exposure. Very preterm infants (VPIs), born before 28 weeks' gestation, who receive supplemental oxygen in the neonatal intensive care unit (NICU) may have dangerously high pulse oximeter readings at intervals, which are known to lead to long-term sequelae.

Background

Hyperoxia is a toxic, unintended consequence of respiratory therapy that produces tissue damage because it triggers production of reactive oxygen species (ROS) and circulating oxygen free radicals (OFRs; Auten & Davis, 2009). VPIs lack sufficient antioxidant levels required to protect cells and organs from the damage free radicals produce. As a result, they are susceptible to negative outcomes when management of oxygen fails to achieve steady control within the target range.

Target oxygen saturation for VPIs receiving supplemental oxygen in this NICU has been set from 88% to 92%. Unit-specific pulse oximetry data (SpO2) for VPIs show blood oxygenation levels above the target range greater than 45% of the time.

Aims

This project had two aims:

1. To increase caregiver knowledge of the pathophysiology and sequelae of hyperoxia for VPIs
2. To reduce exposure to hyperoxia among VPIs in a Level-II NICU

Translation Framework

The Ottawa Model of Research Use (OMRU) provided the structure for knowledge translation, including implementation and evaluation of outcomes. According to the OMRU, translation is interactive, multidirectional, and dynamic. Translation proceeds through three interactive elements: evidence-based innovation (education and rounds), potential adopters (transprofessional team), and practice environment (technology and environment of the NICU). Each was addressed in this project (Logan & Graham, 1998).

Translation Methods

Two methods were used for this quality-improvement (QI) project. They included instructional design and audit and feedback.

Instructional Design

Education was designed and provided for the full NICU team. First, a retrospective chart review was conducted to identify opportunities to improve performance. Then, a thorough search of the evidence was conducted. Evidence was evaluated and practices supported as effective by the evidence were identified. Then, a program was designed to teach the full NICU team about hyperoxia, its pathophysiology, the associated sequelae, and the interventions supported as effective by strong evidence.

Caregiver knowledge was evaluated at baseline and again following the program ($N = 59$).

Audit and Feedback

Audit and feedback were conducted by the project team. Graphic output from pulse oximetry was posted at each bedside to increase awareness of both the amount of time per day that each VPI spent above the target range and progress within the NICU as a whole toward achieving the project aims. Collaborative rounds were also used to provide feedback to the NICU team and to increase engagement of the full interdisciplinary team in efforts to reduce hyperoxia.

Audits of chart and bedside monitor data were completed for two groups of VPIs: those receiving care in the unit before the educational program (retrospective infant data $N = 31$) and those receiving care in the unit after the educational intervention (prospective infant data, $N = 24$).

Results

Caregiver Knowledge

After the educational intervention, caregiver knowledge increased across disciplines from a pretest average of 15.9 to a posttest average of 20.78, paired *t*-test

(p = .000, df = 57). The first aim, to increase caregiver knowledge of hyperoxia in VPIs, was achieved.

Exposure to Hyperoxia

Exposure to hyperoxia did not improve the following project interventions. The average time spent with SpO2 above the target range was higher in cohort 2 than in cohort 1 (p = .047, df = 53). The second aim, to reduce exposure to hyperoxia, was not attained.

The greater average percentage of time cohort 2 infants spent with SpO2 above the target range prompted the consideration of confounding variables. Birth weight and gestational age were normally distributed in both infant cohorts; measures of central tendency and dispersion were similar in each cohort; and p values for these variables did not reach statistical significance (p = .156 and .081, respectively).

Caregiver knowledge did not reduce the time VPIs were exposed to SpO2 readings above the target range.

Impact

Change in knowledge did not lead to change in behavior or the time infants spent above target oxygenation levels. The educational intervention combined with audit and feedback was not sufficient to achieve the desired outcome.

Many factors can influence the target outcome, including human response, judgment time, and competing priorities. All of them can prevent or impede timely, effective response to hyperoxia as evidenced by oxygen saturation readings above the target range.

Dissemination

Deuber, C., Abbasi, S., Schwoebel, A., & Terhaar, M. (2013). The toxigen initiative: Targeting oxygen saturation to avoid sequelae in very preterm infants. *Advances in Neonatal Care, 13*(2), 139–145. doi:10.1097/anc.0b013e31828913cc

Deuber, C., & Terhaar, M. (2011). Hyperoxia in very preterm infants: A systematic review. *Journal of Perinatal and Neonatal Nursing, 25*(3), 1–7. doi:10.1097/jpn.0b013e318226ee2c

Additional References

Auten, R. L., & Davis, J. M. (2009). Oxygen toxicity and reactive oxygen species: The devil is in the details. *Pediatric Research, 66*(2), 121–127. doi:10.1203/pdr.0b013e3181a9eafb

Logan, J., & Graham, I. (1998). Toward a comprehensive interdisciplinary model of health care research use. *Science Communication, 20*(2), 227–246. doi:10.1177/1075547098020002004

■ EXEMPLAR 20.2: PREVENTING CATHETER-ASSOCIATED URINARY TRACT INFECTIONS IN CRITICALLY ILL CHILDREN USING A BUNDLE APPROACH

Judith A. Ascenzi

Team

Clinical nurse specialist
Chief quality officer
Nursing staff
Medical residents
Multidisciplinary pediatric intensive care unit (PICU) team
Johns Hopkins Hospital
John Hopkins Medicine
Johns Hopkins School of Nursing

Problem

The PICU is a 32-bed medical–surgical ICU that cares for patients from newborns to 22 years of age with multiple diagnoses related to cardiac surgery, neurosurgery, general pediatric surgery, transplants, extracorporeal membrane oxygenation (ECMO), oncology, and multisystem failure, which are some of the most common diseases seen in infants, children, and young adults. All patients are managed by the PICU service, which is divided into two physician teams that change on a weekly basis. Each team consists of one PICU attending, one PICU fellow, and two pediatric residents. The unit has dedicated unit-based nurse practitioners (NPs); however, staffing permits NPs only to be part of one of the two rounding teams. Because of the unit's expansive size, per shift it is staffed with approximately 25 nurses of varying experience levels. Multidisciplinary rounds occur every morning.

The use of indwelling urinary catheters (IUCs) is common; the incidence of positive cultures is 6.1%; and there is no evidence-based standard of care for the child with an IUC.

Background

The IUC is a device used to accurately measure urine output in children receiving shock resuscitation, life-sustaining medications, nutrition support, and blood products in the PICU. These catheters disrupt skin integrity, which can lead to bacterial and/or fungal infections referred to as *catheter-associated urinary tract infections (CAUTI)*. CAUTI can lead to longer hospital stays, increased costs, and, in more serious cases, urosepsis, multisystem organ dysfunction, and death.

The incidence of catheter-associated bacteremia is 26% among patients who have an indwelling catheter for 2 to 10 days, and 24% of patients with bacteriuria will advance to a CAUTI (Greene, Marks, & Oriola, 2008). Urinary tract infections (UTIs) are the second most common cause of bacteremia and represent one of the largest breeding grounds for antibiotic-resistant organisms (Gould et al., 2009).

Approximately 24 million IUCs are sold in the United States each year (Saint et al., 2000), and 25% of all hospitalized patients have a urinary catheter placed during their hospital stay (Saint, Kaufman, Thompson, Rogers, & Chenoweth, 2005). Data from the 2010 National Healthcare Safety Network (NHSN) showed a range of pooled mean CAUTI rates of 1.5 to 4.7 infections per 1,000 catheter days and a range of pooled mean CAUTI rates of 2.2 to 3.9 infections per 1,000 catheter days for pediatric critical care units (Dudeck et al., 2005).

Evidence supports the following interventions as effective to reduce both risk and severity of CAUTI: antibiotic- and antiseptic-impregnated urinary catheters (Apisarnthanarak et al., 2007; Cardenas & Hoffman, 2009; Goetz, Kedzuf, Wagener, & Muder, 1999), mitigating risk factors associated with adult urinary catheter infections (Andreessen, Wilde, & Herendeen, 2012; Meddings, Rogers, Macy, & Saint, 2010), educational programs to decrease urinary catheter infections and other complications, and urinary catheter care bundles. Among all risks for CAUTI, duration of catheterization is the most important.

The purpose of this patient safety QI project was to determine whether best practice care bundles for the management of IUCs for adult patients can be tailored and translated to the PICU population in order to reduce CAUTI. Despite the success of efforts to reduce adult CAUTI, it remains unknown which adult CAUTI best practice interventions will improve outcomes in pediatric patients.

Aims

There were two specific aims for this QI project:

1. To decrease the number of urinary catheter days
2. To decrease the number of positive urine cultures in critically ill children with IUCs

Translation Framework

The Knowledge-to-Action Framework guided this project. Figure 20.2.1 relates the details of the project to the components of the framework.

Translation Methods

Two methods were used in this project: a bundle and a decision-support algorithm.

CAUTI Bundle

A clinical bundle was developed based on strong evidence indicating that catheters should be removed as early as possible,; care bundles have been effective in accomplishing similar aims in adults, risk for UTI can be assessed based on patient factors, and silver- or antibiotic-coated catheters reduce risk (Figure 20.2.2).

The Daily Maintenance Bundle included all the strategies supported as effective by strong evidence. The bundle included the following evidence-based strategies:

- Hand hygiene and gloves
- Proper securement
- Maintain closed system

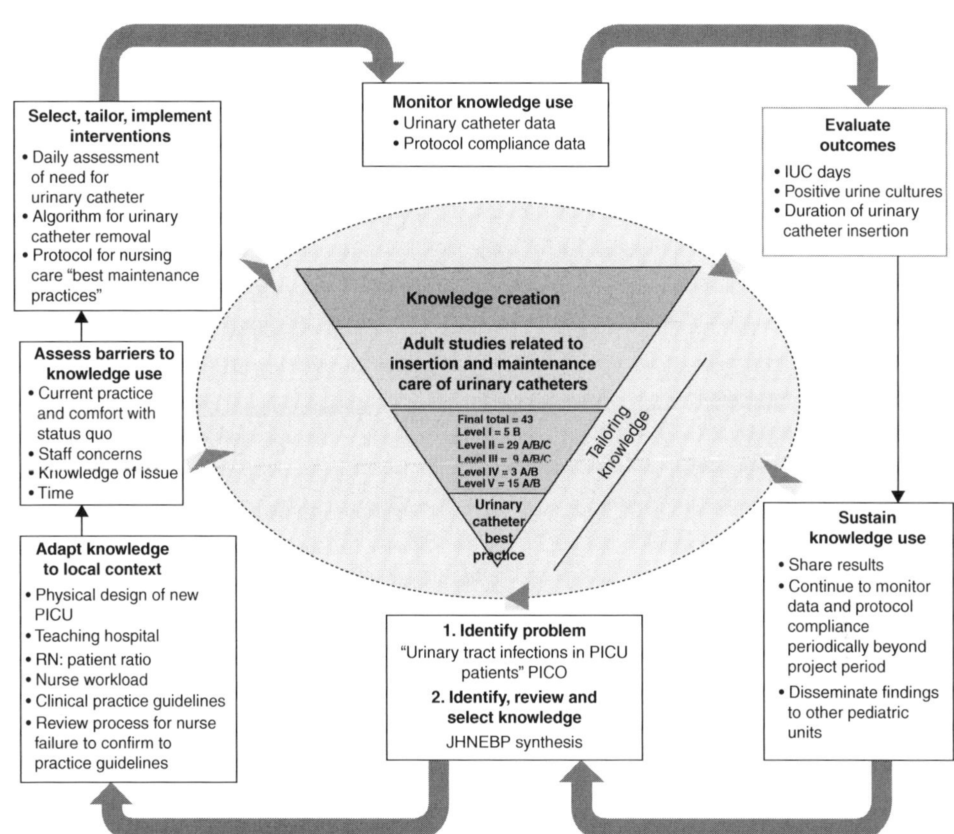

FIGURE 20.2.1 Knowledge-to-Action Framework adapted to CAUTI.

CAUTI, catheter-associated urinary tract infection; IUC, indwelling urinary catheters; JHNEBP, Johns Hopkins Nursing evidence-based practice; PICO, patient/problem, intervention, comparison, outcome; PICU, pediatric intensive care unit.

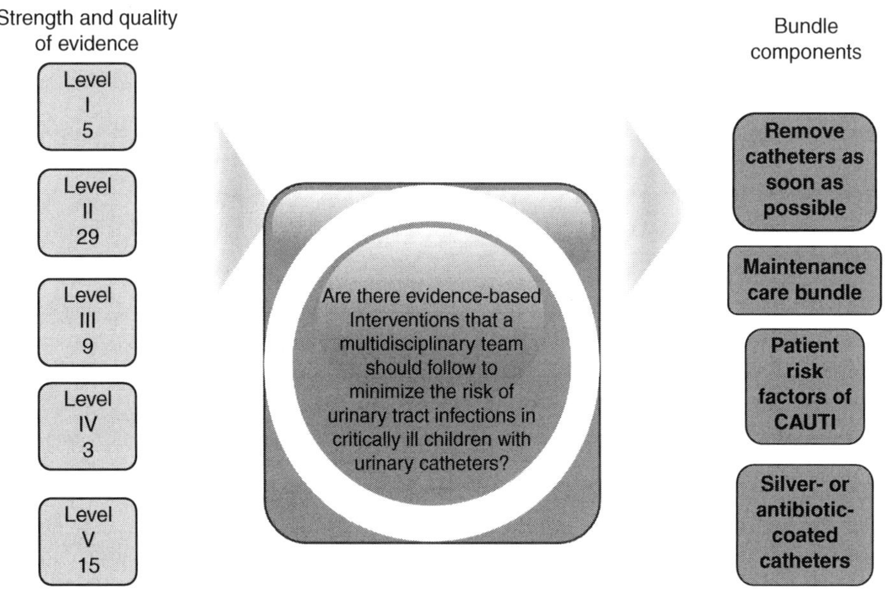

FIGURE 20.2.2 Synthesis of the evidence as the basis for a bundle.

CAUTI, catheter-associated urinary tract infection.

- Maintain unobstructed urine flow
- Keep collection bag below the level of the bladder
- Empty urimeters at least every 4 hours
- Empty urine collection bags every 8 hours
- Perineal care

In addition, an algorithm was developed to facilitate decisions about continuation or discontinuation of urinary catheters (Figure 20.2.3). Both the algorithm and bundle were reviewed on morning rounds. According to criteria, need was evaluated for each catheter in place and prompt removal followed if those criteria were not met.

Evaluation

This prospective QI project uses historical control data and a convenience sample of nurses, authorized prescribers, and patients in the PICU of a large academic medical center. Data collection occurred in two phases: Phase 1, conducted from January 1 to March 31, 2012, comprised the baseline data-collection period and Phase 2, conducted from October 1 to December 31, 2012, comprised the intervention data-collection period.

To evaluate the effectiveness of the change in IUC management, 3 months of retrospective baseline data were obtained by auditing medical records of all patients admitted to the PICU from January 1 to March 31, 2012. Variables retrieved included: total number of patients per day on the unit, total number of patients per day with a urinary catheter, patient's age in months, diagnosis, date of IUC insertion, date of IUC removal, immune status, isolation status, presence of femoral central or arterial line,

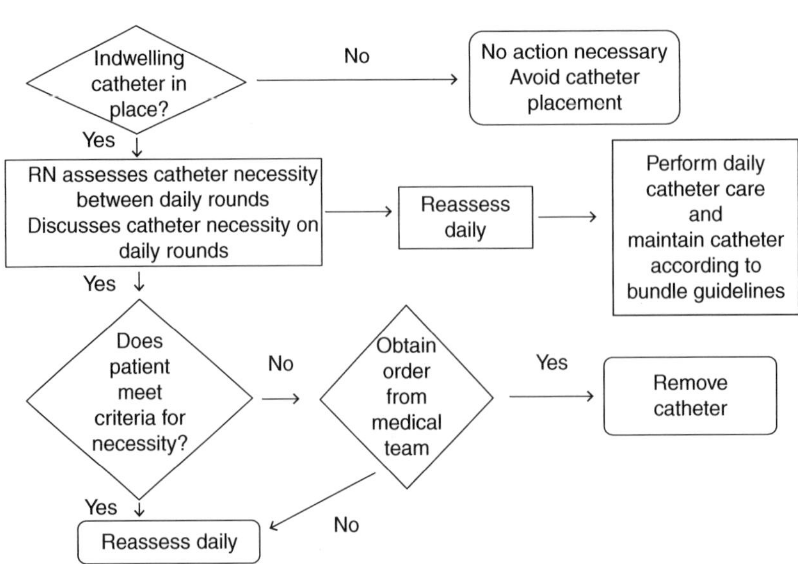

FIGURE 20.2.3 Algorithm for assessment related to urinary catheters.

organism from urine culture, and necessity for IUC reinsertion. Outcome variables included: (a) IUC days (device days), (b) length of time in days IUC remains in place, and (c) number of positive urine cultures. *IUC days* are defined as "the total number of days of exposure to the IUC divided by all of the patients in the selected population during a selected time period." An additional metric to use to analyze IUC use is the device utilization ratio (DUR). This is calculated monthly using the following formula: IUC DUR = number of indwelling urinary device days/number of patient days (Dudeck et al., 2005). The same data were collected after implementation of the nurse-driven IUC maintenance care bundle from October 1 to December 31, 2011 (Figure 20.2.4).

Once the intervention was implemented, the PICU clinical nurse specialist collected the daily bedside checklists completed by the nurse for each patient. This information was used to assess compliance with daily IUC need assessment. Variables included on this checklist included: (a) presence of order, (b) IUC necessity per the nurse-driven algorithm (NDA), and (c) IUC removal per NDA.

In addition, during the intervention period, self-audits were performed weekly by each nurse caring for a patient with an IUC. Audits were performed weekly on random days and shifts. Self-audit completion was anonymous and was placed in the PICU clinical nurse specialist's mailbox when completed. Process variables collected during weekly audits included: (a) use of hand hygiene/clean gloves prior to manipulation of the IUC/drainage system, (b) IUC system maintained as a closed system, (c) IUC drainage bag kept below patient's bladder, (d) IUC drainage bag emptied during shift, (e) perineal care performed daily and after each bowel movement, and (f) assessment of intermittent bladder irrigation (IBI).

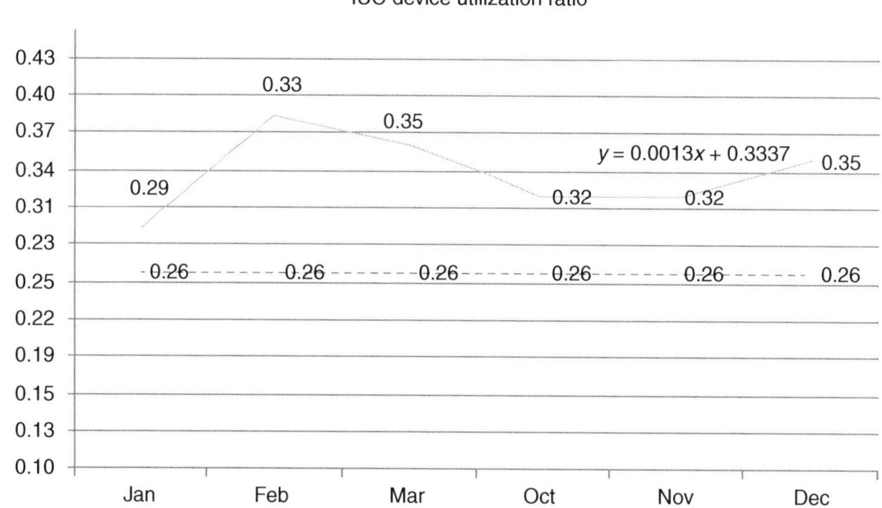

FIGURE 20.2.4 IUC utilization days.

*Device utilization ratio is calculated using formula IUC days/patient days.

IUC, indwelling urinary catheter.

Results

Duration of Catheter Utilization

DUR remained above the national reported PICU mean DUR of .26 for all months in both measurement periods. A comparison of groups on length of time in days that an IUC remains in place showed a reduction in the mean from 4.4 days (standard deviation [*SD*] = 5.8) in the baseline group to 3.58 days (*SD* = 5.1) in the intervention group.

Positive Cultures

Four CAUTI infections were recorded during the baseline phase and two CAUTI infections were reported during the intervention phase (Figure 20.2.5). A chi-square test for significance, using a 2 × 2 table, was performed yielding a Yates's correction for continuity of $p = .637$. Results were not statistically significant. However, the 50% downward change between baseline and the intervention period was clinically significant. The slope of the regression line is −0.7557 per data point.

Impact

The goal of this QI project was to test feasibility, safety, and effectiveness of a nurse-driven IUC maintenance care bundle translated from evidence found in adults. This was accomplished through the implementation of a nurse-driven IUC maintenance care bundle that emphasized: (a) education for both PICU nurses and authorized prescribers related to the assessment of daily IUC need, (b) prompt IUC removal,

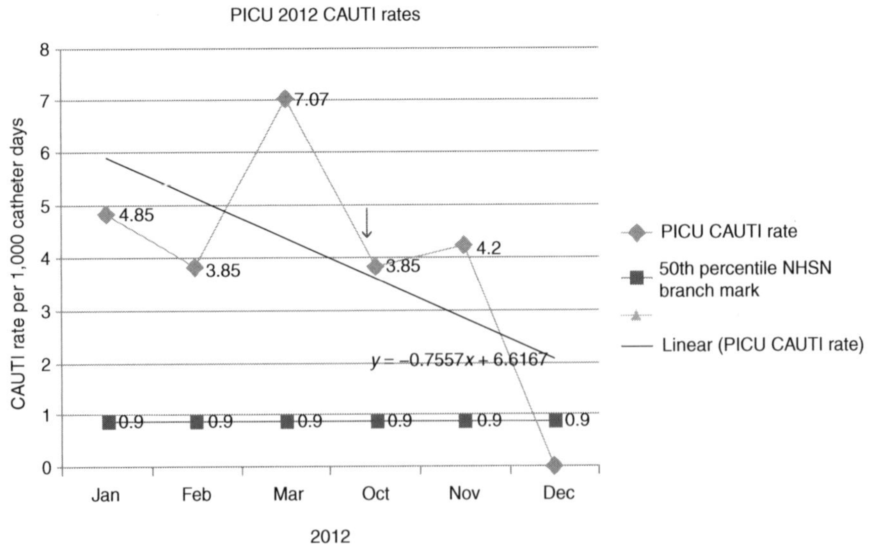

FIGURE 20.2.5 Positive IUC cultures.

CAUTI, catheter-associated urinary tract infection; NHSN, National Healthcare Safety Network; PICU, pediatric intensive care unit.

and (c) routine best maintenance care practices. Although there were no statistically significant differences in the numbers of CAUTIs and positive urine cultures, IUC days, or DUC in the PICU during the intervention measurement period, there was clinical significance in that the PICU experienced a 50% reduction in the number of confirmed CAUTI cases during the intervention period as compared to the baseline period. Another positive clinical finding was the reduction in IUC days in surgical PICU patients. Interventions that were used to routinely prompt the multidisciplinary team to remove unnecessary IUCs have been shown to decrease the rate of CAUTI. This feasibility study resulted in no harm, achieved target change in practice, despite lacking statistically significant reduction in PICU CAUTI.

The clinical findings of this project support the feasibility, utility, and effectiveness of the nurse-driven IUC maintenance bundle that encompasses education, process measurement, and surveillance to positively impact patient outcomes.

Dissemination

Ascenzi, J. (2014, March). *Preventing CAUTIs in critically ill children using a bundle approach. Sixth National Doctors of Nursing Practice Conference*. Phoenix, AZ.

Additional References

Andreessen, L., Wilde, M. H., & Herendeen, P. (2012). Preventing catheter-associated urinary tract infections in acute care: The bundle approach. *Journal of Nursing Care Quality, 27*(3), 209–217. doi:10.1097/ncq.0b013e318248b0b1

Apisarnthanarak, A., Rutjanawech, S., Wichansawakun, S., Ratanabunjerdkul, H., Patthranitima, P., Thongphubeth, K., . . . Fraser, V. J. (2007). Initial inappropriate urinary catheters use in a tertiary-care center: Incidence, risk factors, and outcomes. *American Journal of Infection Control, 35*(9), 594–599. doi:10.1016/j.ajic.2006.11.007

Cardenas, D. D., & Hoffman, J. M. (2009). Hydrophilic catheters versus noncoated catheters for reducing the incidence of urinary tract infections: A randomized controlled trial. *Archives of Physical Medicine Rehabilitation, 90*, 1668–1671. doi:10.1016/j.apmr.2009.04.010

Dudeck, M. A., Horan, T. C., Peterson, K. D., Allen-Bridson, K., Morrell, G., Pollock, D. A., & Edwards, J. R. (2005). National Healthcare Safety Network (NHSN) Report, data summary for 2010, device associated module. *American Journal of Infection Control, 39*, 798–816. doi:10.1016/j.ajic.2011.10.001

Goetz, A. M., Kedzuf, S., Wagener, M., & Muder, R. R. (1999). Feedback to nursing staff as an intervention to reduce catheter associated urinary tract infections. *American Journal of Infection Control, 27*(5), 402–404. doi:10.1016/s0196-6553(99)70005-2

Gould, C. V., Umscheid, C. A., Agarwal, R. K., Kuntz, G., Pegues, D. A., & Healthcare Infection Control Practices Advisory Committee. (2009). Guideline for prevention of catheter associated urinary tract infections. *Infection Control and Hospital Epidemiology, 31*(4), 319–326. doi:10.1086/651091

Greene, L., Marks, J., & Oriola, S. (2008). *Guide to the elimination of catheter-associated urinary tract infections (CAUTIs)*.Washington, DC: Association for Professionals in Infection Control.

Meddings, J., Rogers, M. A. M., Macy, M., & Saint, S. (2010). Systematic review and meta-analysis: Reminder systems to reduce catheter-associated urinary tract infections and urinary catheter use in hospitalized patients. *Clinical Infectious Diseases, 51*(5), 550–560. doi:10.1086/655133

Saint, S., Kaufman, S., Thompson, M., Rogers, M., & Chenoweth, C. A. (2005). A Reminder reduces urinary catheterization in hospitalized patients. *Journal on Quality and Patient Safety, 31*(8), 455–462. doi:10.1016/s1553-7250(05)31059-2

Saint, S., Wiese, J., Amory, J. K., Bernstein, M. I., Patel, U. D., Zemencutt, J. K., . . . Hofer, T. P. (2000). Are physicians aware of which of their patients have catheters? *American Journal of Medicine, 109*(6), 476–480. doi:10.1016/s0002-9343(00)00531-3

■ EXEMPLAR 20.3: PREVENTING HYPERBILIRUBINEMIA IN LATE PRETERM INFANTS USING EVIDENCE-BASED PRACTICES

Suzanne Rubin

Team

Nursing staff

Advanced practice nurses

Lactation services

Maryland Regional Transport Team

Johns Hopkins Hospital

Johns Hopkins University School of Nursing

Problem

Late preterm newborns, between 34 0/7 and 36 6/7 weeks' gestational age, are at risk for hyperbilirubinemia and subsequent kernicterus as compared to full-term infants. This condition is rare (one in 10,000 infants) but considered preventable.

Currently these late preterm infants receive care in the well-baby nursery, but may manifest the feeding and self-regulatory challenges common to preterm babies.

Careful and ongoing evaluation for rising bilirubin levels together with feeding assistance, support for thermoregulation, increased monitoring, family education, and early discharge follow-up are required.

Background

Thorough prosecution of the evidence revealed the following:

1. Excessive bilirubin accumulation is toxic to the brain, especially to the late preterm infant.
2. Severe hyperbilirubinemia and kernicterus are considered preventable.
3. Elimination of unconjugated bilirubin occurs primarily through the gut and can be accelerated by early and adequate feeding.
4. Feeding difficulties are universal in late preterm infants.
5. Lactation evaluation and support (early and often) can enhance feeding adequacy.
6. Poor caloric intake and dehydration contribute to the development of hyperbilirubinemia.
7. American Academy of Pediatrics (AAP) guidelines apply to the late preterm infant, but they should be considered for proposed interventions on the high-risk nomogram curve.
8. Early follow-up after discharge is critical—to address any feeding issues and follow serum values (which peak later than those of a full-term infant).

Aims

There were two aims for this project:

1. To reduce peak bilirubin levels among late preterm infants
2. To increase adherence to best practices for the care of late preterm infants

Translation Framework

Loma's Linear Coordination Model was adapted to guide this project (Figure 20.3.1).

Translation Methods

This project relied on two methods for translation: order sets and a bundle.

Late Preterm Order Set

The newborn nursery NPs reviewed the evidence and developed an order set to be used for all preterm infants on the NP service. These orders translated best practices from strong evidence into standard practice in order to reduce variability and error.

The evidence-based order set comprised the following:

Breastfeeding

- First feeding at 0 to 4 hours of life
- Ad lib or at least every 3 hours thereafter
- Mother to pump breasts for 15 minutes after each breastfeeding
- Offer pumped breast milk after each breastfeeding
- Supplement with formula per prescriber order if no colostrum or pumped milk is obtained
    - Breastfeeding supplementation
    - Feeding method
        - Supplementation at the breast
        - Paced bottle feeding
        - Cup feeding
        - Spoon or dropper feeding
        - Finger feeding
- Weigh twice a day
- Notify provider of jaundice, weight loss greater than 7%, inadequate oral feeding, or decreased urine output
- Patient education: Review handout "Late Pre-Term Infant: What Parents Need to Know"

Bundle

A special bundle was created and printed on a crib card, which was placed with every infant (Figure 20.3.2).

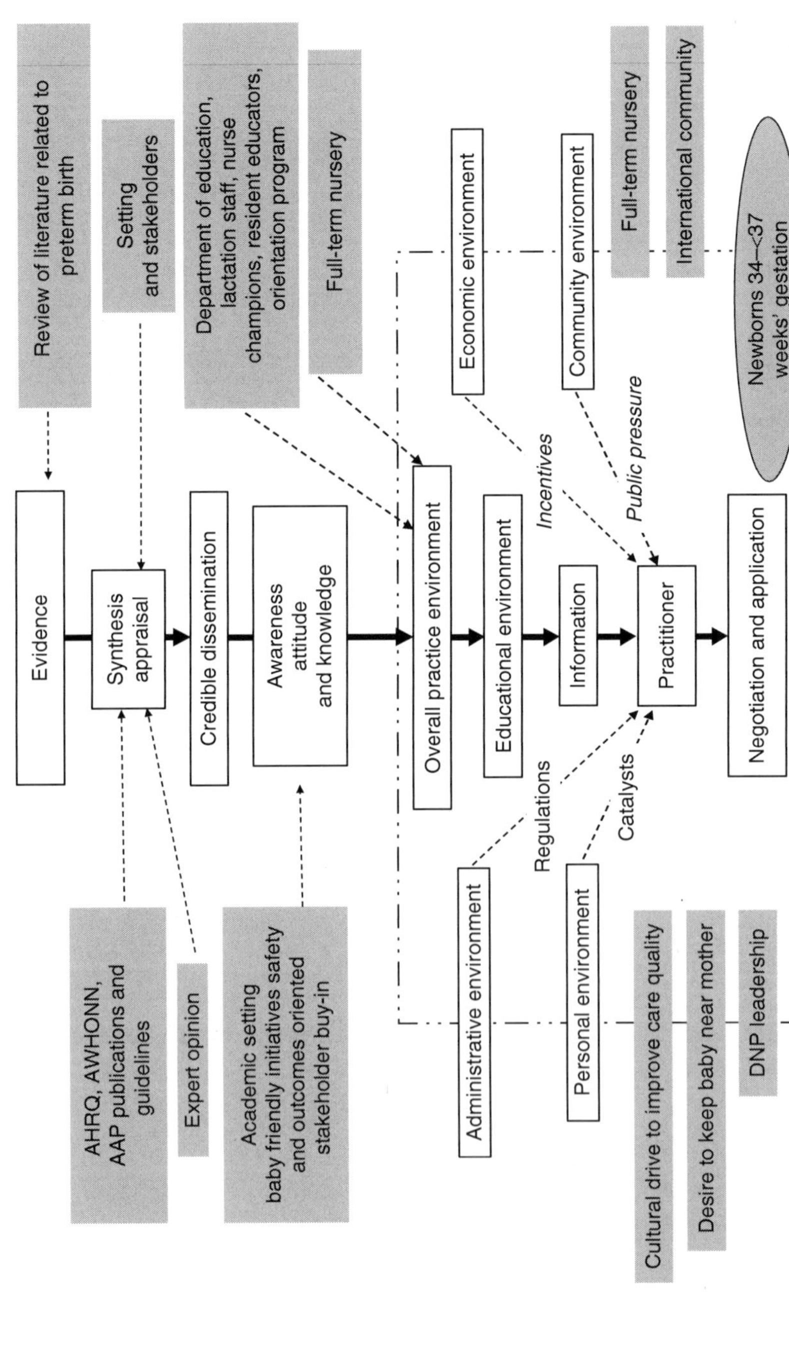

FIGURE 20.3.1 Adaptation of Loma's Linear Coordination Model.

AAP, American Academy of Pediatrics; AHRQ, Agency for Healthcare Research and Quality; AWHONN, Association of Women's Health, Obstetric, and Neonatal Nurses.

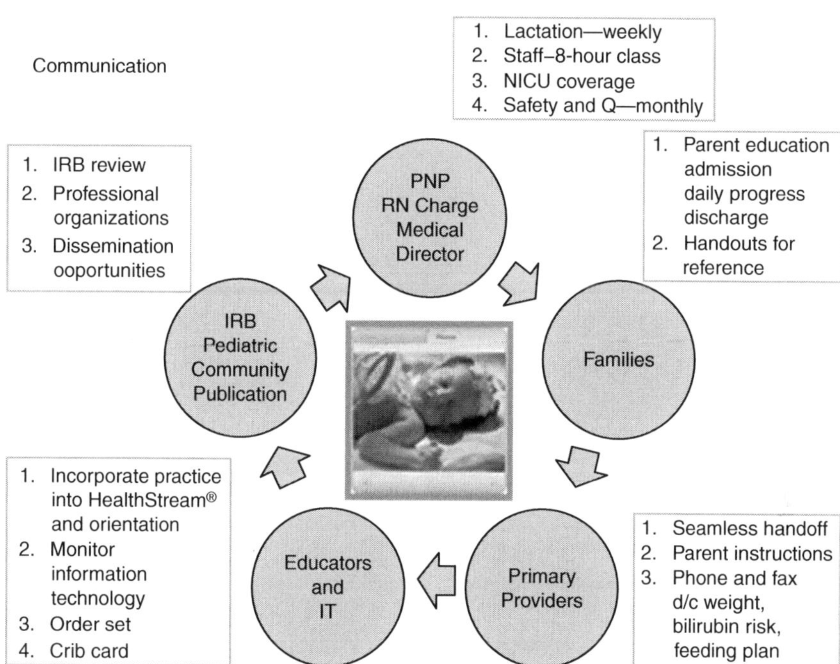

FIGURE 20.3.2 Communication within the team.

IRB, institutional review board; IT, information technology; NICU, neonatal intensive care unit; PNP, pediatric nurse practitioner; Q, quality.

It reminded family members and all staff of the critical, evidence-based practices to be followed for all late preterm infants.

Kangaroo Care

All elements of the bundle can easily be integrated into skin-to-skin or kangaroo care as a best practice supported by strong evidence.

- Undress; head covered with hat; diaper on
- Upright position, skin to skin, on the parent's chest
- Cover with a receiving blanket
- Hold infant for 1 hour for maximum benefit

Results

Peak bilirubin values among infants in cohort 2 (μ = 7.72 mg/dL) were not found to be significantly lower than the peak bilirubin values among infants in cohort 1 (μ = 8.66 mg/dL). No statistical difference was found using the independent samples *t*-test (SD = 2.4–3.3, $t(112) = 1.8$, $p < .05$, $d = .33$). See Figure 20.3.3.

Anecdotally, there were no infants in the treatment group (cohort 2) who had bilirubin levels in the toxic range. The same was not true for cohort 1.

Impact

The incidence of severe hyperbilirubinemia (since the AAP's comprehensive prevention and screening recommendations were released in 2004) has been greatly reduced

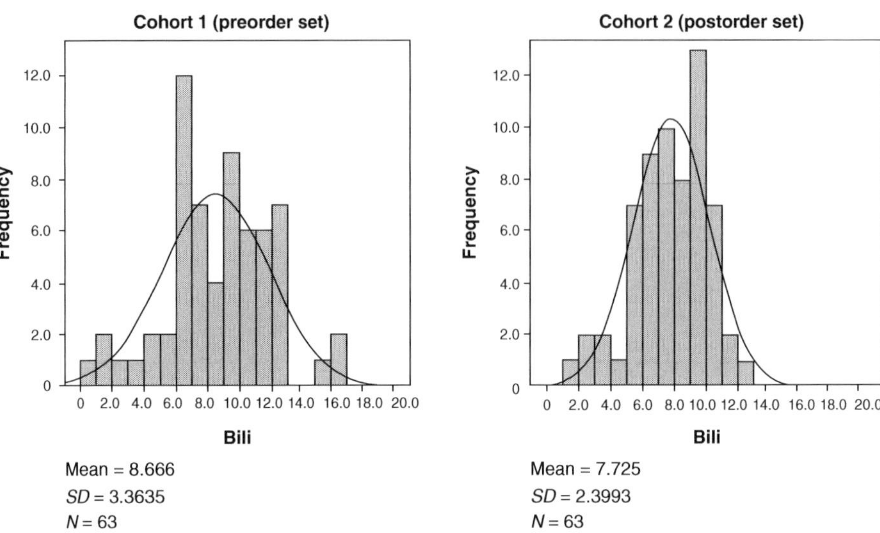

FIGURE 20.3.3 Bilirubin levels by cohort.
Note: Bilirubin values reported as mg/dL.

by a team of providers who became increasingly aware of the significant risk it presents: a team that selected strategies worth implementing consistently for the population they serve, based on a critical review of evidence.

Additional References

Agency for Healthcare Research and Quality. (2002, March). *Management of neonatal hyperbilirubinemia, summary. Evidence report/technology assessment: Number 65.* (AHRQ Publication No. 03-E005). Washington, DC: U.S. Department of Health and Human Services. Retrieved from http://www.ahrq.gov/clinic/epcsums/neonatalsum.htm

American Academy of Pediatrics Subcommittee on Hyperbilirubinemia. (2005). Management of hyperbilirubinemia in the newborn infant 35 or more weeks of gestation. *Pediatrics, 114*, 297–316. doi:10.1542/peds.114.1.297

Bhutani, V. K., & Johnson, L. (2006). Kernicterus in late preterm infants cared for as term healthy infants. *Seminars in Perinatology, 30*, 89–97. doi:10.1053/j.semperi.2006.04.001

Bhutani, V. K., & Johnson, L. H. (2009). Kernicterus in the 21st century: Frequently asked questions. *Journal of Perinatology, 29*(Suppl 1), S20–S24. doi:10.1038/jp.2008.212

Bhutani, V. K., Johnson, L. H., Maisels, M. J., Newman, T. B., Phibbs, C., Stark, A. R., & Yeargin-Allsopp, M. (2004). Kernicterus: Epidemiological strategies for its prevention through systems-based approaches. *Journal of Perinatology, 24*, 650–662. doi:10.1038/sj.jp.7211152

BiliTool™. Retrieved from www.bilitool.org

Centers for Disease Control and Prevention. (2009). *Jaundice/Kernicterus.* Retrieved from www.cdc.gov/ncbddd/dd/kernichome.htm

Engle, W. A., Tomashek, K. M., Wallman, C., & Committee on Fetus and Newborn. (2007). "Late-preterm" infants: A population at risk. *Pediatrics, 120*, 1390–1401. doi:10.1542/peds.2007-2952

Gennaro, S., Schwoebel, A., Hall, J. Y., & Bhutani, V. (2006). *Hyperbilirubinemia: Identification and management in the healthy term and near-term newborn* (2nd ed.). Washington, DC: Association of Women's Health, Obstetrical and Neonatal Nursing.

Lenth, R. V. (2001). Some practical guidelines for effective sample size determination. *The American Statistician, 55*, 187–193. doi:10.1198/000313001317098149

Lomas, J. (2000). Connecting research and policy. *ISUMA, 1*, 140–144. Retrieved from http://www.isuma.net/v01n01/lomas//lomas.html

Ludwig, S. M. (2007). Oral feeding and the late preterm infant. *Newborn and Nursing Infant, 7*(2), 72–75. doi:10.1053/j.nainr.2007.05.005

Meier, P., Furman, L., & Degenhardt, M. (2007). Increased lactation risk for late preterm infants and mothers: Evidence and management strategies to protect breastfeeding. *Journal of Midwifery &Women's Health, 53*(6), 579–587. doi:10.1016/j.jmwh.2007.08.003

Statistical Package for Social Sciences. (2008, September). *PASW Statistics 17.0.3—Description*. Chicago, IL: Author.

The Joint Commission on Accreditation of Healthcare Organizations. (2001, April 1). Kernicterus threatens healthy newborns. *Sentinel Event Alert, 18*. Retrieved from www.jointcommission.org/SentinelEvents/SentinelEventAlert/sea_18.htm

EXEMPLAR 20.4: SEDATION IN THE ICU: CHANGING TRADITIONAL PATTERNS OF PRACTICE

Juliane Jablonski

Team

Clinical nurse specialist

Nursing

Pharmacy

Medicine

Critical care services

University of Pennsylvania Hospital

Johns Hopkins University School of Nursing

Problem

Unnecessary variation in the assessment and treatment of pain, agitation, and delirium (PAD) in the mechanically ventilated surgical critical care patient leads to patient distress and unintended consequences.

Background

Sedatives and analgesics are among the most commonly administered medications in mechanically ventilated ICU patients (Reade, Phil, & Finfer, 2014). The compassionate intent is to ensure comfort and reduce anxiety, while supporting ventilator synchrony (Egerod, 2002; Guttormson, Chlan, Weinert, & Savik, 2009; Reade et al., 2014). Sedative use in the United States has increased from 39.7% of ICU patients in 2001 to 66.7% in 2007 (Wunsch, Kahn, Kramer, & Rubenfield, 2009). Available data from contemporary ICU surveys suggest a high incidence of deep sedation in ICUs across the United States (Jackson, Proudfoot, Cann, & Walsh, 2009). Only a small number of critically ill patients have a clinical indication for continuous, deep sedation, such as refractory intracranial hypertension or severe respiratory failure. Sedation requirements can vary between patients depending on clinical circumstances; however, targeting lighter levels of sedation may lead to better patient outcomes (Girard et al., 2008; Kress, Pohlman, O'Connor, & Hall, 2000; Mehta et al., 2010; Strom, Martinussen, & Toft, 2010).

A growing body of evidence demonstrates that maintaining a deep level of sedation is associated with a longer duration of mechanical ventilation, longer ICU length of stay (Girard et al., 2008; Kress et al., 2000; Mehta et al., 2010; Strom et al., 2010), and ICU-acquired weakness from immobility (Schweickert, Pohlman, & Pohlman, 2009). For patients with a deep level of sedation, assessment for pain and delirium is limited, leading to a potential delay in diagnosis and treatment (Honiden, & Siegel, 2010; Jackson et al., 2009; Reade et al., 2014). Pain and delirium in critically ill patients may cause patient distress and require individualized interventions for treatment (Fraser et al., 2013; Girard et al., 2008; Honiden, & Siegel, 2010; Kress et al., 2000; Mehta et al., 2010; Schweickert et al., 2009; Strom et al., 2010). Delirium occurs in up to 50% to 70% of critically ill patients and is associated with an increased incidence of post-ICU syndrome, with patients suffering from posttraumatic stress disorder up to 1 year after discharge from the hospital (Bienvenu et al., 2013; Davydow, Gifford, Desai, Needham, & Bienvenu, 2008; Ely et al., 2004; Pandharipande et al., 2006; Salluh et al., 2010). Uncontrolled pain, among other factors, has been shown to be a risk factor for the development of delirium (Fraser et al., 2013; Girard et al., 2008; Honiden, & Siegel, 2010; Kress et al., 2000; Mehta et al., 2010; Schweickert et al., 2009; Strom et al., 2010), and early ICU deep sedation levels and delirium have been shown to be predictors of mortality (Bienvenu et al., 2013; Davydow et al., 2008; Ely et al., 2004; Pandharipande et al., 2006; Salluh et al., 2010; Shehabi et al., 2012).

In a research setting, protocols using validated pain and sedation scales with targeted light levels of sedation are shown to maintain patient comfort while decreasing practice variation and cumulative sedative exposure (Awissi, Bégin, Moisan, Lachaine, & Skrobik, 2012; Brook et al., 1999; Fraser et al., 2013; Mehta et al., 2010; Robinson et al., 2008). Many protocols operationalize spontaneous awakening trials once daily during which all continuous sedative infusions are held to evaluate the patients' neurological status (Girard et al., 2008; Kress et al., 2000; Mehta et al., 2010; Strom et al., 2010). National survey data have demonstrated that many providers identify the availability of practice guidelines and sedation protocols within their institutions, but report challenges of low adherence levels, inconsistent use of ICU assessment tools, and gaps in communication among caregivers (Egerod, 2002; Guttormson et al., 2009).

Practice guidelines from the Society of Critical Care Medicine (SCCM) recommend institutions implement an evidence-based ICU PAD bundle (Fraser et al., 2013). The evidence-based goal is to focus on systematically identifying and managing PAD in an integrated fashion. Clinicians are to use validated assessment tools to achieve "lighter sedation" levels (Hughes, Girard, & Pandharipande, 2013) and target specific, individualized treatment for PAD. Strategies for management incorporate an analgesia-first approach (Strom et al., 2010), the judicious use of benzodiazepine sedatives (Frazier et al., 2013; Pandharipande et al., 2006; Pisani et al., 2009), reduction of continuous infusions, and the promotion of early physical therapy (Mah, Staff, Fichnadler, & Butler, 2013; Morris et al., 2008; Strom et al., 2010).

The purpose of this study is to evaluate the efficacy of the SCCM PAD bundle in a high-acuity trauma and surgical patient population. The hypothesis is that patients will have lighter sedation scores, better analgesia, lower incidence of delirium, increased physical therapy sessions, and fewer days spent on mechanical ventilation and in the ICU.

Aims

This project had two aims:

1. To provide comfort, reduce sedation, and reduce days of delirium in mechanically ventilated critical care patients
2. To reduce the time to initiation and increase the frequency of activity sessions for mechanically ventilated critical care patients

Translation Framework

The Knowledge-to-Action Framework was used for this translation project.

Translation Methods

A multidisciplinary team, including physicians, nurses, advanced practice providers, pharmacists, physical therapists, and respiratory care therapists, was created to review routine sedation and analgesia practice. Baseline patient data collection occurred between May 1, 2013, and July 31, 2013. Variation in pharmacological agents, overall management, communication, nursing assessment, and titration practices were identified. A multidisciplinary guideline and protocol was developed through a review of the literature and adaptation of the SCCM PAD bundle. Postintervention data were collected from December 2, 2013 to March 1, 2014.

Two methods were used to accomplish translation in this project: an algorithm and a bundle.

Algorithm

Clinical decision algorithms were designed for the focused assessment and treatment of PAD. Evidence-based assessment tools, including the Richmond Agitation Sedation Scale (RASS), Behavioral Pain Scale (BPS), Numeric Pain Scale (NPS), and the Confusion Assessment Method for the ICU (CAM-ICU), were implemented by the clinical nurses. Frequency of nursing assessments for pain and sedation/agitation is a minimum of every 4 hours and for delirium every 12 hours. An analgesia-first approach was taken, with a goal BPS/NPS score less than 5. Targeted "light sedation," with a goal RASS of 0 to −1, was the standard goal for all intubated patients, unless deep sedation was clinically indicated. According to the protocol, clinical indications for deep sedation include the following: life-threatening hypoxia, hemodynamic instability, unstable airway, intracranial pressure (ICP) management, uncontrolled seizures, severe alcohol withdrawal syndrome, and use of neuromuscular blockade. Pharmacological treatment emphasized utilization of intermittent doses before beginning continuous infusions, use of propofol for initial sedation, and judicious use of benzodiazepines unless clinically indicated for alcohol or benzodiazepine withdrawal syndrome. For patients positive for delirium, nonpharmacological management was preferred; however, patients could receive haloperidol or an atypical antipsychotic for hyperactive delirium.

Bundle

The multidisciplinary team in the surgical/intensive care unit (SICU) implemented the PAD bundle intervention in a stepwise manner. Physician and advanced practice provider support was obtained through presentations at faculty meetings. Pocket cards with the clinical decision algorithms were made available to all staff members. The SICU clinical nurses completed a pre-education survey to evaluate attitudes and baseline knowledge regarding PAD. After the initial survey, the unit-based clinical nurse specialist provided educational sessions for all clinical nurses. Components of the education included accuracy in application of RASS, BPS/NPS, and CAM-ICU, emphasizing "light sedation," target RASS of 0 to −1, for intubated patients (unless criteria met clinical need indicating heavier sedation), the importance of differentiating among pain, agitation, and delirium, and the identification of underlying causes. The clinical nurses then completed the same survey after education. Education was provided to the ICU residents by the physicians who attended and unit-based clinical pharmacists through discussions on daily patient care rounds. Physical and occupational therapists provide a total of 40 hours per week consultation services. The charge nurse and clinical nurse specialist round with the physical and occupational therapists daily and in collaboration with the physician teams to determine patients' activity levels.

Results

There were a total of 54 patients in the preintervention and 52 patients in the postintervention group.

Aim 1—Provide Comfort, Reduce Oversedation, and Reduce Days of Delirium

Mean percentage of scores within the goal BPS of 3 to 5 or goal NPS less than 3 remained stable from 86% to 83% ($p = .16$).

Mean percentage of ventilator days spent on a continuous opioid infusion decreased from 65% to 47% ($p < .01$).

Percentage of ventilator days spent on a continuous sedative remained the same, 44% versus 45% ($p = .86$), in the pre- and postintervention group, respectively.

Mean percentage of scores within the goal RASS of 0 to −1 increased from 38% in the preintervention to 50% in the postintervention group ($p <.02$).

Aim 2—Reduce the Time to Initiation and Increase the Frequency of Activity Sessions

Mean percentage of ICU days with a physical therapy session increased from 24% to 41% ($p <.001$).

Mean day of first physical activity session trended downward from day 5.85 to day 4.75 ($p = .31$).

Mean ventilator days trended downward from 6.9 to 5.1 days ($p = .32$) and mean ICU length of stay trended downward from 11.75 to 9.5 days ($p = .20$) in the pre- and postintervention groups, respectively.

There was no difference in the incidence of delirium, 56% versus 63% ($p = .68$).

Impact

Implementation of the SCCM PAD bundle in a large, academic surgical ICU resulted in decreased use of continuous opioid infusions and improved time spent at target RASS of 0 to –1, while maintaining stable analgesia. Further, physical activity sessions increased and there was a downtrend in ICU length of stay (LOS) and days spent on mechanical ventilation. There was no difference in patient falls or accidental extubations. Implementation of the PAD bundle can be successful and should be considered in all ICUs.

Dissemination

Jablonski, J. (2014). *Winner of 2014 University of Pennsylvania Health System Quality and Safety Honorable Mention Award.* Unpublished manuscript.

Jablonski, J. (2015). *Sedation in the ICU: Changing traditional patterns of practice.* Poster session presented at the Society for Critical Care Medicine National Conference.

Additional References

Awissi, D. K., Bégin, C., Moisan, J., Lachaine, J., & Skrobik, Y. (2012). Impact of sedation, analgesia, and delirium protocols evaluated in the intensive care unit: An economic evaluation. *Annals of Pharmacotherapy, 46*, 21–28. doi:10.1345/aph.1q284

Bienvenu, O. J., Gella, R. J., Althouse, B. M., Colatuoni, E., Sricharoenchai, T., Mendez-Tellez, P. A, . . . Needham, D. M. (2013). Post-traumatic stress disorder symptoms after acute lung injury: A 2-year prospective longitudinal study. *Psychological Medicine, 43*(12), 2657–2671. doi:10.1017/S0033291713000214

Brook, A. D., Ahrens, T. S., Schaiff, R., Prentice, D., Sherman, G., Shannon, W., & Kollef, M. H. (1999). Effect of a nursing-implemented sedation protocol on the duration of mechanical ventilation. *Critical Care Medicine, 27*, 2609–2615. doi:10.1097/00003246-199912000-00001

Davydow, D. S., Gifford, J. M., Desai, S. V., Needham, D. M., & Bienvenu, J. (2008). Posttraumatic stress disorder in general intensive care unit survivors: A systematic review. *General Hospital Psychiatry, 30*, 421–434. doi:10.1016/j.genhosppsych.2008.05.006

Egerod, I. (2002). Uncertain terms of sedation in ICU: How nurses and physicians manage and describe sedation for mechanically ventilated patients. *Journal of Clinical Nursing, 11*, 831–840. doi:10.1046/j.1365-2702.2002.00725.x

Ely, W. E., Shintani, A., Truman, B., Speroff, T., Gordon, S. M., Harrell, F. E., . . . Dittus, R. S. (2004). Delirium as a predictor of mortality in mechanically ventilated patients in the intensive care unit. *Journal of the American Medical Association, 291*(4), 1753–1762. doi:10.1001/jama.291.14.1753

Fraser, G. L., Devlin, J. W., Worby, C. P., Alhazzani, W., Barr, J., Dasta, J. F., . . . Spencer, F. A. (2013). Benzodiazepine versus non-benzodiazepine-based sedation for mechanically ventilated critically ill adults: A systematic review and meta-analysis of randomized controlled trials. *Critical Care Medicine, 41*(9 Suppl. 1), S30–S38. doi:10.1097/ccm.0b013e3182a16898

Fraser, G. L., Puntillo, K., Ely, E. W., Gelinas, C., Dasta, J. F., Davidson, J. E., . . . American College of Critical Care. (2013). Clinical practice guidelines for the management of pain, agitation, and delirium in adult patients in the intensive care unit. *Critical Care Medicine, 41*(1), 263–306. doi:10.1097/ccm.0b013e3182783b72

Girard, T. D., Kress, J. P., Fuchs, B. D., Thomason, J. W., Schweickert, W. D., Pun, B. T., . . . Ely, E. W. (2008). Efficacy and safety of a paired sedation and ventilator weaning protocol for mechanically ventilated patients in intensive care (Awakening and Breathing Controlled Trial): A randomized controlled trial. *Lancet, 371*, 126–134. doi:10.1016/s0140-6736(08)60105-1

Guttormson, J. L., Chlan, L., Weinert, C., & Savik, K. (2009). Factors influencing nurse sedation practices with mechanically ventilated patients: A U.S. national survey. *Intensive and Critical Care Nursing, 26*, 44–50. doi:10.1016/j.iccn.2009.10.004

Honiden, S., & Siegel, M. D. (2010). Managing the agitated patient in the ICU: Sedation, analgesia, and neuromuscular blockade. *Journal of Critical Care Medicine, 25*(4), 187–204. doi:10.1177/0885066610366923

Hughes, C. G., Girard, T. D., & Pandharipande, P. P. (2013). Daily sedation interruption versus targeted light sedation strategies in ICU patients. *Critical Care Medicine, 41*, S39–S45. doi:10.1097/ccm.0b013e3182a168c5

Jackson, D. L., Proudfoot, C. W., Cann, K. F., & Walsh, T. S. (2009). The incidence of sub-optimal sedation in the ICU: A systematic review. *Critical Care, 13*, R204. doi:10.1186/cc8212

Kress, J. P., Pohlman, A. S., O'Connor, M. F., & Hall, J. B. (2000). Daily interruption of sedative infusions in critically ill patients undergoing mechanical ventilation. *New England Journal of Medicine, 342*(20), 1471–1477. doi:10.1056/nejm200005183422002

Mah, J., Staff, I., Fichnadler, D., & Butler, K. L. (2013). Resource-efficient mobilization programs in the intensive care unit: Who stands to win? *American Journal of Surgery, 206*, 488–493. doi:10.1016/j.amjsurg.2013.03.001

Mehta, S., Burry, L., Cook, D., Fergusson, D., Steinberg, M., Granton, J., . . . Canadian Critical Care Trials Group. (2010). Daily interruption in mechanically ventilated critically ill patients cared for with a sedation protocol: A randomized controlled trial. *Journal of the American Medical Association, 308*(19), 1985. doi:10.1001/jama.2012.13872

Morris, P. E., Goad, A., Thompson, C., Taylor, K., Harry, B., Passmore, L., . . . Haponik, E. (2008). Early intensive care unit mobility therapy in the treatment of acute respiratory failure. *Critical Care Medicine, 36*(8), 2238–2243. doi:10.1097/ccm.0b013e318180b90e

Pandharipande, P. P., Girard, T. D., Jackson, J. C., Morandi, A., Thompson, J. L., Brummel, N. E., . . . BRAIN-ICU Study Investigators. (2013). Long-term cognitive impairment after critical illness. *New England Journal of Medicine, 369*, 1306–1316. doi:10.1056/nejmoa1301372

Pandharipande, P., Shintani, A., Peterson, J., Pun, B. T., Wilkinson, G. R., Dittus, R. S., . . . Ely, E. W. (2006). Lorazepam is an independent risk factor for transitioning to delirium in intensive care unit patients. *Anesthesiology, 104*(1), 21–26. doi:10.1097/00000542-200601000-00005

Pisani, M. A., Murphy, T. E., Araujo, K. L. B., Slattum, P., Van Ness, P. H., & Inouye, S. K. (2009). Benzodiazepine and opioid use and the duration of ICU delirium in an older population. *Critical Care Medicine, 37*(1), 177–183. doi:10.1097/CCM.0b013e318192fcf9

Reade, M. C., Phil, D., & Finfer, S. (2014). Sedation and delirium in the intensive care unit. *New England Journal of Medicine, 370*, 444–454. doi:10.1056/nejmra1208705

Robinson, B. R., Mueller, E. W., Henson, K., Branson, R. D., Barsoum, S., & Tsuei, B. J. (2008). An analgesia-delirium-sedation protocol for critically ill trauma patients reduces ventilator days and hospital length of stay. *Journal of Trauma Injury, Infection, and Critical Care, 65*, 517–526. doi:10.1097/ta.0b013e318181b8f6

Salluh, J. I., Soares, M., Teles, J. M., Ceraso, D., Raimondi, N., Nava, V. S., . . . Delirium Epidemiology in Critical Care Study Group. (2010). Delirium epidemiology in critical care (DECCA): An international study. *Critical Care, 14*, R210. doi:10.1186/cc9333

Schweickert, W. D., Pohlman, M. C., & Pohlman, J. (2009). Early physical and occupational therapy in mechanically ventilated, critically ill patients: A randomized controlled trial. *Lancet, 373*, 1874–1882. doi:10.1016/s0140-6736(09)60658-9

Shehabi, Y., Bellomo, R., Reade, M. C., Shehabi, Y., Bellomo, R., Reade, M. C., . . . Sedation Practice in Intensive Care Evaluation (SPICE) Study Investigators; ANZICS Clinical Trials Group. (2012). Early intensive care sedation predicts long-term mortality in ventilated critically ill patients. *American Journal of Respiratory Critical Care Medicine, 186*(8), 724–731. doi:10.1164/rccm.201203-05220C

Strom, T., Martinussen, T., & Toft, P. (2010). A protocol of no sedation for critically ill patients receiving mechanical ventilation: A randomized trial. *Lancet, 375*, 475–480. doi:10.1016/s0140-6736(09)62072-9

Wunsch, H., Kahn, J. M., Kramer, A. A., & Rubenfield, G. D. (2009). Use of intravenous infusion sedation among mechanically ventilated patients in the United States. *Critical Care Medicine, 37*(12), 3031–3039. doi:10.1097/ccm.0b013e3181b02eff

■ EXEMPLAR 20.5: IMPROVING CONTINUOUS POSITIVE AIRWAY PRESSURE COMPLIANCE AMONG PATIENTS

Christina DiNapoli

Team

Advanced practice nurse

Physician

Weill Cornell Medical College

Johns Hopkins University School of Nursing

Problem

Poor adherence to a treatment regimen among adult patients with obstructive sleep apnea can lead to decreased quality of life and increased risk for poor outcomes.

Background

Continuous positive airway pressure, also known as *CPAP*, is used to treat obstructive sleep apnea (OSA). OSA is characterized by repetitive apneas and hypopneas during sleep, associated with oxygen desaturations, which lead to sleep disruptions and excessive daytime sleepiness. It has been estimated that approximately 24% of the U.S. population experience sleep apnea; however, only about 4% of the population have been diagnosed (Epstein et al., 2009; Siccoli et al., 2008; Weaver & Sawyer, 2010). Growing patient awareness and practitioner training are rapidly increasing the pool of diagnosed patients, which is growing at 15% per year (Epstein et al., 2009; Siccoli et al., 2008; Weaver & Sawyer, 2010).

CPAP is widely accepted as the most efficacious therapy for the treatment of moderate to severe OSA as it provides a pneumatic splint to prevent nocturnal airway collapse (Epstein et al., 2009; Weaver & Sawyer, 2010). For the purpose of this project, compliance was defined as CPAP use for more than 4 hours per night, for over 70% of each month. These metrics are tracked inside all CPAP machines.

Although CPAP is an effective treatment for OSA, compliance is a critical problem and is widely recognized as a significant limiting factor in the treatment of OSA (Weaver et al., 2007). Noncompliance with CPAP reduces effectiveness of treatment and leaves patients at an increased risk for comorbid conditions, decreased quality of life, and decreased daily functioning (Siccoli et al., 2008). Studies have shown that 30% to 50% of patients diagnosed with OSA reject CPAP immediately and approximately 80% of OSA patients are noncompliant within a year of starting therapy (Weaver et al., 2007).

The Weill Cornell Center for Sleep Medicine is an outpatient sleep center in an academic medical center. Currently it employs two full-time physicians, two part-time physicians, two psychologists, and one NP. On average, clinicians see approximately

12 to 15 patients daily and 30% to 60% are prescribed to use CPAP. The center's CPAP compliance rate is 54.6% and recent QI data revealed great variation in CPAP compliance among providers.

Noncompliance with CPAP reduces the overall effectiveness of treatment, which leaves patients at increased risk for comorbid conditions, decreased quality of life, and decreased daily functioning (Young, Peppard, & Gottlieb, 2002). Patients with untreated sleep apnea are at an increased risk for poor health outcomes. Untreated OSA increases the risk of hypertension, diabetes, and stroke threefold (Siccoli et al., 2008). Untreated patients are also at risk for ischemic heart disease, cardiac arrhythmias, and peripheral vascular disease as well as decreased quality of life, impaired cognition and memory, decreased functional and occupational capacity, and mood alterations (Simon-Tuval et al., 2009). In addition to affecting the quality of life and health outcomes, OSA has been credited with doubling healthcare costs as compared with patients without OSA (Wittmann & Rodenstein, 2004).

Because the snoring and breathing disturbances associated with OSA can be scary and disruptive, the sleep partner often suffers, too. The patient's bed partner also experiences fragmented sleep and experiences a related decrease in quality of life and daytime functioning (Young et al., 2002).

The community as a whole is also affected because patients with untreated sleep apnea are 3 to 7 times more likely to have motor vehicle accidents and other unintentional injuries (Rodenstein, 2009) . Patients with sleep apnea have decreased occupational function and productivity, which also affect the community as a whole (Rodenstein, 2009; Wittmann & Rodenstein, 2004).

Aims

This project had two aims:

1. To increase provider knowledge of the importance of CPAP compliance among patients diagnosed with OSA
2. To increase the number of patients who are effectively managing their OSA—*effectively managing* is defined as "using CPAP for over 4 hours per night for more than 70% of each month"

Translation Framework

The Quality Enhancement Research Initiative (QUERI) translational framework describes a process for improving patient care by implementing the best evidence-based practice. This is a good fit for this project, which is intended to improve CPAP compliance among patients diagnosed with OSA.

The QUERI model has six steps. The first step is to identify a high-risk patient population; in this case, it is patients with OSA. The significance and risk are presented in the background section of this exemplar. The second step is to identify evidence-based practice. A search of the evidence identified several interventions that improve CPAP compliance. The third step is to measure quality and performance

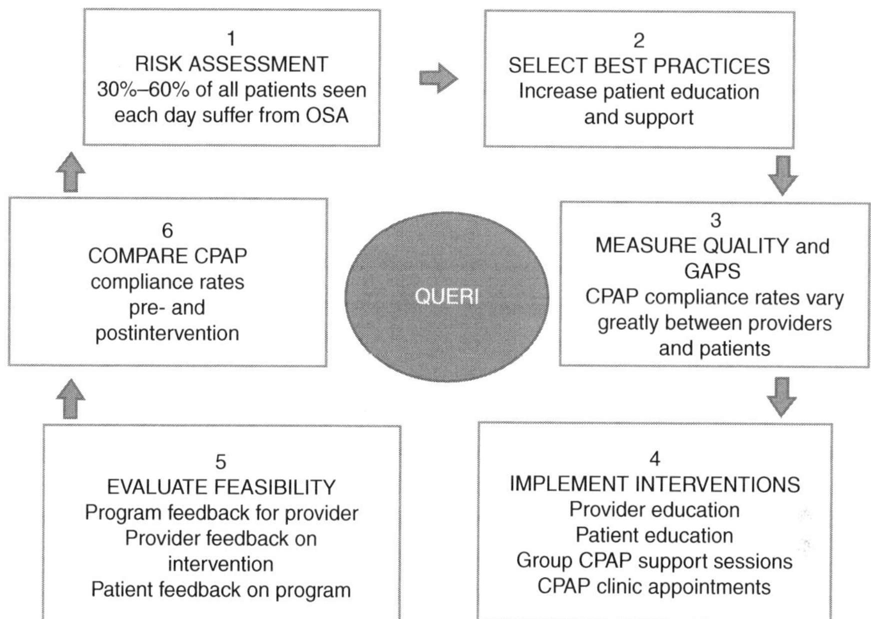

FIGURE 20.5.1 Adaptation of QUERI framework.

CPAP, continuous positive airway pressure; OSA, obstructive sleep apnea; QUERI, Quality Enhancement Research Initiative.

gaps. CPAP compliance rates were found to vary greatly among providers, which identifies a variation in care and predicts variation in outcome. The fourth step is to implement improvement. Education and intensive support both have been shown to improve CPAP compliance and were the methods applied. An OSA/CPAP support group as well as individual CPAP clinic appointments were implemented. The fifth step was to evaluate the feasibility of implementing the program as well as getting feedback. Finally, the sixth step was to evaluate the effects of the intervention, and the team looked at CPAP compliance rates and compared them to the rates recorded before the project was implemented (Figure 20.5.1).

Translation Methods

Two methods were used for this project: instructional design and process redesign.

Instructional Design

The main method used for translation was instructional design. Separate programs of instruction were developed for providers and patients because their needs were different.

Provider Education

Because of the considerable variability in approach to care found among providers, and the lack of evidence-based practice in the care of patients with OSA, this project began with professional development for the providers. The intent was to ensure that all providers understood the most recent evidence regarding OSA, its management, and the outcomes of unmanaged or ineffectively managed OSA. The instruction was designed to accomplish understanding and engagement with the evidence. The goal was to increase knowledge and change practice.

Patient Education

A set of patient education materials was developed for the practice. These materials translated evidence for patients to support effective self-care. A pilot study (1 week) was conducted to establish feasibility of this approach, level of content, usefulness for clinicians, and feedback from patients who were provided education supported by evidence. These materials were then published in a pamphlet and made available for all providers to use in patient care and education. The knowledge of patients would be increased, with the overall goal of improving CPAP compliance among adult patients diagnosed with OSA.

Process Redesign

The second method used in this project was practice redesign. The project leader began to receive additional referrals for assistance with OSA patient management. This evolved into a full day in the clinic when the project leader scheduled OSA patients. An OSA patient support group was then established to provide these individuals with the opportunity to discuss self-care and the challenges of adhering to the CPAP treatment regimen. It has evolved further to several full clinic days when the project leader sees OSA patients, provides education, and refines the approach to care based on patient feedback.

Results

Provider Knowledge

The first aim was to increase provider knowledge of the importance of CPAP compliance among patients with OSA. The mean knowledge assessment score was 70% preintervention and 86.67% postintervention. The mean score increased by 16.67 points, which constitutes a 23.8% increase.

Patient Compliance

The second aim was to increase the number of patients who were effectively managing (using CPAP for more than 4 hours per night for more than 70% of the month) their OSA. A chi-square test was used to compare the CPAP compliance data for patients in the comparison and intervention groups. CPAP compliance was 54.6% in the comparison group and 65.9% in the intervention group. There was an 11.3-point increase in CPAP compliance postintervention, which constitutes a 21% increase ($p = .005$).

Logistic regression was used to adjust for the length of time on CPAP, mask type, as well as provider. After adjusting for confounders, patients with OSA in the intervention were twice as likely to comply with the CPAP treatment plan than patients in the comparison group.

Impact

CPAP compliance increased by 21% in the group whose care was informed by evidence.

Interventions were aimed at both providers and patients. The intent was to increase knowledge, to provide materials useful to providers in their education of patients, and to make available to patients a variety of support options. Together, these methods led to increased CPAP compliance among adult patients diagnosed with OSA.

Improving CPAP compliance improves the overall outcome for the patient diagnosed with OSA. Effective treatment and education of OSA patients decreases the comorbid conditions associated with untreated OSA. It may also decrease healthcare costs as well as increase daily functioning—improving the quality of life in these patients overall.

Dissemination

DiNapoli, C. (2014). Strategies to improve continuous positive airway pressure compliance: A review. *Journal of Nursing Education and Practice, 4*(7), 62–72.

DiNapoli, C. (2015). Improving continuous positive airway pressure adherence among adults. *Journal of Nursing Education and Practice, 5*(2), 110–116.

Additional References

Epstein, L., Kristo, D., Strollo, P., Friedman, N., Malhotra, A., Patil, S., . . . Weinstein, M. (2009). Clinical guideline for evaluation, management and long-term care of obstructive sleep apnea in adults. *Journal of Clinical Sleep Medicine, 5*(3), 263–276.

Rodenstein, D. (2009). Sleep apnea: Traffic and occupational accidents: Individual risks, socioeconomic and legal implications. *Respiration, 78*, 241–248. doi:10.1159/000222811

Siccoli, M., Pepperell, J., Kohler, M., Craig, S., Davies, R., & Stradling, J. (2008). Effects of continuous positive airway pressure on quality of life in patients with moderate to severe obstructive sleep apnea: Data from a randomized control trial. *Sleep, 31*(11), 1551–1558. doi:10.1093/sleep/31.11.1551

Simon-Tuval, T., Reuveni, H., Greenberg-Dotan, S., Oksenberg, A., Tal, A., & Tarasiuk, A. (2009). Low socioeconomic status is a risk factor for CPAP acceptance among adult OSAS patients requiring treatment. *Sleep, 32*(4), 545–552. doi:10.1093/sleep/32.4.545

Weaver, T., Maislin, G., Dinges, D. F., Bloxham, T., George, C. F., Greenberg, H., . . . Pack, A. I. (2007). Relationship between hours of CPAP use and achieving normal levels of sleepiness and daily functioning. *Sleep, 30*(6), 711–719. doi:10.1093/sleep/30.6.711

Weaver, T., & Sawyer, A. (2010). Adherence to continuous positive airway pressure treatment for obstructive sleep apnea: Implications for future interventions. *Indian Journal of Medical Research, 131*, 248–258.

Wittmann, V., & Rodenstein, D. (2004). Health care costs and sleep apnea syndrome. *Sleep Medical Reviews, 4*, 269–279. doi:10.1016/j.smrv.2004.01.002

Young, T., Peppard, P., & Gottlieb, D. (2002). Epidemiology of obstructive sleep apnea. *American Journal of Respiratory Critical Care Medicine, 165*, 1217–1239. doi:10.1164/rccm.2109080

■ EXEMPLAR 20.6: MINIMIZING RISK OF LYMPHEDEMA AMONG BREAST CANCER SURVIVORS

Judy Phillips

Team

Nurse practitioners

Oncologists

Nursing staff
Administrative staff
Nutritionists
Pharmacists
Physical therapists
Occupational therapists
Nursing faculty
Cancer Care of Western North Carolina
Johns Hopkins University School of Nursing

Problem

Healthcare professionals and patients are unaware of the best evidence-based practices to prevent lymphedema among breast cancer patients. As a result, women do not take simple steps to reduce risk.

Background

The diagnosis of breast cancer produces fear for the women who face it. After investigating treatment options, these women quickly receive surgery, radiation, chemotherapy, and/or hormone blockers. Once the initial surgery and treatment are in the past, women go on to face many lifelong challenges, including depression, fear, anxiety, and the risk of lymphedema.

Lymphedema is swelling of the arm, hand, fingers, chest, and/or back that develops on the side or sides affected by breast cancer. Soran et al. (2011) performed a case-control study to estimate the probability of lymphedema after breast cancer surgery. The estimated probability of lymphedema is as low as 6.8%, when the body mass index (BMI) is less than 25, when there is no infection, and when there is a low level of hand use. The estimated probability of lymphedema is as high as 93.7% for patients who engage in a high level of hand use, have an infection, and have a BMI above 25.

At the time this project was conducted, no evidence-based risk reduction strategies to prevent lymphedema had been reported. As a result, practice among providers was inconsistent and not based on evidence. Careful review of evidence regarding lymphedema and its management revealed that certain conditions increase the probability of lymphedema.

Aims

This project had three aims:

1. To increase nurses' knowledge of evidence-based lymphedema prevention
2. To increase breast cancer patients' knowledge of strategies to prevent lymphedema
3. To increase self-care behaviors among postoperative breast cancer patients

Translation Framework

Pender's Health Promotion Model served as a conceptual framework for this project because it fit well with preventive care. Individual characteristics, experiences, and patients' knowledge, including cognition and affect, were all addressed.

The Iowa Model for evidence-based nursing practice was used to structure development, implementation, and evaluation of the lymphedema educational program (Titler et al., 2011). This project focused on the knowledge triggers. Because there are no national guidelines for the management of lymphedema, the team assembled, critiqued, and synthesized the evidence as the model directed. Because strong evidence was available but not practiced, the team developed a program to resolve this component of the problem. Staff education, patient education, and materials to be used in staff education were developed, tested, and refined according to the model. The Iowa Model guided change in teaching patients about self-care and served as a framework for improving patient outcomes, enhancing nursing practice, and monitoring healthcare costs.

Translation Methods

Two educational programs were designed and implemented to achieve the aims of this project. One was for the patients and another was for the professionals providing care for these women at risk.

Evidence to Support the Prevention of Lymphedema

A thorough prosecution of the evidence was conducted to reveal that 10 conditions have been associated with lymphedema. These conditions became the focus of education for professionals and patients, and were used to develop a tool for ongoing criterion-referenced assessment and monitoring. The risk-associated conditions are:

1. BMI—Risk increases when BMI exceeds 25%
2. Lymph node removal—Risk increases if lymph node dissection is performed
3. Chemotherapy—Risk increases if chemotherapy is used
4. Radiation—Risk increases if radiation therapy is used
5. Positive lymph nodes—Risk increases if lymph nodes test positive
6. Infection after surgery—Risk increases if there is infection after surgery
7. Injury after surgery—Risk increases if there is injury after surgery
8. Mastectomy—Risk increases after mastectomy
9. Repetitive hand/arm motions on the affected side—Risk increases if the patient engages in repetitive hand and arm movements after surgery
10. Being African American—Risk increases if the patient is African American

Four of the 10 conditions associated with risk for lymphedema can be influenced by self-care and the rest can be carefully monitored. As a result, two educational programs and an assessment tool were developed and deployed based on findings from the prosecution of the evidence.

Curriculum for Providers

The first program was offered to professionals and all members of the healthcare team. They were introduced to adult learning principles and the self-care practices supported by high-quality evidence.

Curriculum for Patients

The second program of education along with educational materials to help clinicians to teach effective, evidence-based self-care was developed for patients. The program began with a patient knowledge assessment to evaluate each woman's understanding of risk and lymphedema. Nurses then reviewed test results and reinforced knowledge necessary to promote effective self-care and diminish risk. Risk assessment scores were tallied and recorded in the medical record to guide care and future education.

A booklet was developed to review the evidence, reinforce the education, and serve as a resource after women returned home. Nurses were available by phone to answer questions. Three weeks later, a posttest was administered to each patient. In this way, a consistent approach to patient and family education could be implemented.

Behavioral outcomes of decreased anxiety and fear were monitored before and after this project.

As a result, clinicians were able to help patients plan to manage potential barriers and challenges in changing their self-care. This was considered essential to increase the impact of health-promotion behaviors (Peterson & Bredow, 2009).

The Johns Hopkins University and Mission Hospital institutional review boards and the Research Institute approved this QI project and the quasi-experimental design was used to evaluate its outcomes. A convenience sample of 26 nurses and 37 patients participated.

Results

Nurses' Knowledge of Lymphedema

Paired-samples *t*-test established a statistically significant increase in nurses' knowledge of lymphedema: $M = 25.00$, $SD = 9.49$, $df(25)$, $t = -13.43$, and $p < .00$ (two-tailed). Mean increase in test scores was 25 with a 95% confidence interval ranging from −28.83 to −21.17. The eta-squared statistic (.88) indicates a large effect size. Refer to Table 20.6.1.

TABLE 20.6.1 Knowledge of Lymphedema

Aim	Mean Differences or Percentages	Outcome
Increase nurses' knowledge ($N = 26$)	25.00	$p = .00$
Increase patients' knowledge ($N = 37$)	20.27	$p = .00$
Improved patients' behaviors ($N = 37$)		Improved
Risk assessment performed with high-risk intervention ($N = 37$)	100%	100%
Satisfaction of pathway, risk assessment, and booklet ($N = 26$, $N = 37$)	100%	No issues found

Patients' Knowledge of Lymphedema

Paired-samples *t*-test established a statistically significant increase in patients' knowledge of lymphedema: $M = 20.27$, $SD = 17.12$, df (36), $t = -7.20$, and $p <.00$ (two-tailed). The eta-squared statistic (.59) indicates a large effect size.

Findings indicate that patient knowledge of lymphedema, including its definition, risk factors, signs and symptoms, and the importance of BMI, was increased. Awareness of the importance of prompt intervention, weight control, exercise, limited repetitive hand/arm movement, weight lifting, and skin care was also increased in patients.

Evidence of Lymphedema

Patients' hand, wrist, and arm circumferences were measured bilaterally, 4 cm from the hand to the shoulder. Lymphedema was considered present if there was an increase of 2 cm in the before and after measurements. Among 37 participants, no one was determined to have developed lymphedema.

Anecdotal Data Regarding Repetitive Hand Motion

Prior to the intervention, several participants reported performing different repetitive hand motions. For example, one patient described working in a school for the deaf and signing with her affected hand and arm all day. Another patient was a marksman who reported shooting guns for many hours each day. Another patient liked to play video games that required the use of a hand-operated controller device for many hours each day. Others at risk included a hairdresser, a secretary who typed many hours each day, and a concert pianist. All were able to modify behavior based on early evidence-based education.

Anecdotal Data Regarding Exercise

Patient reports of number of exercise minutes increased from pre- to postintervention. Many reported an increased desire to exercise, control their weight, and use proper skin care precautions.

Other Anecdotal Data

- One patient experienced increased pain in her arm, reported it promptly (according to evidence and education), and then reported it resolved quickly.
- BMIs decreased slightly from postintervention.
- Patients and nurses evaluated the educational materials and programs as appropriate and reported high satisfaction scores for word choice, ease of use, and empowerment. No problems or complaints were identified.

Impact

Breast cancer is a devastating diagnosis. If lymphedema complicates recovery, then women experience even greater discomfort and difficulty with daily living. At the time this project was conducted, the evidence to support effective self-care for this vulnerable population had not been assembled into a coherent and comprehensive plan. It could be found only in the scientific literature and was a challenge to interpret even for professionals. As a result, it was not consistently used to help patients make informed decisions. The team involved in this project assembled the evidence; created resources to help clinicians and patients; and demonstrated improved caregiver knowledge, patient knowledge, and self-care behaviors among women at risk.

The patient education materials created in conducting this project have been adopted for publication for Mission Hospital's Breast Program, Cancer Care of Western North Carolina, and the Oncology Nursing Society. They are now available to clinicians and women who receive the diagnosis of breast cancer across the United States and globally.

Dissemination

Phillips, J., Belcher, A., & Terhaar, M. (2012). *Evidence-based practices for lymphedema risk reduction*. 23rd International Research Congress. Brisbane, Australia: Sigma Theta Tau International.

Phillips, J., Belcher, A., & Terhaar, M. (2012). *Evidence-based practices for lymphedema risk reduction*. Phoenix, AZ: Oncology Nursing Society Cancer Connections.

Additional References

Peterson, S., & Bredow, T. (2009). *Middle range theories application to nursing research*. Philadelphia, PA: Lippincott Williams & Wilkins.

Soran, A., Wu, W. C., Dirican, A., Johnson, R., Andacoglu, O., & Wilson, J. (2011). Estimating the probability of lymphedema after breast cancer surgery. *American Journal of Clinical Oncology, 34*(5), 506–510. doi:10.1097/COC.0b013e3181f47955

Titler, M. G., Kleiber, C., Steelman, V. J., Rakel., B. A., Budreau, G., Everett, L. Q., . . . Goode, C. (2001). The Iowa model of evidence-based practice to promote quality care. *Critical Care Nursing Clinics of North America, 13*(4), 497–509. doi:10.1016/s0899-5885(18)30017-0

■ EXEMPLAR 20.7: IMPROVING THE PAIN EXPERIENCE FOR HOSPITALIZED PATIENTS WITH CANCER

Suzanne M. Cowperthwaite

Team

Project lead

Nurse educator

Patient educator

Pain and palliative care nurse

Patient representative

Three clinical RNs

Clinical nurse specialist

Problem

Composite pain satisfaction Hospital Consumer Assessment of Healthcare Providers and Systems (HCAHPS) scores reported by patients with solid tumors on the adult medical oncology inpatient unit measure 58%, which indicates an opportunity to reduce suffering in this vulnerable population.

Background

The HCAHPS survey (Centers for Medicare & Medicaid Services, 2017; Giordano, Elliott, Goldstein, Lehrman, & Spencer, 2010) sought to measure patient satisfaction with pain management by asking discharged patients requiring pain medication during their admission to answer "always," "usually," "sometimes," or "never" to two pain-related questions: "How often was your pain well controlled?" and "How often did the hospital staff do everything they could to help you with your pain?" Composite pain satisfaction HCAHPS scores on an adult medical oncology inpatient unit caring for patients with solid tumors were 58% at baseline, indicating an opportunity to reduce suffering in this vulnerable population. Nurses, in the role of patient caregiver, advocate, and educator, are in a unique position to impact the pain experience of individuals with cancer, therefore, an evidence-based nursing intervention to improve pain management on this unit was sought.

Pain is a significant and multidimensional problem for individuals diagnosed with cancer. The National Comprehensive Cancer Network ([NCCN], 2018) adult pain guidelines advise providers to consider hospitalization of patients suffering from "acute, severe pain or pain crisis" (p. MS-7). Cancer pain has several potential causes. Most often pain is caused by tumor burden, but cancer treatments and unrelated, comorbid conditions may also produce pain (American Cancer Society, 2018). Inadequate management of cancer pain denies comfort and acceptable quality of life, and may even reduce survival (NCCN, 2018). Cancer pain may produce emotional distress, with prolonged duration and higher pain intensity associated with depression (National Cancer Institute, 2018). Patients with cancer may fear addiction, developing tolerance, side effects, or the implications of needing opioid analgesics (National Institute of Health and Care Excellence, 2014). These many features of cancer pain impact the patient's pain experience and the professional caregiver's ability to influence this experience.

Aims

This project had two aims:

1. To increase patient rating on HCAHPS question, "How often did staff do everything to help with your pain?"
2. To increase patient rating on HCAHPS question, "How often was your pain well controlled?"

Translation Framework

The Ottawa Model of Research Use was chosen to guide translation of the evidence into practice because of its emphasis on the patient and its focus on the interaction among the innovation, adopters, and the environment (Graham & Logan, 2004). In keeping with the model, the implementation team reviewed barriers and supports, developed the innovation during the assessment phase of the model, monitored and evaluated outcomes across all phases of the work, ensured fidelity with the intervention, communicated regularly with the team, and shared results with staff.

Translation Methods

Two methods were used for this QI project. These included a pain stoppers tool kit as well as design and deployment of education programming for staff.

Pain Stoppers Tool Kit

A tool kit of materials was developed for use by patients. The Pain Stoppers Kit contained education resources and some note taking materials developed to assist patients to advocate for themselves. Based on the evidence, patients were encouraged to become full participants in their care and to advocate for themselves with respect to pain management.

The Pain Stoppers Kit education materials addressed common misconceptions regarding pain medications and pain management, encouraged patients to notify staff immediately when they experience pain (even if not time for pain medication), informed patients about the availability of the Pain and Palliative Care Team, and encouraged patients to alert staff if they wished to see a pain team member. These materials were packaged together with a small notebook and pen to support note taking that would promote recording of questions or notes regarding their care and pain management.

Staff were asked to record placement of these patient education materials on a centralized document located at the unit secretary's desk. Placement of the Pain Stoppers Kit in patient rooms was initially sporadic, but greatly improved after 1 month and for the remainder of the postintervention period. In addition, the institution's two-page, patient education pain document was placed in frames in each patient room. Clinical technicians (CTs) were instructed to call nurses immediately when patients reported a pain score of 5 or greater on routine screening. Prior to implementing the intervention, CTs would record high pain scores in the electronic health record (EHR), but would not immediately inform the nurse. Pain Stoppers visual aids were placed in staff work areas and medication stations (Figure 20.7.1).

HCAHPS surveys were mailed to a random sample of discharged patients through Press Ganey, a patient experience consulting company.

Pain intensity scores, retrieved from the electronic medical record of all eligible patients admitted to the unit during the pre- and postintervention periods, were measured on an 11-point Likert-type scale ranging from 0 (no pain) to 10 (worst pain

Positive attitude and pain validation
Assess and reassess for pain
Individualize patient education
No waiting for meds

Set expectations
Team approach
Oral transitions
Probing questions
Prepare for pain discussion
Eliminate misconceptions
Round the clock and overnight dosing
Scripted and caring language

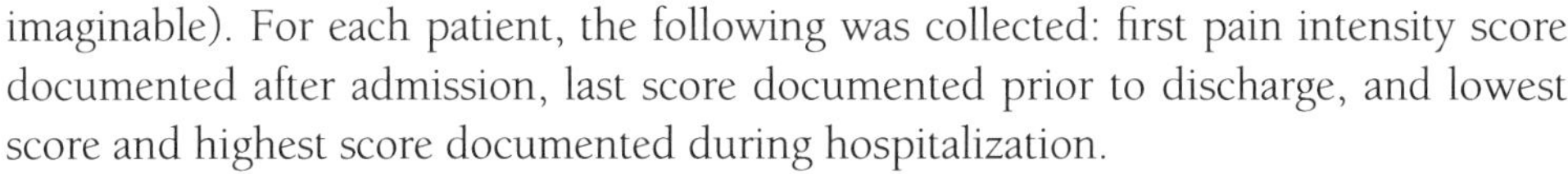

FIGURE 20.7.1 Pain stoppers materials.

imaginable). For each patient, the following was collected: first pain intensity score documented after admission, last score documented prior to discharge, and lowest score and highest score documented during hospitalization.

Unit RNs received email invitations to complete the Knowledge and Attitudes on Pain (KAP) assessment electronically using Qualtrics both pre- and postintervention (Ferrell & McCarthy, 2014).

Instructional Design—Staff Education

Education programs were developed for staff. They provided information regarding strong evidence to support effective management of cancer pain and described the intervention planned for all patients. The project lead presented this education to all RNs and CTs and facilitated a highly engaged discussion about the evidence, its application, and its potential to improve outcomes.

Handouts used for instruction remained available following the program to reinforce education (Exhibit 20.7.1). A series of six follow-up communications were emailed to RNs and CTs spanning 2 months following the education programs, with the intent to review the intervention and expectations, maintain attention and encouragement, provide additional information regarding NCCN Pain Guidelines, and provide additional information related to the five KAP questions with low mean preintervention scores.

Results

Staff Responsiveness to Pain

Aim 1 was met. Patient HCAHPS score on item "How often did staff do everything to help with your pain?" improved from 62% at baseline to 90% following implementation of the Pain Stoppers materials (Figure 20.7.2).

EXHIBIT 20.7.1 Interventions for Improving Pain Management

Communication, Caring Behaviors, and Timely Responses	Patient Education	Maintain Analgesic Levels
Technicians immediately report pain scores ≥5	Utilize a variety of patient education materials	Work with the team to optimize analgesic plan
Utilize caring language with patients	Address myths and misconceptions	Encourage around-the-clock dosing of analgesics
Prepare in advance for pain discussions	Provide continuous and individualized patient education	Consider maintaining analgesic dosing overnight
Ask probing questions about pain	Provide prepackaged educational materials to every patient	Carefully manage parenteral to oral analgesic transitions
Maintain a positive attitude		
Validate patients' pain		
Provide timely responses to patients' requests		
Discuss and set expectations with patients		
Utilize tools to facilitate communication		

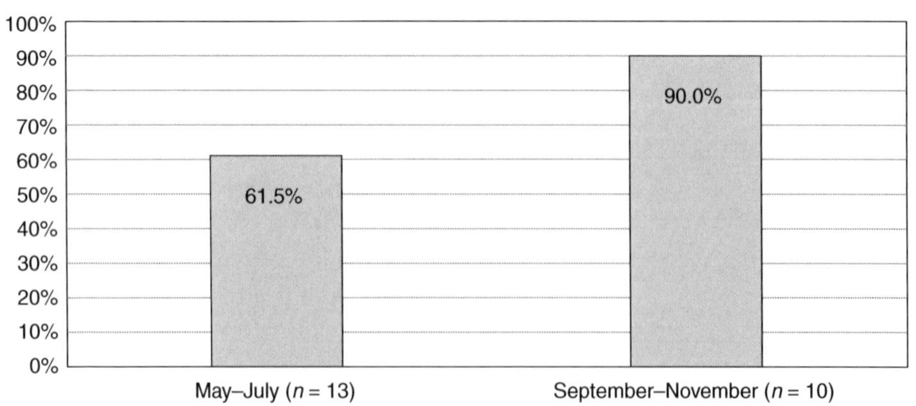

FIGURE 20.7.2 How often did staff do everything they could to help with your pain?

Pain Control

Aim 2, to increase patient rating on the HCAHPS question, "How often was your pain well controlled?" was met. In response to this question, seven of 13 (54%) members in the preintervention group and five of nine (56%) in the postintervention group answered "always." One patient in the postintervention group did not answer the "pain well controlled" question.

RN Knowledge and Attitudes on Pain Scores

Because the success of the intervention relied on staff understanding of the evidence to support it, staff education was provided for everyone on the unit and an evaluation of knowledge pre- and postintervention was conducted. Eleven (31%) RNs returned preintervention KAP surveys and nine (25%) returned postintervention surveys. The mean number of questions answered correctly on the KAP survey by the 11 RNs in the preintervention group was 30.6 ($SD = 2.46$) compared with 30.9 ($SD = 2.42$) for the nine RNs representing the postintervention group.

Two of the five items on which staff scored poorly on the preintervention showed meaningful improvement using Fisher's exact test. Nurses' knowledge of the effectiveness of nonsteroidal anti-inflammatory agents and aspirin on painful bone metastases (Question 5) improved significantly with nurses scoring 36% on the preintervention test and 89% on the postintervention test ($p = .025$). Nurses' knowledge of analgesic dose equivalencies (question 16) also improved from a preintervention score of 46% to a postintervention score of 89% ($p = .058$).

Discussion

Cancer diagnoses are varied as are the characteristics of the patients who experience them and receive treatment in acute care. The demographics of the two samples (before and after intervention) are presented in Tables 20.7.1 and 20.7.2. These data will be useful for clinicians seeking to understand the findings in relation to populations in their care.

Impact

This QI project supports the findings of previous studies indicating that nurses are able to improve patients' pain experience without affecting actual pain intensity scores, and that nurses can influence patients' satisfaction with how their pain is managed. HCAHPS scores improved following implementation of the Pain Stoppers intervention. Although the sample size was small during the 3 months preintervention and 3 months postintervention, the main aim of the project was to improve these scores, and this was achieved. Nurses, in their roles as caregivers, educators, and advocates, can improve the pain experience of hospitalized patients who are diagnosed with a solid tumor cancer.

Dissemination

"Improving the Pain Experience for Hospitalized Patients with Cancer" was published in the *Oncology Nursing Forum* in March 2019 (Cowperthwaite & Kozachik, 2019) and a poster presentation was delivered at the Oncology Nursing Society's 44th Annual Congress in Anaheim, California, in April 2019.

TABLE 20.7.1 Patient Demographics

	Preintervention $n = 173$	Postintervention $n = 157$
Characteristic	**N (%)**	**N (%)**
Gender		
Male	90 (52.0)	86 (54.8)
Female	83 (48.0)	71 (45.2)
Race		
White	123 (71.1)	103 (65.6)
Black	33 (19.1)	41 (26.1)
Asian	7 (4.0)	5 (3.2)
Hispanic	3 (1.7)	1 (0.6)
Other	7 (4.0)	7 (4.5)
Chemotherapy within 30 days	132 (76.3)	102 (65.0)
Radiation within 30 days	18 (10.4)	18 (11.5)
Age (years)		
Range	19–90	26–85
Mean (*SD*)	58.7 (14.96)	57.6 (13.03)
Length of stay (days)		
Range	1–39	1–29
Mean (*SD*)	6.71 (5.34)	6.14 (4.79)

Notes: There were no statistically significant differences among groups in terms of age, gender, race, length of stay, or those receiving radiation therapy within the past 30 days. Patients in the postintervention groups were less likely to have been receiving chemotherapy within the past 30 days (x^2 (1) = 5.12, p = .024).

TABLE 20.7.2 Patient Diagnoses

	Preintervention $n = 173$	Postintervention $n = 157$
Characteristic	***n* (%)**	***n* (%)**
Cancer diagnosis		
Pancreas/liver/gallbladder	35 (20.2)	18 (11.5)
Sarcoma	23 (13.3)	15 (9.6)
Colorectal/gastric	22 (12.7)	22 (14.0)

(continued)

TABLE 20.7.2 Patient Diagnoses (*continued*)

	Preintervention *n* = 173	**Postintervention** *n* = 157
Characteristic	***n* (%)**	***n* (%)**
Head and neck/larynx/thyroid	22 (12.7)	21 (13.4)
Breast	14 (8.1)	14 (8.9)
Lung/mesothelioma	10 (5.8)	16 (10.2)
Bladder/kidney	11 (6.4)	9 (5.7)
Brain	10 (5.8)	11 (7.0)
Melanoma/other skin	9 (5.2)	7 (4.5)
Prostate/testicle	8 (4.6)	9 (5.7)
Leukemia/lymphoma	4 (2.3)	2 (1.3)
Gynecologic	1 (0.6)	4 (2.5)
Other/unknown primary	4 (2.3)	9 (5.7)
Primary admitting diagnosis		
Fever/infection	25 (14.5)	38 (24.2)
Chemotherapy	26 (15.0)	13 (8.3)
Respiratory problems	14 (8.1)	24 (15.3)
Liver problems	14 (8.1)	3 (1.9)
Neurologic problems	12 (6.9)	14 (8.9)
Gastrointestinal problems	13 (7.5)	4 (2.5)
Pain	13 (7.5)	8 (5.1)
Thrombus/coagulopathy	7 (4.0)	8 (5.1)
Renal failure	6 (3.5)	5 (3.2)
Dehydration/electrolyte imbalance	4 (2.3)	3 (1.9)
Failure to thrive/decline	6 (3.5)	7 (4.5)
Cardiac problems	2 (1.2)	2 (1.3)
Gastrointestinal bleeding	3 (1.7)	4 (2.5)
New cancer/disease progression	4 (2.3)	7 (4.5)
Other	24 (13.9)	17 (10.8)
Length of stay (days)		
Range	1–39	1–29
Mean (*SD*)	6.71 (5.34)	6.14 (4.79)

Notes: There were minor differences in cancer diagnoses between the groups, although this was not statistically significant. More patients in the postintervention group were admitted for fever/infection and respiratory problems and fewer were admitted for chemotherapy administration.

Additional References

American Cancer Society. (2018). Facts about cancer pain. Retrieved from https://www.cancer.org/treatment/treatments-and-side-effects/physical-side-effects/pain/facts-about-cancer-pain.html

Centers for Medicare & Medicaid Services. (2017). CAHPS hospital survey. Retrieved from https://www.cms.gov/Research-Statistics-Data-and-Systems/Research/CAHPS/hcahps1.html

Cowperthwaite, S. M., & Kozachik, S. L. (2019). Improving the pain experience for hospitalized patients with cancer. *Oncology Nursing Forum, 46*(2), 198–207. doi:10.1188/19.onf.198-207

Ferrell, B., & McCaffery, M. (2014). Knowledge and attitudes survey regarding pain. Retrieved from http://prc.coh.org/Knowldege%20%20&%20Attitude%20Survey%207-14%20(1).pdf

Giordano, L. A., Elliott, M. N., Goldstein, E., Lehrman, W. G., & Spencer, P. A. (2010). Development, implementation, and public reporting of the HCAHPS survey. *Medical Care Research and Review, 67*(1), 27–37. doi:10.1177/1077558709341065

Graham, I. D., & Logan, J. (2004). Innovations in knowledge transfer and continuity of care. *Canadian Journal of Nursing Research, 36*(2), 89–103.

National Cancer Institute. (2018). Cancer pain: Health professional version. Retrieved from http://www.cancer.gov/about-cancer/treatment/side-effects/pain/pain-hp-pdq#link/_15_toc

National Comprehensive Cancer Network. (2018). Adult cancer pain. Retrieved from https://www.nccn.org/professionals/physician_gls/pdf/pain.pdf

National Institute of Health and Care Excellence. (2014). Palliative care for adults: Strong opioids for pain relief. Retrieved from https://www.nice.org.uk/guidance/cg140/chapter/1-recommendations

■ EXEMPLAR 20.8: INCREASING COMPETENCE IN PRESSURE INJURY PREVENTION USING COMPETENCY-BASED EDUCATION IN ADULT INTENSIVE CARE UNIT

Carla Aquino

Team

Chief nursing officer

Senior director of clinical quality

Central Staff Education Committee

Hospital Pressure Injury Prevention Subcommittee

Hospital ICU Standards of Care Committee

Department of Medicine director of nursing

Department of Medicine Clinical Quality Committee

The medical intensive care unit (MICU) Wound Care Team

MICU staff

Informatician

Problem

A pressure injury quarterly prevalence survey showed the adult ICU patients accounted for more than half of the pressure injury prevalence in the hospital.

Background

Preventing unit-acquired pressure injuries (UAPI) is a strategic priority for nursing at one Magnet-designated, academic medical center that aims to promote optimal patient outcomes, control healthcare costs, and maintain exemplary nursing practice (American Nurses Credentialing Center, 2011). The academic medical center where this work was conducted had demonstrated serious commitment to reducing UAPI and had already implemented pressure injury prevention interventions based on the National Pressure Ulcer Advisory Panel (NPUAP) recommendations (National Pressure Ulcer Advisory Panel, European Pressure Ulcer Advisory Panel, Pan Pacific Pressure Injury Alliance, 2014). At baseline, an organization-wide provider survey that included the ICU staff nurses revealed a positive perception of the importance of pressure injury prevention (Wong, Walia, Bello, Aquino, & Sacks, 2018). However, staff compliance with implementing the recommended prevention interventions continued to be a challenge in the ICUs where the prevalence of pressure injury persisted, accounting for 58% of the pressure injury prevalence in the hospital. A review of quarterly prevalence data pointed to opportunities to improve nursing critical thinking skills in selecting and documenting appropriate UAPI prevention interventions based on identified risks.

More than 2.5 million people develop pressure injury in the United States annually, contributing up to $11 billion in cost for direct treatment and resulting in some 60,000 deaths per year (Agency for Healthcare Research and Quality, 2014). These pressure injuries have become increasingly detrimental to institutions just as they have always been for patients because of recent changes in compensation and disclosure requirements. Because they are now classified as a never event, The Centers for Medicare & Medicaid Services no longer provides reimbursement for care attributed to the treatment of hospital-acquired pressure injuries (HAPI; Padula, Makic, Wald, et al., 2015). Low occurrence of HAPI staged as 2 or greater (HAPI 2+) is recognized by the American Nurses Credentialing Center's Magnet Recognition Program as a nurse-sensitive metric of exemplary professional practice (Shepherd & Hawthorne, 2017).

Strong evidence suggests that competency-based education serves as a foundation for pressure injury prevention (National Pressure Ulcer Advisory Panel, 2013). Competency, not just knowledge, can reduce HAPI prevalence (Henry & Foronda, 2015). The use of pressure injury prevalence data can guide QI initiatives, such as education and leadership initiatives, skin care, and nutrition, with success (Padula, Makic, & Mishra, et al., 2015; Tayyib & Coyer, 2016; VanGilder, Lachenbruch, Algrim-Boyle, & Meyer, 2017). The adult MICU initiated an evidence-based competency development education program to reduce UAPI (Wright, 2005).

Aims

This QI project had two aims:

1. To increase compliance with NPUAP prevention guidelines as evidenced in nursing documentation
2. To reduce the rate of stage 2 UAPIs

Translational Framework

The project utilized the Johns Hopkins Quality and Research Group (JHQSRG) Translating Evidence into Practice Model as the translational framework. Figure 20.8.1 shows the four stages of JHQSRG, which include: (a) summarizing the evidence, (b) identifying local barriers to implementation, (c) measuring performance, and (d) ensuring all patients receive the intervention (Poe, Abbott, & Pronovost, 2011; Pronovost, Berenholtz, & Needham, 2008).

The project lead involved all stakeholders across all phases of the project. Active stakeholders included the chief nursing officer, senior director of clinical quality, Central Staff Education Committee, Hospital Pressure Injury Prevention Subcommittee, Hospital ICU Standards of Care Committee, Department of Medicine director of nursing, Department of Medicine Clinical Quality Committee, and the MICU Wound Care Team.

Stage 1: Summarizing the Evidence

A expert group composed of wound care nurses, ICU clinical nurse specialists, and educators gathered and synthesized the evidence and developed the online education module and competency verification tools.

Stage 2: Identifying Local Barriers to Implementation

The director of nursing approved the project aims and measures by approving 4 hours a month of dedicated time for unit champions to spearhead the implementation of competency-based education implementation and evaluation in the MICU.

Stage 3: Measuring Performance

The established wound care team identified process measures and patient outcomes to determine the effectiveness of the competency education. The group agreed to use the existing monthly pressure injury prevalence survey process conducted by the MICU unit champion, considered the expert in the unit in pressure injury prevention. To measure the effectiveness of the competency education, the project compared the staff documentation of prevention interventions 24 to 48 hours prior to the survey against the unit champion's identified prevention interventions during the survey. The group agreed to evaluate agreement between the documentation of the staff prior to the survey and the unit champion during the survey. The project also monitored the UAPI 2+ rates in the MICU as the patient outcome. The project lead evaluated the percentage agreement between staff nurses' documentation and unit champion and documentation of prevention interventions.

Stage 4: Ensuring All Patients Receive the Intervention

The JHQSRG implementation stage uses what is known as the 6Es: (1) engage, (2) educate, (3) execute, (4) evaluate, (5) endure, and (6) extend (Daly, Speedy, & Jackson,

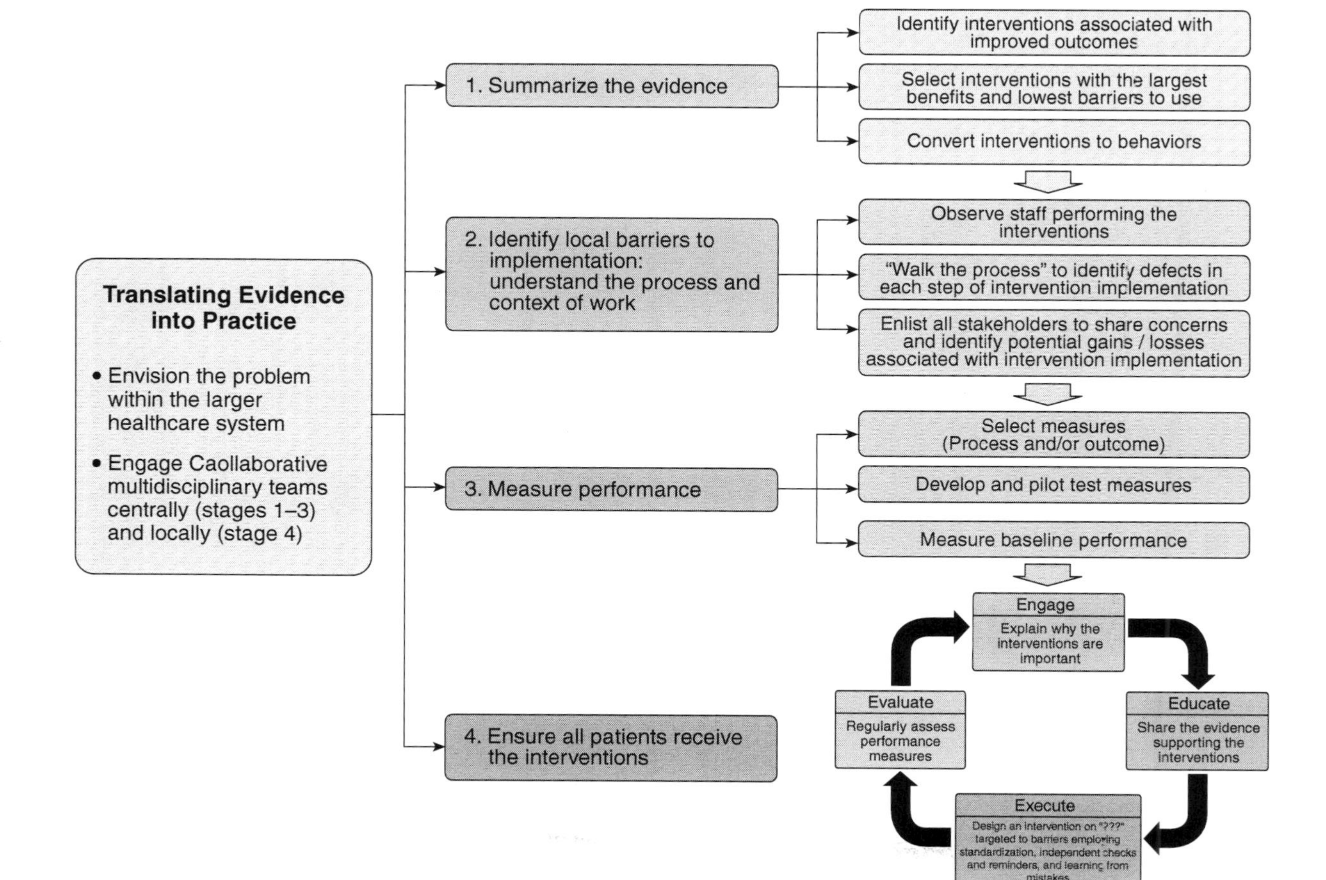

FIGURE 20.8.1 The JHQSRG Translating Evidence Into Practice Model.

Source: From Pronovost, P. J., Berenholtz, S. M., & Needham, D. M. (2008). Translating evidence into practice: A model for large scale knowledge translation. *British Medical Journal, 337*, a1714.

2015). The group of engaged wound care nurses, ICU nurses, and educators defined competency goals, built an online competency-based education module, and developed competency verification methods to educate MICU staff and execute the competency-verification process based on the Donna Wright model (Wright, 2005). The project used the monthly prevalence surveys to evaluate both process and patient outcomes.

■ FINDINGS

Descriptive statistics summarized staff engagement in the development and completion of the online education module and verification tools. At least one educator, wound care nurse, and/or staff champion attended each of the seven meetings and actively contributed in developing an online education module and accompanying verification tools. Fully 98% of the MICU nursing staff competed the online education module. Ninety-one percent of the MICU nursing staff competed the first competency verification tool.

Aim 1 was met. A chi-square test was used to evaluate the difference in percentage agreement between the staff nurse and the unit champion documentation of prevention intervention (Table 20.8.1). Significant improvement was documented for three of the five prevention interventions, including skin assessment (p = .015), repositioning (p = .001), and nutrition support (p = .020).

TABLE 20.8.1 Percentage Agreement of Documented Necessary Prevention Intervention Between Staff and Unit Champion by Implementation Period

Prevention Intervention	Percentage Agreement of Necessary Intervention Documentation		Percentage Increase in Percentage Agreement of Necessary Intervention Documentation	*p* Value*
	Preimplementation (N = 57)	Postimplementation (N = 60)		
Skin assessment	82%	96%	18%	0.015†
Pressure redistribution	96%	100%	4%	0.124‡
Repositioning	63%	91%	44%	0.001
Nutritional support	45%	71%	58%	0.020
Moisture management	86%	87%	1%	0.937

*Significant at p value <.05.

†Fisher exact test p = .016.

‡Fisher exact test p = .211.

Aim 2 was not met. Although the UAPI 2+ rate was reduced by 5.7%, the finding did not reach statistical significance.

Impact

The results suggest that competency-based education can be effective in increasing documentation of PI prevention intervention, which the project team asserts will lead to improved staff compliance with best practices in the MICU. The MICU continued to reduce the UAPI 2+ prevalence rate by 86% from the fiscal year 2016 to the fiscal year 2018.

For dissemination, the project used the last two "Es" of the implementation framework of JHQRSG Translation into Practice model: (5) endure and (6) expand (Armstrong Institute, 2011; Daly et al., 2015). The sustainability and endurance plan for this project included the MICU staff completion of the second competency verification sign-off 3 months after the first verification sign-off. The wound care nurse administered a posttest 6 months after the first verification sign-off. The unit established the same procedure and timeline for each new staff member oriented in the MICU.

The project team has kept stakeholders and committees updated, presented at the organization's scholar's day, and submitted a manuscript for national publication to expand the knowledge garnered from the project.

Dissemination

Aquino, C., Owen, A., Predicce, A., Poe, S., & Kozachik, S. (2019). Increasing competence in pressure injury prevention using competency-based education in adult intensive care unit. *Journal of Nursing Care Quality, 34*, 312–317. doi:10.1097/NCQ.0000000000000388

Additional References

Agency for Healthcare Research and Quality. (2014). *Preventing pressure ulcers in hospitals: A toolkit for improving quality of care*. Rockville, MD: Author.

American Nurses Credentialing Center. (2011). *Magnet teaching tips*. Retrieved from http://www.nursecredentialing.org/Documents/Magnet/MagTeachTips.pdf

Armstrong Institute. (2011). Two more Es. Retrieved from https://www.hopkinsmedicine.org/armstrong_institute/improvement_projects/infections_complications/stop_bsi/educational_sessions/national_content_calls/two_more_es.html

Daly, J., Speedy, S., & Jackson, D. (2015). *Leadership and nursing: Contemporary perspectives*. New York, NY: Elsevier Health Sciences.

Henry, M., & Foronda, C. (2017). Evaluation of evidence-based nursing education of hospital acquired pressure injury prevention in clinical practice: An integrative review. *Journal of Nursing Education and Practice, 8*, 1–9.

National Pressure Ulcer Advisory Panel. (2013). *Nursing curriculum: Registered nurse competency-based curriculum: Pressure ulcer prevention*. Retrieved from http://www.npuap.org/resources/educational-and-clinical-resources/nursing-curriculum/

National Pressure Ulcer Advisory Panel, European Pressure Ulcer Advisory Panel, Pan Pacific Pressure Injury Alliance. (2014). *Prevention and treatment of pressure ulcers: Clinical practice guideline* (2nd ed.). Perth, Australia: Cambridge Media.

Padula, W. V., Makic, M. B. F., Mishra, M. K., Campbell, J. D., Nair, K. V., Wald, H. L., Valuck, R. J. (2015). Comparative effectiveness of quality improvement interventions for pressure ulcer prevention in academic medical centers in the United States. *The Joint Commission Journal on Quality and Patient Safety, 41*(6), 246–256. doi:10.1016/s1553-7250(15)41034-7

Padula, W. V., Makic, M. B. F., Wald, H. L., Campbell, J. D., Nair, K. V., Mishra, M. K., & Valuck, R. J. (2015). Hospital-acquired pressure ulcers at academic medical centers in the united states, 2008–2012: Tracking changes since the CMS nonpayment policy. *The Joint Commission Journal on Quality and Patient Safety, 41*(6), 257–263. doi:10.1016/s1553-7250(15)41035-9

Poe, S. S., Abbott, P., & Pronovost, P. (2011). Building nursing intellectual capital for safe use of information technology: A before-after study to test an evidence-based peer coach intervention. *Journal of Nursing Care Quality, 26*(2), 110–119. doi:10.1097/ncq.0b013e31820b221d

Pronovost, P. J., Berenholtz, S. M., & Needham, D. M. (2008). Translating evidence into practice: A model for large scale knowledge translation. *British Medical Journal, 337*, a1714. doi:10.1136/bmj.a1714

Tayyib, N., & Coyer, F. (2016). Effectiveness of pressure ulcer prevention strategies for adult patients in intensive care units: A systematic review. *Worldviews on Evidence-Based Nursing, 13*(6), 432–444. doi:10.1111/wvn.12177

VanGilder, C., Lachenbruch, C., Algrim-Boyle, C., & Meyer, S. (2017). The international pressure ulcer prevalence™ survey: 2006–2015. *Journal of Wound, Ostomy and Continence Nursing, 44*(1), 20–28. doi:10.1097/won.0000000000000292

Wong, A. L., Walia, G. S., Bello, R., Aquino, C. S., & Sacks, J. M. (2018). Pressure ulcer prevalence and perceptions on prevention: A hospital-wide survey of health professionals. *Journal of Wound Care, 27*(Suppl. 4), S29–S35. doi:10.12968/jowc.2018.27.sup4.s29

Wright, D. (2005). *The ultimate guide to competency assessment in healthcare*. Minneapolis, MN: Creative Health Care Management.

CHAPTER TWENTY-ONE

Healthcare System Exemplars

Mary F. Terhaar

SYSTEMS ARE COMPLEX AND COMPLICATED ORGANISMS. To *accomplish impactful, sustainable change requires meticulous planning, execution, and tending. Much has been written here about the theory of change and the process of translationto guide individuals and teams engaged in that work. This chapter presents a set of projects that accomplished change through the translation of evidence. Some took place at the microsystem level and others targeted the meso- or macrosystem. The methods, analytics, and execution varied with the scope and complexity of the work.*

In this chapter, you find eight examples of translation projects that focus on achieving the Triple Aim of delivering quality care, a positive experience, and value (Berwick, Nolan, & Worthington, 2008). Each exemplar summarizes scholarship conducted by a DNP in partial fulfillment of requirements for graduation. These students are the authors of the work presented here and the primary sources are provided within the text. Each exemplar addresses a different clinical challenge, engages different members of the healthcare team, employs different methods, and uses different approaches to evaluation. Each exemplar provides the following:

- *The* **title** *of the project*
- *The* **team** *that participated in the work*
- *A* **statement of the problem** *in a particular site or setting*
- **Background** *describing a brief overview of the problem, including baseline data*
- **Aims**, *which are measurable, directional statements of what will be better once the project is complete*
- **Translation framework**, *which provides an overview of the framework(s) used to conceptualize the work and process*
- **Translation method(s)**, *which explains the strategy or approach used to accomplish change while ensuring fidelity with the evidence and adaptation to the setting*
- **Results**, *which describe whether the aims were achieved*
- **Impact**, *which explains the significance, implications, and sustainability of the work*
- **Dissemination**, *which credits the primary publication of the work and conferences at which it has been presented*
- **Additional references**, *which cite translated evidence*

■ EXEMPLAR 21.1 USING BEST-FIT INTERVENTIONS TO IMPROVE THE NURSING INTERSHIFT HANDOFF PROCESS AT A MEDICAL CENTER IN LEBANON

Lina A. Younan

Team

Nursing director

Three nurse managers

Five staff nurses

Floor physician

Quality coordinator

Clinical educator

Labib Medical Center

Johns Hopkins University School of Nursing

Problem

Incidents have been caused by the omission of pertinent patient information during RN intershift handoffs on medical, surgical, and cardiac units of a 130-bed hospital.

Background

The nursing intershift handoff is a process that takes place daily at the beginning of every shift. This handoff involves communication of essential patient information between the outgoing and the incoming nurses (Strople & Ottani, 2006). Any omission, misinterpretation, or incongruence has the potential to lead to deficient or inappropriate care (Arora & Johnson, 2006; Dracup & Morris, 2008; Ong & Coiera, 2011).

The Joint Commission has identified communication failures as the leading cause of sentinel events in the United States, and shift reports are a contributing factor (Riesenberg, Leiztsch, & Cunningham, 2010). The Institute of Medicine reported that inadequate nursing handoffs are the first shortfall in patient safety (Friesen, White, & Byers, 2008). The Canadian Ontario Hospital Association estimates that 70% of all sentinel events are linked to communication breakdown (Ontario Hospital Association, 2006).

An assessment of patient safety culture in 68 Lebanon hospitals conducted in 2009 revealed that 57% of 6,807 responding hospital employees (including physicians, nurses, and other clinical and nonclinical staff) agreed that pertinent patient information, such as abnormal vital signs, laboratory values or radiology test findings, pain management, allergy, fall risk, and functional status, is often lost during shift change (El-Jardali, Jaafar, Dimassi, Jamal, & Hamdan, 2010). Adequacy of communication at shift change was a concern for 17 (23%) of the 76 nurses who responded to a survey (Labib Medical Center, Quality Department, 2009). A subsequent review of patient safety incidents showed medication errors, delay in treatment, wrong treatment, duplication of lab tests, and near-miss events resulted when important patient information was omitted at intershift handoff (Labib Medical Center, 2010).

Aim

This project had a single aim: to improve the quality of RN intershift handoff on the medical, surgical, and cardiac units as a way to enhance patient safety and continuity of care.

Translation Framework

Two conceptual frameworks were used in this work. The first was systems theory and the second was the Ottawa Model of Research Use (OMRU).

Systems theory provides a framework for understanding many kinds of systems, natural and man-made, as being composed of components that together result in function that exceeds the sum of the parts (Theorieenoverzicht, n.d.). It suggests assessment and optimization of the performance of variables, and relationships between variables and the environment within and surrounding a system (Henriksen, Battles, Marks, & Lewin, 2005). In the conduct of this project, attention will focus on relationships and structures to facilitate the flow of information.

Within a systems framework, the handoff process is a dynamic open system that includes interconnected variables (the nurse, patient information, the communication method, and the environment); the relationships between those variables are circular with feedback loops. Adopting a systems approach led the team to assess barriers and optimize the performance of systems' variables.

The Ottawa Model prescribes that research use requires an initial assessment of potential barriers and supporters followed by monitoring of the intervention and outcomes evaluation.

Translation Methods

This project relied on communication-centered methods to improve accuracy and completeness of intershift handoffs. A task force was charged with developing a process and tool to structure communication in order to standardize handoffs and reduce error. The situation, history, assessment, recommendation, and questions (SHARQ) approach was used as a guide for both the process and the tool to support it (Arora & Johnson, 2006). The clinical educator and manager provided education and coaching to introduce the change and made rounds to support transition.

Results

The mean number of omissions per handoff across the three units decreased from 4.96 to 2.29 ($t = 6.29$, $p = .000$).

The mean number of interruptions per intershift report decreased from 2.17 to 1.26 ($t = 2.7$, $p = .008$).

Training sessions helped nurses communicate not only on what physicians need to know but also patient safety criteria.

Impact

Greater precision and focus in communicating information have been achieved. Evaluation of completeness of handoff report using the new tool is ongoing. Data available for the follow-up period were reported as:

98.5% (n = 133) in the first quarter
96% (n = 127) in the second quarter
98.5% (n = 133) in the third quarter (Labib Medical Center, Nursing Executive Committee, 2012a)

Semiannual reports revealed one incident related to a communication breakdown in 2012, as compared to 11 in 2010 (Labib Medical Center, Nursing Executive Committee, 2012a).

Omission of patient information was included as a patient safety indicator in the 2013 to 2015 nursing department strategic plan (Labib Medical Center, Nursing Executive Committee, 2012b).

Dissemination

Younan, L. A., & Fralic, M. F. (2013). Using best-fit interventions to improve the nursing inter-shift handoff process at a medical center in Lebanon. *The Joint Commission Journal on Quality and Patient Safety, 39*(10), 460–467. doi:10.1016/s1553-7250(13)39059-x

Additional References

Arora, V., & Johnson, J. (2006). A model for building a standardized handoff protocol. *The Joint Commission Journal on Quality and Patient Safety*, 32(11), 646–655. doi:10.1016/S1553-7250(06)32084-3

Berwick, D. M., Nolan, T. W., & Whittington, J. (2008). The Triple Aim: Care, health, and cost. *Health Affairs,* 27(3), 759–769.

Dracup, K., & Morris, P. E. (2008). Passing the torch: The challenge of handoffs. *American Journal of Critical Care, 17*(2), 95–97.

El-Jardali, F., Jaafar, M., Dimassi, H., Jamal, D., & Hamdan, R. (2010). The current state of patient safety culture in Lebanese hospitals: A study at baseline. *International Journal of Quality in Healthcare.* 22(5), 386–395. doi:10.1093/intqhc/mzq047

Friesen, M. A., White, S. V., & Byers, J. F. (2008, April). Handoffs: Implications for nurses. In R. G. Hughes (Ed.), *Patient safety and quality: An evidence-based handbook for nurses*. Rockville, MD: Agency for Healthcare Research and Quality. Retrieved from http://www.ncbi.nlm.nih.gov/books/NBK2649

Henriksen, K., Battles, J. B., Marks, E. S., & Lewin, D. I. (Eds.). (2005). *Advances in patient safety: From research to implementation* (Vol. 2: Concepts and Methodology). Rockville, MD: Agency for Healthcare Research and Quality. Retrieved from http://www.ncbi.nlm.nih.gov/books/NBK20523

Labib Medical Center. (2010). *Hospital executive committee: Strategic plan* (internal document). Saida, Lebanon: Author.

Labib Medical Center, Nursing Executive Committee. (2012a). *Nursing department quarterly report*. Saida, Lebanon: Author.

Labib Medical Center, Nursing Executive Committee. (2012b). *Nursing department strategic plan*. Saida, Lebanon: Author.

Labib Medical Center, Quality Department. (2009). *Patient safety survey report* (internal document). Saida, Lebanon: Author.

Ong, M. S., & Coiera, E. (2011). A systematic review of failures in handoff communication during intrahospital transfers. *The Joint Commission Journal on Quality and Patient Safety*. 37(6), 274–284. doi:10.1016/S1553-7250(11)37035-3

Ontario Hospital Association. (2006). *Inspiring ideas and celebrating successes: A guidebook to leading patient safety practices in Ontario hospitals*. Toronto, Ontario: Author.

Riesenberg, L. A., Leiztsch, J., & Cunningham, J. M. (2010). Nursing handoffs: A systematic review of the literature. *American Journal of Nursing, 110*(4), 24–34. doi:10.1097/01.NAJ.0000370154.79857.09

Strople, B., & Ottani, P. (2006). Can technology improve intershift report? What the research reveals. *Journal of Professional Nursing*, 22(3), 197–204. doi:10.1016/j.profnurs.2006.03.007

Theorieenoverzicht, T. C. W. (n.d.). *System theory*. University of Twenty. Retrieved from http://www.utwente.nl/cw/theorieenoverzicht/Theory%20Clusters/Communication%20Processes/System_Theory

EXEMPLAR 21.2 MITIGATION OF INTRAVENOUS MEDICATION ADMINISTRATION BARRIERS: A COMPREHENSIVE UNIT-BASED SAFETY PROGRAM (CUSP) INITIATIVE

Laura J. Wood and Rhonda Wyskiel

Team

Johns Hopkins Medicine

Armstrong Institute for Patient Safety and Quality

Johns Hopkins University School of Nursing

Johns Hopkins Hospital Office of Nursing Practice and Nursing Research

Johns Hopkins Hospital's Weinberg Intensive Care Unit (WICU) Nursing Staff

Problem

Infusion pump-related performance barriers associated with intravenous (IV) medication administration are commonly experienced by nurses within ICU settings. These barriers can result in a high rate of error as well as significant risk of preventable harm, resulting in humanistic and financial burden for patients, families, nurses, and healthcare delivery systems (Bates, Vanderveen, Seger, Yamaga, & Rothschild, 2005; Bosk, Dixon-Woods, Goeschel, & Pronovost, 2009). The oncological ICU within a leading academic health system noted increased complexity in the provision of care and the administration of medications as evidenced by data captured within Patient Safety Network (PSN) reports. Nursing and an extended network of interprofessional team members committed to evaluate the situation and mitigate the risk for untoward events and outcomes for this vulnerable population of patients (Carayon, Hundt, & Wetterneck, 2010).

Background

A systematic review of the literature related to IV medication administration and infusion pump-related workflow challenges was conducted in three phases. The first phase focused on cognitive failure, cognitive systems engineering, cognitive stacking, cognitive workload, critical thinking, healthcare microsystem, human factors framework, intensive care nursing, ICUs, interprofessional practice, nursing workload,

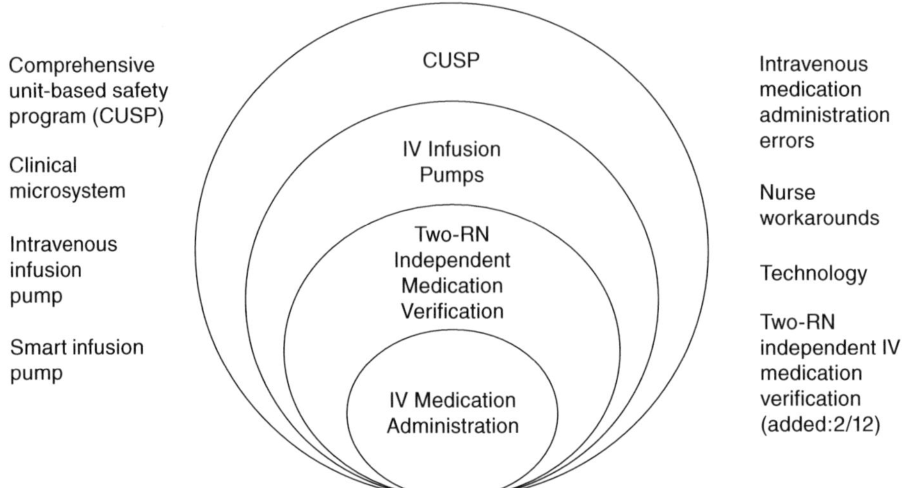

FIGURE 21.2.1 Concept map: mitigating IV medication administration barriers.
IV, intravenous.

performance obstacles, verbal protocol analysis, and work complexity. The second phase focused on technology and included infusion pumps, intensive care nursing, ICU, medication management, medication safety, smart pumps, and workarounds. The third and final phase focused on cognitive stacking, cognitive workload, distractions, interruptions, interruption management, medication administration, patient safety, and prospective memory.

Findings were organized according to the inductively developed concept map shown in Figure 21.2.1.

Aims

Two aims guided the conduct of the project:

1. To improve IV medication administration via infusion pump
2. To guide the use of at least one potentially significant evidence-based practice improvement developed by the unit-based team

Translation Framework

Two translational models guided this work. The first model was Titler's Middle-Range Nursing Conceptual Framework, which focused on organizational adoption of evidence-based practice. The second model applied was the Johns Hopkins Quality and Safety Research Group's Model for Translating Evidence Into Practice, already established within this practice setting (Pronovost, Berenholtz, & Needham, 2008).

Translation Methods

Two methods were also used in the conduct of this project. The first was audit and feedback and the second was rapid cycle performance improvement (RCPI).

Audit and Feedback

First, a set of interviews, a direct observation study of IV medication administration workflow, and a questionnaire to better understand nurses' acceptance of smart IV pump technology were administered to understand current perceptions as well as actual use case challenges nurses face during the administration of IV medications via infusion pumps. Then, unit-level quality data were synthesized and presented to the CUSP team for discussion, interpretation, and analysis of the findings. A review of the Safety Attitude Questionnaire (SAQ) and PSN event data was discussed together with the results of key stakeholder interviews, IV medication administration observations, and the findings identified through the administration of the IV infusion pump perceived usability survey (Carayon et al., 2010). These conversations led to the development of an action plan for RCPI.

Rapid Cycle Performance Improvement

The CUSP team determined that the evidence and data supported the establishment of a two-RN, independent verification process for the administration of high-alert medications.

Unit-based nursing leaders guided staff in the design of this process within the participating unit. The initial design prototype was created by the unit-based clinical nurse specialist (CNS) and patient safety RN. Adoption followed in accordance with unit-based governance practices consistent with CUSP and American Nurses Credentialing Center (ANCC) Magnet professional practice initiatives.

A pilot study was conducted; data were gathered according to the evaluation plan; and the CUSP team then met to evaluate the outcomes, communicate results through the unit, and disseminate findings in both the WICU and via the intensive care and medication safety microsystem workgroups to follow.

Results

Aim 1: To Improve IV Medication Administration Via Infusion Pump

Staff reported high satisfaction with pump usability relative to that reported in a benchmark study by Carayon et al. (2010) as presented in Figure 21.2.2.

Aim 2: To Guide the Use of at Least One Potentially Significant Evidence-Based Practice Improvement Developed by the Unit-Based Team

Nursing staff reported overall satisfaction with the two-RN, independent verification of high-risk medications protocol as presented in Figure 21.2.3.

Impact

- Nursing staff and interprofessional team members affirmed unit-based data-collection methods and CUSP meetings illuminated "known" practice challenges thought to contribute to future safety and quality risks.
- The CUSP-informed process enhanced problem definition and served as a catalyst to advance both a strategic planning process and concomitant intervention.
  - The first ever, unit-based PharmD/clinical pharmacist role was created.

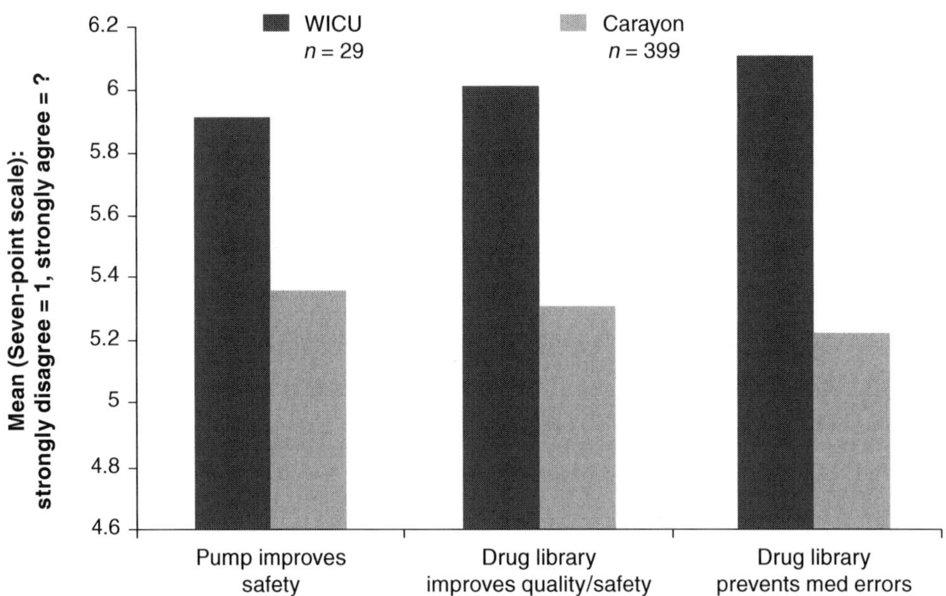

FIGURE 21.2.2 Infusion pump usability survey: means of key outcome variables.

WICU, Weinberg intensive care unit.

Source: Adapted with permission from Carayon, P., Hundt, A., & Wetterneck, T. (2010). Nurses' acceptance of smart IV pump technology. *International Journal of Medical Informatics, 79*, 401–411.

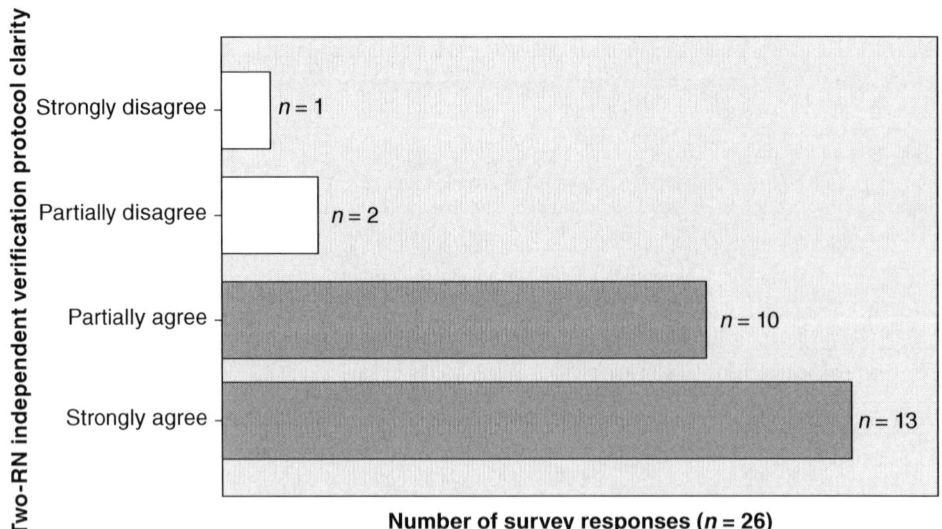

FIGURE 21.2.3 Perceived clarity of the two-RN, independent verification of high-risk medications protocol.

Note: Survey Question: Do you agree the existing hospital protocol related to two-RN verification of high-alert medications (e.g., insulin, heparin, and opiates) is clear and specifically outlines each required step in the two-RN verification process?

  - Association among drug library utilization by RNs, clinical pharmacist productivity with regard to drug library maintenance, wireless network capability, and related infrastructure planning requirements, including radio frequency identification (RFID)
  - Information technology (IT) requirements, for example, rules-based electronic drug calculator and planning for anticipated bar-coded medication administration (BCMA) implementation
- Significant opportunity exists in this setting to provide national leadership related to IV medication administration safety, given safety-focused culture and available resources.

Dissemination

Wood, L. J. (2012). *Nursing grand rounds*. Philadelphia, PA: Children's Hospital of Philadelphia.

Wood, L. J. (2012). *Patient safety exemplars* [Film]. Baltimore, MD: Johns Hopkins Hospital.

Wood, L. J., & Wyskiel, R. (2012). *Building clinical practice knowledge: research, evidence-based practice, quality improvement*. Baltimore, MD: The Johns Hopkins University, School of Nursing. Consultation to Flinders University and Adelaide-affiliated hospitals, South Australia. Evidence-based Practice Exemplars, Doctor of Nursing Practice Program.

Wood, L. J., & Wyskiel, R. (2012). *Creating an evidence-based practice translation plan: Bringing quality and safety innovations to scale via rapid cycle performance improvement*. (Course lecture: JHUSON RN 210 805). Baltimore, MD: Johns Hopkins University School of Nursing.

Additional References

Bates, D. W., Vanderveen, T., Seger, D., Yamaga, C., & Rothschild, J. (2005). Variability in intravenous medication practices: Complications for medication safety. *The Joint Commission Journal of Quality and Patient Safety, 31*(4), 203–210. doi:10.1016/S1553-7250(05)31026-9

Bosk, C. L., Dixon-Woods, M., Goeschel, C. A., & Pronovost, P. J. (2009). The art of medicine: Reality check for checklists. *Lancet, 374*(9688), 444–445. Retrieved from http://download.thelancet.com/pdfs/journals/lancet/PIIS0140673609614409.pdf

Carayon, P., Hundt, A., & Wetterneck, T. (2010). Nurses' acceptance of smart IV pump technology. *International Journal of Medical Informatics, 79*, 401–411. doi:10.1016/j.ijmedinf.2010.02.001

Fahimi, F., Ariapanah, P., Faizi, M., Shafaghi, B., Namdar, R., & Ardakani, M. T. (2008). Errors in preparation and administration of intravenous medications in the intensive care unit of a teaching hospital: An observational study. *Australian Critical Care, 21*(2), 110–116. doi:10.1016/j.aucc.2007.10.004

FDA launches initiative to reduce infusion pump risks. (2010, April). *Agency calls for improvements in device design*. Retrieved from U.S. Food & Drug Administration website http://www.fda.gov/NewsEvents/Newsroom/PressAnnouncements/ucm209042.htm

Harding, A. D. (2012). Increasing the use of 'smart' pump drug libraries by nurses: A continuous quality improvement project. *American Journal of Nursing, 112*(1), 26–35. doi:10.1097/01.NAJ.0000410360.20567.55

Husch, M., Sullivan, C., Rooney, D., Barnard, C., Fotis, M., Clarke, J., & Noskin, G. (2005). Insights from the sharp end of infusion medication errors: Implications for infusion pump technology. *Quality and Safety in Health Care, 14*, 80–86. doi:10.1136/qshc.2004.011957

Infusing Patients Safely. (2010, October). *Priority issues from the AAMI/FDA infusion device summit* (pp. 14–16). Retrieved from http://www.aami.org/infusionsummit/AAMI_FDA_Summit_Report.pdf

Manias, E., Williams, A., & Liew, D. (2012). Interventions to reduce medication errors in adult intensive care: A systematic review. *British Journal of Clinical Pharmacology, 74*, 411–422. doi:10.1111/j.1365-2125.2012.04220.x

Murdoch, L., & Cameron, V. (2008). Smart infusion technology: A minimum safety standard for intensive care? *British Journal of Nursing, 17*(10), 630–636. doi:10.12968/bjon.2008.17.10.29476

Nieva, V. F., Murphy, R., Ridley, N, Donaldson, N., Combes, J., Mitchell, P., . . . Carpenter, D. (2005). From science to service: A framework for the transfer of patient safety research into practice. In K. Henriksen, J. Battles, E. Marks, & D. I. Lewin (Eds.), *Advances in patient safety: From research to implementation* (Vol. 2, Concepts and methodology, pp. 441–453, AHRQ Publication No. 05-00221-2). Rockville, MD: Agency for Healthcare Research and Quality.

Phelps, P. K. (2011). *Smart infusion pumps: Implementation, management and drug libraries.* Bethesda, MD: American Society of Health-System Pharmacists.

Pronovost, P., Berenholtz, S., & Needham, D. (2008). Translating evidence into practice: A model for large scale knowledge translation. *British Medical Journal, 337*, 963–965. doi:10.1136/bmj.a1714

Romig, M., Goeschel, C., Pronovost, P., & Berenholtz, S. (2010). Integrating CUSP and TRIP to improve patient safety. *Hospital Practice, 38*(4), 114–121. doi:10.3810/hp.2010.11.348

Titler, M. (2010). Translation science and context. *Research and Theory for Nursing Practice, 24*(1), 35–55. doi:10.1891/1541-6577.24.1.35

Westbrook, J., Rob, M., Woods, A., & Parry, D. (2011). Errors in the administration of intravenous medications in hospital and the role of correct procedures and nurse experience. *British Medical Journal of Quality and Safety, 20,* 1027–1034. doi:10.1136/bmjqs-2011-000089

White, R. E., Trbovich, P. L., Easty, A. C., Savage, P., Trip, K., & Hyland, S. (2010). Checking it twice: An evaluation of checklists for detecting medication errors at the bedside using a chemotherapy model. *Quality and Safety in Health Care, 19*, 562–567. doi:10.1136/qshc.2009.032862

Wilson, K., & Sullivan, M. (2004). Preventing medication errors with smart infusion technology. *American Journal of Health-System Pharmacists, 61*, 177–183. doi:10.1093/ajhp/61.2.177

■ EXEMPLAR 21.3 RAPID ACCESS TO TERTIARY CARE: MITIGATING BARRIERS IMPACTING CLINICAL, FINANCIAL, AND OPERATIONAL OUTCOMES

Scott M. Newton

Team

Transport nurses

Admissions

Finance

Discharge coordinators

Administrator

Johns Hopkins Hospital

Johns Hopkins University School of Nursing

Problem

Delays of interhospital patient transfers are attributable to barriers, including complex transfer processes, lack of available beds, and awaiting availability of transport teams. These delays result in 8% higher mortality, $9,600 increased care cost, and 23% longer length of stay.

Background

Approximately 500,000 interhospital patient transfers occur each year, including 50% of all acute myocardial infarctions, and nearly 5% of all admissions to one of three critical care units: ICUs 1, 2, and 3. At the time this project was conducted, the project implementation facility reported an average time to patient transfer was 15 hours, 13 minutes, and an average of 16 patients were turned away each week due to transfer system barriers.

Aims

This project had two aims:

1. Primary aim: Decrease interhospital transfer time by 20%
2. Secondary aim: Reduce the proportion of lost transfers by 10%

Translation Framework

The Pronovost Model for large-scale knowledge translation was used to drive this project (Jaynes, Werman, & White, 2013).

The project began with a clear statement of the problem and thorough review and critique of the evidence focused on transport processes and outcomes. Barriers to timely and effective transport were identified, and outcome measures to evaluate performance were selected. This model directs engagement of the full transdisciplinary team across the cycle of education, execution, and evaluation. Fit between this model and the solution for this problem is further explained in the methods section that follows.

Translation Methods

Three methods were used to implement the project. These included a dashboard, infrastructure redesign, and a pathway (Figure 21.3.1).

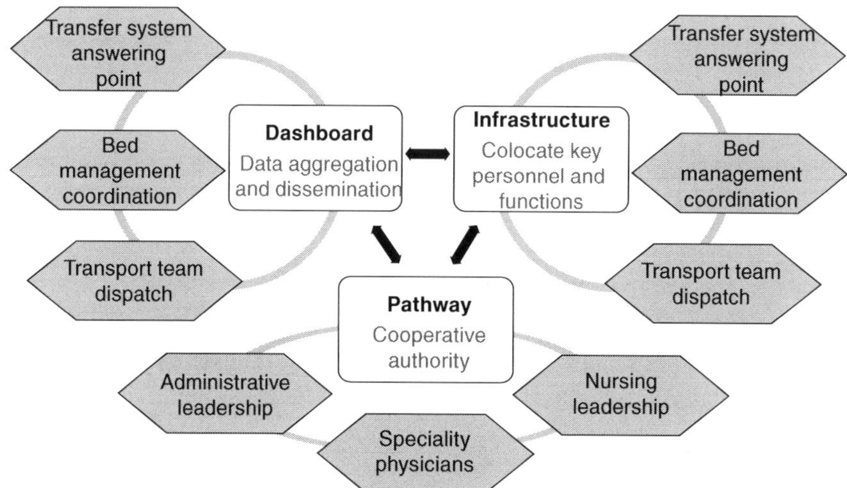

FIGURE 21.3.1 Conceptual model for interhospital transfer system.

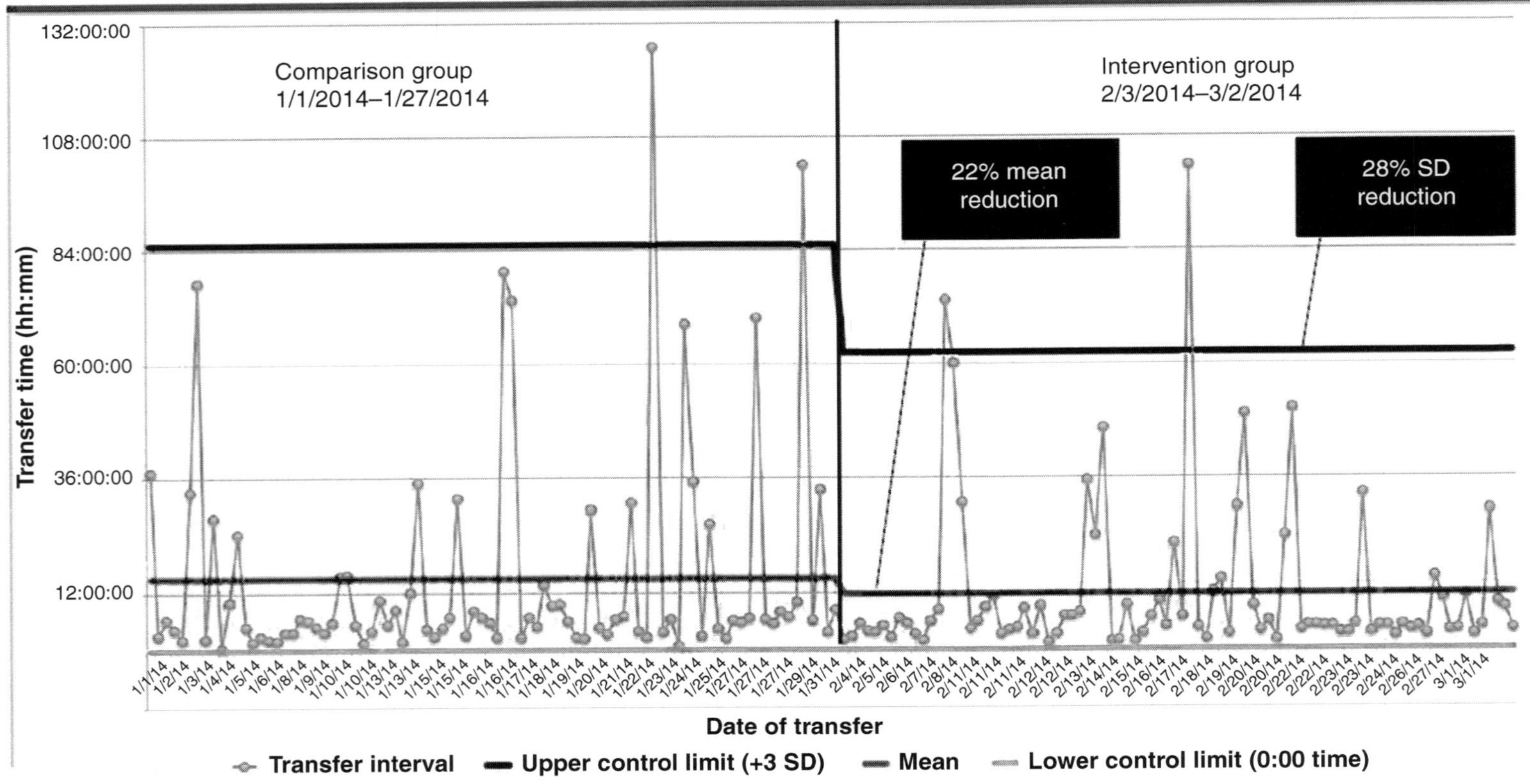

FIGURE 21.3.2 Statistical process control chart.

SD, standard deviation.

First, an extensively interprofessional transfer process workgroup was established.

Key data elements to monitor transfer system performance and outcomes were identified, aggregated using information systems and monitors, and disseminated using a dashboard. As a result, all team members were aware of performance targets and the impact of delays on patients and community partners seeking to arrange transfer.

A pathway was designed to improve the process. The interprofessional team described workflows and then collaborated to eliminate variables identified as barriers to achieving optimal outcomes.

In addition, a comprehensive redesign of the physical workspace was executed to colocate essential functions and personnel. This approach was used to enhance interprofessional communication within the host facility as well as interhospital communication and coordination to expedite transfer.

Results

- Interhospital patient transfer time was reduced by 22%.
- Lost admissions were not affected.
- Workspace redesign project plan was approved for $12 million, and is currently under construction.
- Progress over time was captured and reported using statistical process control methods, which clearly capture and communicate sustained improvement (Figure 21.3.2).

Impact

This translation project reduced interhospital transfer time and workflow variability. The improved process and responsiveness are significant to patients and families, community hospitals, and healthcare systems.

Dissemination

Newton, S. M. (2014, July). *Barriers impacting rapid access to tertiary care for time sensitive critically ill patients.* Podium presentation at Sigma Theta Tau 25th International Nursing Research Congress, Hong Kong.

Newton, S. M., & Fralic, M. (2015). Inter-hospital transfer center model: Components, themes, and design elements. *Air Medical Journal, 34*(4), 207–212. doi:10.1016/j.amj.2015.03.008

Additional References

Barratt, H. (2012). Critical care transfer quality 2000–2009: Systematic review to inform the ICS guidelines for transport of the critically ill adult (3rd ed.). *Intensive Care Society, 13*(4), 309–313. doi:10.1177/175114371201300409

Bosk, E. A., Veinot, T., & Iwashyna, T. J. (2011). Which patients and where: A qualitative study of patient transfers from community hospitals. *Medical Care, 49*(6), 592–598. doi:10.1097/MLR.0b013e31820fb71b

Catalano, A. R., Winn, H. R., Gordon, E., & Frontera, J. A. (2012). Impact of interhospital transfer on complications and outcome after intercranial hemorrhage. *Neurocritical Care, 17,* 324–333. doi:10.1007/s12028-012-9679-z

Fanara, B., Manzon, C., Barbot, O., Desmettre, T., & Capellier, G. (2010). Recommendations for the intrahospital transport of critically ill patients. *Critical Care, 14,* R87. Retrieved from http://ccforum.com/content/14/3/R87

Golestanian, E., Scruggs, J. E., Gangnon, R. E., Mak, R. P., & Wood, K. E. (2007). Effect of interhospital transfer on resource utilization and outcomes at a tertiary care referral center. *Critical Care Medicine, 35*(6), 1470–1476. doi:10.1097/01.CCM.0000265741.16192.D9

Hill, A. D., Fowler, R. A., & Nathens, A. B. (2011). Impact of interhospital transfer on outcomes for trauma patients: A systematic review. *Journal of Trauma, 71*(6), 1885–1901. doi:10.1097/TA.0b013e31823ac642

Iwashyna, T. J., Christie, J. D., Moody, J, Kahn, J. M., & Asch, D. A. (2009). The structure of critical care transfer networks. *Medical Care, 47*(7), 797–793. doi:10.1097/MLR.0b013e318197b1f5

Jaynes, C. L., Werman, H. A., & White, L. J. (2013). A blueprint for critical care transport research. *Air Medical Journal, 32*(1), 30–35. doi:10.1016/j.amj.2012.11.001

Pronovost, P., Berenholtz, S., & Needham, D. (2008). Translating evidence into practice: A model for large scale knowledge translation. *British Medical Journal, 337,* 963–965. doi:10.1136/bmj.a1714

■ EXEMPLAR 21.4 IMPROVING EFFECTIVE COMMUNICATION WITHIN THE NEONATAL INTERDISCIPLINARY TEAM

Jenelle M. Zambrano

Team

- Physicians
  - Neonatologists
  - Fellows
  - Residents/interns
- Nursing
  - Nurse manager
  - Clinical nurse specialist
  - Neonatal intensive care unit (NICU) RNs
- Respiratory therapists (RTs)
  - RT supervisor
  - NICU RTs

Problem

Ineffective communication interferes with development of the best, most comprehensive care plan for complex neonatal patients and their families. Breakdown in communication and collaboration prevents healthcare team members from functioning at their full capacity, working together, exchanging innovative ideas, or having open discussions about patient care management. Lack of effective communication increases staff moral distress and decreases patient advocacy. These three forms of poor communication can contribute to incivility, unprofessional behavior, lack of teamwork, passive aggressive behavior, insecurity, and frustration within the multidisciplinary team (Bosque, 2011). All can detract from the safety and quality of care.

Background

Communication breakdown can result in fragmented care, compromised patient safety, and increased morbidity and mortality. Each of these consequences is unacceptable in any patient care setting. Given the fragility of the neonates as they transition to extrauterine life, the unintended consequences of poor communication are unacceptable. Breakdown in teamwork can increase the neonate's risk for unnecessary patient procedures, pain, hospital-acquired infections (HAIs), and expense (Capella et al., 2010; Hoff et al., 2011; Okah, Wolff, Boos, Haney, & Oshodi, 2012). HAIs extend treatment and care, and lengthen stay. HAIs can cost an institution a nonreimbursable $3,700 to $29,000 per infection and threaten the financial stability of any NICU (Hoff et al., 2011).

Ineffective communication within the multidisciplinary team is likely to result in medical errors and place patients in direct harm (Sengupta, Lehmann, Diener-West, Perl, & Milstone, 2010). In close to 75% of all neonatal mortality and morbidity situations reported to The Joint Commission (TJC), ineffective team communication was a significant factor (American Academy of Pediatrics & American Heart Association, 2011). The complexity and stress of NICU care can contribute to communication breakdown (The Joint Commission, 2013). In 2012, TJC identified communication failure as the third leading root cause of sentinel events, which accounted for approximately 59% of all sentinel events (Leonard & Frankel, 2011). In addition, ineffective team communication compromises patient safety and can lead to potentially devastating consequences for the patients and families (Nadzam, 2009).

Aims

The purpose of this project was to improve communication within the neonatal interdisciplinary team.

There were three aims:

1. To improve communication, defined as shared agreement on patient daily goals
2. To increase staff satisfaction with patient care rounds (PCRs)
3. To improve staff perception of communication within the interdisciplinary team

Translation Framework

Donabedian's Quality of Care Framework was adapted to translate the evidence into practice and was used as the foundation for this project (Avanian & Markel, 2016). The Quality of Care Framework focuses on three main components: structure, process, and outcome to determine quality of care. Donabedian's original framework was conceptualized as a linear process within which structure and process were modifiable as a means to impact outcome (White & Dudley-Brown, 2012). By contrast, the adapted model presents the processes as nonlinear and was selected for that reason. The adapted Donabedian Quality of Care Framework helped to identify structure–affected process and outcome and to conceptualize these as interrelated and impactful on the other. The adapted model brought clarity to the complexities of ineffective communication.

Awareness of the structures in place helped the team understand the reasons for ineffective communication within the NICU. This awareness helped the team to identify evidence suited to addressing the problem in this NICU (Exhibit 21.4.1). As a result, the team implemented a communication advisory board (structure) and the standardized neonatal interdisciplinary rounds (process), as directed by the evidence. The team also set outcomes to be achieved.

Structure

- Inefficient flow of information
- Barriers to address patient care issues
- Lack of staff accountability
- Conflict avoidance
- Blameful and disrespectful team interactions
- Ineffective communication
- Minimal collaboration

Process

- Leadership collaborative advisory board (LCAB)
- Standardization of PCRs

Outcome

- Increased effective communication
- Increased staff satisfaction with PCRs
- Increased staff perception of communication

Translation Methods

This project focused on the interdisciplinary team and used three methods to accomplish improvement: formation of a collaborative interdisciplinary advisory board, daily rounds, and a toolkit.

Structure

Collaborative Interdisciplinary Advisory Boards. Two advisory boards were established to ensure that all stakeholders were engaged and informed of work and any additional information that flowed from the project. These groups were active throughout the project and remain active and effective after its completion.

Leadership Collaborative Advisory Board. A NICU interdisciplinary LCAB was established and included leadership from all disciplines and functional units. LCAB consisted of an attending neonatologist, neonatal fellow, nurse manager, CNS, respiratory therapist, and pediatric chief resident. This group had the authority to institute practice changes. Its charge was to support and guide the neonatal collaborative advisory board (NCAB) in the development of standardized, abbreviated daily shift PCRs,

EXHIBIT 21.4.1 Key Themes From the Evidence

Level	Article	PCR	Team building	Perception	Measurement
Level II B	Brodsky et al., 2013		X		Components of teamwork
	Phipps & Thomas, 2007	X			Understanding pt's daily goals
	Pronovost et al., 2003	X			Understanding pt's daily goals
	Rehder et al., 2012	X			Shared agreement daily goals
	Vats et al., 2012	X			Rounding time, discharge time
	Zwarenstein et al., 2009	X			Length of stay
Level III B	Al-Doghaiter et al., 2001			X	Perception of open communication
	Anderson et al., 1996			X	Perception of open communication
	Chang et al., 2010			X	Perception of open communication
	Manojlovich et al., 2008			X	Perception of open communication
	Okah et al., 2012			X	Comfort of expressing distress
	Reader et al., 2007			X	Perception of open communication
	Stern et al., 1991			X	Perception of open communication
	Thomas et al., 2003			X	Perception of open communication
	Vats et al., 2011	X			Rounding time

PCR, patient care rounds; pt, patient.

which were not in place at the beginning of this project. The LCAB was also responsible to help promote interprofessional collaboration, learning, and understanding between team members.

Clinician Advisory Board. The NCAB included direct care providers, pediatric residents, RNs, and respiratory therapists. The NCAB was charged with determining the practice changes and processes, and with implementation of the standardized PCRs.

Process

The NCAB developed the process for conduct of the PCRs including time, frequency, focus, and participants based on the evidence. They developed tools to facilitate PCRs including a daily goals sheet and script. Two sets of rounds were planned including those at the beginning of each shift and those with the full team.

The LCAB then created awareness among the NICU interdisciplinary team, explained the new process, and clearly stated support prior to implementation.

Abbreviated PCRs. Abbreviated PCRs occurred at the beginning of each shift. Participants included oncoming shift nurses, the assigned NICU respiratory therapist, and fellow (during dayshift PCRs) or resident (during nightshift PCRs). Each patient's outgoing bedside nurse followed a standardized script to provide a brief, yet complete overview of the condition, active concerns, and daily goals for each patient as they had been discussed during full PCRs. Respiratory therapists provided additional information on respiratory status and events as well as recommendations to help improve respiratory status. Frequent assessment and constant refinement of the abbreviated, standardized shift PCRs occurred to ensure the PCRs met the needs and were beneficial to the interdisciplinary team.

Comprehensive Team PCRs. Comprehensive daily PCRs occurred midmorning. Participants included an attending physician, fellow, residents, interns, CNS, charge nurse, bedside nurse, and respiratory therapist when available. During these PCRs, detailed discussion of the patient's current condition, status, plan of care, and anticipated needs were discussed. Each team member was given the opportunity and encouraged to voice any concerns, ask questions, and make recommendations to the patient's care plan. The attending physician then addressed each of these concerns, questions, or recommendations. At the end of the PCR, the fellow or senior resident verbally recapped the plan, goals, and new orders for the patients to the team to which the attending physician would confirm or clarify the plan.

Results

Communication Defined As Shared Agreement on Patient Daily Goals

Shared agreement among staff on daily patient goals was ascertained following 56 PCRs preintervention and 168 PCRs postintervention. A total of 513 questionnaires were completed, 155 (30.2%) preintervention and 358 (69.8%) postintervention. Mean shared agreement improved from .5164 (SD = .22581) preintervention to .6153 (SD = .23165) postintervention, p = .006.

Staff Satisfaction With PCRs

Staff satisfaction with PCRs increased.

Staff Perception of Communication

Perception of communication accuracy, understanding, and satisfaction increased. Perception of communication openness and timeliness decreased.

Impact

Change in Culture

- Open communication and collaboration
- Respectful of other interdisciplinary members
- Willing to participate/make a change
- Improved unit morale

Dissemination

Zambrano, J. M. (2014, June). *Improving effective communication within the neonatal interdisciplinary team: A journey to the problem.* Paper presented at the Johns Hopkins University, School of Nursing.

Zambrano, J. M. (2014, September). *Effective communication within the neonatal interdisciplinary team: A systematic review—Creating the leadership collaborative team.* Paper presented at the Los Angeles Department of Health Services Patient Safety Conference.

Zambrano, J. M. (2014, September.) *Interprofessional crisis mode communication within a neonatal multidisciplinary team: A systematic review.* Paper presented at the Academy of Neonatal Nursing 14th Annual Conference.

Zambrano, J. M. (2014, October.) *Interprofessional communication within a neonatal multidisciplinary team.* Paper presented at the American Academy of Pediatrics Conference.

Zambrano, J. M. (2015, April). *Improving communication within the NICU team: A comparison of strategies to improve interprofessional communication infrastructure & crisis mode communication.* Paper presented at the International Forum on Quality and Safety in Healthcare.

Zambrano, J. M. (2015, June). *Improving effective communication within the neonatal interdisciplinary team: A journey to the problem.* Paper presented at the Johns Hopkins University, School of Nursing.

Zambrano, J. M. (2015, July). *Improving effective communication within the neonatal interdisciplinary team: A project design.* Paper presented at Sigma Theta Tau International 26th International Nursing Research Congress.

Additional References

American Academy of Pediatrics & American Heart Association. (2011). In J. Zaichkin (Ed.), *Simulation* (6th ed.). Media, PA: Author.

Ayanian, J. Z., & Markel, H. (2016). Donabedian's lasting framework for health care quality. *New England Journal of Medicine, 2016*(375), 205–207.

Bosque, E. (2011). A model of collaboration and efficiency between neonatal nurse practitioner and neonatologist: Application of collaboration theory. *Advances in Neonatal Care, 11*(2), 108–113. doi:10.1097/ANC.0b013e318213263d

Capella, J., Smith, S., Philip, A., Putnam, T., Gilbert, C., Fry, W., . . . ReMine, S. (2010). Teamwork training improves the clinical care of trauma patients. *Journal of Surgical Education, 67*(6), 439–443. doi:10.1016/j.jsurg.2010.06.006

Hoff, T., Hartmann, C. W., Soerensen, C., Wroe, P., Dutta-Linn, M., & Lee, G. (2011). Making the CMS payment policy for healthcare-associated infections work: Organizational factors that matter. *Journal of Healthcare Management, 56*(5), 319–335. doi:10.1097/00115514-201109000-00007

Leonard, M. W., & Frankel, A. S. (2011). Role of effective teamwork and communication in delivering safe, high-quality care. *Mount Sinai Journal of Medicine, 78*(6), 820–826. doi:10.1002/msj.20295

Nadzam, D. M., (2009). Nurses' role in communication and patient safety. *Journal of Nursing Care Quality, 24*(3), 184–188. doi:10.1097/01.NCQ.0000356905.87452.62

Okah, F. A., Wolff, D. M., Boos, V. D., Haney, B. M., & Oshodi, A. A. (2012). Perceptions of a strategy to prevent and relieve care provider distress in the neonatal intensive care unit. *American Journal of Perinatology, 29*(9), 687–691. doi:10.1055/s-0032-1314889

Sengupta, A., Lehmann, C., Diener-West, M., Perl, T. M., & Milstone, A. M. (2010). Catheter duration and risk of CLABSI in neonates with PICCs. *Pediatrics*, *125*(4), 648–653. doi:10.1542/peds.2009-2559
The Joint Commission. (2013, February 7). *Sentinel event data root causes by event type 2004–2012*. Retrieved from http://www.jointcommission.org/assets/1/18/Root_Causes_Event_Type_04_4Q2012.pdf
White, K. M., & Dudley-Brown, S. (2012). *Translation of evidence into nursing and health care practice*. New York, NY: Springer Publishing Company.

■ EXEMPLAR 21.5 USE OF PAGERS WITH AN ALARM ESCALATION SYSTEM TO REDUCE CARDIAC MONITOR ALARM SIGNALS

Maria M. Cvach

Team

Nursing
Biomedical engineering
Johns Hopkins Hospital
Johns Hopkins University School of Nursing

Problem

Clinicians rely on monitor alarms to notify them of impending problems. When there are excessive quantities of alarms, most of which are false or nonactionable, clinicians develop mistrust toward medical device alarm systems. This may lead to staff apathy resulting in errors of omission, distraction, or ignoring warning signals intended to keep patients safe. Known as "alarm fatigue," the excessive noise from false and nonactionable alarm signals makes it difficult for staff to identify the alarms that are true and actionable. Missed medical device alarms have resulted in patient injury and death (The Joint Commission, 2013).

Background

Over the past 30 years, the use of clinical alarms has become more widespread, bringing the number of different alarms in an ICU from six in 1983 to 40 in 2011 (Borowski et al., 2011; Kerr & Hayes, 1983). From 2005 to 2008, the Food and Drug Administration, Manufacturer and User Facility Device Experience (MAUDE) database received 566 reports of patient deaths related to inappropriate actions toward monitoring device alarms (Weil, 2009). TJC reported 98 alarm-related events between January 2009 and June 2012. Eighty of these resulted in death and 13 in permanent loss of function (Kerr & Hayes, 1983; The Joint Commission, 2013). The Emergency Care Research Institute (ECRI) publishes an annual top 10 technology hazards list. Alarm hazards have been at the top of their list since its inception in 2007 and have been the number one technology hazard for the past 4 years (ECRI, 2014).

Cardiac monitor alarms are purposefully designed for high sensitivity, not to miss a true monitor event. Studies indicate that 68% to 99% of monitor alarms are false and/or nonactionable (Chambrin et al., 1999; Gross, Dahl, & Nielsen, 2011; Lawless,

1994; Schmid et al., 2011; Siebig et al., 2010; Tsien & Fackler, 1997). A false alarm occurs when there is no true event, but the monitor elicits a signal. A nonactionable alarm is real, but does not require clinician intervention. Nonactionable alarms occur due to momentary alarm limit breaches caused by staff manipulating patients during routine care or patient movement. Caregivers view these alarms as "nuisance" alarms and may take inappropriate actions toward these alarm signals.

Research indicates that adding slight delays can reduce alarm burden, thereby decreasing false and nonactionable alarms (Gross et al., 2011; Siebig et al., 2010). By reducing alarm burden and by using an algorithm to send meaningful alarm signals to care providers through notification devices, the likelihood of a missed alarm can be reduced.

Aims

The purpose of this quality improvement (QI) project was to determine whether a reduction in alarm burden and use of a cardiac monitor alarm escalation algorithm that filters monitor alarm signals before sending them to a nurse's wireless device is an effective method to notify nurses of high-priority monitor alarm signals.

There were two specific aims:

1. To decrease the average frequency and duration of high-priority monitor alarms per monitored bed
2. To improve nurses' attitudes about clinical alarms, including perceptions of effectiveness of notification devices

Translation Framework

The Johns Hopkins Nursing Evidence-Based Model (Dearholt & Dang, 2012) was used to search and rate the evidence related to the background problem, intervention, comparison, outcome question referred to as the *PICO question*, which is used to begin the evidence-based practice (EBP) process in this model: Does the amount of noise (false alarms) as context to signal (true alarms) interfere with the nurses' response to physiologic monitor alarms? The Knowledge-to-Action (KTA) Framework (Graham et al., 2006) was used to translate the selected evidence into practice.

Translation Methods

Technology

This project used technology-related solutions to address a technology-related problem.

This project was implemented on two surgical progressive care units at the Johns Hopkins Hospital. Both units were similar in size, staffing, and had a similar layout. Monitor default parameters were adjusted identically for both units.

Unit A, a cardiac progressive care unit, implemented the alarm escalation algorithm and acknowledgment arrhythmia pager slightly differently than did unit B, a noncardiac progressive care unit. Because most patients on unit A were on a cardiac monitor, each nurse received an arrhythmia pager and responded to his or her own patient's alarms.

Unit B had fewer patients on a monitor. Unit B decided that only the charge nurse would carry the arrhythmia pager and respond to monitor alarms transmitted via the algorithm. Prior to beginning the project, nurses on both units were invited to take a national clinical alarm survey to measure their perception of alarms.

Nurses were asked to repeat the survey 4 months postimplementation of the alarm escalation algorithm. Monitor alarm quantity and duration for three (7-day) time frames were extracted and analyzed as follows: T0—prior to alarm algorithm implementation, T1–2 months postimplementation, T2–4 months postimplementation.

Results

The average number of alarms/bed/day and alarm duration was measured and trended for the three (7-day) time frames. A linear regression line demonstrated that the slope of the trend line decreased by 0.75 alarms/bed/day and 0.33 seconds/day when each nurse carried an arrhythmia pager. When only one person on the unit was assigned the arrhythmia pager, the trend line increased by 0.07 alarms/bed/day but the alarm duration decreased by 0.27 seconds/day. Based on these results, it was decided that providing nurses with their own arrhythmia pager was a more effective method than having a single person carry the alarm notification pager.

Seven questions on the clinical alarm survey were used to determine nurse perception of alarms. A paired *t*-test was used to compare nurse responses pre/post-implementation of the alarm escalation algorithm. There was a statistically significant change in sensitivity to alarms and quickness of response from preintervention ($p = .045$, two-tailed). Although there was a change in a positive direction in nurses' perception of adequacy of alarm notification and devices, the results were not statistically significant (Cvach, Frank, Doyle, & Stevens, 2014).

Impact

As a result of this project, reduction of alarm burden and implementation of the alarm escalation algorithm, with each nurse carrying a notification device, has become standard practice on most monitored units at the Johns Hopkins Hospital.

Dissemination

Cvach, M. M., Frank, R. J., Doyle, P., & Stevens, Z. K. (2014). Use of pagers with an alarm escalation system to reduce cardiac monitor alarm signals. *Journal of Nursing Care Quality, 29*(1), 9–18. doi:10.1097/NCQ.0b013e3182a61887

Additional References

Borowski, M., Görges, M., Fried, R., Such, O., Wrede, C., & Imhoff, M. (2011). Medical device alarms. *Biomedizinische Technik [Biomedical Engineering], 56*(2), 73–83. doi:10.1515/BMT.2011.005

Chambrin, M. C., Ravaux, P., Calvelo-Aros, D., Jaborska, A., Chopin, C., & Boniface, B. (1999). Multicentric study of monitoring alarms in the adult intensive care unit (ICU): A descriptive analysis. *Intensive Care Medicine, 25*(12), 1360–1366. doi:10.1007/s001340051082

Dearholt, S., & Dang, D. (2012). *Johns Hopkins nursing evidence-based practice: Models and guidelines*. Indianapolis, IN: Sigma Theta Tau.

ECRI. (2014, November). Alarm hazards: Inadequate alarm configuration policies and practices. In *Top 10 health technology hazards for 2015* (pp. 3–6). Retrieved from https://www.ecri.org/Pages/2015-Hazards.aspx

Graham, I. D., Logan, J., Harrison, M. B., Straus, S. E., Tetroe, J., Caswell, W., & Robinson, N. (2006). Lost in knowledge translation: Time for a map? *Journal of Continuing Education in the Health Professions, 26*(1), 13–24. doi:10.1002/chp.47

Gross, B., Dahl, D., & Nielsen, L. (2011). Physiologic monitoring alarm load on medical/surgical floors of a community hospital. *Biomedical Instrumentation & Technology*, 45, 29–36. doi:10.2345/0899-8205-45.s1.29

Kerr, J. H., & Hayes, B. (1983). An "alarming" situation in the intensive therapy unit. *Intensive Care Medicine, 9*(3), 103–104. doi:10.1007/BF01772574

Lawless, S. (1994). Crying wolf: False alarms in a pediatric intensive care unit. *Critical Care Medicine, 22*(6), 981–985. doi:10.1097/00003246-199406000-00017

Schmid, F., Goepfert, M. S., Kuhnt, D., Eichhorn, V., Diedrichs, S., Reichenspurner, H., & Reuter, D. A. (2011). The wolf is crying in the operating room: Patient monitor and anesthesia workstation alarming patterns during cardiac surgery. *Anesthesia and Analgesia, 112*(1), 78–83. doi:10.1213/ANE.0b013e3181fcc504

Siebig, S., Kuhls, S., Imhoff, M., Gather, U., Scholmerich, J., & Wrede, C. E. (2010). Intensive care unit alarms—How many do we need? *Critical Care Medicine, 38*(2), 451–456. doi:10.1097/CCM.0b013e3181cb0888

The Joint Commission. (2013). The joint commission announces 2014 national patient safety goals. *The Joint Commission Perspectives, 33*(7), 1–4.

Tsien, C. L., & Fackler, J. C. (1997). Poor prognosis for existing monitors in the intensive care unit. *Critical Care Medicine, 25*(4), 614–619. doi:10.1097/00003246-199704000-00010

Weil, K. M. (2009). Alarming monitor problems. *Nursing, 39*(9), 58. doi:10.1097/01.NURSE.0000360252.10823.b8

■ EXEMPLAR 21.6 IMPROVING THE PRACTICE ENVIRONMENT OF THE BEDSIDE NURSE USING MASLOW'S HIERARCHY OF HUMAN NEED, NATIONAL DATABASE OF NURSING QUALITY INDICATORS DATA, AND A TOOL KIT FOR CHANGE

Lisa Groff Reuschling

Team

Newborn Nursery Pilot Steering Committee

- Night-shift nurse (1)
- Day-shift nurses (2)

Nursing faculty

Greater Baltimore Medical Center

Johns Hopkins University School of Nursing

Problem

Institution-specific workforce planning data revealed issues with nurse retention:

- Sixteen percent turnover among bedside nurses
- Average age of nurses on staff ranges from 25 to 29
- Average tenure of nurses is 1 to 5 years (52.4%)
- More than half the nurses will be lost within 5 years

These internal data concur with external evidence that newer nurses leave much faster than seasoned nurses (Aiken, Clarke, & Sloane, 2002).

Background

Healthcare in the United States is in crisis due to escalating cost, challenging access to care, and instability within the nursing workforce. As a result, reducing staff turnover has been the focus of reform. In one study, 37% of newly licensed registered nurses were ready to change or leave their jobs (Kovner et al., 2007). At the time of this work, a report released by Price Water House Cooper's Health Research Institute found that the average voluntary turnover for first-year nurses was 27.1% (Block, Claffey, Korow, & McCaffrey, 2005).

The strongest predictors of nurse job dissatisfaction and intent to leave are related to job stress in the practice environment (Zangaro & Soeken, 2007). Many conditions are associated with job stress, but the most common include patient acuity, nurse–patient ratios, work schedules, poor MD–RN interactions, new technology, staff shortages, unpredictable workload or workflow, and the perception that the care offered was unsafe (Bowles & Candela, 2005; Leurer, Donnelly, & Domm, 2007; Shader Broome, Broome, West, & Nash, 2001; Zangaro & Soeken, 2007). Conversely, good communication, control over practice, decision-making at the bedside, teamwork, and nurse empowerment are aspects of the practice environment that increase satisfaction and decrease nurse turnover (DiMiglio et al., 2005; Heath, Johanson, & Blake, 2004; Kalisch, Curley, & Stefanov, 2007). Although much can be gleaned from the literature and the experience of others, care must be taken to critically assess the perceptions of the nurses at each individual facility, and each unit within that facility, to determine which practice environment improvement strategies would be most effective.

The National Database of Nursing Quality Indicators (NDNQI) practice survey is a nationally applied, valid, and reliable tool that measures the perceptions of the nurse within the practice environment. Currently over 200,000 nurses participate across the country, which allows for national benchmarking in addition to unit- and facility-specific comparisons. The survey is based on Lake's (2002) Practice Environment Scale of the Nursing Work Index, which measures five parameters: nurse participation in hospital affairs, nursing foundations for quality care, nurse manager ability and support of nurses, staffing and resource adequacy, and collegial nurse–physician relationships. Aiken's work, mentioned earlier, is reflected in the survey in the work context items related to job plans and quality of care within the practice environment. Demographics and job enjoyment are also collected within the survey (Aiken et al., 2002; Lake, 2002).

Hospital and nursing leaders frequently include nurse retention as a metric in their strategic goals. A successfully implemented survey will equip hospitals and nurse leaders with the information to create, implement, and evaluate evidence-based practice environment improvement projects and nurse retention strategies.

Aims

The aims of this project were:

1. To increase engagement of nurses in activities to retain staff
2. To facilitate effective application of NDNQI data

Translation Framework

Two frameworks undergirded this project: Havelock and Zlotolow's (1995) planned change framework and Maslow's hierarchy of needs (1943).

The theory of planned change describes six successive cycles of action that repeat as change advances: relating, examining, acquiring, trying, extending, and renewing. Much relationship building (*relating*) was involved in this project and in retaining nurses. *Examining* was key to understanding the data and the reasons for poor retention. *Acquiring* involved efforts to help staff master skills for processing and interpreting data. *Trying* would describe cycles to implement the best solutions for positive change. *Extending* would describe diffusion of change throughout the unit and *renewing* describes efforts to stabilize the improved practice setting. This cycle will require continued repetition to achieve quality and RN job satisfaction.

Maslow conceptualized human needs as a pyramid with five levels ascending from physiologic needs at the base, to safety, belonging, esteem, and self-actualization at the apex. The unmet need at the lowest level of the hierarchy takes the highest priority. As each lower level need is satisfied, the next higher need occupies one's main attention until it is satisfied. The highest level need is that of "becoming all that one is capable of becoming in terms of talents, skills and abilities" (Hoffman, 2008, p. 36). Maslow posits that people are innately motivated toward psychological growth and self-development. Tools, such as the NDNQI Practice Environment Scale, are critical in assisting nurses to achieve empowerment and self-actualization. Applying this model to nursing practice suggests that when nurses do not feel that their basic needs are being met, they will be less motivated and less likely to progress to higher level functions (Chinnis, Summers, Doer, Paulson, & Davis, 2001; Figure 21.6.1).

Translation Methods

The project progressed in two phases. The first phase involved deployment of the NDNQI survey across the entire facility (macrosystem level) and the second phase involved performance improvement activities on a single patient care unit, which were conducted as a pilot test of the approach (microsystem level) based on the NDNQI data.

Phase I: Macrosystem Deployment of NDNQI

The project began with the implementation of the online NDNQI survey with the Practice Environment Scale as a baseline measurement across all nursing units. All NDNQI guidelines for implementation were strictly adhered to. Executive support

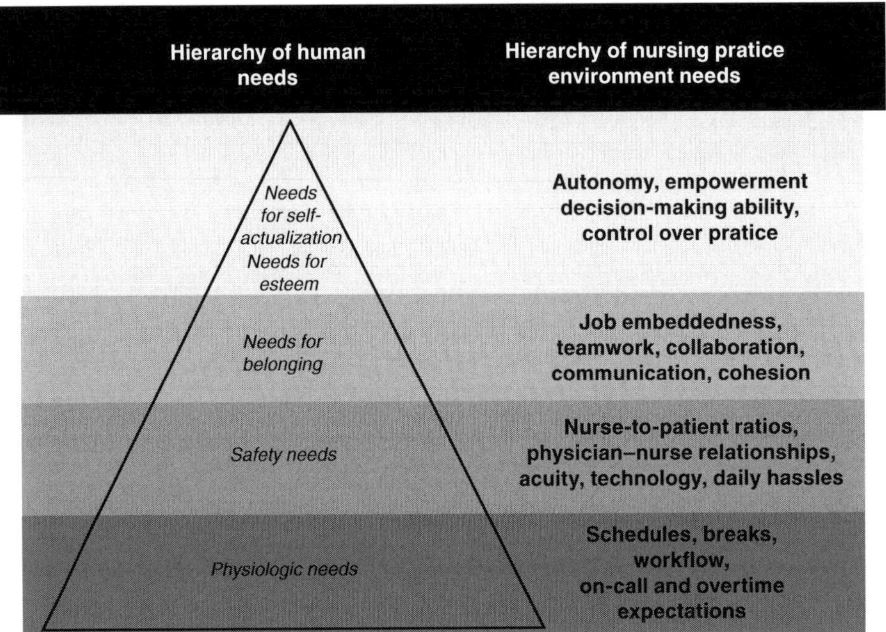

FIGURE 21.6.1 Hierarchy of nursing practice environment needs.

Source: From Groff Paris, L., & Terhaar, M. (2010). Using Maslow's pyramid and the National Database of Nursing Quality Indicators to attain a healthier work environment. *OJIN: The Online Journal of Issues in Nursing, 16*(1), 6. Copyright by the American Nurses Association, Inc.

was obtained and a communication strategy was developed. This included ongoing communication to the nursing leadership council, and both the house-wide divisional and unit-level practice councils. An overall response rate of 62% was obtained.

Phase II: Microsystem Performance Improvement

This translation project was embedded in phase II of the NDNQI rollout and two methods were used, including RCPI and a tool kit (Figure 21.6.2).

The newborn nursery was selected to serve as a pilot unit. This approach was intended to ensure full participation of staff in development, deployment, and refinement of a set of tools to support RCPI. These tools would subsequently be used by staff across the house in data-driven RCPI work.

Tool Kit

Once NDNQI data became available, staff on the pilot unit met with the project leader to discuss the data. The group discussed the reports and their own readiness to make use of them. The group then decided it needed a few tools that had yet to be developed. The project leader then created a set of new tools to guide the staff in reading, analyzing, prioritizing, and deciding, based on data.

A discussion guide was developed to facilitate meaningful and productive conversations about large amounts of data. In addition, resources for reviewing measures of central tendency, distribution, and common analytics were provided. These guides

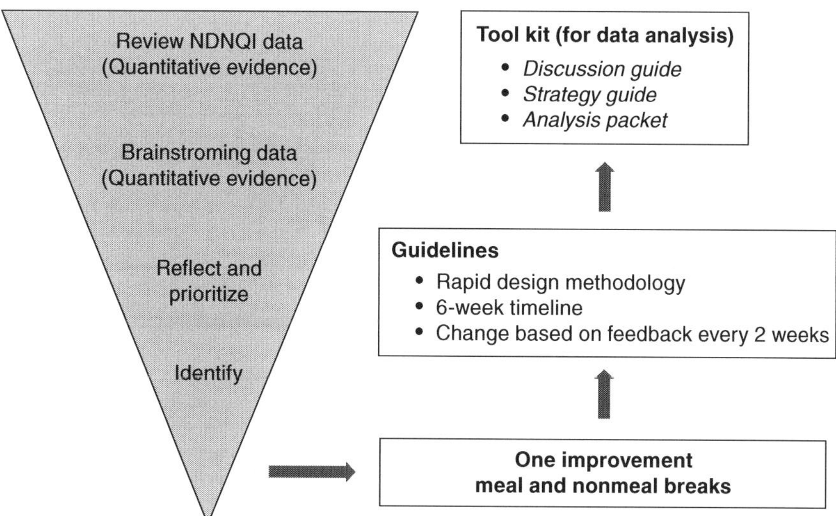

FIGURE 21.6.2 Process improvement and tool kit development.
NDNQI, National Database of Nursing Quality Indicators.

helped focus conversations and organize input so that staff could select numbers with meaning. For instance, the discussion guide directed participants to select the highest and the lowest numbers and then consider the meaning and relevance of the data.

Rapid Cycle Performance Improvement

Once staff became more facile with the data, they identified areas for improvement as indicated by the data. The pilot unit selected breaks as an important concern supported by the data and then began to develop strategies to address the problem.

The group formed partnerships and helped each other get time away from direct care. They helped each other plan for and then follow through on plans for breaks. They monitored performance on a metric that they cared about and observed progress.

Results

Quantitative Findings

- At baseline, only 25% of the nurses on the pilot unit took breaks.
- The number of nurses who took a *meal break lasting 30 minutes or longer increased* from 29% to 39%.
- The number of nurses *unable to take any meal breaks during their shift decreased* from 25% to 22%.
- The number of nurses *able to sit down free of patient care responsibility for meal breaks increased* from 0% to 26%.
- One-hundred percent of the steering committee identified the tool kit and rapid design process as *very helpful*.

Qualitative Findings

- Some nurses remained reluctant to leave their patients to take a break, or to call on their equally busy colleagues to "double their patient load" to cover for them while on a break.
- Staff nurses felt empowered by their participation. One nurse stated it was "exciting to be part of making a difference" on their unit.
- One nurse stated that it was "good to be part of the solution rather than stating issues but seeing no change."
- The tools were considered very helpful in the problem-solving process.

Impact

NDNQI is a powerful tool that can be useful at the microsystem as well as at the macrosystem level. Nurses can benefit from both interpretative tools and coaching to evaluate and understand data.

In this case, the staff selected a low-performing metric. They scored low on taking breaks and they themselves valued taking breaks. This became the focus of the RCPI work. And there was measurable improvement. This group learned that nurses want and need to take breaks, but require structure and guidance to change the old behavior, which has led nurses not to take the breaks they want and need.

Participation in performance improvement activities at the unit level in this pilot test increased staff engagement, peer support, and accountability.

Dissemination

Groff Paris, L. (2009). *Improving the practice environment.* National Database of Nursing Quality Indicators.

Groff Paris, L. (2011). *Engaging the staff nurse at the bedside.* National Database of Nursing Quality Indicators.

Groff Paris, L. (2011). *Orienting to outcomes in today's complex environment.* Academy of Neonatal Nursing.

Groff Paris, L., & Terhaar, M. (2010, December 7). Using Maslow's pyramid and the National Database of Nursing Quality Indicators to attain a healthier work environment. *OJIN: The Online Journal of Issues in Nursing, 16*(1), 6.

Additional References

Aiken, L. H., Clarke, S. P., & Sloane, D. M. (2002). Hospital staffing, organization, and quality of care: Cross-national findings. *International Journal for Quality in Health Care, 14*, 4–13. doi:10.1093/intqhc/14.1.5

Block, L. M., Claffey, C., Korow, M. K., & McCaffrey, R. (2005). The value of mentorship within nursing organizations. *Nursing Forum, 40*(4), 134–140. doi:10.1111/j.1744-6198.2005.00026.x

Bowles, C., & Candela, L. (2005). First job experiences of recent RN graduates: Improving the work environment. *Journal of Nursing Administration, 35*(3), 130–137. doi:10.1097/00005110-200503000-00006

Chinnis, A. S., Summers, D. E., Doer, C., Paulson, D. J., & Davis S. M. (2001). Q methodology: A new way of assessing employee satisfaction. *Journal of Nursing Administration, 31*(5), 252–259. doi:10.1097/00005110-200105000-00005

DiMiglio, K., Padula, C., Piatek, C., Korber, S., Barrett, A., Ducharme, M., . . . Corry, K. (2005). Group cohesion and nurse satisfaction: Examination of a team-building approach. *Journal of Nursing Administration, 35*(3), 110–120. doi:10.1097/00005110-200503000-00003

Havelock, R. G., & Zlotolow, S. (1995). *The change agent's guide* (2nd ed.). Englewood Cliffs, NJ: Educational Technology Publications.

Heath, J., Johanson, W., & Blake, N. (2004). Healthy work environments: A validation of the literature. *Journal of Nursing Administration, 34*(11), 524–530. doi:10.1097/00005110-200411000-00009

Hoffman, E. (2008). The Maslow effect: A humanist legacy for nursing. *American Nurse Today, 3*(8), 36–37.
Kalisch, B. J., Curley, M., & Stefanov, S. (2007). An intervention to enhance nursing staff team work and engagement. *Journal of Nursing Administration, 37*(2), 77–84. doi:10.1097/00005110-200702000-00010
Kovner, C. T., Brewer, C. S., Fairchild, S., Poornima, S., Kim, H., & Djukic, M. (2007). Newly licensed RNs' characteristics, work attitudes, and intentions to work. *American Journal of Nursing, 107*(9), 58–70. doi:10.1097/01.NAJ.0000287512.31006.66
Lake, E. T. (2002). Development of the practice environment scale of the nursing work index. *Research in Nursing & Health, 25*, 176–188. doi:10.1002/nur.10032
Leurer, M. D., Donnelly, G., & Domm, E. (2007). Nurse retention strategies: Advice from experienced registered nurses. *Journal of Health Organization and Management, 21*(3), 307–319. doi:10.1108/14777260710751762
Shader, K., Broome, M. E., Broome, C. D., West, M. E., & Nash, M. (2001). Factors influencing satisfaction and anticipated turnover for nurses in an academic medical center. *Journal of Nursing Administration, 31*(4), 210–216. doi:10.1097/00005110-200104000-00010
Zangaro, G. A., & Soeken, K. L. (2007). A meta-analysis of studies of nurses' job satisfaction. *Research in Nursing & Health, 30*, 445–458. doi:10.1002/nur.20202

■ EXEMPLAR 21.7 RETENTION OF CARDIOPULMONARY RESUSCITATION SKILLS AND PRIORITIES

Nancy Sullivan

Team

Nursing staff
Public health staff
Health educators
Simulation lab coordinator
Medical faculty
Nursing faculty
Professional development
Vice provost for digital initiatives
Johns Hopkins School of Medicine
Johns Hopkins University School of Nursing

Problem

Poor retention of CPR skills and priorities in all healthcare providers is well documented in the literature (Leary & Abella, 2008). In addition, it has been observed that nurses neglect the initial priorities essential in the first 5 minutes in an attempt to be ready for the arrival of the code team by readying drugs, intubation equipment, and intravenous fluids.

Background

CPR done correctly can restore circulation 40% to 60% of the time (Thel & O'Connor, 1999). Survival to hospital discharge is much lower with some studies reporting approximately 20% (Meaney et al., 2010; Peberdy et al., 2003). Although there are many nonmodifiable variables that influence survival to discharge, such as the patient's age, gender, race, morbidity, and first monitored rhythm, there are modifiable variables as well. They include speed and appropriateness of response. Immediate initiation of quality compressions has been documented to improve the effectiveness of arrest medications and defibrillation (Dichtwald, Matot, & Einav, 2009; Leary & Abella, 2008). If CPR is started within the first minute of an arrest, survival improves significantly (Herlitz, Bang, Alsen, & Aune, 2002). Defibrillation occurring within 3 minutes is also associated with improved survival to discharge (Herlitz et al., 2005; Peberdy et al., 2003). It is clear the two variables, immediate initiation of compressions and quick defibrillation, impact survival after cardiac arrest. These actions are directly associated with the prompt response of the initial responder, typically the nurse in the hospital setting. The nurse's performance of correct CPR priorities is crucial.

Aims

This project had two aims.

1. To improve nurses' retention and performance of the initial CPR priorities in the management of an in-hospital cardiac arrest
2. To determine the most efficient training interval necessary to improve performance of CPR priorities

Translation Framework

The KTA Framework was used as the foundation for this project. A critical evaluation of the evidence informed all work to follow and determined the approach to solving the problem.

The search began broadly. Through refinement and evaluation, only strong evidence was retained. The base of the funnel represents only the strong evidence, which includes American Heart Association guidelines already in place. Additional strong evidence informed the revised guidelines developed as a result of this project.

The action cycle provided clear guidance through the steps necessary for successful translation. The evidence summary clearly identified the problem of poor retention of CPR skills and priorities completing the first step.

Identifying and adapting to local context is extremely important. For this problem, local context related to nursing staff as first responders to cardiac arrest in the hospital setting. Additional context was the construction of a large new building on campus, which had the potential to add considerable transport time for the hospital code team when responding to arrests. This would require nursing staff to manage arrests for a longer period of time. This situation as context helps provide perspective on the need to change and provide better training.

The next step was to identify potential barriers. This helped the project team plan strategies to diminish the impact of potential barriers, and there were many.

Because multiple changes were already occurring at the hospital related to the new building, time, money, and personnel for training could also have become issues.

After identifying the problem, adapting to context, and identifying barriers, an intervention was selected and tailored to meet the needs of the project. The intervention for this project was identified through synthesis of the literature. The highest level evidence suggested frequent, short, deliberate practice simulation training. Testing of knowledge retention focused on specific critical accomplishments and skills such as compression depth and rate and sequencing and timing of arrest priorities.

Evaluation was conducted through performance comparison of individuals trained with frequent deliberate practice as compared with individuals trained via standard practice: CPR recertification every 2 years and annual or biannual mock codes.

Finally, sustaining knowledge use was evaluated through identifying barriers to institution-wide adoption of the training strategy, establishing unit champions, enlarging the pilot, and continuing evaluation.

Translation Methods

The method used for this project was instructional design using simulation.

Instructional Design

The intervention included deliberate practice in the form of a simulated cardiac arrest teaching session, which was conducted in three steps (Hunt et al., 2014; Oermann, Kardong-Edgren, & Odom-Maryon, 2011; Sutton et al., 2011).

Step one involved a skills assessment that evaluated performance in a simulated cardiac arrest, which lasted until the patient was defibrillated or until 4 minutes had elapsed, whichever came first. To facilitate accurate assessment of the participant's knowledge of the initial CPR priorities, each participant was told staff would respond to a call for help but would not initiate any emergency procedures without first being directed.

Step two involved a structured debriefing session, which started with a demonstration of the immediate initiation of compressions and a discussion of the correct use of the defibrillator. This was followed by viewing a video depicting the ideal choreography of an arrest response and a brief discussion of priorities.

Step three involved a repetition of the scenario followed by a brief review of priorities. The study coordinator who acted as a staff nurse confederate was always present to facilitate consistent staging and debriefing of the simulated arrest. Each participant was assessed and trained individually with nonparticipant coworkers functioning as members of the responding team.

Assignment to Groups for Evaluation. Participants trained every 2, 3, or 6 months. There was also a control group of participants who did not receive the intervention at all but were current in their CPR certification. Participants were nurses working on general medicine and neuroscience units. ICU and intermediate care unit nurses, nurses in orientation, and nurses not current in CPR certification were excluded from the project.

A parallel block randomization was accomplished by filling opaque envelopes with paper slips labeled *training every 2 months (2M), 3 months (3M)*, or *6 months (6M)*. Participants blindly chose a slip from the envelope thus enrolling themselves in a specific training group. Because there was no guarantee that individuals who volunteered would be available for a particular training session, randomization was completed just prior to the first session. Envelopes were limited to three slips at a time noting the three training options to ensure equal group sizes. Once enrolled, participants were no longer blinded to their group. The project coordinator scheduled all subsequent training sessions and thus was also not blinded to the group assignments.

Statistical Analysis

Statistical analysis was performed utilizing Statistical Package for Social Sciences (SPSS) version 20 software. Descriptive analyses were carried out on demographics, baseline, and outcome measures. Comparisons of the groups on demographic characteristics were performed using Fisher's exact test. Evaluation of the distribution of data on continuous variables revealed the presence of outliers. As a result, continuous data was reported as medians and interquartile ranges (IQRs). Analysis was completed using the Kruskal–Wallis test due to the small sample size (18 per group). When a significant difference was indicated, multiple comparisons between pairs of the four groups were evaluated, using a Bonferroni adjustment of the *p* values for an experiment-wise error rate of .05. Comparisons of categorical variables between groups and the control were evaluated using the chi-square statistic. Because of the small group sample sizes, Fisher's exact test was also performed. When a significant difference was indicated, multiple comparisons between pairs of the four groups were evaluated using a Bonferroni correction for an experiment-wise error rate of .05.

Results

Seventy-two participants were enrolled in the project, 18 in each group. Sixty-six participants completed all training sessions conducted and were evaluated in the final sessions conducted at 6 months. Statistical analysis revealed no significant differences among the groups' demographics.

Nurses' Retention and Performance of Initial CPR Priorities

Significant differences were noted among the groups trained every 2 and 3 months versus the control. Median ± IQR seconds to compressions decreased as the time between training sessions was decreased [2M: 13 (9–20) vs. C: 33 (25–40.5); $p < .001$, $r = .68$, 3M: 14 (10.5–20) vs. C: 33 (25–40.5); $p < .001$, $r = .63$].

Similarly, when evaluating seconds to defibrillation, significant differences were noted between the groups that trained every 2 and 3 months versus the control. Median (IQR) seconds to defibrillation decreased as the time between training sessions was decreased [2M: 109 (98–129) vs. C: 152 (131–177); $p < .001$, $r = .67$, 3M: 115 (100.7–188.7) vs. C: 152 (131–177); $p <$ 001, $r = .71$].

Median (IQR) percentage no-flow fraction also decreased as the time between training intervals decreased. Again, significant differences were noted between the groups that trained every 2 and 3 months versus the control, but not for the every-6-month group: [C: 0.59 (0.67–0.40) vs. 6M: .56 (0.70–0.46) vs. 3M: .72 (0.76–0.66) vs. 2M: 0.72 (0.77–0.62); $p < .02$].

The percentage of participants successfully initiating compressions by 10 seconds increased steadily as the training sessions increased, but most participants had trouble reaching that goal. Although performance was improved in the 2M group, no statistical differences were revealed between the groups.

When evaluating compressions by 15 seconds, significant differences were found between the groups that trained every 2 months and the control [2M: 67% (10) vs. C: 11% (2); $p = .001$, $phi = .575$].

When evaluating compressions by 20 seconds, significant differences were found between the groups that trained every 2 months and the control [2M: 87% (13) vs. C: 17 % (3); $p = .001$, $phi = .697$] and the groups that trained every 3 months and the control [3M: 75% (12) vs. C: 17% (3); $p = .001$, $phi = .586$].

Overall Pass Rates

Evaluating the ability to pass an overall assessment combined the initiation of compressions within a predetermined time frame (10, 15, or 20 seconds), defibrillating by 180 seconds, and using a backboard. For example, "pass 10" included initiating compressions within 10 seconds, defibrillating by 180 seconds, and using a backboard. This outcome also revealed improved performance as the time between training intervals decreased: "pass 15" [2M: 53% (8) vs. C: 5% (1); $p = .004$, $phi = .534$], "pass 20" [2M: 73% (11) vs. C: 5% (1); $p = .000$, $phi = .702$, 3M: 56% (9) vs. C: 5% (1); $p = .002$, $phi = .555$].

Defibrillation

No significant differences were identified among any of the groups in the defibrillation by 180 seconds measure. This goal was reached 67% to 100% of the time in all participant groups. Although not statistically significant, clinically, it is desirable to reach this goal more than 67% of the time. The final variable, refining compressions, revealed poor performance by all groups. Full refinement was accomplished only between 11% and 20% of the time.

Impact

This project does not attempt to define a training modality to replace traditional American Heart Association training. Rather, the primary aim was to define a realistic adjunct to that training to improve the initial timing and sequencing of response. This project reveals an overall improved performance in participants trained with this intervention as compared to standard CPR training.

The secondary aim was to evaluate the most efficient training interval. The groups that trained every 2 and 3 months demonstrated significantly improved performance over the control but there were no significant differences between those groups. Also, there were no statistical differences between the group that trained every 6 months and the control. These two findings indicate training is needed more frequently than every 6 months; every 3 months may be an efficient training interval.

Dissemination

Sullivan, N. (2014). An integrative review: Instructional strategies to improve nurses' retention of cardiopulmonary resuscitation priorities. *International Journal of Nursing Education Scholarship, 12*(1). doi:10.1515/ijnes-2014-0012.

Sullivan, N. J., Duval-Arnould, J., Twilley, M., Smith, S. P., Aksamit, D., Boone-Guercio, P., . . . Hunt, E. A. (2015). Simulation exercise to improve retention of cardiopulmonary resuscitation priorities for in-hospital cardiac arrests: A randomized controlled trial. *Resuscitation, 86*, 6–13. doi:10.1016/j.resuscitation.2014.10.021

Additional References

Dichtwald, S., Matot, I., & Einav, S. (2009). Improving the outcome of in-hospital cardiac arrest: The importance of being earnest. *Seminars in Cardiothoracic and Vascular Anesthesia, 13*, 19–30. doi:10.1177/1089253209332212

Herlitz, J., Aune, S., Bång, A., Fredriksson, M., Thorén, A., Ekström, L., & Holmberg, S. (2005). Very high survival among patients defibrillated at an early stage after in-hospital ventricular fibrillation on wards with and without monitoring facilities. *Resuscitation, 66*, 159–166. doi:10.1016/j.resuscitation.2005.03.018

Herlitz, J., Bang, A., Alsen, B., & Aune, S. (2002). Characteristic outcomes among patients suffering from in-hospital cardiac arrest in relation to whether the arrest took place during office hours. *Resuscitation, 53*, 127–133. doi:10.1016/S0300-9572(02)00014-X

Hunt, E. A., Duval-Arnould, J. M., Nelson-McMillan, K. L., Bradshaw, J. H., Diener-West, M., Perretta, J. S., & Shilkofski, N. A. (2014). Pediatric resident resuscitation skills improve after "rapid cycle deliberate practice" training. *Resuscitation, 85*(7), 945–951. doi:10.1016/j.resuscitation.2014.02.025

Leary, M., & Abella, B. (2008). Challenge of CPR quality: Improvement in the real world. *Resuscitation, 77*, 1–3. doi:10.1016/j.resuscitation.2008.02.005

Meaney, P. A., Nadkarni, V. M., Kern, K. B., Indik, J. H., Halperin, H. R., & Berg, R. A. (2010). Rhythms and outcomes of adult in-hospital cardiac arrest. *Critical Care Medicine, 38*, 101–108. doi:10.1097/CCM.0b013e3181b43282

Oermann, M. H., Kardong-Edgren, S. E., & Odom-Maryon, T. (2011). Effects of monthly practice on nursing students' CPR psychomotor skill performance. *Resuscitation, 82*(4), 447–453. doi:10.1016/j.resuscitation.2010.11.022

Peberdy, M. A., Kaye, W. Ornato, J. P., Larkin, G. L., Nadkarni, V., Mancini, M. E., & Lane-Trultt, T. (2003). Cardiopulmonary resuscitation of adults in the hospital: A report of 14,720 cardiac arrests from the National Registry of Cardiopulmonary Resuscitation. *Resuscitation, 58*, 297–308. doi:10.1016/S0300-9572(03)00215-6

Sutton, R. M., Niles, D., Meaney, P. A., Aplenc, R., French, B., Abella, B. S., . . . Nadkarni, V. (2011). Low-dose, high-frequency CPR training improves skill retention of in-hospital pediatric providers. *Pediatrics, 128*(1), e145–e151. doi:10.1542/peds.2010-2105

Thel, M. C., & O'Connor, C. M. (1999). Cardiopulmonary resuscitation: Historical perspective to recent investigations. *American Heart Journal, 137*, 39–48. doi:10.1016/S0002-8703(99)70458-8

■ EXEMPLAR 21.8 IMPLEMENTATION OF A COMPREHENSIVE EVIDENCE-BASED OUTPATIENT REHABILITATION PROGRAM FOR POST-ACUTE AND CHRONIC CLINICAL MANAGEMENT OF VETERANS WITH POLYTRAUMA AND TRAUMATIC BRAIN INJURY AT REMOTE VETERANS AFFAIRS FACILITIES

Jemma Ayvazian

Team

Nursing

Physical therapy

Medicine
Pharmacy
Occupational therapy
Administration
Social work
Kinesthesiology
Biomedical engineering
Veterans
Veterans' families
Department of Veterans Affairs (VA), Dayton Ohio
VA, national office
Johns Hopkins University School of Nursing

Problem

Traumatic brain injury (TBI) and polytrauma are pressing issues for veterans of the Iraq and Afghanistan conflicts. Over the past several years, there has been increasing interest in developing effective, integrated rehabilitation models of care that offer systematic and structured approaches to the postacute and chronic rehabilitation of veterans with polytrauma.

The majority of polytrauma services for veterans are provided near large metropolitan areas (Box 21.8.1). Veterans living outside those areas are disadvantaged in being able to access these services. Many are required to travel 60 to 400 miles to access care (Ripley, 2008).

Background

Since 2000, 2.3 million service members have been deployed to combat regions. More than 30% of all veterans come from rural areas and return to their hometowns after separation. More than 1 million soldiers who served in Operation Iraqi Freedom (OIF) and Operation Enduring Freedom (OEF) are eligible to receive services through the VA. The signature injuries of these conflicts complicate care, rehabilitation, and recovery and place significant demands for coordination of care and evidence-based services to support soldiers suffering from TBI and posttraumatic stress disorder (PTSD) and their families.

Blast-related injuries are the most common combat-related injury among OIF/OEF veterans (U.S. Department of Veterans Affairs, 2013). Both research and practice show a high prevalence of polytrauma among veterans who are affected by TBI, which causes multisystem sequelae, including complex musculoskeletal injuries, amputations, spinal cord injuries, and injuries to internal organs (Meyer, Marion, Coronel, & Jaffee, 2010; Schultz, Cifu, McNamee, Nichols, & Carne, 2011). Three out of four OIF/OEF veterans with TBI have a concurrent diagnosis of PTSD (Congressional

BOX 21.8.1 Locations for Polytrauma Services for Veterans in the United States

Polytrauma Rehabilitation Center	Polytrauma Network Site
Minneapolis, MN	Augusta, GA
Palo Alto, CA	Boston, MA
Richmond, VA	Bronx, NY
Tampa, FL	Cleveland, OH
	Dallas, TX
	Denver, CO
	Hines, IL
	Houston, TX
	Indianapolis, IN
	Lexington, KY
	Philadelphia, PA
	Seattle, WA
	St. Louis, MO
	Syracuse, NY
	Tucson, AZ
	Washington, DC
	West Los Angeles, CA

Budget Office, 2012). Studies have found a high prevalence of comorbid pain and PTSD in TBI patients (Hoge et al., 2008; Otis, McGlinchey, Vasterling, & Kerns, 2011; Sayer et al., 2009). Lew et al. (2009) showed that more than 42% of veterans with polytrauma suffer from overlapping multisymptom conditions that are associated with TBI, PTSD, and chronic pain.

Aims

The purpose of this project was to use a variety of practical clinical rehabilitation interventions identified in the literature and strongly supported by evidence in order to:

1. Decrease the length of time polytrauma veterans spend in postacute/chronic care
2. Promote recovery and help veterans successfully transition back to their communities

Translation Framework

Elements of the Chronic Care Model (CCM), the Johns Hopkins Evidence-Based Practice (JHEBP) Model, and the VA's Quality Enhancement Research Initiative (QUERI) were utilized to synthesize evidence, develop recommendations, and implement clinical interventions.

Translation Methods

A systematic review was used to identify the essential components of rehabilitation care for veterans diagnosed with polytrauma. Clinical experts were consulted to augment findings from the thorough analyses of the evidence to ensure that proposed interventions would be feasible, relevant to the specific needs of military and veteran populations, and likely to produce positive outcomes.

After soliciting recommendations from specialists involved in polytrauma and TBI care, an integrated model of rehabilitation care was designed to simultaneously treat chronic pain, TBI, PTSD, depression, anxiety, substance use disorder (SUD), and other co-occurring conditions within the context of polytrauma, while promoting self-management skills and self-reliance. This integrated outpatient polytrauma rehabilitation care model was pilot tested in three phases: comprehensive evaluation by the interdisciplinary team and identification of treatment goals, active treatment, and community reintegration (Figure 21.8.1).

Focus groups with veterans and caregivers were then conducted to evaluate satisfaction with the rehabilitation care model. Approval was obtained from an institutional review board (IRB) to conduct focus groups with the veterans and caregivers to assess four main areas of interest: satisfaction with care, essential components of care, family involvement, and patient and family education.

Results

Thirty-four veterans and seven caregivers (n = 41) participated in focus groups. The results are organized according to the four main predetermined thematic categories.

Thematic Category 1: Satisfaction

The veterans and caregivers noted several reasons they were satisfied with the piloted model of rehabilitation care: (a) the integrated approach to treatment, (b) the genuine care and concern that the providers had for the veterans, and (c) inclusivity in the decision-making process. The theme that emerged from the data was that the veterans were satisfied with the rehabilitation model because of its integrated and holistic approach to treatment (Figure 21.8.2).

Thematic Category 2: Essential Components of Treatment

Several essential components of treatment were cited by the veterans: (a) the integrated approach, (b) education and information, (c) TBI treatment, (d) pain management, (e) mental healthcare, and (f) respect and understanding. Pain management

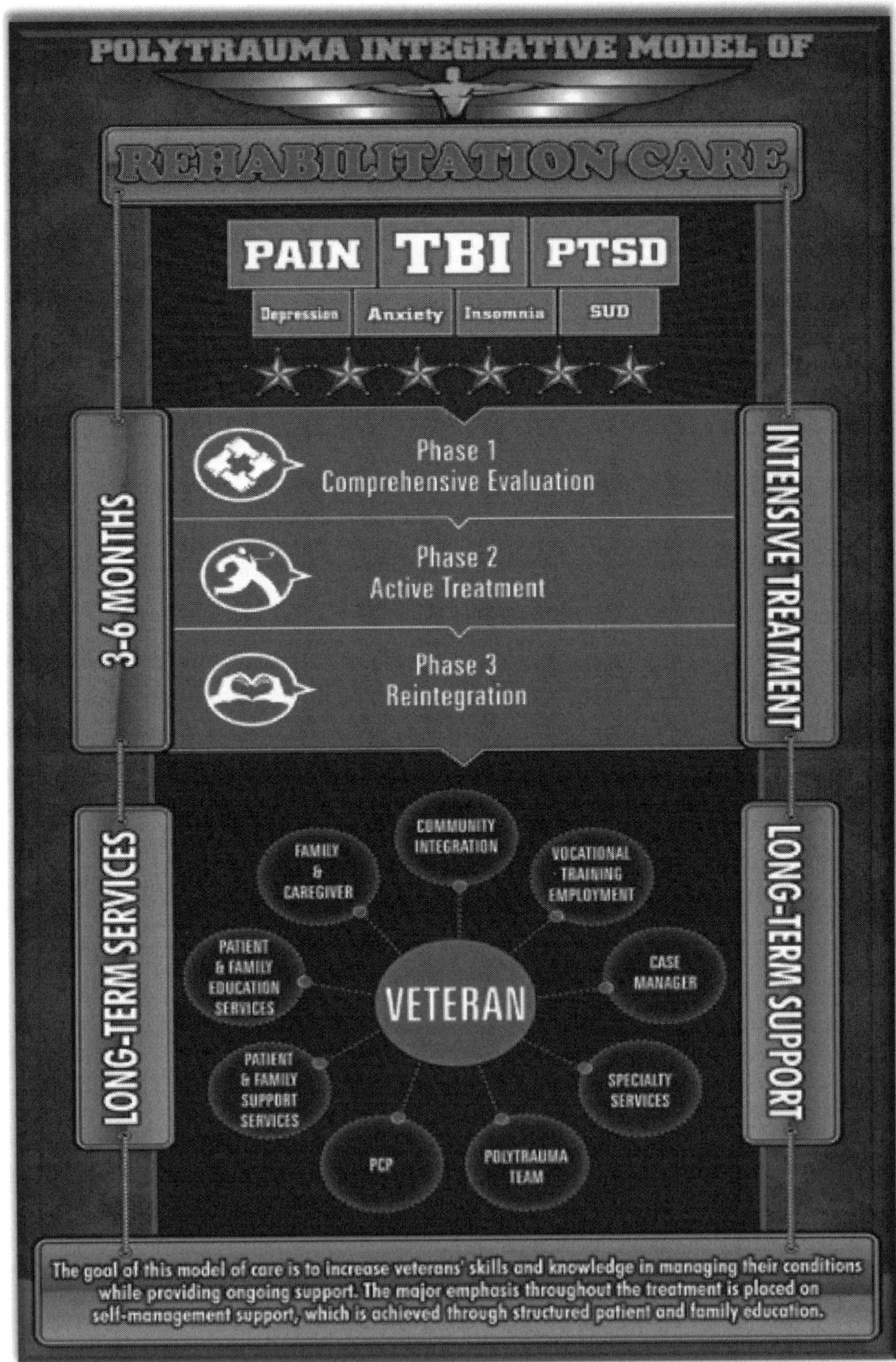

FIGURE 21.8.1 Integrated outpatient polytrauma rehabilitation care model.

PCP, primary care provider; PTSD, posttraumatic stress disorder; SUD, substance use disorder; TBI, traumatic brain injury.

and associated treatments were one of the most commonly discussed subjects. The veterans voiced their satisfaction with the nonpharmacological strategies available

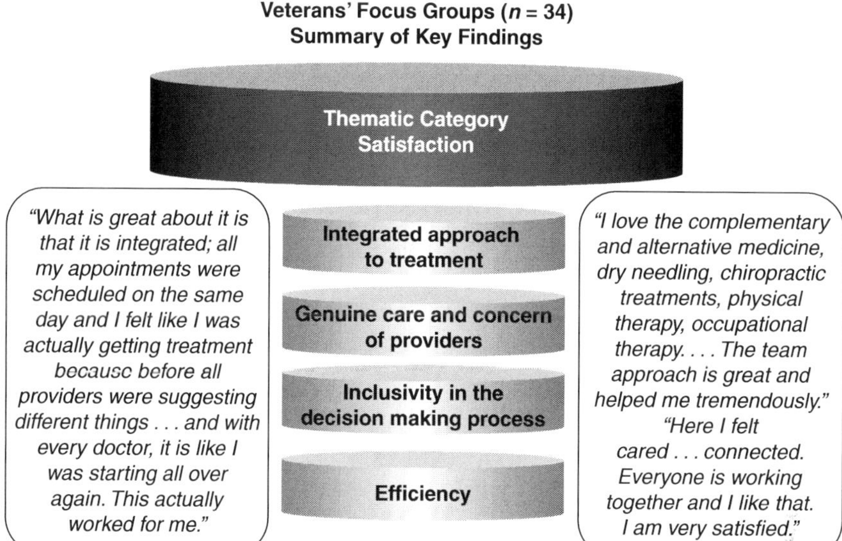

FIGURE 21.8.2 Thematic category 1: Satisfaction among veterans and caregivers.

to treat chronic pain, especially trigger-point dry needling therapy and chiropractic treatment. Most veterans claimed that they significantly benefited from kinesiotherapy, which provided numerous exercise options for veterans with physical limitations. Treatment that focused on the veteran's cognitive or psychological health was also considered an essential component. Both groups, the veterans and caregivers, recognized the importance of addressing veterans' mental health needs as a priority. Effective patient and family education emerged as an important component of a successful rehabilitation program. Other aspects of care that the veterans identified as essential components were peer support, family involvement and support, couples counseling, speech therapy, individualized treatment, qualified and experienced staff, substance abuse treatment, medication management, and coordination of care among multiple providers.

Thematic Category 3: Family Involvement

Regarding family involvement in the treatment process, veterans noted that family support is essential and identified that family members should be more aware of the complexity of their conditions. Familial and occupational obligations were recognized as the major barriers preventing family members from being more involved in the treatment process.

Thematic Category 4: Patient and Family Education

The veterans and caregivers identified several acceptable learning methods, including face-to-face interactions with healthcare providers, group discussions, text messaging, and email. The majority of veterans believed that face-to-face interaction with a healthcare provider was the most effective method of delivering healthcare information.

Impact

Polytrauma injuries are the most common injuries sustained by service members in Iraq and Afghanistan. It is essential to design innovative strategies using evidence-based treatment interventions and to pilot test integrated models of care to decrease the length of time that veterans with polytrauma/TBI spend receiving postacute and chronic care. The nearly unanimous positive feedback that the veterans and their caregivers gave regarding the integrated model of rehabilitation care supports the future development and evaluation of such models. We found that veterans were highly satisfied with the piloted integrated polytrauma rehabilitation approach and believed that integrated treatment was more successful than systems that aim to manage specific conditions or symptoms.

Dissemination

Ayvazian, J. (2014, October). *Implementation of a comprehensive evidence-based outpatient rehabilitation program for post-acute and chronic clinical management of veterans with polytrauma and traumatic brain injury at remote veterans affairs facilities.* Presented at STTI Region 12 Chesapeake Consortium, Washington, DC .

Ayvazian, J., Hamilton, S., Welch, J., Williams, D., Venkat, S., Bendel, E., . . . Dudley-Brown, S. (2012, Septmber). *Clinical management of veterans with traumatic brain injury within the context of polytrauma.* Poster presented at theTenth Annual Conference on Brain Injury, Miami, FL. Granted Best Poster Abstract Presentation Award.

Additional References

Congressional Budget Office. (2012). *The Veterans Health Administration's treatment of PTSD and traumatic brain injury among recent combat veterans.* Washington, DC: U.S. Government Printing Office.

Hoge, C. W., McGurk, D., Thomas, J. L., Cox, A. L., Engel, C. C., & Castro, C. A. (2008). Mild traumatic brain injury in U.S. soldiers returning from Iraq. *New England Journal of Medicine, 358*, 453–463. doi:10.1056/NEJMoa072972

Lew, L. H., Otis, D. J., Tun, C., Kerns, D. R., Clark, E. M., & Cifu, X. D. (2009). Prevalence of chronic pain, post-traumatic stress disorder, and persistent postconcussive symptoms in OIF/OEF veterans: Polytrauma clinical triad. *Journal of Rehabilitation Research and Development, 46*, 697–702. doi:10.1682/JRRD.2009.01.0006

Meyer, K. S., Marion, D. W., Coronel, H., & Jaffee, M. S. (2010). Combat-related traumatic brain injuries and its implication to military healthcare. *Psychiatric Clinics of North America, 33*, 784–796. doi:10.1016/j.psc.2010.08.007

Otis, J. D., McGlinchey, R., Vasterling, J. J., & Kerns, R. D. (2011). Complicating factors associated with mild traumatic brain injury: Impact on pain and posttraumatic stress disorder treatment. *Journal of Clinical Psychology in Medical Settings, 18*, 145–154. doi:10.1007/s10880-011-9239-2

Ripley, D. C. (2008). VA to play role in defense-funded research on PTSD, TBI. *VA Research Currents.* Washington, DC: U.S. Department of Veterans Affairs.

Sayer, N. A., Cifu, D. X., McNamee, S., Chiros, C. E., Sigford, B. J., Scott. S., & Lew, H. L. (2009). Rehabilitation needs of combat-injured service members admitted to the VA polytrauma rehabilitation centers: The role of PM&R in the care of wounded warriors. *Physical Medicine and Rehabilitation Journal, 1*, 23–28. doi:10.1016/j.pmrj.2008.10.003

Schultz, B. A., Cifu, D. X., McNamee, S., Nichols, M., & Carne, W. (2011). Assessment and treatment of common persistent sequelae following blast induced mild traumatic brain injury. *NeuroRehabilitation, 28*, 309–320.

U.S. Department of Veterans Affairs. (2013, October). *Polytrauma and blast-related injuries.* Minneapolis, MN: Department of Veterans Affairs, Office of Research and Development, Health Services Research and Development Service. Retrieved from http://www.queri.research.va.gov/about/factsheets/polytrauma_factsheet.pdf

Index